Hoffman and Abeloff's

HEMATOLOGY-ONCOLOGY REVIEW

Hoffman and Abeloff's HEMATOLOGY-ONCOLOGY REVIEW

Editor

Claudine Isaacs, MD
Professor of Medicine and Oncology
Co-Director, Breast Cancer Program
Medical Director, Fisher Center for Hereditary
*   Cancer and Clinical Genomics Research*
Georgetown University
Washington, District of Columbia

Section Editors

Sanjiv S. Agarwala, MD
Professor and Chief
Department of Oncology and Hematology
St. Luke's Cancer Center
Temple University
Bethlehem, Pennsylvania

John L. Marshall, MD
Chief, Division of Hematology/Oncology
MedStar Georgetown University Hospital
Associate Director, Clinical Research
Lombardi Comprehensive Cancer Center
Georgetown University
Washington, District of Columbia

Naiyer A. Rizvi, MD
Director of Thoracic Oncology and
*   Immunotherapeutics*
Division of Hematology and Oncology
Columbia University Medical Center
New York, New York

Bruce D. Cheson, MD
Professor of Medicine
Head of Hematology
Director of Hematology Research
Lombardi Comprehensive Cancer Center
Georgetown University
Washington, District of Columbia

Alice D. Ma, MD
Professor of Medicine
Hemophilia and Thrombosis Center
University of North Carolina – Chapel Hill
Chapel Hill, North Carolina

ELSEVIER

ELSEVIER

1600 John F. Kennedy Blvd.
Ste 1800
Philadelphia, PA 19103-2899

HOFFMAN AND ABELOFF'S HEMATOLOGY-ONCOLOGY REVIEW   ISBN: 978-0-323-42975-7

Notices

Knowledge and best practice in this field are constantly changing. As new research and experience broaden our understanding, changes in research methods, professional practices, or medical treatment may become necessary.

Practitioners and researchers must always rely on their own experience and knowledge in evaluating and using any information, methods, compounds, or experiments described herein. In using such information or methods they should be mindful of their own safety and the safety of others, including parties for whom they have a professional responsibility.

With respect to any drug or pharmaceutical products identified, readers are advised to check the most current information provided (i) on procedures featured or (ii) by the manufacturer of each product to be administered, to verify the recommended dose or formula, the method and duration of administration, and contraindications. It is the responsibility of practitioners, relying on their own experience and knowledge of their patients, to make diagnoses, to determine dosages and the best treatment for each individual patient, and to take all appropriate safety precautions.

To the fullest extent of the law, neither the Publisher nor the authors, contributors, or editors, assume any liability for any injury and/or damage to persons or property as a matter of products liability, negligence or otherwise, or from any use or operation of any methods, products, instructions, or ideas contained in the material herein.

Library of Congress Cataloging-in-Publication Data

Names: Isaacs, Claudine, editor.
Title: Hoffman and Abeloff's hematology-oncology review / editor, Claudine
   Isaacs ; section editors, Sanjiv Agarwala, John Marshall, Naiyer Rizvi,
   Bruce Cheson, Alice Ma.
Other titles: Hematology-oncology review
Description: First edition. | Philadelphia, PA : Elsevier, [2018] | Includes
   bibliographical references and index.
Identifiers: LCCN 2017029350 | ISBN 9780323429757 (pbk. : alk. paper)
Subjects: | MESH: Neoplasms | Hematologic Diseases | Examination Questions
Classification: LCC RC266.5 | NLM QZ 18.2 | DDC 616.99/40076--dc23 LC
   record available at https://lccn.loc.gov/2017029350

Content Strategist: Kayla Wolfe
Content Development Specialist: Lisa Barnes
Publishing Services Manager: Patricia Tannian
Senior Project Manager: Cindy Thoms
Book Designer: Ashley Miner

Printed in the United States of America

Last digit is the print number: 9   8   7   6

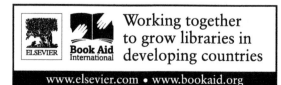

To all of our colleagues, contributors, trainees,
and patients who have taught us so much

The Editors

The authors would like to thank Lisa Barnes and Kayla Wolfe
for their valuable contributions in publishing this book.

CONTRIBUTORS

Ghassan K. Abou-Alfa, MD
Assistant Attending Physician
Memorial Sloan Kettering Cancer Center
Assistant Professor
Weill Medical College at Cornell University
New York, New York

Sanjiv S. Agarwala, MD
Professor and Chief
Department of Oncology and Hematology
St. Luke's Cancer Center
Temple University
Bethlehem, Pennsylvania

Jeanny B. Aragon-Ching, MD, FACP
Clinical Program Director of Genitourinary Cancers
Inova Schar Cancer Institute
Associate Professor of Medicine
Virginia Commonwealth University
Fairfax, Virginia

Nilofer Azad, MD
Associate Professor
Department of Gastrointestinal Oncology
Johns Hopkins Medical Institutions
Baltimore, Maryland

Julie Brahmer, MD, MSc
Associate Professor of Oncology
Department of Medical Oncology
Johns Hopkins Kimmel Cancer Center
Baltimore, Maryland

Susana Campos, MD, MPH
Medical Oncology
Dana-Farber Cancer Institute
Assistant Professor of Medicine
Harvard Medical School
Boston, Massachusetts

Edward Chu, MD, MMS, BS
Professor and Chief
Division of Hematology-Oncology
University of Pittsburgh School of Medicine
Deputy Director
University of Pittsburgh Cancer Institute
University of Pittsburgh School of Medicine
Pittsburgh, Pennsylvania

Corey Cutler, MD, MPH, FRCP(C)
Associate Professor of Medicine
Harvard Medical School
Senior Physician
Department of Medical Oncology
Dana-Farber Cancer Institute
Boston, Massachusetts

Don S. Dizon, MD
Head of Women's Cancers
Lifespan Cancer Institute
Director of Medical Oncology
Rhode Island Hospital
Associate Professor of Medicine
Warren Alpert Medical School of Brown University
Providence, Rhode Island

Nathan Fowler, MD
Associate Professor of Medicine
Co-Director, Clinical and Translational Research
Lead, New Drug Development Program
Department of Lymphoma/Myeloma
University of Texas – MD Anderson Cancer Center
Houston, Texas

Geoffrey Gibney, MD
Co-Leader Melanoma Program
Lombardi Comprehensive Cancer Center
MedStar Georgetown University Hospital
Washington, District of Columbia

Ann Gramza, MD
Medical Oncology Director of Head and Neck Cancer
Lombardi Comprehensive Cancer Center
Medical Oncologist
Head and Neck and Endocrine Cancers
Washington Cancer Institute
MedStar Washington Hospital Center
Washington, District of Columbia

Peter Hammerman, MD, PhD
Dana-Farber Cancer Institute
Boston, Massachusetts

Christine L. Hann, MD, PhD
Assistant Professor
Department of Oncology
Johns Hopkins University School of Medicine
Baltimore, Maryland

Steven Horwitz, MD
Medical Oncologist
Memorial Sloan Kettering Cancer Center
New York, New York

David Ilson, MD, PhD
Attending physician
Gastrointestinal Oncology Service
Department of Medicine
Memorial Sloan Kettering Cancer Center
New York, New York

Fabio M. Iwamoto, MD
Columbia University Medical Center
New York, New York

Marc J. Kahn, MD, MBA
Peterman-Prosser Professor, Sr. Associate Dean
Department of Medicine
Section of Hematology/Medical Oncology
Tulane University School of Medicine
New Orleans, Louisiana

Nikhil I. Khushalani, MD
Vice-Chair and Associate Member
Cutaneous Oncology
H. Lee Moffitt Cancer Center
Associate Professor
Department of Oncological Sciences
Morsani College of Medicine
University of South Florida
Tampa, Florida

Ann Steward LaCasce, MD, MMSc
Assistant Professor of Medicine
Medical Oncology
Dana-Farber Cancer Institute
Boston, Massachusetts

Andrew B. Lassman, MS, MD
Chief, Neuro-Oncology Division
Department of Neurology
Columbia University Medical Center
Medical Director
Clinical Protocol & Data Management Office
Herbert Irving Comprehensive Cancer Center
New York, New York

Christopher H. Lieu, MD
Assistant Professor
Division of Medical Oncology
University of Colorado Denver
Denver, Colorado

Caio Max Rocha Lima, MD
Associate Director for Translational Research
Gibbs Cancer Center and Research Institute,
Spartanburg, South Carolina

Filipa Lynce, MD
Assistant Professor
Department of Medicine
Lombardi Comprehensive Cancer Center
MedStar Georgetown University Hospital
Washington, District of Columbia

Alice D. Ma, MD
Professor of Medicine
Hemophilia and Thrombosis Center
University of North Carolina – Chapel Hill
Chapel Hill, North Carolina

Ravi A. Madan, MD
Clinical Director, Genitourinary Malignancies Branch
National Cancer Institute Center for Cancer Research
Bethesda, Maryland

Molly Weidner Mandernach, MD, MPH
Assistant Professor, Hematology/Oncology
Department of Medicine
University of Florida
Gainesville, Florida

Erica Mayer, MD, MPH
Assistant Professor of Medicine
Susan F. Smith Center for Women's Cancers
Dana-Farber Cancer Institute
Assistant Professor in Internal Medicine
Harvard Medical School
Boston, Massachusetts

Jason Meadows, MD
Assistant Attending, Supportive Care Service
Memorial Sloan Kettering Cancer Center
New York, New York

Ara Metjian, MD
Assistant Professor
Division of Hematology
Department of Medicine
Duke University
Durham, North Carolina

Pashna N. Munshi, MD
Assistant Professor
Blood and Marrow Transplantation
MedStar Georgetown University Hospital
Lombardi Comprehensive Cancer Center
Washington, District of Columbia

Jarushka Naidoo, MB BCh
Assistant Professor
Department of Oncology
The Sidney Kimmel Comprehensive Cancer Center at Johns
Hopkins University
Baltimore, Maryland

Kiran Naqvi, MD, MPH
Assistant Professor
Department of Leukemia
University of Texas
MD Anderson Cancer Center
Houston, Texas

Beth Overmoyer, MD
Assistant Professor of Medicine
Susan F. Smith Center for Women's Cancers
Dana-Farber Cancer Institute
Assistant Professor of Medicine
Harvard Medical School
Boston, Massachussetts

Michael J. Pishvaim, MD, PhD
Assistant Professor
Lombardi Comprehensive Cancer Center
Georgetown University
Washington, District of Columbia

Paula R. Pohlmann, MD, MSc, PhD
Assistant Professor
Department of Medicine
Lombardi Comprehensive Cancer Center
MedStar Georgetown University Hospital
Washington, District of Columbia

Dennis Priebat, MD
Director, Medical Oncology
Department of Medicine
Washington Cancer Institute
Medstar Washington Hospital Center
Washington, District of Columbia

Anita Rajasekhar, MD, MS
Associate Professor
Department of Medicine
Division of Hematology/Oncology
University of Florida
Gainesville, Florida

Farhad Ravandi, MD
Associate Professor of Medicine
University of Texas - MD Anderson Cancer Center
Houston, Texas

Brandi Reeves, MD
Assistant Professor
Department of Internal Medicine/Hematology-Oncology
University of North Carolina – Chapel Hill
Chapel Hill, North Carolina

Gregory J. Riely, MD, PhD
Memorial Sloan Kettering Cancer Center
New York, New York

Erin Roesch, MD
Assistant Clinical Professor of Medicine
Division of Hematology and Oncology
University of California–San Diego
Moores Cancer Center
San Diego, California

Jonathan Strosberg, MD
Associate Professor
GI Oncology
Moffitt Cancer Center
Tampa, Florida

Antoinette Tan, MD, MHSc, FACP
Chief, Section of Breast Medical Oncology
Co-Director of Phase I Program
Department of Solid Tumor Oncology and Investigational
Therapeutics
Levine Cancer Institute
Carolinas HealthCare System
Charlotte, North Carolina

David H. Vesole, MD, PhD
Co-Chief
Myeloma Division
John Theurer Cancer Center
Hackensack, New Jersey
Professor of Medicine
Department of Medicine
Georgetown University
Washington, District of Columbia

Benjamin A. Weinberg, MD
Assistant Professor of Medicine
Division of Hematology and Oncology
Lombardi Comprehensive Cancer Center
Georgetown University Medical Center
Washington, District of Columbia

Marc S. Zumberg, MD
Professor and Section Chief, Non-Malignant Hematology
Department of Medicine
Division of Hematology/Oncology
University of Florida
Gainesville, Florida

PREFACE

The fields of medical oncology and hematology have witnessed dramatic advances over the past decade.

When I was preparing for my second board recertification examination in medical oncology a couple of years ago, I searched without success for a comprehensive, practical, and well-written multiple choice question review book to serve as my study aid. This experience provided the original impetus for creating this review book.

As I continued to conceptualize the book, I envisioned creating a stand-alone resource to serve as an intuitive and easy-to-follow review for those preparing for board examinations in medical oncology or hematology. Realizing the high rate of dual-certification and close relationship between hematology and medical oncology, it was ultimately decided to include study material for both examinations in a single publication.

In these early stages, I was fortunate to recruit an outstanding group of co-editors and authors from Georgetown University Medical Center, Columbia University Medical Center, Dana-Farber Cancer Institute, Memorial Sloan Kettering Cancer Center, St. Luke's University, University of North Carolina, and other leading institutions across the United States. It is with the help of these experts across the broad spectrum of medical oncology and hematology that this book has been made possible.

The result of this careful planning and fruitful collaboration is a practical review book with board-style questions focusing on all relevant aspects of medical oncology and hematology, including an emphasis on case-based questions. The content, style, distribution, and format of the questions are modeled on the ABIM blueprints for the medical oncology and hematology boards. Questions are presented in multiple-choice format with the answer listed along with a rationale explaining both the correct and incorrect answers options for a complete and thorough understanding.

The organization of the book by chapter corresponding to the topic tested in each exam enables the user to easily locate specific questions for more efficient review. A unique feature of this book is the online version, which provides a total of three simulated exams per specialty that can be taken in an untimed study mode or timed assessment mode to portray the experience of the real examination. Using both the print version and electronic version of the book in tandem is intended to provide the user with several options for studying the material for optimal understanding and preparation.

Whether used as a stand-alone review or as a study companion to *Abeloff's Clinical Oncology* and *Hematology: Basic Principles and Practice*, I believe this comprehensive and practical book will be a valuable resource for first-time board examinations in addition to those going through the recertification process.

Claudine Isaacs, MD

CONTENTS

SECTION **1** Cancer Biology, Genomics, and Immunology

CHAPTER

1

Cancer Biology

Nikhil I. Khushalani and Sanjiv S. Agarwala

QUESTIONS

1. According to the "cancer stem cell" hypothesis, which of the following characteristics does a subpopulation of cancer cells in a tumor have?
   - **A.** Maintenance of self-renewal
   - **B.** Capacity for unlimited growth
   - **C.** Ability to differentiate into other more specialized cancer cell types
   - **D.** A, B, and C
   - **E.** All cells within a tumor are capable of self-renewal and differentiation

2. Which of the following accurately describes the process of splicing?
   - **A.** Forming a copy of the gene using messenger RNA (mRNA)
   - **B.** Transporting an mRNA transcript into the cytoplasm of the cell
   - **C.** Removal of introns to produce a continuous chain of coding exons
   - **D.** Translation of coding sequences into proteins
   - **E.** The addition of polyadenylyl moiety to mRNA

3. All of the following are methods to detect single nucleotide polymorphisms except:
   - **A.** Polymerase chain reaction
   - **B.** Allele-specific hybridization
   - **C.** Single nucleotide primer extension
   - **D.** Western blot
   - **E.** Invasive signal amplification

4. Which of the following is the correct sequence of gene expression?
   - **A.** Transcription, splicing, translation
   - **B.** Splicing, transcription, translation
   - **C.** Translation, transcription, splicing
   - **D.** Splicing, translation, transcription
   - **E.** Transcription, translation, splicing

5. Which of the following was the first antiangiogenic agent to receive regulatory approval for use in patients with cancer?
   - **A.** Axitinib
   - **B.** Sunitinib
   - **C.** Bevacizumab
   - **D.** Aflibercept
   - **E.** Pazopanib

6. Which of the following is/are cellular mechanisms involved in the vascularization of tumors?
   - **A.** Co-option
   - **B.** Intussusception
   - **C.** Sprouting
   - **D.** Vasculogenesis
   - **E.** All of the above

7. Which of the following are class effects of antiangiogenic agents?
   - **A.** Hypertension
   - **B.** Thromboembolism
   - **C.** Myocardial ischemia
   - **D.** Nausea and vomiting
   - **E.** A, B, and C

8. In the invasion process of cancer metastasis, cells need to detach themselves from neighboring cells. Which of the following mediates the function of cell-cell adhesion?
   - **A.** E-cadherin
   - **B.** Vascular endothelial growth factor (VEGF)
   - **C.** Epidermal growth factor receptor (EGFR)
   - **D.** HER-2
   - **E.** Fibroblast growth factor (FGF)

9. Which of the following cancers metastasizes primarily via the transcoelomic route?
   A. Non-small cell lung cancer
   B. Ovarian cancer
   C. Thyroid cancer
   D. Melanoma
   E. Bladder cancer

10. Metastases to the brain is common in all of the following cancers except:
    A. Melanoma
    B. Lung cancer
    C. Prostate cancer
    D. Breast cancer
    E. A and B

11. Which of the following is the correct sequence of events in cellular division?
    A. G0, S, G1, G2, M
    B. G0, G1, G2, S, M
    C. S, M, G2, G1, G0
    D. G0, G1, S, G2, M
    E. S, G0, G1, G2, M

12. Which of the following is an example of a protooncogene?
    A. P53
    B. RB1
    C. MYC
    D. BRCA1
    E. CDH1

13. Which of the following cancers are associated with the Li-Fraumeni syndrome?
    A. Breast cancer
    B. Bone and soft-tissue sarcoma
    C. Brain tumors
    D. Adrenocortical carcinoma
    E. All of the above

14. A knockout mouse model of carcinogenesis is characterized by all of the following attributes, except:
    A. Being an excellent method to study "loss-of-function" mutations in tumor suppressor genes
    B. Requiring both alleles of a gene to be inactivated for phenotypic expression
    C. Being ideal for understanding "gain-of-function" oncogene biology

   D. Utilizing gene disruption in the embryonic stem cell to effect changes in the progeny
   E. Being useful for studying gene replacement as a therapeutic strategy

15. Which of the following is an incorrect statement regarding *RET* (rearranged during transfection) signaling?
    A. *RET* plays an important role in the normal development of the nervous system.
    B. Germ-line mutations in *RET* are responsible for the multiple endocrine neoplasia (MEN) type 2 syndromes.
    C. The endogenous ligands for *RET* are glial cell line-derived neurotrophic factors.
    D. Loss of function mutations in *RET* can cause Hirschsprung disease.
    E. Inhibitors of *RET* have not proven to be useful in clinical practice.

16. Which of the following molecular abnormalities are found in gastrointestinal stromal tumors (GISTs)?
    A. CKIT
    B. PDGFR
    C. IGF1R
    D. A and B
    E. All of the above

17. What does the process of anoikis refer to?
    A. Ability of a cell to survive immune attack by CD-8 T-cells
    B. Development of tumor cell emboli in the process of metastasis
    C. Exit of tumor cells from the circulation into surrounding stroma
    D. Programmed cell death resulting from detachment and loss of adhesion
    E. Apoptosis resulting from anaerobic and hypoxic conditions

18. What is the primary function of cyclin-dependent kinases (CDKs) in the regulation of the cell cycle?
    A. Repression of gene transcription
    B. Phosphorylation of proteins to drive progression within the phases of the cell cycle
    C. Segregation of chromosomes
    D. Initiate proapoptotic signaling
    E. Regulation of centrosome functioning

ANSWERS

1. D
The cancer stem cell hypothesis postulates that only a subpopulation of cancer cells can maintain self-renewal, proliferation, and specialized differentiation within a heterogeneous tumor. This is in contrast to the clonal evolution hypothesis, that every cell within a neoplastic mass was capable of these listed traits. Cancer stem cells have characteristic stem cell markers that are not present on other cancer cells within the tumor. These have been described in solid tumors and hematological malignancies.

2. C
Splicing refers to the process of removal of the noncoding sequences of DNA to form a continuous chain of exons to eventually undergo translation into protein. This process

requires precision as any alteration can result in aberrant protein formation and disease, including cancer.

3. D
Single nucleotide polymorphisms (SNPs) constitute the most common form of genetic variation in humans. Modern methods in molecular biology have the capability of detecting a large number of SNPs that exist within the genome. All of the tests listed can detect SNPs, except Western blotting, which is used to detect proteins within the analyzed sample.

4. A
Gene expression is a highly regulated process that starts with transcription of mRNA to form a copy of the gene, followed by removal of the noncoding sequences called introns (splicing), and finally translation into proteins. Alternate splicing can result into translation of multiple isoforms of protein from the same gene.

5. C
Bevacizumab was first approved for patients with metastatic colorectal cancer in combination with chemotherapy. Since then, several other agents have entered the clinic and are used commonly in the management of kidney cancer, non-small cell lung cancer, hepatocellular carcinoma, glioblastoma, and others.

6. E
All of the listed mechanisms are involved with the vascularization of tumors. Initially, tumor cells grow around existing vasculature (co-opt) to form cuffs around the micro-circulation. Intussusception refers to the enlargement of tumor vessels in response to tumor-related growth factors and the creation of an interstitial tissue column in the enlarged lumen. Expansion of the existing vascular network and proliferation of the endothelial cells to form a "bridge" or "sprout" with subsequent canalization constitutes the process of sprouting. Finally, mobilization of endothelial precursor cells from the bone marrow by the process of vasculogenesis also contributes to vascularization within tumors.

7. E
Hypertension, arterial and venous thrombosis, and myocardial ischemia can be seen with all available inhibitors of angiogenesis. In addition, proteinuria can be seen with this class of agents as well. Several other side effects are unique to each agent. However, gastrointestinal toxicity is not a commonly reported adverse event from these drugs.

8. A
E-cadherin proteins are responsible for mediated adhesion between cells through protein-protein interactions at the cell surface. An alteration of the expression of E-cadherin permits disassociation of cells and initiates the process of metastatic invasion. Truncating mutations in the E-cadherin gene (*CDH1*) have been associated with hereditary diffuse gastric cancer, an autosomal dominant familial syndrome.

9. B
This pattern of metastasis involving the surface of the peritoneal cavity is most commonly observed with ovarian cancer. Hematogenous and lymphatic dissemination also occur in ovarian cancer, though less frequently. In the transcoelomic metastatic process, tumor cells first detach from the primary tumor site to enter the peritoneal fluid where they must resist anoikis and immune-mediated destruction. This is followed by peritoneal implantation and metastatic growth. If uncontrolled, this is a major cause of morbidity and mortality in ovarian cancer and certain gastrointestinal cancers, such as colon cancer.

10. C
Metastasis to the brain is distinctly an uncommon pattern of spread in prostate cancer where osteoblastic bone metastases are the norm. In all of the other cancers listed, spread to the brain is a major cause of morbidity and mortality. The etiology of this preferred landing zone for these tumors is not entirely clear.

11. D
Cell division is a tightly regulated process. This is initiated by transition from the G0 (or quiescent) phase to the G1 (first gap) phase. Once the cell crosses the point of "no return" (restriction point), it enters the S (synthesis) phase where chromosome replication takes place. This is followed by the G2 (second gap) phase, and finally mitosis (M phase).

12. C
MYC is a typical protooncogene and is implicated in the genesis of many cancers, most notably Burkitt lymphoma. All of the others listed are classic tumor suppressor genes.

13. E
The Li-Fraumeni syndrome is an autosomal dominant inherited disorder characterized by mutations in the *P53* tumor suppressor gene. In addition to the malignancies listed, leukemia is also seen with higher frequency in this disorder. Some patients with this syndrome lack *P53* mutations. Mutations of CHK2 have been observed in a subset of these patients.

14. C
Gain-of-function mutations are best studied by a transgenic model of cancer where an oncogene is introduced into the mouse genome to further propagate in a dominant pattern of inheritance. All of the other answers are traits for a knockout model of cancer, which is ideal to understand recessive genetic disorders.

15. E
RET is a proto-oncogene required for normal development of the enteric nervous system and the kidney. Following ligand binding, *RET* dimerization occurs, resulting in phosphorylation of tyrosine residues and subsequent cellular signaling. Mutations in *RET* for the molecular basis for the spectrum of MEN type 2 syndromes. This is also seen in sporadic medullary thyroid carcinoma. There are several inhibitors of *RET* that are approved in clinical practice, including vandetanib and cabozantinib for medullary thyroid cancer.

16. E
All of those listed are correct. The vast majority (85%) of GISTs harbor activating mutations in CKIT or the platelet-derived growth factor receptor. In the remaining "wild-type" adult GISTs, recent molecular developments have identified low levels of mitochondrial succinate dehydrogenase and high expression of insulin-like growth factor 1 receptor (IGF1R). Activation of IGF1R eventually leads to increased cellular proliferation through intermediate activation of the mitogen-activated protein kinase and PI3K-AKT-mTOR pathways.

17. D
Anoikis refers to apoptotic cell death induced by detachment of the cell from the extracellular matrix (ECM). This is an important process in the development of metastasis as tumor cells overcome adverse proapoptotic interactions with the matrix. These cells have to circumvent other adverse features, including immune attack, hypoxia, etc., in order to survive and propagate. This process was first described in 1993–94.

18. B
CDKs are responsible for the phosphorylation of proteins in various phases of the cell cycle. The retinoblastoma (Rb) gene controls repression of gene transcription, while the chromosome passenger complex and polo-like kinases (Plk1-5) control chromosome segregation. The polo-like kinases are also involved in centrosome function along with NIMA-related kinases.

CHAPTER

2

Tumor Immunology

Nikhil I. Khushalani and Sanjiv S. Agarwala

QUESTIONS

1. Which of the following cells can suppress the antitumor immune response?
   A. Regulatory T-cells (T$_{regs}$)
   B. CD8+ T lymphocytes
   C. Myeloid-derived suppressor cells (MDSCs)
   D. A and C
   E. All of the above

2. All of the following cancers are known to have an etiological association with microbial infection except:
   A. Kaposi sarcoma
   B. Prostate cancer
   C. Angioimmunoblastic T-cell lymphoma
   D. Stomach cancer
   E. Merkel cell carcinoma

3. Which of the following statements accurately describes the process of "immunoediting"?
   A. The initial recognition of the cancer cell by the immune system
   B. Active destruction of the neoplastic cell by T-lymphocytes
   C. Adaptive response of the tumor to pressure from the immune system in order to enable it to survive
   D. Creation of a local microenvironment that is inhibitory to the effects of the immune system
   E. Recruitment of inflammatory cells to the site of tumor or infection

4. Which of the following is an anticytotoxic T-lymphocyte associated antigen-4 (CTLA-4) antibody?
   A. Pembrolizumab
   B. Nivolumab
   C. Avelumab
   D. Ipilimumab
   E. Atezolizumab

5. Which of the following are immunological (antigenic) differences between normal tissues and tumors?
   A. Genetic instability is a primary characteristic of tumors
   B. The majority of mutations in tumors occur in intracellular proteins
   C. Tumor-specific antigens are often unique to individual tumors
   D. Tumors overexpress a large number of genes relative to normal cells
   E. All of the above

6. Which of the following cells has the capacity to directly kill antigen-presenting cells?
   A. CD8+ T-cells
   B. CD4+ T-cells
   C. MDSCs
   D. T$_{regs}$
   E. None of the above

7. Which of the following statements is true regarding immune surveillance?
   A. The immune system recognizes and eliminates tumors based on tumor-associated antigens.
   B. In animal models of carcinogenesis, "progressor tumors" develop through an intact immune surveillance mechanism.
   C. Nude mice demonstrate a dramatic increase in tumor incidence due to impaired immune surveillance.
   D. Transplant recipients on immunosuppression have a decreased incidence of virus-associated tumors secondary to an intact immune surveillance mechanism.
   E. The NKG2D receptor does not play a role in immune surveillance.

8. On which of the following cells is the CTLA-4 checkpoint receptor located?
   A. B-cells
   B. Neutrophils
   C. Dendritic cells
   D. T-cells
   E. All of the above

9. Which of the following immune checkpoint—ligand combination is correct?
   A. TIM-3—Galectin-9
   B. PD1—PD-L1
   C. LAG-3—MCHII
   D. BTLA—HVEM
   E. All the above are correct

10. Which of the following statements is accurate regarding transforming growth factor-beta (TGF-β)?
    A. TGF-β stimulates angiogenesis and promotes matrix metalloproteinase activity.
    B. TGF-β functions as an inhibitory cytokine and blunts antitumor immune response.
    C. In most normal epithelial cells, TGF-β causes G1 cell cycle arrest and inhibits cellular proliferation.
    D. All of the above are correct.
    E. Only A and B are correct.

11. What is the mechanism by which indoleamine-2,3 dioxygenase (IDO) effects unresponsiveness in T-cells?
    A. Increased production of IL-2
    B. Through catabolism of tryptophan
    C. Suppression of γ-interferon
    D. Decreased regulatory T-cell activation
    E. Increased TGF-β production

12. Which of the following are mediators of T-cell unresponsiveness?
    A. IDO
    B. Reactive oxygen species (ROS) and reactive nitrogen
    species (RNS)

    C. Nitrous oxide (NO)
    D. TGF-β
    E. All of the above

ANSWERS

1. D

There exists a complex interplay between the cancer cell
and the tumor microenvironment. Regulatory T-cells and
MDSCs can inhibit antitumor cytotoxic T-cell responses,
thus allowing tumor propagation. A high level of MDSCs
has been shown to be a negative prognostic indicator in
several tumor subtypes.

2. B

All of the cancers listed, except prostate cancer, are associated
with an infectious organism. Kaposi's sarcoma results from
infection with human herpes virus 8 (HHV8). Several lymphoproliferative disorders (both B- and T-cell) are associated
with the Epstein-Barr virus (EBV). Angioimmunoblastic lymphoma is a peripheral T-cell lymphoma where EBV has been
identified in the B-cells present within the tumor as well as
within some of the neoplastic T-cells. Gastric carcinoma has
been linked to infection with *Helicobacter pylori* while the Merkel cell polyomavirus is found in the majority of cases of Merkel cell carcinoma, a rare but aggressive form of skin cancer.

3. C

There exists a dynamic interaction between the cancer cell and
the host immune response that results in the shaping of the
tumor, both in biology and behavior; this constitutes the hypothesis of immunoediting and consists of three phases (elimination, equilibrium, and escape). Recent advances in our
understanding of this interaction have enabled pre-clinical
and clinical development of therapeutic strategies to restore
immune control and elicit an antitumor immune response.

4. D

Ipilimumab is the first and only anti-CTLA-4 antibody to receive regulatory approval in the immune therapy of cancer.
All of the other agents listed, either target the programmed
death receptor-1 (PD-1; pembrolizumab, nivolumab) or its
ligand PD-L1 (avelumab, atezolizumab). These agents have
received approval in the United States for the management
of one or more cancers.

5. E

All of the tenets listed are typically seen in tumors compared to normal cells. Genetic instability results in a large
number of mutations within exons of tumor cells, resulting in the production of neoantigens. These effects occur
more frequently within the intracellular proteins; circulating antibodies do not readily recognize the resulting neoantigens. Similarly, epigenetic differences between tumor
cells and normal cells results in the overexpression of a
large number of genes in the former relative to the latter.

6. A

Cytotoxic CD8+ T-cells have T-cell receptors (TCRs) that recognize antigens on a foreign cell, such as a cancer cell or an
infected cell, and initiate the process of destruction of that
cell. CD4+ helper T-cells play a prominent role in modulat-
ing the immune response through the secretion of a variety

of cytokines. Regulatory T-cells and myeloid-derived suppressor cells play important roles in the down-regulation of
the immune response to pathogens and cancer.

7. A

The systematic identification and destruction of tumor cells
through the recognition of tumor-specific antigens is referred
to as an immune surveillance. Defects in immune surveillance
are purported to result in the development of tumors, so
called "progressor" tumors through immune escape or
resistance. While inherently it would be assumed that im-
munodeficient nude mice would have a higher incidence of
tumors, this has not proven to be the case, which is likely
from a compensatory increase in innate immunity and the
production of T-cells via pathways that are independent of
the thymus. The NKG2D receptor is expressed on NK cells,
select T-cells, and on subsets of intraepithelial lymphocytes,
where it plays a role against invading pathogens in contact
with epithelial linings of the gut, the respiratory tract, and
the skin, thus being involved with immune surveillance.

8. D

The CTLA-4 is an immune checkpoint expressed exclusively on several subtypes of T-cells including CD4+, CD8+,
and T_{reg} cells. It functions as a negative regulator of the immune response. Inhibition of CTLA-4 by antibodies, such
as ipilimumab and tremelimumab, can trigger an immune
response with the potential for therapeutic benefit. Ipilimumab is approved for use in patients with advanced unresectable melanoma, and as adjuvant therapy for stage III
melanoma, based on the results from phase III trials.

9. E

Maintenance of an immunological homeostasis is a closely
regulated process with immune checkpoints playing an important role. Each of the immune checkpoints listed in the
question can inhibit lymphocyte activity. TIM-3 is selectively expressed on cytokine-producing CD4+ helper cells (Th1)
and CD8+ cytotoxic T-cells and functions to limit responses
from these cells, both in duration and extent. Galectin-9 is
a ligand for TIM-3. There are two known ligands for PD-1:
PD-L1 and PD-L2. Following ligand binding, PD-1 inhibits
T-cell activation through several mechanisms. Inhibition
of PD-1 activity has been one of the major therapeutic advances in cancer immunotherapy in the last decade. LAG-3
(CD223) enhances T_{reg} activity and inhibits CD8+ effector
T-cell function; MHC class II is the only known ligand for
LAG-3. The herpes virus entry mediator (HVEM) is the ligand for B- and T-lymphocyte attenuator (BTLA); binding
can negatively modulate the function of the T-cell.

10. D

TGF-β is an important cytokine for normal physiological
functioning and in pathological states with a variety of effects on the microenvironment. Mutations in TGF-β can
promote the invasive phenotype through the mechanisms
outlined. TGF-β can effect T_{reg}-mediated suppression of CD8
T-cell antitumor response. Elevated serum levels of TGF-β
have been associated with poor prognosis in several cancers.

11. B

Within the tumor microenvironment, numerous molecules can blunt the immune response. IDO is one of the rate-limiting enzymes of the catabolic pathway of tryptophan causing its depletion. This deficiency of tryptophan inhibits T-cell responses by causing an arrest in proliferation. A number of IDO inhibitors are currently under investigation in clinical trials, typically in combination with other immune checkpoint inhibitors, in an attempt to restore and enhance the antitumor response.

12. E

All of the molecules listed can inhibit the immune response within the tumor microenvironment. IDO depletes tryptophan and thus blocks T-cell proliferation as this process requires an adequate supply of tryptophan. The production of ROS and RNS by myeloid cells can inhibit T-cell response. Similar effects are seen with nitrous oxide production by immature myeloid cells and myeloid-derived suppressor cells. The inhibitory cytokine TGF-β plays a role in the suppression of cytotoxic T-cell responses mediated by T_{regs}.

CHAPTER

3

Cancer Chemotherapy

Edward Chu

QUESTIONS

1. The multidrug resistance (mdr) phenotype is a well-established mechanism of cellular drug resistance. Which one of the following statements is true regarding this resistance mechanism?
   A. Decreased drug efflux
   B. Decreased drug influx
   C. Enhanced drug influx
   D. Enhanced intracellular drug accumulation
   E. Enhanced drug efflux with reduced intracellular drug accumulation

2. A 55-year-old male with newly diagnosed stage IV colorectal cancer and widespread metastatic involvement of the liver and lungs has been started on FOLFIRI chemotherapy in combination with the anti-VEGF antibody bevacizumab. Within 4 days of receiving his first cycle of therapy, he begins to note increased oral discomfort with a number of new mouth sores, —six to seven loose stools per day, repeat CBC shows significant myelosuppression with neutropenia, and the patient's wife states that her husband's mental status appears to be markedly altered from his normal baseline. Which of the following enzymes is most likely altered in this patient?
   A. Dihydrofolate reductase
   B. UDP glucuronyltransferase
   C. Dihydropyrimidine dehydrogenase
   D. Thymidylate synthase (TS)
   E. Thiopurine methyltransferase

3. Which one of the following statements is correct?
   A. All dihydropyrimidine dehydrogenase (DPD) mutations are associated with DPD deficiency
   B. The absence of DPD mutations rules out DPD deficiency
   C. DPD*2A is associated with inactive DPD protein and DPD deficiency
   D. All of the above
   E. None of the above

4. Bevacizumab exerts its antiangiogenic effects by binding to which one of the following VEGF ligands?
   A. VEGF-A
   B. VEGF-B
   C. VEGF-C
   D. PlGF
   E. All of the above

5. Treatment with panitumumab is associated with which electrolyte abnormality?
   A. Hyponatremia
   B. Hypokalemia
   C. Hypophosphatemia
   D. Hypomagnesemia
   E. Hypouricemia

6. A 49-year-old white female is diagnosed with stage III colon cancer. She is diabetic and has impaired kidney function with a creatinine clearance (CrCl) of 35 mL/min. She has decided to be treated with the XELOX combination regimen. Which of the following statements is correct?
   A. Give full dose of capecitabine with no dose reduction
   B. Reduce the capecitabine dose by 25%
   C. Reduce the capecitabine dose by 30%
   D. Reduce the capecitabine dose by 50%
   E. Capecitabine should not be given

7. A 49-year-old white female is diagnosed with stage III colon cancer. She is diabetic and has impaired kidney function with a CrCl of 35 mL/min. She has decided to be treated with the XELOX combination regimen. Which of the following is true relating to oxaliplatin dosing?
   A. No dose reduction is necessary
   B. Reduce the oxaliplatin dose by 25%
   C. Reduce the oxaliplatin dose by 33%
   D. Reduce the oxaliplatin dose by 50%
   E. Oxaliplatin should not be given

8. Which of the following statements about the platinum agents is correct?
   A. Cisplatin is effective for upper gastrointestinal (GI) cancers, while oxaliplatin is only effective in colorectal cancer.
   B. The mechanisms of resistance to cisplatin, carboplatin, and oxaliplatin are identical.
   C. The DNA lesions associated with oxaliplatin are different than those associated with cisplatin and carboplatin.
   D. Carboplatin is less nephrotoxic, less emetogenic, and less myelosuppressive than cisplatin.
   E. Oxaliplatin can be safely administered to patients with moderate impaired renal function (CrCl, 20–39 mL/min).

9. A 64-year-old patient with early-stage node-positive ER+ breast cancer is about to start on tamoxifen for her adjuvant therapy. She has a long-standing history of depres-

sion for the past 18 years and has been on paroxetine. Her depressive symptoms have been well controlled, and she believes that she needs to continue with antidepressive therapy. Which one of the following liver microsomal enzymes is responsible for tamoxifen metabolism?

A. CYP3A4
B. CYP2C8
C. CYP2D6
D. CYP1A2
E. CYP3A5

10. In a breast cancer patient who is on adjuvant tamoxifen therapy, which one of the following is the most appropriate treatment option for her depression?

A. St. John's wort
B. Duloxetine
C. Fluoxetine
D. Continue with paroxetine
E. Venlafaxine

11. Which one of the following statements is true relating to sorafenib therapy?

A. Drugs such as rifampin, phenytoin, and phenobarbital reduce the metabolism of sorafenib leading to increased drug levels.
B. Drugs such as ketoconazole and other CYP3A4 inhibitors increase the metabolism of sorafenib leading to reduced drug levels.
C. Sorafenib is an inducer of UGT1A1.
D. Avoid Seville oranges and grapefruit products while on sorafenib therapy.
E. The oral bioavailability of sorafenib is not affected by food.

12. A 56-year-old male patient with advanced renal cell cancer was treated with sunitinib for 5 months. He now presents with disease progression with widespread involvement of both lobes of the liver. The decision is made to now switch over to everolimus therapy and to use a daily dose of 10 mg PO. In reviewing his various laboratory results, his total serum bilirubin level is 2.5 mg/dL, serum albumin is 2.6 g/dL, prothrombin time is elevated to 18 seconds, and there is no ascites. Overall, he is determined to have moderate liver impairment (Child-Pugh class B). Which one of the following statements is true?

A. Grapefruit products can be taken while on therapy.
B. St. John's wort can be safely taken, as there is no drug-drug interaction with everolimus.
C. The dose of everolimus should be reduced to 5 mg daily.
D. Oral bioavailability is not affected by food content.
E. There is no increased risk of opportunistic infections.

13. A 65-year-old female patient with metastatic HER2-positive disease is being treated with the combination of capecitabine and trastuzumab. Of note, she has a history of ischemic heart disease, but she has not had any cardiac symptoms for the past 2 years. She has been on therapy for 8 months and is tolerating this combination regimen well with no symptoms. Computed tomography (CT) scans were just performed, and they confirm a nice response to therapy. A follow-up multigated acquisition scan to assess her cardiac status shows a 20% reduction in the left ventricular ejection fraction (LVEF) from a normal baseline. Which one of the following statements is true?

A. Continue with current dose of trastuzumab
B. Reduce dose of trastuzumab by 25%
C. Reduce dose of trastuzumab by 50%

D. Withhold trastuzumab therapy and continue with capecitabine
E. Stop trastuzumab and capecitabine and switch to a new treatment regimen

14. A patient with metastatic osteogenic sarcoma is about to start treatment with high-dose methotrexate (MTX). With respect to the extent of his disease, the patient has multiple pulmonary nodules, mediastinal lymph node, and a malignant left pleural effusion. He complains of lower back pain, unrelated to his underlying cancer, which is well controlled on indomethacin. Which one of the following is the most appropriate intervention?

A. Administer intravenous fluids with alkalinization of the urine to a pH > 6
B. Continue with indomethacin
C. Leucovorin rescue should be continued even when serum MTX levels are less than 50 nM
D. Drainage of the left pleural effusion prior to initiation of MTX infusion
E. Discontinue indomethacin and begin patient on a different nonsteroidal agent

15. Which one of the following statements is true relating to pertuzumab?

A. Immunologic mechanisms are not involved in antitumor activity.
B. Binds to subdomain II of the HER2-neu growth factor receptor.
C. Main biological effect is inhibition of homodimerization of HER2.
D. Patients with prior exposure to anthracyclines or radiation therapy to the chest are not at increased risk for developing cardiac toxicity.
E. Infusion reactions are usually observed with prolonged therapy.

16. A patient with metastatic nonsquamous non-small cell lung cancer is being treated with pemetrexed and cisplatin. Which one of the following is the most appropriate treatment option?

A. Supplementation with folic acid and vitamin B6
B. Supplementation with folinic acid and vitamin B6
C. Supplementation with folic acid and vitamin B3
D. Supplementation with folic acid and vitamin B12
E. Supplementation with vitamin B6 and dexamethasone

17. A 45-year-old male patient with metastatic colorectal cancer is being treated in the second-line setting with FOLFIRI plus cetuximab. One week after his initial treatment, the patient presents with a 2-day history of increasing fatigue and an absolute neutrophil count of 500/μL. What is the most likely diagnosis?

A. DPD deficiency
B. FOLFIRI-associated myelosuppression
C. UGT1A1*28
D. UGT2B4
E. UGT2B7

18. A 46-year-old male patient with primary CNS lymphoma is presently receiving high-dose MTX. He receives leucovorin rescue according to protocol, and serum MTX levels are being closely monitored. Which one of the following best describes when leucovorin rescue can be safely stopped?

A. Serum MTX levels <500 nM
B. Serum MTX levels <100 nM
C. Serum MTX levels <250 nM
D. Serum MTX levels <5×10^{-8} M
E. Serum MTX levels <1×10^{-8} M

19. A patient with non-Hodgkin lymphoma is being treated with the combination of fludarabine, cyclophosphamide, and rituximab. Which one of the following statements is true?
    A. Dose modification of fludarabine is not required in the setting of renal dysfunction.
    B. Dose modification of cyclophosphamide is not required in the setting of renal dysfunction.
    C. Dose modification of fludarabine is required in the setting of liver dysfunction.
    D. Prophylaxis with bactrim to prevent *Pneumocystis carinii* is required.
    E. Fludarabine is active in its parent form.

20. A patient with end-stage renal disease and multiple myeloma is being treated with single-agent bortezomib. Which one of the following statements is true?
    A. Bortezomib should be administered before dialysis.
    B. Dose modifications are not required in the setting of moderate to severe hepatic impairment.
    C. Green tea products should be avoided.
    D. St. John's wort does not alter the metabolism of bortezomib.
    E. Bortezomib can only be administered via the intravenous route.

21. A 38-year-old female with stage IV Hodgkin lymphoma is being treated with ABVD chemotherapy. She has been treated with 4 cycles, and repeat CT scans show a nice response to therapy. Review of her serum chemistries are notable for a serum sodium of 125 mEq/L, potassium of 3.7 mEq/L, bicarbonate of 25 mEq/L, chloride of 100 mEq/L, blood urea nitrogen of 10 mg/dL, creatinine of 1.1 mg/dL, and uric acid less than 4 mg/dL. Which one of the following is the most appropriate cause of her hyponatremia?
    A. Dehydration
    B. Adrenal insufficiency
    C. Renal tubular acidosis
    D. Syndrome of inappropriate antidiuretic hormone secretion (SIADH)
    E. Underlying kidney disease

22. A deficiency in thiopurine methyltransferase (TPMT) results in significantly increased toxicity to which one of the following agents?
    A. MTX
    B. Nelarabine
    C. 6-Mercaptopurine
    D. Fludarabine
    E. Cladribine

23. A 38-year-old male with newly diagnosed metastatic colorectal cancer is started on mFOLFOX6 plus bevacizumab. There was a miscalculation in the chemotherapy orders, and he was given a 20-fold higher dose of 5-FU in the 46-hour infusion. Which of the following is the most appropriate treatment intervention?
    A. Administer high-dose leucovorin
    B. Administer glucarpidase
    C. Immediate hemodialysis
    D. Administer uridine triacetate
    E. Wait for symptoms to occur and then institute appropriate supportive care measures

24. Which of the following tyrosine kinases are inhibited by crizotinib?
    A. c-Met
    B. ALK
    C. RON
    D. ROS1
    E. All of the above

25. Which reduced folate is part of the TS ternary complex?
    A. 5,10-Methlenetetrafolate
    B. 5-Formyltetrahydrofolate
    C. 10-Formyltetrahydrofolate
    D. Folic acid
    E. 5-Methyltetrahydrofolate

ANSWERS

1. **E**
The multidrug resistance (mdr) gene encodes a P-170 glycoprotein whose function is to cause efflux of drug out of the cell, which results in reduced intracellular accumulation of drug within the cell. This mechanism is a well-established mechanism for a wide range of unrelated classes of drugs, which include anthracyclines, taxanes, camptothecins, and the vinca alkaloids.

2. **C**
This is a classic presentation of the DPD deficiency in which there is either partial or complete deficiency in DPD. In this setting, patients present with severe toxicities in the form of myelosuppression, GI toxicity with diarrhea, mucositis, nausea/vomiting, and neurotoxicity with altered mental status, lethargy, and/or encephalopathy.

3. **C**
To date, more than 30 sequence variations in the DPD gene have been identified, with the most well-established variant being DPD*2A (c.1905 + 1G > A; IVS14+11G.A; rs3918290). This is a single nucleotide variant at the intron boundary of exon 14 that results in a splicing defect, skipping of the entire exon, and a completely inactive protein. The other *DPD* variants that are associated with reduced DPD enzyme activity and increased 5-FU toxicity include *DPD*5, *DPD*6, *DPD*9A, *DPD*13 (c.1679T > G; I560S; rs55886062), c.2846A > T (D949V; rs67376798), c.1236G > A (E412E; rs56038477). It has now been well established that not all DPD mutations are associated with DPD deficiency. In fact, there are some mutations that lead to increased DPD expression and activity. In up to 40% of patients who present with the class symptoms of DPD deficiency, mutations in the DPD gene have yet to be identified.

4. **A**
Bevacizumab binds to only the VEGF-A ligand, of which there are 6 isoforms. In contrast, ziv-aflibercept binds to VEGF-A, VEGF-B, and PlGF.

5. **D**
Treatment with anti-EGFR antibodies, cetuximab and panitumumab, is associated with magnesium wasting with inappropriate urinary excretion, which then leads to

hypomagnesemia. EGFR is strongly expressed in the kidney, especially in the ascending limb of the loop of Henle, where up to 70% of filtered magnesium is reabsorbed. In patients being treated with anti-EGFR antibody therapy, serum magnesium levels need to be routinely measured and repleted as necessary.

6. B

Capecitabine and capecitabine metabolites are cleared by the kidneys, and increased toxicity has been observed with capecitabine therapy in the presence of renal impairment. The capecitabine dose does not need to be dose-reduced when the CrCl is greater than 50 mL/min. The dose of capecitabine needs to be reduced by 25% when the CrCl is between 30 and 50 mL/min. Capecitabine is contraindicated and should not be administered when the CrCl is less than 30 mL/min.

7. A

As with other platinum agents, oxaliplatin is excreted by the kidneys. However, renal dysfunction studies have shown no increase in pharmacodynamic drug-related toxicities in patients with mild or moderate renal dysfunction and CrCl down to 20 mL/min. No formal studies have been conducted to date in patients with CrCl <20 mL/min, and in this setting of severe renal dysfunction, oxaliplatin should not be administered

8. E

The DNA lesions are similar for cisplatin, carboplatin, and oxaliplatin with formation of both inter- and intrastrand crosslinks. With respect to safety profile, carboplatin is less nephrotoxic and less emetogenic than cisplatin, but significantly more myelosuppressive than cisplatin. The resistance mechanisms for cisplatin and carboplatin are identical. However, in the presence of mismatch repair defects where cisplatin and carboplatin resistance develops, sensitivity to oxaliplatin is maintained, which explains the efficacy of oxaliplatin in colorectal cancer and other GI cancers where mismatch repair defects have been identified. Oxaliplatin can be safely administered to patients with abnormal function with CrCl down to as low as 20 mL/min

9. C

Tamoxifen is a prodrug that is activated by the liver microsomal system and specifically CYP2D6 to form endoxifen and other active metabolites. In patients, the activity of this enzyme can be highly variable leading to variations in the levels of the active metabolites of tamoxifen. Patients can have reduced CYP2D6 activity because of their genotype of by coadministration of drugs that inhibit CYP2D6 function. In both cases, there is reduced formation of endoxifen, an active metabolite of tamoxifen, which then leads to inferior clinical benefit from tamoxifen.

10. E

Tamoxifen is a prodrug that is activated by the liver microsomal system and specifically CYP2D6 to form the active metabolite endoxifen. Inhibitors of CYP2D6 can lead to a reduced formation of the active metabolites. Antidepressant agents, including St. John's wort, duloxetine, fluoxetine, paroxetine, bupropion, and sertraline, are inhibitors of CYP2D6, which can then interfere and inhibit tamoxifen metabolism, leading to lower blood levels of the active tamoxifen metabolites.

11. D

Sorafenib is metabolized in the liver primarily by the CYP3A4 microsomal enzymes. As a result, there are a number of important drug-drug interactions with sorafenib therapy.

Drugs that inhibit CYP3A4, such as ketoconazole, may reduce the metabolism of sorafenib leading higher drug levels and potentially increased toxicity. Drugs, such as rifampin, phenytoin, phenobarbital, and carbamazepine, increase the metabolism of sorafenib leading to reduced drug levels and potentially reduced clinical benefit. Seville oranges, grapefruit products, starfruit, and pomelos contain substances that inhibit the liver metabolism of sorafenib, which can then lead to increased drug levels and potentially increased toxicity. Sorafenib is an inhibitor of UGT1A1, and caution must be used when sorafenib is administered with agents that are metabolized by UGT1A1, such as irinotecan. Sorafenib is rapidly absorbed after an oral dose. The general recommendation is to take sorafenib without food at least 1 hour before or 2 hours after eating, as oral bioavailability is affected by food. In particular, foods with a high fat content reduce oral bioavailability by as much as 30%.

12. C

Grapefruit products, Seville oranges, starfruit, and pomelos should be avoided, as these food products can impair liver metabolism of everolimus, which then leads to increased drug levels. There is a drug-drug interaction between St. John's wort and everolimus where St. John's wort can increase everolimus metabolism in the liver, resulting in lower effective drug levels. Food with a high fat content reduces oral bioavailability by up to 20%. Patients are at increased risk for developing opportunistic infections, including fungal infections, while on everolimus therapy. Metabolism of everolimus occurs mainly in the liver the CYP3A4 enzymes, and elimination of drug is mainly hepatic with excretion in feces. In patients with moderate liver impairment (Child-Pugh class B), the everolimus dose should be reduced to 5 mg daily, and in the setting of severe liver impairment (Child-Pugh class C), everolimus therapy should not be given.

13. D

Careful baseline assessment of cardiac function (LVEF) must be done prior to the start of trastuzumab therapy with frequent monitoring (every 2–3 months) while on therapy. Trastuzumab should be held if there is an absolute reduction in LVEF by greater than 16% from a normal baseline value. Trastuzumab should be stopped immediately in any patient who develops clinically significant symptoms of congestive heart failure.

14. D

MTX is cleared by the kidneys, and the process of renal excretion is inhibited in the presence of aspirin, nonsteroidal antiinflammatory agents, penicillins, cephalosporins, and probenecid. MTX distributes in to third-space fluid collections, such as pleural effusions and ascites, and the fluid collections should be drained prior to the start of MTX, as they can cause a delay in drug clearance. In the presence of these fluid collections, patients may experience increased toxicity. Vigorous intravenous hydration with alkalinization of the urine to a pH of greater than 7.0 is required to prevent precipitation of MTX and MTX polyglutamates in acidic urine, which can then lead to renal failure. The rationale for leucovorin rescue is to protect normal cells from MTX toxicity. Leucovorin should be given until the serum MTX levels are down to 50 nM, and once below that threshold level, leucovorin rescue can be stopped.

15. B

Pertuzumab is a recombinant humanized IgG1 monoclonal antibody direct against the extracellular domain (subdomain II) of the HER2-neu growth factor receptor. It binds to a different epitope on HER2-neu receptor than trastuzumab, which binds to subdomain IV. Binding of pertuzumab to the HER2-neu receptor leads to inhibition of heterodimerization of HER2 with other HER family members, including EGFR, HER3, and HER4. As pertuzumab is an IgG1 antibody, immunologic mechanisms may also be involved in its antitumor activity, including antibody-dependent cellular cytotoxicity. The main side effects of pertuzumab are cardiac toxicity and infusion-related reactions. Patients with a prior history of anthracycline treatment or radiotherapy to the chest and/or mediastinal region may be at increased risk of developing cardiac toxicity, which is usually manifested by a reduction in LVEF.

16. **D**

Patients who receive pemetrexed-based therapy should receive vitamin supplementation with folic acid (350 µg/day) and vitamin B12 (1000 µg IM every 3 cycles) to reduce the risk and severity of toxicity while on therapy. Steroids have been shown to reduce the development of skin rash, and dexamethasone (4 mg PO bid) can be given for 3 days beginning the day before starting pemetrexed.

17. **C**

DPD deficiency presents with severe toxicity to 5-FU with the classic triad of myelosuppression, GI toxicity, and neurotoxicity. This patient presents with isolated myelosuppression, which would be unusual for DPD deficiency. Irinotecan is metabolized by UDP glucuronyltransferase, and the process of glucuronidation leads to inactive metabolites of both irinotecan and SN-38. In patients with the UGT1A1*28 genotype, there is significant reduction in irinotecan and SN-38 glucuronidation, which then leads to increased myelosuppression and/or GI toxicity. Approximately 10% of the North American population is homozygous for this specific genotype.

18. **D**

The rationale for leucovorin rescue is to protect normal cells from MTX toxicity. Leucovorin should be given until the serum MTX levels below 50 nM (5×10^{-8} M), and once below that threshold level, leucovorin rescue can be stopped.

19. **D**

Fludarabine is a prodrug, and following administration, it is rapidly dephosphorylated to 2-fluoro-ara-adenosine. This nucleoside then enters the cells via a nucleoside-mediated process, and it is then initially phosphorylated to the monophosphate form and eventually metabolized to the fludarabine triphosphate form, which is the active cytotoxic metabolite. Both fludarabine and cyclophosphamide are renally excreted. In the presence of renal dysfunction, the doses of fludarabine and cyclophosphamide need to be modified. Dose modification of fludarabine is not required in the setting of liver dysfunction. Fludarabine therapy is associated with an increased risk of opportunistic infections, including *Pneumocystis carinii*, and patients should be empirically placed on bactrim prophylaxis.

20. **C**

Bortezomib can be administered via the IV or SC routes with both administration routes providing similar total systemic exposure. Bortezomib is metabolized by the liver cytochrome P450 system, and dose modification is recommended in the setting of moderate to severe hepatic impairment. St. John's Wort along with other CYP3A4 inducers can increase the liver metabolism of bortezomib, resulting in reduced drug levels. Bortezomib is dialyzed out via hemodialysis so in patients with end-stage renal disease who require dialysis, the drug should be administered after dialysis. Green tea products and supplements have been shown to inhibit the clinical activity of bortezomib and other boron-containing proteasome inhibitors, such as ixazomib. Such a food-drug interaction does not exist with carfilzomib as this agent does not contain a boron moiety. (Golden EB et al. Green tea polyphenols block the anticancer effects of bortezomib and other boronic acid-based proteasome inhibitors. Blood 2009;113:5927-5937; Chu E and DeVita VT, Physicians' Cancer Chemotherapy Drug Manual 2016, Jones & Bartlett Learning, 2016)

21. **C**

In patients with dehydration and underlying kidney disease, the blood urea nitrogen (BUN) and/or creatinine levels should be elevated. With adrenal insufficiency, patients present with hyponatremia and hyperkalemia. In renal tubular acidosis, the bicarbonate levels are reduced along with an elevation in chloride levels and a reduction in potassium levels. SIADH presents with hyponatremia and normal potassium, chloride, BUN/creatinine levels. Several anticancer agents are associated with SIADH, including the vinca alkaloids, cyclophosphamide, cisplatin, and melphalan. While SIADH has been observed with certain tumor types, the most common being small cell lung cancer, Hodgkin lymphoma is not normally associated with SIADH.

22. **C**

A partial or complete deficiency of TPMT results in excessive, severe toxicity with myelosuppression, GI toxicity, and/or neurotoxicity, in response to the thiopurines, 6-mercaptopurine and 6-thioguanine. TPMT is not involved in the metabolism of other purine analogs, such as nelarabine, cladribine, and fludarabine.

23. **D**

The administration of uridine triacetate (vistonuridine), an oral prodrug form of uridine, has been shown to be a safe and effective antidote to 5-FU overdose, and this agent was recently approved by the US Food and Drug Administration. 5-FU cannot be removed by hemodialysis, and it is not known whether peritoneal dialysis can be used to remove circulating 5-FU. Leucovorin and glucarpidase are two agents that have been used to prevent and/or rescue against MTX-associated toxicities but would not be able to prevent the toxicities of 5-FU.

24. **E**

Crizotinib inhibits the tyrosine kinases associated with c-Met, ALK, RON, and ROS1. This agent is now approved in the United States to treat patients with metastatic non-small cell lung cancer whose tumors are ALK-positive or ROS1-positive.

25. **A**

The TS ternary complex is made up of the 5-FU metabolite FdUMP, the reduced folate 5,10-methylenetetrahydrofolate, and the TS enzyme. The role of the reduced folate is to enhance the inhibitory effect of the 5-FU metabolite in inhibition of TS. When TS is bound in this ternary complex, TS enzymatic activity is optimally inhibited, leading to inhibition of thymidylate synthesis and subsequent inhibition of DNA biosynthesis. Leucovorin is 5-formyltetrahydrofolate, which is eventually metabolized within the cell to 5,10-methylenetetrahydrofolate.

REFERENCES

Question 1

1. Chu E, Sartorelli AC. Cancer chemotherapy. In: Katzung BG, ed. *Basic and Clinical Pharmacology*. 13th ed. New York, NY: McGraw-Hill; 2014.

Question 2

1. van Kuilenberg AB. Dihydropyrimidine dehydrogenase and the efficacy and toxicity of 5-fluorouracil. *Eur J Cancer*. 2004;40:939–950.
2. Chong CR, Zirkelbach JF, Diasio RB, Chabner BA. Pharmacogenetics. In: Chabner BA, Longo DL, eds. *Cancer Chemotherapy and Biotherapy: Principles and Practice*. 5th ed. Philadelphia: Lippincott Williams & Wilkins; 2010.

Question 3

1. van Kuilenberg AB. Dihydropyrimidine dehydrogenase and the efficacy and toxicity of 5-fluorouracil. *Eur J Cancer*. 2004;40:939–950.
2. Saif MW, Chu E. Antimetabolites. In: DeVita VT, Lawrence T, Rosenberg SA, eds. *Cancer: Principles and Practice of Oncology*. 10th ed. Philadelphia: JB Lippincott Co.; 2015.

Question 4

1. Ferrara N. VEGF as a therapeutic target in cancer. *Oncology*. 2005;69(suppl 3):11–16.
2. Ferrara N, Adamis AP. Ten years of anti-vascular endothelial growth factor therapy. *Nat Rev Drug Discov*. 2016;15(6):385–403.

Question 5

1. Schrag D, Chung KY, Flombaum C, Saltz L. Cetuximab therapy and symptomatic hypomagnesemia. *J Natl Cancer Inst*. 2005;97:1221–1224.

Question 6

1. Walko CM, Lindley C. Capecitabine: a review. *Clin Ther*. 2005;27:23–44.
2. Mikhail SE, Sun JF, Marshall JL. Safety of capecitabine: a review. *Expert Opin Drug Saf*. 2010;9:831–841.

Question 7

1. Takimoto CH, Graham MA, Lockwood G, et al. Oxaliplatin pharmacokinetics and pharmacodynamics in adult cancer patients with impaired renal function. *Clin Cancer Res*. 2007;13:4832–4839.

Question 8

1. O'Dwyer PJ, Calvert AH. Platinum analogs. In: DeVita VT, Lawrence T, Rosenberg SA, eds. *Cancer: Principles and Practice of Oncology*. 10th ed. Philadelphia: JB Lippincott Co.; 2015.

Question 9

1. Jin Y, Desta Z, Stearns V, et al. CYP2D6 genotype, antidepressant use, and tamoxifen metabolism during adjuvant breast cancer treatment. *J Natl Cancer Inst*. 2005;97(1):30–39.
2. Hoskins JM, Carey LA, McLeod HL. CYP2D6 and tamoxifen: DNA matters in breast cancer. *Nat Rev Cancer*. 2009;9:576–586.

Question 10

1. Jin Y, Desta Z, Stearns V, et al. CYP2D6 genotype, antidepressant use, and tamoxifen metabolism during adjuvant breast cancer treatment. *J Natl Cancer Inst*. 2005;97(1):30–39.
2. Hoskins JM, Carey LA, McLeod HL. CYP2D6 and tamoxifen: DNA matters in breast cancer. *Nat Rev Cancer*. 2009;9:576–586.

Question 11

1. Chu E, DeVita VT. *Physicians' Cancer Chemotherapy Drug Manual 2016*. Burlington, MA: Jones & Bartlett Learning; 2016.

Question 12

1. Chu E, DeVita VT. *Physicians' Cancer Chemotherapy Drug Manual 2016*. Burlington, MA: Jones & Bartlett Learning; 2016.

Question 13

1. Martin M, Esteva FJ, Alba E, et al. Minimizing cardiotoxicity while optimizing treatment efficacy with trastuzumab: review and expert recommendations. *Oncologist*. 2009;14:1–11.

Question 14

1. Chu E, Sartorelli AC. Cancer chemotherapy. In: Katzung BG, ed. *Basic and Clinical Pharmacology*. 13th ed. New York, NY: McGraw-Hill; 2014.
2. Saif MW, Chu E. Antimetabolites. In: DeVita VT, Lawrence T, Rosenberg SA, eds. *Cancer: Principles and Practice of Oncology*. 10th ed. Philadelphia: JB Lippincott Co.; 2015.

Question 15

1. McCormack PL. Pertuzumab: a review of its use for first-line combination treatment of HER2-positive metastatic breast cancer. *Drugs*. 2013;73:1491–1502.

2. Chu E, DeVita VT. *Physicians' Cancer Chemotherapy Drug Manual 2016*. Burlington, MA: Jones & Bartlett Learning; 2016.

Question 16

1. Chu E, DeVita VT. *Physicians' Cancer Chemotherapy Drug Manual 2016*. Burlington, MA: Jones & Bartlett Learning; 2016.

Question 17

1. Toffoli G, Cecchin E, Corona G, et al. The role of UGT1A1*28 polymorphism in the pharmacodynamics and pharmacokinetics of irinotecan in patients with metastatic colorectal cancer. *J Clin Oncol*. 2006;24:3061–3068.
2. Shulman K, Cohen I, Barnett-Griness O, et al. Clinical implications of UGT1A1*28 genotype testing in colorectal cancer patients. *Cancer*. 2011;117:3156–3162.

Question 18

1. Chu E, Sartorelli AC. Cancer chemotherapy. In: Katzung BG, ed. *Basic and Clinical Pharmacology*. 13th ed. New York, NY: McGraw-Hill; 2014.
2. Saif MW, Chu E. Antimetabolites. In: DeVita VT, Lawrence T, Rosenberg SA, eds. *Cancer: Principles and Practice of Oncology*. 10th ed. Philadelphia: JB Lippincott Co.; 2015.

Question 19

1. Anaissie EJ, Kontoyiannis DP, O'Brien S, et al. Infections in patients with chronic lymphocytic leukemia treated with fludarabine. *Ann Intern Med*. 1998;129:559–566.
2. Byrd JC, Hargis JB, Kester KE, Hospenthal DR, Knutson SW, Diehl LF. Opportunistic pulmonary infections with fludarabine in previously treated patients with low-grade lymphoid malignancies: a role for *Pneumocystis carinii* pneumonia prophylaxis. *Am J Hematol*. 1995;49:135–142.

Question 20

1. Golden EB, Lam PY, Kardosh A, et al. Green tea polyphenols block the anticancer effects of bortezomib and other boronic acid-based proteasome inhibitors. *Blood*. 2009;113:5927–5937.
2. Chu E, DeVita VT. *Physicians' Cancer Chemotherapy Drug Manual 2016*. Burlington, MA: Jones & Bartlett Learning; 2016.

Question 21

1. Adrogue HJ, Madias NE. Hyponatremia. *N Engl J Med*. 2000;342:1581–1589.
2. Chu E, DeVita VT. *Physicians' Cancer Chemotherapy Drug Manual 2016*. Burlington, MA: Jones & Bartlett Learning; 2016.

Question 22

1. Lennard L. Clinical implications of thiopurine methyltransferase—optimization of drug dosage and potential drug interactions. *Ther Drug Monit*. 1998;20:527–531.

Question 23

1. von Borstel R, O'Neil J, Bamat M. Vistonuridine: an orally administered, life-saving antidote for 5-fluorouracil overdose. *J Clin Oncol*. 2009;27:15S, abstract 9616.

Question 24

1. Gridelli C, Peters S, Sgambato A, Casaluce F, Adjei AA, Ciardiello F. ALK inhibitors in the treatment of advanced NSCLC. *Cancer Treat Rev*. 2014;40:300–306.
2. Farina F, Gambacorti-Passerini C. ALK inhibitors for clinical use in cancer therapy. *Front Biosci*. 2016;8:46–60.

Question 25

1. Chu E, Callender MA, Farrell MP, Schmitz JC. Thymidylate synthase inhibitors as anticancer agents: from bench to bedside. *Cancer Chemother Pharmacol*. 2003;52(suppl 1):S80–S89.
2. Chu E, DeVita VT. *Physicians' Cancer Chemotherapy Drug Manual 2016*. Burlington, MA: Jones & Bartlett Learning; 2016.

CHAPTER

4

Immunotherapy and Pathway Inhibitors

Geoffrey Gibney

QUESTIONS

1. A 60-year-old male with metastatic BRAF V600E mutant melanoma is treated with dabrafenib plus trametinib. He tolerates treatment well with intermittent mild fevers and fatigue. On restaging scans, he has a deep partial response with reduction in disease burden in the lungs and liver. Lytic bone areas remain stable. His blood work shows a hemoglobin of 9, which is stable from his baseline. There are no other significant abnormalities on the complete blood count (CBC) or comprehensive metabolic panel. Four weeks later on treatment, he develops swelling in his legs, mild dyspnea on exertion, and more fatigue but is still active. He has no chest pain. Blood work, including CBC and comprehensive metabolic panel, are similar to his last visit. What would you recommend for the management in this patient?
   A. Perform restaging scans for disease progression
   B. Continue dabrafenib and trametinib and monitor symptoms closely
   C. Hold trametinib and order an echocardiogram
   D. Hold dabrafenib and order an echocardiogram
   E. Discontinue dabrafenib and trametinib

2. A 40-year-old female with a history of resected stage IIIA melanoma from a left arm primary site presents to her oncologist with restaging computed tomography (CT) scans of the chest, abdomen, and pelvis. Unfortunately, there were three new pulmonary lesions, the largest measuring 1.5 cm at the left lower lung. No other areas of metastatic disease were identified. Labs were normal including the lactate dehydrogenase (LDH) level. Biopsy of the left lower lung lesion confirmed metastatic melanoma. BRAF testing on the tumor specimen identified a BRAF V600E mutation. Treatment options were reviewed, and the patient chose to pursue BRAF-targeted therapy based on the recent data showing improved outcomes in patients with low disease burden and normal LDH. Her oncologist gets approval for vemurafenib plus cobimetinib and brings her back to clinic to start treatment and review a magnetic resonance imaging (MRI) of the brain to complete her staging workup. The MRI shows a 2-mm lesion in the left frontal cortex that is a possible metastasis, but there is no prior comparison. The patient wants to start vemurafenib plus cobimetinib today. What would be the most appropriate recommendation?
   A. Proceed with vemurafenib plus cobimetinib and repeat MRI in a short interval
   B. Hold vemurafenib plus cobimetinib and refer to neurosurgery
   C. Hold vemurafenib plus cobimetinib and refer to radiation oncology
   D. Change treatment to anti-PD-1 therapy
   E. Change BRAF therapy to dabrafenib plus trametinib

3. A 56-year-old male with stage IV transitional cell bladder cancer is treated with atezolizumab after progression platinum-based chemotherapy. At the start of treatment, he has an ECOG performance status of 1 and has minimal symptoms related to his disease. He tolerates therapy well except for a minor rash that is controlled with topical corticosteroids. A restaging scan is performed at 9 weeks, which shows regression in the pelvic adenopathy and stable liver lesions. However, there is an increase in size of two small lung nodules. He continues to have an ECOG performance status of 1 and has no new pulmonary symptoms. What would you recommend for the management of this patient?
   A. Increase the dose of atezolizumab
   B. Change therapy to gemcitabine
   C. Continue atezolizumab
   D. Monitor off treatment
   E. Change therapy to pemetrexed

4. A 35-year-old female with a history of depression is diagnosed with T4aN2bM0 (stage IIIB) melanoma from a primary site on her left shoulder. She is status post wide-local excision, sentinel lymph node biopsy, and completion lymph node dissection. She has recovered well from her surgeries, and staging CT scan of the neck, chest, abdomen, and pelvis and MRI of the brain show no evidence of metastatic disease. She is concerned about the risk of disease relapse and is interested in pursuing adjuvant immunotherapy. Which immunotherapy that has demonstrated improvement in relapse-free survival and overall survival would you recommend to this patient?
   A. High dose interferon
   B. Ipilimumab
   C. GM-CSF
   D. Interleukin (IL)-2
   E. Nivolumab

5. A 60-year-old male with stage IIIB non-small cell lung cancer (NSCLC) was initially treated with combined chemotherapy and radiation. On restaging scans 6 months later, he is noted to have new and progressive disease in the lungs and new liver metastases. He is asymptomatic and working full-time. A decision is made to start treatment with the anti-PD-1 therapy pembrolizumab based on his tumor's PD-L1 status. After 12 weeks of therapy, restaging CT scans show disease regression. The radiologist also comments on a few areas of nonspecific ground glass opacities in both lungs. On questioning, the patient does endorse mild dyspnea on exertion and a dry cough that is new, but he is still able to work. He denies fevers, sweats, chest pain, or other new symptoms. His resting

and ambulatory oxygen saturation is 98%, and his cardiac and lung exams are unrevealing. The patient is eager to continue with pembrolizumab. What is the most appropriate course in this patient?

A. Discontinue pembrolizumab and monitor off treatment
B. Hold pembrolizumab until the respiratory symptoms improve
C. Hold pembrolizumab and administer systemic corticosteroids
D. Continue pembrolizumab but at a 20% dose reduction
E. Continue pembrolizumab and monitor closely for worsening respiratory symptoms and hypoxia

6. A 70-year-old patient with resected stage II melanoma at the left arm now presents with palpable adenopathy at the left axilla. Biopsy confirms metastatic melanoma. Staging CT scans of the torso show pulmonary nodules consistent with distant metastatic disease. MRI of the brain is negative for CNS disease. He is asymptomatic from his melanoma disease, but he does have a history of coronary artery disease, type 2 diabetes, and peripheral neuropathy. This limits his activities, but he is able to complete his activities of daily living. His tumor is BRAF wild type. He wishes to receive effective treatment for his metastatic melanoma, but he is concerned about the risks of serious side effects. Which immune therapy would you recommend for this patient?

A. Ipilimumab
B. Nivolumab
C. IL-2
D. Nivolumab plus ipilimumab
E. High-dose interferon

7. A 50-year-old male with a significant smoking history and resected stage I NSCLC patient presents with weight loss, chest pains, and shortness of breath. He undergoes a staging CT scan of the chest, abdomen, and pelvis, which shows mediastinal lymphadenopathy and lung and liver metastases. Biopsy of a liver lesion demonstrates metastatic adenocarcinoma consistent with recurrent disease. PD-L1 immunohistochemistry is performed, and over 50% of tumor cells stain positive. The anti-PD-1 agent pembrolizumab is offered to the patient based on the high clinical activity seen in patients whose tumors are strongly positive for PD-L1. What other molecular markers or clinical features are associated with greater clinical activity of anti-PD-1 therapy in patients with NSCLC and other malignancies?

A. High tumor mutational burden
B. Nonsmoker status
C. BRAF mutation
D. History of brain metastases
E. Low tumor infiltrating lymphocyte density

8. A 45-year-old female is diagnosed with metastatic melanoma of unknown primary after presenting with seizures and undergoing craniotomy to resect a 2 cm right parietal mass. She recovered from her surgery and has no further seizures or neurologic deficits. Staging scans of the torso show metastatic disease in the liver and several lytic bone lesions. She reads her pathology report and sees that the tumor stained positive for GP100, MART-1, and S100—all common melanoma markers. She wishes to be aggressive in the treatment of her cancer and receive immunotherapy that is specific to targeting her tumor type. She inquires if she could receive a GP100 vaccine combined with an anti-PD-1 drug after reading about this on the internet. Based on the available information, which statement is true about human studies of vaccines in combination with immune checkpoint blockade therapy?

A. GP100 vaccine has demonstrated improved survival when combined with ipilimumab.
B. Vaccine therapy alone is effective treatment in metastatic melanoma patients.
C. Vaccines in combination with checkpoint therapy do not increase toxicity risks.
D. A multipeptide vaccine with nivolumab enhances clinical responses in melanoma patients.
E. Patients should be tested for HLA-A2 status prior to treating with vaccines.

9. The development of immune agents as therapeutic strategies have ranged from vaccine- and cytokine-based treatments to more focused approaches to manipulate targets within the adaptive immune system in order to modify antitumor T-cell responses. This can be direct antibody mediated stimulation or inhibition of immune checkpoints that augment immune responses, such as the anti-CTLA-4 and anti-PD-1/PD-L1 agents that are now approved for a range of malignancies. However, many of these mechanisms are important for maintaining appropriate checks and balances within the immune system for normal functions, such as defending against infection, wound healing, and maternal-fetal tolerance. It is important for providers to understand these mechanisms when making treatment recommendations, as they differ significantly from standard chemotherapy agents and have different implications on patient monitoring. Which of the following is believed to be the correct mechanism of action for anti-PD-1 therapies in cancer?

A. Depletion of regulatory T-cells via antibody-dependent cellular toxicity
B. Enhancement of natural killer cell function through via stimulation of the PD-1 pathway
C. Priming of CD4+ T-cells in response to dendritic cell presentation of tumor antigen
D. Blocking CD8+ T-cell exhaustion in the tumor microenvironment
E. Allow CD28 co-stimulatory signaling on T-cells for enhanced cytotoxic activity

10. A 65-year-old male with metastatic prostate cancer comes to your office with evidence of progressive disease while on treatment with leuprolide and bicalutamide. Laboratory values and scans show a rising PSA and increased bone metastases. His testosterone level is less than 50 ng/dL. Despite these findings, he feels well. He denies any bone pain, fatigue, or other symptoms related to his cancer. He wishes to discuss further treatment options, in particular immunotherapy options. He is aware of other non-immunotherapy options, such as abiraterone and enzalutamide from past discussions. In your discussion with the patient, you mention the impressive activity of anti-PD-1 and anti-PD-L1 therapies in a range of cancers, but not so far in prostate cancer patients. The only approved immunotherapy in prostate cancer is sipuleucel-T, which works by a different mechanism of action. Which of the following is appropriate to tell the patient, based on available information?

A. Overall survival, but not progression-free survival, is prolonged with sipuleucel-T.
B. Sipuleucel-T is a checkpoint inhibitor that activates cytotoxic T-cell function.
C. Significant declines in PSA are typically seen with sipuleucel-T administration.
D. Sipuleucel-T is a peptide vaccine administered to patients as subcutaneous injections.
E. Peripheral blood lymphocytes are collected for the preparation of sipuleucel-T.

11. A 58-year-old female with a history of resected stage II melanoma at the left ankle presents to your office with multiple dark subcentimeter nodules over the left shin. These appear to be in the dermal layer and are nontender. The patient's exam shows no other disease. At the left groin, the surgical scar from the sentinel lymph node biopsy is well healed, and there is no palpable adenopathy. A biopsy of one of the dermal nodules demonstrates metastatic melanoma. Staging scans show no distant disease. The patient is active and works full-time. She does not have any limitations or other significant medical problems. Surgery is not practical given the number and extent of disease. After a discussion of systemic therapy versus intralesional therapy, she is most interested in receiving talimogene laherparepvec (TVEC). You explain this is an immunotherapy, but works by a different mechanism of action than the anti-PD-1 therapies frequently used in patients with advanced melanoma. What is most appropriate to tell the patient?
    A. The majority of responses occur within the first month of treatment.
    B. All patients are at substantial risk of developing a disseminated herpes infection with treatment.
    C. TVEC is safe to administer to patients with compromised immune systems.
    D. The therapy only works in tumor sites that are directly injected.
    E. Durable responses are seen in one-third of stage III melanoma patients treated with TVEC.

12. A 40-year-old male with resected stage IIIB melanoma is treated with adjuvant ipilimumab at 10 mg/kg every 4 weeks. Prior to the third dose of ipilimumab, he develops watery bowel movements and abdominal cramping. He denies any history of sick contacts. There is no blood in the stool. His usual pattern is one formed bowel movement per day. The frequency escalates from three bowel movements in a 24-hour window to six bowel movements over 2 days. The consistency is now more watery, and there has been no improvement with loperamide. He comes to the clinic for evaluation. His vital signs are stable, and he is afebrile. Bowel sounds are more active than usual, but there is no abdominal pain with palpation, distention, or other concerning signs. Overall, he appears well despite the symptoms. A CT scan of the abdomen and pelvis is performed and shows inflammatory changes in the descending colon. Stool studies are positive for leukocytes, but the *Clostridium difficile* (*C. difficile*) antigen is negative and cultures preliminarily are negative for infectious source. Oral prednisone 1 mg/kg daily is started. Two days later, his symptoms are worsened and he is admitted to the hospital. What are the next appropriate steps?
    A. Increase oral prednisone to 2 mg/kg daily and monitor
    B. Switch to intravenous methylprednisolone 1 mg/kg q12 hours, test for latent tuberculosis and monitor
    C. Switch to intravenous methylprednisolone 1 mg/kg q12 hours and add mycophenolate 1 gram q12 hours

    D. Continue oral prednisone at 1 mg/kg daily and add antibiotic coverage with oral vancomycin and intravenous levofloxacin and metronidazole
    E. Hold corticosteroids and schedule urgent gastrointestinal consultation for colonoscopy

13. In viral-associated malignancies, such as HPV-associated head and neck squamous cell carcinoma (HNSCC) and polyomavirus-associated Merkel cell carcinoma (MCC), antitumor immune responses with dense T-cell infiltrate can be observed. T-cell-specific responses against viral antigens that are present in tumor cells have been identified. This suggests a particularly important role that immunotherapies could play in viral-associated malignancies. Anti-PD-1 and PD-L1 therapies have now been studied in nonselected patient populations with advanced HNSCC and MCC. Which of the statements most accurately represents the activity of anti-PD-1/PD-L1 therapies in viral associated malignancies compared to their nonviral counterparts?
    A. Anti-PD-1/PD-L1 therapies are significantly more effective in viral-associated HNSCC and MCC than in nonviral HNSCC and MCC.
    B. There is a trend of higher response rates in polyomavirus-associated MCC that is not seen in HPV-associated HNSCC.
    C. There is a trend of higher response rates in HPV-associated HNSCC that is not seen in polyomavirus-associated MCC.
    D. Anti-PD-1/PD-L1 therapies have lower response rates in viral-associated HNSCC and MCC due to lower low mutational burden.
    E. Patients with HNSCC and MCC should be screened for viral status prior to the recommendation of immunotherapies.

14. A 55-year-old male with renal cell carcinoma (RCC; clear cell subtype) develops recurrence 2 years after nephrectomy for localized disease. Staging scans show numerous pulmonary lesions with the largest measuring 2 cm in the right lower lobe. A biopsy confirms the diagnosis. He is not interested in targeted therapies, such as pazopanib and sunitinib. He wishes to be treated upfront with immunotherapy. He feels well overall with a good performance status. In his past medical history, it is noted that he has ischemic cardiomyopathy from a prior coronary artery event. He has no active angina symptoms at present, but finds he develops shortness of breath during moderate exertion. His last recorded ejection fraction was 40%–50%. Which immune therapy agent would you recommend?
    A. Ipilimumab
    B. IL-2
    C. Clinical trial with anti-PD-1 therapy
    D. Interferon alpha plus bevacizumab
    E. GM-CSF

ANSWERS

1. C

Hold trametinib and order an echocardiogram. Past studies of MEK inhibitors have reported infrequent but potentially serious events of cardiomyopathy, left ventricular dysfunction, and decreased ejection fraction. In the COMBI-d phase III study of dabrafenib plus trametinib, decreased ejection fraction was reported in 4% of patients on the combination. In a patient with signs of heart failure,

trametinib should be held and an echocardiogram would be most appropriate.

2. A

Proceed with vemurafenib plus cobimetinib and repeat MRI in a short interval. In this patient, a new small brain lesion is identified, which could be an early brain metastasis. Prior phase II studies of vemurafenib and dabrafenib have demonstrated objective responses in active brain metastases in patients with metastatic BRAF V600E/K mutant melanoma.

There is also direct evidence that BRAF agents do penetrate the blood-brain barrier, which is based on cerebrospinal fluid testing. Therefore, in an asymptomatic patient, it would be reasonable to proceed with BRAF-targeted therapy and monitor the brain lesion on serial imaging studies. Furthermore, if the brain lesion did eventually increase in size, this would provide more certainty that it is a brain metastasis, and a radiation oncologist or neurosurgeon should offer definitive treatment. There is no clear data indicating that one BRAF plus MEK inhibitor combination is superior to another.

3. **C**

Continue atezolizumab. In past clinical studies of anti-CTLA-4 and anti-PD-1/PD-L1 therapies, it has been noted that some patients experience initial progressive disease or mixed responses, followed by disease regression. This has been termed "pseudoprogression," originating from studies of ipilimumab in patients with advanced melanoma, which occurred in up to 10% of patients. This may be due to delayed tumor regression based on the mechanism of action by immunotherapies and/or an initial increase in tumor size due to inflammation. In the phase II study of atezolizumab in advanced bladder cancer patients, 20 of the 121 (17%) patients treated beyond progression subsequently demonstrated significant responses. Therefore, in this patient with a mixed response and clinical stability, it would be best to continue with atezolizumab until the next restaging scans.

4. **B**

Ipilimumab. In the EORTC 18071 study, ipilimumab demonstrated superior relapse-free survival and overall survival over placebo in patients with resected stage III melanoma. Of note, grade 3 or higher related adverse events were reported in over 40% of patients in the ipilimumab arm. Patients need to be educated on the potential toxicity risks, and treatment generally should not be offered in patients with active autoimmune disorders or significant comorbidities. In this young patient with only a history of depression, it would be reasonable to offer ipilimumab. The only other option in this list that is Food and Drug Administration approved for this indication demonstrating gains in survival, is high-dose interferon. However, some studies with interferon have failed to show an improvement in overall survival over the control arm, and depression can occur as a related adverse event.

5. **C**

Hold pembrolizumab and administer systemic corticosteroids. In this patient, there are radiographic signs and clinical symptoms of pneumonitis related to the pembrolizumab therapy. This would be grade 2 by CTCAE reporting. Although other possible diagnoses are not fully ruled out, such as heart failure or infectious pneumonia, they would be unlikely in this patient scenario. An electrocardiogram and serum cardiac enzymes could be obtained to rule out a cardiac etiology. Pneumonitis has been reported in approximately 1%–5% of patients treated with anti-PD-1 therapy and may be higher in NSCLC patients previously treated with radiation. For grade 2 pneumonitis, anti-PD-1 therapy should be held and systemic corticosteroids administered, such as an oral prednisone 1 mg/kg daily dose with a 4–5 week taper.

6. **B**

Nivolumab. Anti-PD-1 therapies, including nivolumab and pembrolizumab, have objective response rates of 40%–45% in the front-line setting for patients with advanced melanoma. Clinical activity has proven superior over ipilimumab in randomized phase III studies. Anti-PD-1 monotherapy has been associated with a grade 3 or greater adverse event rate of approximately 15% in most studies, which is lower than other immune therapy regimens listed. Nivolumab plus ipilimumab has demonstrated a higher objective response rate and longer progression-free survival, but also a grade 3 or greater adverse event rate above 50%.

7. **A**

High mutational burden. Overall, immune checkpoint therapies have demonstrated greater clinical activity in tumor types with high mutational burden, such as NSCLC and melanoma. This is thought to be due to the generation of neoantigens that are recognized by the immune system and generate a stronger adaptive immune response. This is supported by data showing greater cytolytic T-cell activity in tumors with higher mutational and neoantigen burden and the identification of specific T-cell subpopulations that recognize individual neoepitopes that are unique to the patient's tumor.

8. **C**

Vaccines in combination with checkpoint therapy do not increase toxicity risks. Efforts so far have failed to demonstrate improved clinical activity of immune checkpoint therapy when combined with a vaccine. In the phase III study of ipilimumab alone, ipilimumab plus GP100, or GP100 alone, in advanced melanoma patients, there was no significant difference in clinical outcomes between the two ipilimumab arms. Furthermore, GP100 monotherapy had minimal clinical activity and the shortest survival. The addition of vaccine in this study and others did not significantly increase the toxicity risks outside of minor local injection site reactions. Similar findings were noted in a phase II single arm study of a multipeptide vaccine plus nivolumab in advanced melanoma patients. In this study, patients were required to be HLA-A2 positive (thought to be required for specific melanoma antigen presentation) and positive by immunohistochemistry for at least one of the vaccine peptides included in the treatment. Newer data are suggesting that antigen recognition may be primarily patient specific towards neoantigens existing in the tumor cells, making global vaccine strategies more difficult.

9. **D**

Blocking CD8+ T-cell exhaustion in the tumor microenvironment. PD-1 is a transmembrane protein expressed on a range of immune cells, including CD8+ T-cells. It serves as an inhibitory pathway to cause tolerance or T-cell exhaustion when it binds to the PD-L1 or PD-L2 ligand. The PD-L1 ligand is frequently expressed on tumor cells in response to cytokines, such as interferon-gamma and IL-12. This leads to tumor cell escape or immune tolerance and T-cell exhaustion when PD-L1 interacts with PD-1 on immune cells. Direct interference of this interaction with anti-PD-1 monoclonal antibodies, such as nivolumab and pembrolizumab, prevents the exhaustion of T-cells and allows for an augmented antitumor response. This is evidenced by posttreatment biopsies where a dense accumulation of cytotoxic T-cells is seen in responding tumor sites.

10. **A**

Overall survival, but not progression-free survival, is prolonged with sipuleucel-T. This is an autologous dendritic cell vaccine strategy approved by the Food and Drug Administration for the treatment of castrate-resistant metastatic prostate cancer. It involves leukapheresis of a patient's peripheral blood mononuclear cells and exposing them *ex vivo* to a recombinant prostatic acid phosphatase (PAP) protein fused with GM-CSF. This is designed to active dendritic cell function. The activated cells are then intravenously administered back to the patient as a series of three treatments. The activated dendritic cells will then induce T-cell immunity against prostate cancer cells expressing PAP. After multiple phase III studies of sipuleucel-T, improvement in overall survival, but not response rate or progression-free survival, has been demonstrated.

11. **E**

Durable responses are seen in one-third of stage III melanoma patients treated with TVEC, which is an oncolytic virus that is based on a modified herpes simplex virus type 1. Functional deletion of the neurovirulence factor gene (ICP34.5) limits its ability to cause a disseminated infection and promotes the tumor-cell-specific replication. It also has insertion of a gene encoding human GM-CSF. When TVEC is injected directly into the tumor site, it locally replicates causing tumor cell death and induction of tumor-specific T-cell responses. Antitumor responses can occur both at the injected and the noninjected tumor sites. In the phase III melanoma study of intralesional TVEC versus subcutaneous GM-CSF, the durable response rate was 16.3% versus 2.1%, respectively. However, in the subgroup analysis, the durable response rate was much higher in stage III patients at 33%. Given the favorable toxicity profile and ability to monitor for delayed responses, offering TVEC to the patient in this question is a reasonable approach.

12. **B**

Switch to intravenous methylprednisolone 1 mg/kg q12 hours, test for latent tuberculosis and monitor. The patient in this question has initially developed grade 2 diarrhea/colitis, which then progresses to a grade 3 level despite appropriate outpatient treatment with prednisone at 1 mg/kg. Grade 3 diarrhea was reported in 10% of patients treated with ipilimumab on the EORTC 18071 trial. Infection and other causes of diarrhea need to be considered, but in a patient treated with ipilimumab 10 mg/kg, immune-mediated diarrhea or enterocolitis is usually the most likely diagnosis and requires prompt treatment. In patients not responding to oral prednisone as an outpatient, admission

to the hospital for supportive care and intravenous corticosteroids is required. If there is no rapid improvement, administration of infliximab is indicated. Because of the potential risk of reactivation of latent tuberculosis with infliximab, ruling this out with assays, such as a commercially available interferon-gamma release test, is a good consideration prior to administration.

13. **C**

There is a trend of higher response rates in HPV-associated HNSCC that is not seen in polyomavirus-associated MCC. In studies of anti-PD-1/PD-L1 therapies in patients with advanced HNSCC and MCC, objective responses are seen in both viral positive and viral negative patients. The absence of the virus component does not limit the immune recognition and potential for immunotherapies in these disease types. Immune infiltrates are seen in both viral positive and viral negative tumors. However, the biology may be different. For example, in MCC, viral positive tumors typically have a low mutational burden, whereas viral negative tumors have a high mutational burden similar to melanoma. In Keynote-012 and Checkmate 141 HNSCC studies with pembrolizumab and nivolumab, respectively, objective response rates and survival were higher in patients with HPV+ tumors. In the studies of pembrolizumab and avelumab (anti-PD-L1 antibody; pending Food and Drug Administration approval) in MCC, there were no clear associations or trends in polyomavirus status and response.

14. **C**

Clinical trial with anti-PD-1 therapy. Currently anti-PD-1 therapy is approved only as a second-line therapy in patients with metastatic RCC. In the phase III study of nivolumab versus everolimus in patients progressing after initial treatment with a vascular endothelial growth factor tyrosine kinase inhibitor, nivolumab was superior with an objective response rate of 25%. Long-term follow up of the phase I study of nivolumab in RCC patients showed a 5-year overall survival rate of 34%. IL-2 is another frontline immunotherapy to consider in appropriately selected patients based on its potential for cure but also its toxicities. In particular, patients can undergo a significant cardiovascular leak syndrome leading to hemodynamic instability. IL-2 would not be a good choice in a patient with coronary artery disease and cardiomyopathy.

CHAPTER

5

Acute Myeloid Leukemia and Myelodysplastic Syndrome

Kiran Naqvi and Farhad Ravandi

QUESTIONS

1. A 78-year-old male presented to his primary care physician reporting weakness for 3 months. His past medical problems include hypertension and BPH. He is currently on lisinopril and tamsulosin. He was also noted to be mildly anemic on a routine blood test that was done a year ago, but no further workup was done at that time. Complete blood profile shows Hb = 7.9 g/dL, MCV = 101, WBC = 5.6, ANC = 2.0, and platelets = 182 K/mm^3. B12, folate, and TSH are all within normal limits. EPO level is 600 mU/mL. A bone marrow biopsy was done that showed hypercellular marrow (80% cellularity) with 2% blasts and dyserythropoiesis. Cytogenetics showed del 5q(q13q33) in all 20 cells. What is the most appropriate next step?
   A. Observation
   B. Start treatment with epoetin
   C. Blood transfusion alone
   D. Start treatment with lenalidomide
   E. Consider a clinical trial

2. A 67-year-old male presents with worsening fatigue. A complete blood count shows Hb = 8.8 g/dL, MCV = 110. White blood cell and platelet counts are normal. Retic count is 1.2%. Serum epo level is 225 mU/mL. Folate, B12, and TSH are within normal limits. Serum ferritin is 185. Direct Coomb test is negative. He denies drinking alcohol. Hepatitis profile is negative. A bone marrow biopsy is done that shows myelodysplasia. Cytogenetics are diploid. What is the most appropriate initial treatment for this patient?
   A. Blood transfusion alone
   B. Start EPO
   C. Start lenalidomide
   D. Start azacitidine
   E. Consider clinical trial

3. A 45-year-old male with a history of Hodgkin lymphoma diagnosed 5 years ago presents to his oncologist with fatigue, dizziness, and easy bruising for the past month. A complete blood count shows Hb = 7.9 g/dL, WBC = 2.2 K/mm3, ANC = 0.9, and platelets of 27 K/mm3. A bone marrow exam shows a hypercellular marrow with trilineage dysplasia with 7% blasts. Karyotype is complex with del5q, monosomy 7, +11, and +8, in 17 out of 20 metaphases. He is transfused with 2 units of packed red blood cells. A donor search for a hematopoietic stem cell transplant is in progress. What should the next step in the management of this patient?
   A. Azacitidine
   B. Supportive care with packed red cells and platelet transfusions
   C. Lenalidomide
   D. Cyclosporine
   E. Hospice

4. A 77-year-old female with prior history of ER/PR positive stage IIIA breast cancer diagnosed 10 years ago was treated with Adriamycin and paclitaxel followed by aromatase inhibitor for 5 years. She was diagnosed with coronary artery disease 5 years ago and had a stent placed. She also suffers from diabetes mellitus, hypertension, and hyperlipidemia. A year ago she was noted to be mildly anemic (Hb = 10.5 g/dL) with mild thrombocytopenia (platelets = 128 K/mm^3). She was observed by her PCP. She now presents with easy bruising and fatigue. A CBC shows WBC = 1.4 K/mm^3, ANC = 0.6 K/mm^3, Hb = 7.5 g/dL, and platelets = 25 K/mm^3. EPO level is 550 mU/mL. She received 2 units of packed red blood cells. A bone marrow biopsy demonstrated an overall cellularity of 50%, trilineage dysplasia especially marked in the erythroid precursors, and 12% blasts with complex karyotype including monosomy 5 and monosomy 7. What is next appropriate step in the management of this patient?
   A. Refer for a hematopoietic stem cell transplant
   B. Hospice
   C. Azacitidine
   D. Epoetin
   E. Supportive care with transfusions

5. An 80-year-old female who has been in fairly good health all her life besides mild hypertension and osteoarthritis presents to her PCP for a routine visit and reports feeling more tired than usual. Her blood work reveals she is anemic with Hb = 8.1 g/dL, MCV = 105, WBC = 5.5 K/mm^3, and platelets = 550 K/mm^3. Iron studies are within normal limits. EPO is 605 mU/L. Direct Coomb test is negative. Stool for guaiac is negative. She undergoes a bm biopsy demonstrating increased marrow cellularity for age, erythroid dysplasia, and an increased number of small, monolobulated megakaryocytes. Blasts are 3%. Cytogenetics reveals an abnormal female karyotype. What does this patient have?
   A. High-risk MDS with complex cytogenetics
   B. Aplastic anemia
   C. Pure red cell aplasia
   D. 5q- syndrome
   E. Autoimmune hemolytic anemia

6. A 45-year-old male reports feeling tired and fatigued for the last 2 months. He presents to his PCP for further evaluation and is noted to be pancytopenic. Hb = 7.7 g/dL (MCV = 101), WBC = 1.2 K/mm^3 (ANC = 0.4), and platelets are 25 K/mm^3. B12, folate, TSH, hepatitis panel, and HIV tests are all within normal limits. EPO level is 546 mU/L. He receives 2 units of packed red cells. He undergoes a bm biopsy that shows a hypocellular marrow for age with no obvious dysplasia. PNH testing shows a small clone at 2%. Cytogenetics shows a +8 and del13q abnormality. What is the next best step in management of this patient?
   A. Decitabine
   B. Low-dose cytarabine
   C. Supportive care with transfusions and antibiotics
   D. Immunosuppressive therapy with horse ATG and cyclosporine
   E. Epoetin

7. A 58-year-old female with pancytopenia was diagnosed with low-risk myelodysplasia 7 months ago with baseline Hb = 10.1 g/dL, WBC = 3.3 (ANC = 1.9), and platelets = 35 K/mm^3. She was started on decitabine and has received four cycles so far without any improvement in her counts. She remains pancytopenic and now requires packed red cells and platelet transfusion once every 4–6 weeks. Repeat bm biopsy shows persistent MDS with 4% blasts and diploid karyotype. What is the most appropriate next step?
   A. Switch to azacitidine
   B. Continue decitabine for another four cycles
   C. Switch to lenalidomide
   D. Switch to supportive care alone with transfusions
   E. Consider clinical trial and discuss hematopoietic stem cell transplantation

8. A 65-year-old female presented with a 2-month history of fatigue and easy bruising. She was noted to be pancytopenic. This led to a bm biopsy that demonstrated 65% cellularity with multilineage dysplasia and 13% blasts. Karyotype showed −7, +8, +11 in 20/20 metaphases. What mutation, if found, would affect the response to hypomethylating agents?
   A. TET2
   B. EZH2
   C. DNMT3A
   D. RUNX1
   E. JAK2

9. A 25-year-old male is noted to have macrocytic anemia on a routine blood test done as part of college sports physical. He recalls being told he was anemic 5 years ago when he was trying to donate blood as part of his school's health fair. He did not follow up with his PCP at that time because he felt great and had no symptoms. On exam he is noted to be short statured but without any other abnormality. He has no rash and leukoplakia. His finger- and toenails appear normal. He has no family history of anemia, and both his parents and siblings are in good health. Workup including iron studies, B12, folate, TSH, and retic count are all within normal limits. His bone marrow exam, however, shows dysplasia with monosomy 7 consistent with a diagnosis of MDS. Besides referring him for hematopoietic stem cell transplant, what is the most appropriate next step in the evaluation of this patient?
   A. Telomere length analysis
   B. Check for mutation in GATA2
   C. Check for mutation in RUNX1
   D. Chromosome breakage analysis when cultured with a DNA crosslinker
   E. Check red blood cell adenosine deaminase level

10. A 72-year-old female was diagnosed with metastatic melanoma 2 years ago and treated with trametinib and dabrafenib. She unfortunately progressed on the regimen and underwent lymphodepletion with fludarabine and cyclophosphamide followed by infusion of tumor infiltrating lymphocytes as part of a clinical trial and then high-dose IL-2. This was close to a year ago. She responded really well to her treatment. However, she has been noted to have a steady decline in her platelet count over the past 6 months that has been ranging between 60 and 70 K for the last 2 months. White cell count and hemoglobin are normal. B12, folate, and TSH are also within normal limits. HIV and hepatitis profile are negative. A bone marrow biopsy was done that shows a mildly hypocellular marrow with no conclusive evidence of dysplasia or melanoma. Karyotype is of a normal female. FISH and flow cytometry for MDS are unremarkable. Molecular mutation panel shows RUNX1 mutation. What is the next best step in this patient's management?
   A. Romiplostim
   B. Close observation
   C. Azacitidine
   D. Revlimid
   E. Stem cell transplant referral

11. A 70-year-old male with low-risk MDS has been on epoetin treatment for the last 6 months. The patient has still been requiring packed red cell transfusions of 1–2 units/month. His most recent hemoglobin is 8.1 g/dL and ferritin is 2500. His renal and liver functions are within normal limits. With the elevated ferritin level, the patient is at high risk for developing cardiac, liver, and pancreatic dysfunction. What step should be taken to reduce the risk of iron overload?
   A. Increase the dose and of epoetin shots
   B. Add G-CSF to epoetin
   C. Start deferasirox
   D. Phlebotomy
   E. Only do blood transfusion when patient is symptomatic

12. A 56-year-old male presents to his PCP with fatigue, dizziness, and easy bruising for a month. On exam, he is noted to have scattered areas of petechiae and bruising. A complete blood count shows Hb = 7.9 g/dL, WBC = 2.8 K/mm^3, ANC = 0.9, and platelets of 27 K/mm^3. A bone marrow exam shows a hypercellular marrow with trilineage dysplasia with 12% blasts. Karyotype is complex with del7, +11, and +8 in 17 out of 20 metaphases. He is

transfused with 2 units of packed red blood cells. The patient has a matched sibling donor. What should be the next step in the management of this patient?

A. Lenalidomide

B. Supportive care with transfusions

C. Azacitidine

D. Growth factor support

E. Proceed with hematopoietic stem cell transplant

13. A 55-year-old morbidly obese female underwent gastric bypass surgery a year ago. She has lost 30 pounds since her surgery. She reports her knee pain has significantly improved with weight loss. She tries to exercise on a daily basis. However, for the last couple of months she gets tired and fatigued easily. She presents to her PCP and is noted have pallor on exam. CBC shows Hb = 8.8 g/dL with MCV = 88. She has mild leukopenia and normal platelets. Her peripheral blood smear is reviewed by the hematopathologist who reports dysplasia and recommends a bone marrow exam. Stool exam is negative for occult blood. Other than MDS, what can be causing dysplasia in this patient?

A. Vitamin B12 excess

B. Zinc deficiency

C. Copper deficiency

D. Lead deficiency

E. Mercury poisoning

14. A 65-year-old female presented with a 2-month history of fatigue and easy bruising. She was noted to be pancytopenic. This led to a bm biopsy that demonstrated 65% cellularity with multilineage dysplasia and 13% blasts. Karyotype showed −7, −5, +11, +8 in 20/20 metaphases. What mutation is likely to be found in this patient?

A. RUNX1

B. GATA2

C. EZH2

D. ASXL1

E. TP53

15. A 78-year-old male with coronary artery disease s/p CABG complicated by ischemic stroke 2 years ago and diabetes mellitus (HbA1c = 10.1). The patient was noted to be pancytopenic on a routine blood test 2 weeks ago. Workup shows high-risk MDS with complex cytogenetics and TP53 mutation. He remains blood and platelet transfusion dependent. He has three younger siblings aged 75, 72, and 68 years of age who are in good health and would like to be tested as a potential match for a stem cell transplant. What should be next step in treating this patient?

A. Refer for stem cell transplant

B. Decitabine

C. Hospice

D. Observation

E. Lenalidomide

ANSWERS

1. D

The patient has myelodysplastic syndrome with symptomatic anemia. CG shows a 5q- abnormality that is sensitive to lenalidomide. The recommended dose of lenalidomide is 10 mg daily 21/28 days or 28 days monthly. Because the EPO level is greater than 500, the chances of responding to epoetin are low. If the patient fails to respond to lenalidomide, certainly a clinical trial should be considered. Blood transfusion alone is only supportive care and would not control the underlying myelodysplasia.

2. B

This patient should be treated with epogen because his serum EPO level is less than 500. EPO dose of 40,000–60,000 IU once to twice weekly is the preferred dose. Darbepoetin can be used at a dose of 150–300 µg subq every 2 weeks. Lenalidomide should be considered in patients with low-risk MDS with low EPO level and diploid karyotype after EPO failure. Azacitidine is considered in a front-line setting in low-risk MDS patients if additional cytopenias are present, which this patient does not have.

3. A

Azacitidine should be used as a bridge to transplant in this case due to high-risk MDS. In the AZA-001 study that compared azacitidine versus conventional care treatment in high-risk MDS, azacitidine improved overall survival with a higher hematological response compared to conventional care. Lenalidomide is a not an appropriate option in this patient with complex cytogenetics and trilineage dysplasia. Cyclosporine in combination with ATG is a potential option in patients with low-risk MDS with a hypocellular marrow, PNH clone, and HLA-DR15+.

4. C

This is an elderly patient with high-risk therapy-related MDS. All cell lines are affected. Azacitidine remains a treatment of choice in this case. In the AZA-001 study in patients with high-risk MDS, azacitidine increased overall survival and hematological response rate compared to conventional care. Hematopoietic stem cell transplantation would have been a valid option if the patient was younger and with fewer comorbidities.

5. D

This patient has 5q- syndrome. 5q- syndrome is usually seen in elderly females. It is characterized by anemia with normal to elevated platelet count. 5q- is the sole cytogenetic abnormality, and the bm demonstrates micromegakaryocytes with monolobulated and bilobulated nuclei. These patients are particularly responsive to lenalidomide therapy.

6. D

This patient has hypoplastic MDS that is characterized by a hypocellular marrow. There is no obvious dysplasia, but there are abnormal cytogenetics differentiating this from aplastic anemia. These patients respond well to immunosuppressive therapy. The patient also has a small PNH clone, making immunosuppressive therapy a better treatment choice in this patient.

7. E

This patient is failing therapy with a hypomethylating agent and now has increasing transfusion requirements. Switching to another hypomethylating agent is of no benefit. The best option for this patient is to proceed to hematopoietic stem cell transplant. Because it can take weeks to identify a donor, it would appropriate to enroll this patient in a suitable clinical trial and proceed to stem cell transplant once a donor is available.

8. A

DNA methylation is a prognostic marker and predictor of response to therapy among patients with MDS and appears to be a mechanism of disease progression to AML.

TET2 belongs to a family of genes that play a role in the epigenetic control of DNA expression through demethylation. Mutations in TET2 are therefore more responsive to therapy with hypomethylating agents.

9. **D**

This patient likely has Fanconi anemia. Chromosome breakage analysis testing should be arranged in this patient to confirm the diagnosis. Once confirmed, the patient should proceed with allogeneic stem cell transplantation. Telomerase length analysis is done in patients where dyskeratosis congentia (DKC) is suspected. DKC patients usually present with a rash, and nail changes are common. Red blood cell adenosine deaminase level is elevated in patients with Diamond-Blackfan anemia, which is usually diagnosed in the first few years of life. Mutations in GATA2 and RUNX1 are familial disorders with a strong family history, which this patient does not have. RUNX1 mutation is associated with familial thrombocytopenia, whereas mutation in GATA2 mostly involves decreased monocytes and increased susceptibility to mycobacterial infections.

10. **B**

More than 30% of patients with unexplained cytopenias who do not meet diagnostic criteria for MDS carry MDS-associated somatic mutations. These mutations are indicative of clonal hematopoiesis. Such cases are referred to as clonal cytopenia of undetermined significance (CCUS). The natural history of such patients is largely unknown. It is recommended that blood counts be closely monitored in such patients.

11. **C**

Iron overload is associated with organ toxicity. Measures should be taken to reduce iron in patients with iron overload to reduce iron-associated organ damage. There are currently three iron chelators that are approved in the United States: deferoxamine, deferasirox, and deferiprone. Patients are recommended to undergo ocular and auditory exams as well as renal and liver function testing prior to starting therapy. Deferiprone is also associated with agranulocytosis. Increasing the dose of epoetin or adding G-CSF may improve the anemia but not help the iron overload. The patient is anemic and phlebotomy will worsen the anemia.

12. **E**

The patient has high-risk MDS given elevated bm blasts, complex karyotype, and all three cell lines affected. This patient should proceed to allogeneic stem cell transplant because he already has a matched sibling donor available. Otherwise, starting azacitidine followed by allogeneic stem cell transplant when a donor is available is the appropriate treatment.

13. **C**

It is important to distinguish between MDS and other conditions that can mimic MDS. Copper deficiency occurs often in patients who have undergone bariatric surgery. Along with B12 deficiency and zinc excess, copper deficiency should be ruled out as a cause of anemia especially in patients having undergone bariatric surgery. Erythroid hyperplasia with decreased myeloid-to-erythroid ratio and dyserythropoiesis including megaloblastic changes may be seen in the bm exam, which can be mistaken for MDS.

14. **E**

The TP53 gene is located on chromosome 17p. It is a tumor suppressor gene and plays a vital role in cell cycle arrest. Mutations in TP53 are commonly seen in MDS with complex cytogenetics (up to 50%) and with 5q- (15%–20%). TP53 mutation confers a poor prognosis independent of the IPSS in MDS.

15. **B**

This patient has high-risk MDS. Allogeneic stem cell transplant is recommended in patients with high-risk MDS and offers a chance to cure the disease. However, given this patient's age and comorbidities, the risks involved in undergoing a transplant outweigh the benefits. This patient should be treated with decitabine. In a phase 3 trial, decitabine was compared to the best supportive care in patients with high-risk MDS not suitable for stem cell transplant. Decitabine was found to be associated with a higher progression-free survival and a lower risk of progression to AML in 1 year. However, there was no difference in overall survival noted. Lenalidomide is not an appropriate choice for patients with high-risk MDS.

REFERENCE

Question 10

1. Brian K, Jeff MH, John SW, et al. MDS-associated somatic mutations and clonal hematopoiesis are common in idiopathic cytopenias of undetermined significance. *Blood.* 2015;126:2355–2361.

Myeloproliferative Disorders

Kiran Naqvi and Farhad Ravandi

QUESTIONS

1. A 55-year-old female presents to her PCP for an annual physical. Her complete blood profile shows leukocytosis = 60 K/mm^3, Hb = 12.5 g/dL, and platelets = 450 K/mm^3. The differential showed metamyelocytes, myelocytes, and basophilia at 5.0%. A bone marrow exam shows CML chronic phase with t(9;22). What is the most likely aberrant fusion protein?
   A. P210 BCR/ABL
   B. P190 BCR/ABL
   C. P230 BCR/ABL
   D. P290 BCR/ABL
   E. PML/RARA

2. A 68-year-old female is diagnosed with chronic myeloid leukemia after having leukocytosis on a routine blood test. She started imatinib 400 mg by mouth daily 3 months ago. Today her WBC = 9 K/mm^3, Hb = 12.5, and platelets are 210 K/mm^3. There is no basophilia. There is no palpable spleen on exam. PCR for BCR/ABL is 2.5%. What is the next appropriate step?
   A. Stop imatinib and switch to dasatinib
   B. Stop imatinib and switch to nilotinib
   C. Increase imatinib to 800 mg daily
   D. Refer for stem cell transplant
   E. Continue the same dose of imatinib

3. A 33-year-old male presented to the emergency center with a 2-week history of fever and sore throat. He reports severe fatigue and left upper quadrant discomfort. His WBC = 250 K/mm^3 with basophilia at 25%, metamyelocytes and myelocytes and no peripheral blasts, Hb = 10.5 g/dL, and platelets = 450 K/mm^3. The spleen is palpable 6 cm below the left costal margin. The patient is started on hydroxyurea. A bone marrow biopsy is done that shows hypercellular marrow with 5% blasts, and FISH is positive for BCR/ABL. What is the most likely diagnosis?
   A. PH + acute lymphoblastic leukemia
   B. Chronic myeloid leukemia, blast phase
   C. Chronic myeloid leukemia, accelerated phase
   D. Chronic myeloid leukemia, chronic phase
   E. Atypical chronic myeloid leukemia

4. A 58-year-old male diagnosed with chronic myeloid leukemia 5 years ago has failed treatment with imatinib and dasatinib. His most recent bone marrow exam shows persistent chronic myeloid leukemia with t(9;22) in 15/20 metaphases. An ABL mutation analysis shows T315I. What should be next TKI of choice?
   A. Ponatinib
   B. Nilotinib
   C. Bosutinib
   D. Sorafenib
   E. Sunitinib

5. A 58-year-old male diagnosed with chronic myeloid leukemia 7 years ago has failed treatment with imatinib, dasatinib, and nilotinib. His most recent bone marrow exam shows persistent chronic myeloid leukemia with t(9;22) in 15/20 metaphases. No ABL mutations are detected. What is the best next step in the management of this patient?
   A. Bosutinib
   B. Ponatinib
   C. Omacetaxine
   D. Interferon alpha
   E. Referral to stem cell transplant

6. A 68-year-old female presents with a 2-month history of fatigue and generalized pruritus that is worse after a hot shower. She also complains of left upper quadrant pain and early satiety. On exam, she is slightly overweight. Spleen is palpable 6 cm below the left costal margin. She does not smoke or drink alcohol. Blood work shows Hb = 17.0 g/dL with WBC = 12.5 K/mm^3, and platelets = 450 K/mm^3. EPO level is low. Peripheral blood shows a mutation in JAK2V617F. What is next step in the management of this patient?
   A. Aspirin alone
   B. Hydroxyurea alone
   C. Phlebotomy alone
   D. Aspirin and hydroxyurea, and phlebotomy
   E. Weight loss

7. A 45-year-old male presents with a 2-month history of fatigue and generalized pruritus with tingling and burning in the hands and feet. For the past 2 days, his left lower extremity has been swollen and tender to the touch. The patient denies smoking or taking anabolic steroids. On examination, the patient has an enlarged spleen. His left lower calf is swollen and erythematous. A CBC is done that shows Hb = 17.8 g/dL, WBC = 13 K/mm^3, and platelets = 400 K/mm^3. EPO level is low, and ferritin is 30. Peripheral blood testing shows a JAK2V617F mutation. Lower extremity Doppler studies show a left lower extremity deep vein thrombosis. Patient is started on anticoagulation with lovenox. What is the next step in managing this patient?
   A. Phlebotomy alone
   B. Phlebotomy with hydroxyurea
   C. Ruxolitinib
   D. Antihistamines
   E. Amitriptyline

8. A 48-year-old male presents to his PCP for an annual physical. Routine blood work shows an elevated platelet count of 800 K/mm^3. The WBC and Hb are within normal limits. The patient denies any excessive bleeding or any chronic infection. He has no history of blood clots. The iron studies are also within normal limits. Test for BCR/ABL from peripheral blood is negative. The presence of which of the following is associated with a lower risk of thrombosis in this patient?
   - **A.** JAK2V617F
   - **B.** MPL
   - **C.** CALR
   - **D.** ASXL1
   - **E.** EZH2

9. A 56-year-old male is found to have thrombocytosis at 750 K/mm^3. WBC and Hb are normal. Stool for occult blood is negative, and iron studies are within normal limits. There is no history of chronic infection or blood clots. He tests positive for JAK2V617F and negative for BCR/ABL. What is the next best step in the management of this patient?
   - **A.** Aspirin alone
   - **B.** Hydroxyurea alone
   - **C.** Aspirin and hydroxyurea
   - **D.** Ruxolitinib
   - **E.** Observation

10. A 68-year-old male with osteoarthritis of his right knee was undergoing a preoperative evaluation for knee replacement. He was noted to have elevated platelet count of 1.1 million K/mm^3. Further workup showed positive JAK2V617F. What is the next appropriate step?
    - **A.** Start aspirin and hydroxyurea
    - **B.** Start aspirin alone
    - **C.** Start hydroxyurea alone
    - **D.** Start ruxolitinib
    - **E.** Observation

11. A 68-year-old male with a long-standing history of essential thrombocythemia was on aspirin. Most recently, he reports feeling fatigued with loss of appetite, early satiety, and weight loss. Blood work shows Hb = 8.0, WBC = 12 K/mm^3 with 1% peripheral blasts, and platelets = 120 K/mm^3. On examination, the spleen is palpable 8 cm below the left costal margin. A bone marrow exam demonstrates fibrotic marrow. Cytogenetics is complex. Mutational analysis shows ASXL1. What is the next best approach?
    - **A.** Continue aspirin and add hydroxyurea
    - **B.** Start ruxolitinib
    - **C.** Start ruxolitinib and refer the patient for hematopoietic stem cell transplant
    - **D.** Supportive care with blood transfusions
    - **E.** Hospice

12. A 67-year-old female is diagnosed with primary myelofibrosis after she presented with a 1-month history of worsening fatigue, weight loss, anorexia, and left upper quadrant fullness. She was noted to be anemic and had 1% circulating blasts. Spleen is palpable 10 cm below the left costal margin. A bone marrow exam shows a fibrotic marrow with a complex karyotype. Workup is negative for JAK2V617F, MPL, and CALR. Prognosis of this patient is expected to be poor mainly due to?
    - **A.** Negative JAK2V617F
    - **B.** Negative CALR
    - **C.** Triple negative disease
    - **D.** Anemia
    - **E.** Constitutional symptoms

13. A 52-year-old female presents with a 3-month history of generalized pruritus. She denies using any new detergent, soap, body lotion, or cream. She denies any new medication including over-the-counter supplements. She has tried antihistamines but with only a temporary relief in her symptoms. She denies having any cough, fever, shortness of breath, or diarrhea. Blood work reveals Hb = 11.5 g/dL, WBC = 16 K/mm^3, neutrophils = 45%, basophils = 1%, eosinophils = 12%, and platelets = 160 K/mm^3. Further testing of peripheral blood shows FIP1L1-PDGFRA by FISH. What is the next step in this patient's management?
    - **A.** Imatinib 100 mg daily
    - **B.** Imatinib 400 mg daily
    - **C.** Imatinib 600 mg daily
    - **D.** Dasatinib 100 mg daily
    - **E.** Sorafenib 400 mg twice daily

14. A 35-year-old male presents with a 4-month history of pruritic rash that comes and goes. The rash mainly involves his upper back. He also reports shortness of breath with wheezing and diarrhea when the rash appears. The rash improves with antihistamines. The patient is concerned that he is developing new allergies despite not being exposed to new detergents, creams, lotions, or soaps. He has cut back on dairy products but with no improvement in diarrhea when it occurs. Workup shows elevated serum tryptase levels. A bone marrow exam is expected to show which of the following by flow cytometry:
    - **A.** CD117+, CD25−, CD2−
    - **B.** CD117+, CD25+, CD2+
    - **C.** CD117+, CD33+, MPO+
    - **D.** CD34+, CD33+, MPO+
    - **E.** CD5+, CD23+ CD20+

15. An 80-year-old male presents to the emergency center feeling weak and tired for the past 2 weeks. On presentation, his WBC = 200 K/mm^3, Hb = 10.1 g/dL, and platelets = 75 K/mm^3. Peripheral blood differential shows marked neutrophilia without any circulating blasts or basophilia. On examination, the spleen is palpable 6 cm below the left costal margin and the liver edge is also palpable. A bone marrow biopsy demonstrates increased myeloid precursors with 3% blasts. There is no evidence of dysplasia. Cytogenetics are negative for t(9;22). What is the most likely mutation to be found in this case?
    - **A.** SETBP1
    - **B.** CSF-3R
    - **C.** EZH2
    - **D.** TP53
    - **E.** RUNX1

16. A 56-year-old male with a past history of alcohol-induced pancreatitis was diagnosed with CML, chronic phase, 2 years ago. He has been maintained on imatinib 400 mg daily without any significant side effects except occasional muscle cramps. His last bm exam 1 year ago showed complete cytogenetic remission. His PCR for BCR/ABL 3 months ago was 0.12%. He comes today for a 3-month follow-up and is noted to have WBC = 9.8 K/mm^3, Hb = 12.5 g/dL, and platelets = 170 K/mm^3. There is no evidence of basophilia. Spleen is not palpable. Peripheral PCR for BCR/ABL drawn 1 week ago is 2.5%. What is the next step in the management of this patient?
    - **A.** Increase dose of imatinib to 800 mg daily
    - **B.** Change therapy to dasatinib

C. Change therapy to nilotinib

D. Monitor PCR levels closely and repeat bm exam to assess loss of cytogenetic response

E. Check ABL kinase domain mutations

ANSWERS

1. A

P210 is the most common fusion protein found in patients with CML-chronic phase produced due to a breakpoint in exon 13 or exon 14 (also called exon b2 and b3) in the BCR gene that is fused to the ABL1 gene on exon a2. P190 is more commonly found in Philadelphia positive ALL, whereas P230 is a larger fusion protein that occurs less commonly in CML (<1%). PML/RARA is found in acute promyelocytic leukemia and not CML.

2. E

There is no indication to switch therapy at this point as the PCR is less than 10%. In the DASISION and ENESTnd trials with dasatinib and nilotinib, respectively, patients achieving less than 10% BCR/ABL at 3 months were associated with a superior PFS and OS. The most important time point is 6 months into therapy, when a PCR for BCR/ABL of greater than 10%, which corresponds to less than a partial cytogenetic response, is considered a failure of therapy. Achievement of a major cytogenetic response (Ph+ metaphases <35%) at 6 months is associated with a superior PFS and OS.

3. C

This is the accelerated phase of CML based on the peripheral blood basophilia of greater than 20%. The WHO criteria defining the accelerated phase of CML includes the presence of one or more of the following features:

- 10%–19% blasts in the peripheral blood or bone marrow
- Peripheral blood basophils greater than 20%
- Platelets less than 100,000/μL, unrelated to therapy
- Platelets greater than 1,000,000/μL, unresponsive to therapy
- Progressive splenomegaly and increasing white cell count, unresponsive to therapy
- Cytogenetic evolution (defined as the development of chromosomal abnormalities in addition to the Philadelphia chromosome)

4. A

Ponatinib is the only available tyrosine kinase inhibitor with activity against the gatekeeper T315I mutation. In the phase II PACE trial of ponatinib, 70% of the patients with CML-chronic phase with T315I mutation achieved a major cytogenetic response.

5. E

In this case, the patient has failed to respond to three different TKIs. The chances of responding to a fourth TKI is much less, and hence the patient should be referred to stem cell transplant if eligible.

6. D

This patient has clinical features consistent with PV including generalized pruritus and enlarged spleen. JAK2V617F positivity further confirms the diagnosis of PV. One of the main goals of treatment is to reduce the risk of thrombosis in these patients. Low-dose aspirin and phlebotomy (aiming at hematocrit <45) reduces this risk. Addition of hydroxyurea is indicated in patients who are at high risk of thrombosis (older than 60 years and prior thrombosis).

7. B

This patient has clinical features consistent with PV including generalized pruritus, erythromelalgia, and enlarged spleen. JAK2V617F positivity further confirms the diagnosis of PV. One of the main goals of treatment is to reduce the risk of thrombosis in these patients. Low-dose aspirin and phlebotomy (aiming at hematocrit <45) reduces this risk. Addition of hydroxyurea is indicated in patients who are at high risk of thrombosis (older than 60 years and prior thrombosis). Addition of hydroxyurea is therefore warranted in this patient due to deep vein thrombosis.

8. C

This patient has findings consistent with ET. The presence of CALR mutation in ET is more commonly associated with male sex, lower WBC count and Hb levels, higher platelet count, and lower risk of thrombosis. There is, however, no clear difference in overall survival or transformation to myelofibrosis in these patients.

9. A

This patient has essential thrombocythemia. Patients younger than 60 years of age and with no prior thrombosis should be maintained on low-dose aspirin to prevent thrombosis.

10. C

This patient has essential thrombocythemia given elevated platelets with positive JAK2V617F. The patient should be started on low-dose aspirin and hydroxyurea to prevent thrombosis. However, because the platelets are greater than 1 million, this puts the patient at risk for acquired von Willebrand disease due to abnormal adsorption of large von Willebrand factor multimers. This increases the risk of bleeding with aspirin. Low-dose aspirin is acceptable if the ristocetin cofactor level is greater than 30%.

11. C

This patient has likely transformed to myelofibrosis from underlying ET. Presence of constitutional symptoms with worsening anemia, peripheral blood blasts, enlarged spleen, fibrotic marrow with complex cytogenetics, and ASXL1 mutation all indicate transformation. Ruxolitinib is a valid option in this patient given constitutional symptoms and splenomegaly. However, he needs a transplant referral due to his high-risk disease and possibility of transformation to acute leukemia. At present, allogeneic hematopoietic cell transplantation constitutes the only treatment modality with a curative potential in myelofibrosis.

12. C

Patients with primary myelofibrosis with triple negative disease (without JAK2, MPL, or CALR mutations) have a poor outcome. Tefferi et al. demonstrated an inferior leukemia-free survival in patients with triple negative myelofibrosis.

13. A

FIP1L1-PDFRA is very sensitive to imatinib. Initial imatinib dose of 100 mg daily has shown to be effective in inducing rapid and durable responses in patients with PDGFRA-associated hypereosinophilic syndromes.

14. B

This is a case of mastocytosis. A typical immunophenotype in mastocytosis is CD117+, CD25+ and CD2 is +/−. Options C and D are consistent with acute myeloid leukemia. Option E is consistent with chronic lymphocytic leukemia.

15. B

This is a case of chronic neutrophilic leukemia (CNL) in which the patient demonstrates an elevated white cell count with mature granulocytic proliferation. The disease involves infiltration of these mature granulocytes into the organs causing enlargement of the spleen and liver. Mutations in CSF-3R have been noted to play a central role in the pathogenesis of patients with CNL.

16. D

Patient has a rise in the PCR level for BCR/ABL. He should therefore be monitored closely, and a bone marrow exam should be done to confirm cytogenetic relapse. Loss of cytogenetic response or hematologic response are the two major indicators of switching therapy in patients with CML. Mutational analyses should be done prior to switching therapy in such patients. Increasing the dose of imatinib would result in more toxicity.

REFERENCES

Question 4

1. Cortes JE, Kim DW, Pinilla-Ibarz J, et al. A phase 2 trial of ponatinib in Philadelphia chromosome-positive leukemias. *N Engl J Med.* 2013;369:1.

Question 8

1. Rotunno G, Mannarelli C, Guglielmelli P, et al. Impact of calreticulin mutations on clinical and hematological phenotype and outcome in essential thrombocythemia. *Blood.* 2014;123:1552–1555.
2. Rumi E, Pietra D, Ferretti V, et al. JAK2 or CALR mutation status defines subtypes of essential thrombocythemia with substantially different clinical course and outcomes. *Blood.* 2014;123:1544–1551.

Question 12

1. Tefferi A, Lasho TL, Finke CM, et al. CALR vs JAK2 vs MPL-mutated or triple-negative myelofibrosis: clinical, cytogenetic and molecular comparisons. *Leukemia.* 2014;28(7):1472–1477.

Question 13

1. Metzgeroth G, Walz C, Erben P, et al. Safety and efficacy of imatinib in chronic eosinophilic leukaemia and hypereosinophilic syndrome: a phase-II study. *Br J Haematol.* 2008;143(5):707.

Chronic Lymphocytic Leukemia, Hairy Cell Leukemia, and Other Chronic Lymphoproliferative Disorders

Kiran Naqvi and Farhad Ravandi

QUESTIONS

1. A 68-year-old female presents to her PCP for a routine physical. Blood work shows leukocytosis at 35 K/mm³, Hb = 12.5 g/dL, and platelets = 188 K/mm³. The differential shows 80% lymphocytes. Exam is unremarkable for palpable lymphadenopathy or hepatosplenomegaly. She denies any fatigue, weight loss, fever, or drenching night sweats. What is the most appropriate next step in the evaluation of this patient?
   A. Obtain CT neck, chest, abdomen, and pelvis
   B. Obtain a bm biopsy
   C. Send peripheral blood for flow cytometry
   D. Obtain ultrasound of the abdomen
   E. Obtain a PET-CT

2. A 70-year-old male is referred to an oncologist after leukocytosis is noted on preoperative workup for right knee replacement. Repeat blood work shows WBC count = 48 K/mm³, with 70% lymphocytes. Hemoglobin and platelets are normal. There is no lymphadenopathy or splenomegaly on examination. Patient denies fatigue, fever, weight loss, or night sweats. Peripheral blood is sent for flow cytometry, which is consistent with chronic lymphocytic leukemia. What profile fits the diagnosis?
   A. CD5+, CD19+, CD23+, CD20 dim, cyclinD1−
   B. CD5+, CD19+, CD23−, CD20 bright, cyclinD1+
   C. CD5+, CD19+, CD20+, sIgM+
   D. CD117+, CD13+, CD33+
   E. CD5−, CD20 bright, CD103+, cyclinD1+

3. A 55-year-old male with newly diagnosed CLL presents to your office for a second opinion. He was diagnosed with CLL 6 months ago after he was noted to have an elevated white count of 33 K/mm³ with an absolute lymphocyte count of 26 K/mm³. Hemoglobin and platelet count were normal. The CLL fluorescent in situ hybridization panel showed del11q as the sole abnormality. IgHV is unmutated, and Zap-70 and CD38 were negative. Today he reports significant fatigue, drenching night sweats, and left upper quadrant fullness for the last 3 weeks. Blood work shows WBC = 55 K, absolute lymphocyte count = 38 K/mm³, Hb = 11.5, and platelets = 90 K/mm³. LDH = 256. He has palpable cervical lymphadenopathy up to

2 cm in size. Spleen is palpable 7 cm below the left costal margin. What is the next step in the management of this patient?
   A. Fludarabine, cyclophosphamide, rituximab
   B. Bendamustine and rituximab
   C. Observation
   D. Idelalisib with rituximab
   E. Revlimid with rituximab

4. A 58-year-old male with newly diagnosed CLL presents to your office for a second opinion. He was diagnosed with CLL 3 months ago after an elevated white count of 33 K/mm³ with an absolute lymphocyte count of 26 K/mm³ were noted. Hemoglobin and platelet count are normal. There is no lymphadenopathy or organomegaly on exam. He denies any constitutional symptoms. CLL fluorescent in situ hybridization panel shows del17p as the sole abnormality. IgHV is unmutated, and Zap-70 and CD38 are negative. What is the next step in the management of this patient?
   A. Fludarabine, cyclophosphamide, rituximab
   B. Bendamustine and rituximab
   C. Observation
   D. Idelalisib with rituximab
   E. Alemtuzumab

5. A 68-year-old female was diagnosed with Rai stage 1 CLL 2 years ago. FISH was positive for del13q as the sole abnormality. She is IgHV mutated and CD38 negative. Her counts have been stable for the last 2 years. She has been on observation. Today she presents with fatigue for past 2 weeks. She states she can barely make it through the day and has been taking afternoon naps. Blood work shows stable WBC = 37 K/mm³ and platelets = 188 K/mm³, but the patient is significantly anemic with Hb = 7.8 g/dL. She denies noticing any blood in her stools. Occult blood testing is negative. Further workup shows retic count = 8%, LDH = 350, and normal iron studies. DAT is positive +3. What is the next appropriate step?
   A. Fludarabine
   B. Bendamustine and rituximab
   C. Ibrutinib
   D. Alemtuzumab
   E. Prednisone

6. A 78-year-old female with TP53 mutated CLL diagnosed 1 year ago was treated with ibrutinib for 9 months. Patient unfortunately progressed with worsening lymphadenopathy. She has now been on idelalisib and rituximab for 2 months. She presents to the ER with 1-day history of worsening shortness of breath, dry cough, and fever. On presentation, she is noted to be hypoxic. CXR shows bilateral fluffy infiltrates. What is the most likely causative agent?
   A. *Mycoplasma pneumoniae*
   B. *Legionella pneumophila*
   C. *Pneumocystis jiroveci*
   D. Human immunodeficiency virus
   E. *Mycobacterium avium* intracellulare

7. A 78-year-old male with significant comorbidities, including history of coronary artery disease s/p–coronary bypass surgery, cerebrovascular accident, hypertension, and history of recurrent bleeding peptic ulcer disease, was diagnosed with CLL 3 years ago. His performance status is 2. He has been on observation alone. More recently he has noticed enlarging cervical and axillary lymphadenopathy. His spleen is enlarged and measures 7 cm below the left costal margin. PET-CT shows multicompartmental lymphadenopathy, the largest one measuring 5 cm in the left axillary chain. It also shows an enlarged spleen measuring 18 cm. The CLL FISH panel shows +12. What is the next step in managing this patient?
   A. Continue observation
   B. Rituximab alone
   C. Chlorambucil + obinutuzumab
   D. Ofatumumab alone
   E. Ibrutinib

8. A 66-year-male is suspected to have CLL after he is noted to have an elevated WBC count with an absolute lymphocyte count greater than 5000. What translocation, if present on FISH testing, would help differentiate CLL from mantle cell lymphoma?
   A. t(14;18)
   B. t(11;14)
   C. t(8;14)
   D. t(1;14)
   E. t(3;14)

9. A 65-year-old female diagnosed with CLL 3 years ago presents to the ER with 1-day history of productive cough, fever, nausea, and vomiting. Blood shows WBC = 65 K/mm^3 with absolute lymphocyte count = 45 K/mm^3. Hemoglobin = 11.5 g/dL and platelets = 150 K/mm^3. On exam, she appears sick and is lethargic. Chest x-ray shows multiple bilateral pulmonary infiltrates consistent with pneumonia. Her serum IgG level is 420. This is her third episode of pneumonia in the last 6 months. On her last episode, the nasal wash was positive for parainfluenza virus. What is the most appropriate next step in the management of this patient?
   A. Start empirical antibiotic therapy
   B. Start empirical antibiotic therapy + IVIG
   C. Start ibrutinib
   D. Start IV ganciclovir
   E. Start IV foscarnet

10. A 54-year-old male was diagnosed with Rai stage 0 CLL 3 years ago and has been under observation since. He presents today for his follow-up and reports feeling significantly fatigued for last 3–4 weeks. He denies any fever, chills, weight loss, or night sweats. He feels dizzy and lightheaded but reports no syncopal episodes. On examination, there is significant pallor noted. No lymphadenopathy or organomegaly is noted. Blood work shows Hb = 7.7 g/dL, WBC = 42 K/mm^3 with 80% lymphocytes, and platelets = 150 K/mm^3. Retic count is 0.1%, LDH and haptoglobin are normal. Liver and kidney function, B12, folate, and TSH are all within normal limits. Serum iron level and saturation are elevated. Direct Coomb test is negative. Stool for occult blood is negative. What should be the next step in the management of this patient?
    A. Start erythropoietin
    B. Start prednisone
    C. Start rituximab
    D. Perform a bone marrow biopsy and send viral PCR for parvo B19, CMV, and EBV
    E. Continue observation

11. A 68-year-old male presents with a 2-month history of worsening fatigue. For the past 1 week, he has been significantly dizzy and lightheaded. Prior to 2 months ago, he was in good health. He reports loss of appetite and feels full all the time. On examination, the spleen is notably enlarged and palpable 8 cm below the left costal margin. Complete blood profile demonstrates Hb = 8.0, WBC = 3.3, and platelets = 35 K. Iron studies, B12, folate, TSH, and serum protein electrophoresis are within normal limits. Hepatitis panel and HIV testing are negative. Peripheral blood shows mature lymphocytes with hair-like projections. A bone marrow biopsy is done. Which option reflects the most likely flow cytometry results?
    A. CD5+, CD19+, CD20 bright, CD23−, cyclin D1+
    B. CD5+, CD19+, CD20 dim, CD23+, cyclinD1−
    C. CD5−, CD11c+, CD20 bright, CD25+, CD103+
    D. CD5+, CD19+, CD20+, sIgM+
    E. CD117+, CD13+, CD33+

12. A 58-year-old male presents with a 2-month history of worsening fatigue. He reports loss of appetite and feels full all the time. On examination, the spleen is notably enlarged and palpable 8 cm below the left costal margin. A complete blood profile demonstrates Hb = 7.8, WBC = 2.5, and platelets = 45 K. Iron studies, B12, folate, TSH, and serum protein electrophoresis are within normal limits. Hepatitis panel and HIV testing are negative. Peripheral blood shows mature lymphocytes with hair-like projections. Tartrate-resistant acid phosphatase activity is positive. A bone marrow biopsy is done. Which mutation is most likely to be found?
    A. TP53
    B. BRAF V6000E
    C. RUNX1
    D. ASXL1
    E. TET2

13. A 65-year-old male presents with low-grade fever and weight loss of 8 pounds over the last 6 weeks. He has been in good health all his life except for hypertension for which he is on amlodipine. Blood work shows pancytopenia with WBC = 3.0, ANC = 1.2, Hb = 8.8 g/dL, and platelets = 68 K/mm^3. On examination, the spleen is palpable 5 cm below the left costal margin. A bone biopsy demonstrates hairy cell leukemia. BRAF V600E is positive. What is the next step in the management of the patient?
    A. Cladribine
    B. Rituximab
    C. Ofatumumab
    D. Stem cell transplant
    E. Observation

14. A 56-year-old female was diagnosed with CLL 2 years ago. On diagnosis, the patient was noted to have bulky lymphadenopathy and splenomegaly. FISH for CLL was positive for 17p deletion with unmutated IgVH. Zap 70 and CD38 were negative. The patient was started on ibrutinib. She responded well with a significant decrease in the size of lymph nodes. However, for the last 3 weeks, she has noticed worsening cervical lymphadenopathy and fatigue. Blood work shows rising WBC = 45 K/mm^3 with 75% lymphocytes, Hb = 9.8, and platelets = 80K. LDH is normal. CT of the neck, chest, abdomen, and pelvis shows multicompartment lymphadenopathy, with the largest lymph node measuring 5 cm in the anterior cervical chain. The patient has now been started on venetoclax. For which of the following is the patient at risk?
A. Cytokine release syndrome
B. Tumor lysis syndrome
C. Infection with *Pneumocystis jiroveci*
D. Gastrointestinal bleed
E. Atrial fibrillation

15. A 48-year-old female with a long-standing history of rheumatoid arthritis presents with pancytopenia. Blood work shows WBC = 3.2 K/mm^3, ANC = 0.8, Hb = 9.0, and platelets = 92 K/mm^3. The patient reports ongoing fatigue and weight loss. Peripheral blood shows cell lymphocytes with abundant cytoplasmic granules. Peripheral blood flow cytometry shows CD3+, CD8+, CD56-, CD57+, TCR α/β+. What is the most likely diagnosis?
A. T-cell ALL
B. NK cell leukemia
C. Plasma cell leukemia
D. T-cell large granular lymphocytic leukemia
E. Hairy cell leukemia

ANSWERS

1. **C**
Per the WHO and IWCLL, the diagnosis of CLL requires the presence of at least 5×10^9 B lymphocytes/L (5000/μL) in the peripheral blood. The clonality of the circulating B lymphocytes needs to be confirmed by flow cytometry. CLL cells co-express the T-cell antigen CD5 and B-cell surface antigens CD19, CD20, and CD23. Although the other tests mentioned may all be used for further evaluation of the CLL, they are not needed in a diagnosis of the disease that includes a bone marrow exam.

2. **A**
The typical CLL immunophenotype demonstrates CD5+, CD20+ (dim), CD23+. CyclinD1 is, however, negative. CLL needs to be differentiated from mantle cell lymphoma that is also CD5+, but typically CD23- and cyclinD1 is + (choice B). Choice C is consistent with Waldenstrom macroglobulinemia with positive surface immunoglobulin for IgM. Choice D is consistent with acute myeloid leukemia, whereas choice is E is hairy cell leukemia.

3. **A**
This patient with CLL meets the criteria to receive treatment including constitutional symptoms and significant splenomegaly. The presence of 11q- on FISH testing and presence of unmutated IgHV indicate poor prognosis in this patient. Treatment with chemoimmunotherapy in patients with 11q- is associated with higher response rate, survival rate, and relapse-free survival. Hence, younger patients who are able to tolerate chemoimmunotherapy should receive the FCR regimen. From the CLL-10 study, FCR is superior to bendamustine and rituximab (BR) regimen in younger patients. In those younger than 65 years, both FCR and BR have similar outcomes, but BR is less toxic. Options D and E are appropriate in the relapse/refractory setting.

4. **C**
It is important to recognize the indications/criteria for treating CLL patients. Not all patients with CLL need to be treated.
The IWCLL defines "active disease" by the presence of one or more of the following criteria:
1. Evidence of progressive marrow failure as manifested by the development of, or worsening of, anemia and/or thrombocytopenia.
2. Massive (at least 6 cm below the left costal margin) or progressive or symptomatic splenomegaly.
3. Massive nodes (at least 10 cm in longest diameter) or progressive or symptomatic lymphadenopathy.
4. Progressive lymphocytosis with an increase of more than 50% over a 2-month period or LDT of less than 6 months.
5. Autoimmune anemia and/or thrombocytopenia that is poorly responsive to corticosteroids or other standard therapy.
Constitutional symptoms, defined as any one or more of the following disease-related symptoms or signs:
- Unintentional weight loss of 10% or more within the previous 6 months
- Significant fatigue (ECOG PS 2 or worse; inability to work or perform usual activities)
- Fevers higher than 100.5°F or 38.0°C for 2 or more weeks without other evidence of infection
- Night sweats for more than 1 month without evidence of infection

The patient in the given scenario does not meet the IWCLL criteria for initiating treatment.

5. **E**
Up to one-third of the patients with CLL can develop autoimmune hemolytic anemia (AIHA) that is unrelated to the type of treatment. These patients are treated in the same manner as other patients with AIHA. Glucocorticoids are the initial treatment of choice. In this scenario, elevated retic count and LDH and DAT + are markers of hemolysis. The remaining choices are appropriate if anemia is a result of disease progression or refractory cases of AIHA.

6. **C**
One should recognize the side effects and toxicity of different treatment modalities. Idelalisib is associated with increased risk of *Pneumocystis jiroveci* and cytomegalovirus infection. Patients are recommended to remain on pneumocystis prophylaxis throughout treatment with idelalisib. If infection is confirmed, the drug should be permanently discontinued.

7. **C**
The patient meets the criteria to initiate treatment. Given multiple comorbidities, the patient is less likely to tolerate purine analogs. In this case, obinutuzumab with chlorambucil and ibrutinib are category 1 choices for treatment. However, ibrutinib is associated with increased bleeding

risk. The patient in this scenario has a history of recurrent bleeding peptic ulcer disease. Ibrutinib is therefore not a good option in this case. The patient should therefore be treated with chlorambucil with obinutuzumab. Both ofatumumab and rituximab can be used in combination with chlorambucil in older patients with CLL in the front-line setting.

8. **B**

Mantle cell lymphoma (MCL) in its rare leukemic form shares some of the immunophenotypic features with CLL. Like CLL, MCL is CD5+, CD19+ and CD20+, but negative for CD23. Unlike CLL, MCL is positive for t(11;14), which helps distinguish between the two entities. Choice A is commonly seen in follicular lymphoma, whereas choices D and E are seen in marginal zone lymphoma. Choice C is seen in Burkitt leukemia/lymphoma.

9. **B**

Recurrent infections are commonly seen in CLL due to hypogammaglobulinemia. This patient has recurrent pneumonia with low levels of serum IgG. Besides coverage with broad-spectrum antibiotics, the patient should receive immunoglobulin replacement. Prophylactic use of immunoglobulin remains controversial. IV ganciclovir and foscarnet are used in patients with confirmed CMV infection, but has yet to be proved in this case. Treating the patient with ibrutinib will not necessarily help boost the immune system to help fight infection.

10. **D**

Patients with CLL are at increased risk for developing pure red cell aplasia (PRCA), most likely considered to be immune mediated. This is the most likely diagnosis in this patient, who presents with severe anemia without any evidence of bleed or nutritional deficiencies. A bone marrow is warranted to rule out anemia from disease progression versus PRCA. Viral studies, however, should also be done in patients with PRCA because viruses are known to be associated with this condition.

Prednisone and rituximab are more commonly used in treating AIHA.

11. **C**

This patient has features of hairy cell leukemia including pancytopenia, enlarged spleen, and a peripheral smear showing cells with hairy projections. Choice C is the correct answer. The mucosal lymphocyte antigen, CD103, is a sensitive marker for HCL. CD103 is a member of the integrin family and is also present on mucosa-associated T cells and some activated lymphocytes. The presence of CD103, when co-expressed with other pan-B cell markers, is highly suggestive of HCL.

12. **B**

The correct answer is BRAF V600E. Most patients with hairy cell leukemia harbor mutation in the BRAF gene. The remaining choices are more commonly seen in MDS, AML, and myelofibrosis.

13. **A**

Cladribine, as a single agent, has been shown to achieve a complete remission rate of 80%–98%. Long-term follow-up of patients treated with cladribine has shown disease-free survival of more than 8 years and a 12-year overall survival rate of 80%–90%. Rituximab, used mainly in the relapse setting, is associated with modest activity.

14. **B**

One should recognize the toxicity that is associated with each treatment modality. Venetoclax, a BCL-2 inhibitor, has been approved by the FDA for the treatment of relapsed/refractory CLL with 17p deletion after failing at least one prior therapy. Venetoclax can lead to a rapid decline in the tumor burden in the first 5 weeks of dose escalation. This increases the risk of tumor lysis syndrome. Patients should be vigilantly watched for possible tumor lysis. Venetoclax may need to be put on hold if there is evidence of tumor lysis.

15. **D**

This is most consistent with a diagnosis of T-cell large granular lymphocytic leukemia (T-LGL). It is very commonly associated with autoimmune disorders like rheumatoid arthritis and Sjogren syndrome. It is most commonly associated with rheumatoid arthritis in up to 25% of the cases of T-LGL. It is characterized by organ infiltration by the LGL cells causing splenomegaly and cytopenias. The most common immunophenotypes associated with this disorder in up to 85% of the cases include CD3+, CD56–, and CD57+.

REFERENCES

Question 1

1. Hallek M, Cheson BD, Catovsky D, et al. Guidelines for the diagnosis and treatment of chronic lymphocytic leukemia: a report from the International Workshop on Chronic Lymphocytic Leukemia updating the National Cancer Institute-Working Group 1996 Guidelines. *Blood*. 2008;111(12):5446.

Question 3

1. Eichhorst B, Fink AM, Bhalo J, et al. First-line chemoimmunotherapy with bendamustine and rituximab versus fludarabine, cyclophosphamide, and rituximab in patients with advanced chronic lymphocytic leukaemia (CLL10): an international, open-label, randomised, phase 3, non-inferiority trial. *Lancet Oncol*. 2016;17(7):928–942.
2. Tsimberidou AM, Tam C, Abrusso LV, et al. Chemoimmunotherapy may overcome the adverse prognostic significance of 11q deletion in previously untreated patients with chronic lymphocytic leukemia. *Cancer*. 2009;115(2):373–380.

Question 13

1. Zinzani PL, Tani M, Marchi E, et al. Long term follow-up of frontline treatment of hairy cell leukemia with 2-chlorodeoxyadenosine. *Hematologica*. 2004;89:309–313.

QUESTIONS

1. A 22-year-old college student presents with unexplained 15-pound weight loss, drenching night sweats, and diffuse pruritus without a rash. On physical exam, she appears tired but otherwise well. She has no peripheral lymphadenopathy or splenomegaly. Chest radiograph reveals a large mediastinal mass. Computerized tomography scans of the chest, abdomen, and pelvis show a 13-cm anterior mediastinal mass without lymphadenopathy in the neck, axilla, or below the diaphragm. What is the next step in her diagnostic evaluation?
   A. Positron emission tomography (PET)
   B. Needle biopsy of the mass
   C. Referral to thoracic surgery for mediastinoscopy and biopsy
   D. Bone marrow biopsy
   E. Echocardiogram

2. A 25-year-old man presents with a right-axillary mass. He is otherwise asymptomatic. Physical exam is notable for normal vital signs. He has a 4-cm right axilla node without other palpable peripheral lymphadenopathy. Incisional lymph node biopsy reveals the node is effaced by large atypical cells with multilobulated nuclei and small, peripheral nucleoli surrounded by predominately small lymphocytes. The large cells express CD20 and are negative for CD15 and CD30. What is the diagnosis?
   A. Mixed cellularity Hodgkin lymphoma (HL)
   B. Gray zone lymphoma
   C. Nodular lymphocyte predominant Hodgkin lymphoma (NLPHL)
   D. Lymphocyte rich HL
   E. Lymphocyte depleted HL

3. A 50-year-old male with human immunodeficiency virus (HIV) on antiretrovirals with a CD4 count of $500/mm^3$ and undetectable viral load presents with fevers, drenching night sweats, and 20-pound weight loss. The positron emission tomography scan reveals fluorodeoxyglucose avid lymphadenopathy above and below the diaphragm with multiple sites of bony involvement. Biopsy of a right neck node reveals mixed cellularity, HL. He has stage IVB disease with four risk factors on the International Prognostic Scale (age >45, male gender, stage IV disease, and lymphopenia). Pretreatment echocardiogram and pulmonary function tests are normal. How would you treat this patient?
   A. Doxorubicin, bleomycin, vinblastine, and dacarbazine (ABVD × 6)
   B. AVD × 6
   C. Escalated bleomycin, etoposide, doxorubicin, cyclophosphamide, vincristine, procarbazine, and prednisone (BEACOPPesc)

   D. Brentuximab vedotin plus ABVD
   E. Nivolumab

4. A 19-year-old male is diagnosed with stage IA NLPHL involving the left neck. Which of the following is an appropriate therapeutic strategy?
   A. ABVD × 4 cycles
   B. Mantle irradiation
   C. Single agent rituximab, followed by maintenance
   D. Involved field radiotherapy
   E. RCHOP × 6 cycles

5. An 18-year-old woman presents with persistent cough and chest pain with alcohol consumption but denies any fevers, night sweats, or weight loss. Chest radiograph and subsequent computed tomography (CT) images demonstrate a 10-cm mediastinal mass. Surgical biopsy reveals nodular sclerosis subtype of classical HL. Which of the following is correct:
   A. The large atypical cells express CD30 and CD25.
   B. PAX-5 is strongly expressed on Reed-Sternberg (RS) cells.
   C. PD-1 is expressed on the RS cells.
   D. The RS cells have frequent copy gain or amplification of 9p24.

6. A 35-year-old woman presents with neck fullness without fevers, night sweats, or weight loss. On physical examination, she has enlarged lymph nodes in the cervical and supraclavicular regions bilaterally. Left axillary lymph node biopsy indicates classical HL, nodular sclerosis subtype. Positron emission tomography/computed tomography (PET-CT) images demonstrate fluorodeoxyglucose avid lymphadenopathy on both sides of the neck and the mediastinum. Which of the following baseline studies is required as part of her pretreatment prognostic evaluation?
   A. Erythrocyte sedimentation rate
   B. Pulmonary function tests
   C. Unilateral bone marrow biopsy
   D. Bilateral bone marrow biopsy
   E. Serum lactate dehydrogenase level

7. A 26-year-old female with stage IIA NS HL is treated with 6 cycles of ABVD and achieves a PET-CT at the end of therapy. After 2 years, she develops recurrent neck lymphadenopathy. Biopsy reveals nodular sclerosis HL. What is the next step in her management?
   A. Radiotherapy
   B. Autologous stem cell transplant
   C. Retreat with ABVD × 4
   D. Second-line chemotherapy with ICE chemotherapy
   E. Gemcitabine monotherapy

8. A 36-year-old male treated with involved-field radiation therapy (IFRT) to the right neck for stage IA lymphocyte predominate Hodgkin lymphoma (NLPHL) presents with fatigue and night sweats. The PET scan reveals FDG avid lymphadenopathy in the abdomen with multiple lesions in the liver and spleen. What is the most likely diagnosis?
   A. Recurrent NLPHL
   B. Diffuse large B-cell lymphoma
   C. Metastatic carcinoma
   D. Classical HL
   E. Sarcoidosis

9. A 20-year-old woman presents with persistent cough without fevers, night sweats, or weight loss. On physical examination, her vital signs are normal. Physical exam is notable for 2–3 cm nodes in the bilateral neck. Excisional lymph node biopsy reveals classical HL, nodular sclerosis. The positron emission tomography images show multiple fluorodeoxyglucose-avid lymph nodes in the bilateral cervical/supraclavicular regions and a 5 cm mediastinal mass. Laboratory values are notable for a normal CBC and ESR of 40 mm/h. After 2 cycles of chemotherapy with ABVD, all the nodes have normalized in size and the uptake in all sites is less than mediastinal blood pool (Deauville criteria 2). Which of the following is the most appropriate next step?
   A. No further therapy
   B. Involved-field radiation therapy at 20 Gy
   C. Two cycles of ABVD
   D. One cycle of ABVD
   E. Two cycles of ABVD plus involved-field radiation therapy at 20 Gy

10. A 68-year-old woman with presents with an asymptomatic left neck mass. Her examination is notable for a 3-cm left supraclavicular node with smaller nodes in the ipsilateral left neck. Incisional lymph node biopsy is performed and reveals mixed cellularity subtype of classical HL. Immunoperoxidase staining demonstrates the RS cells are positive for CD30 and CD15. Epstein-Barr virus (EBV)-encoded RNA (EBER) signal is positive. Staging shows nonbulky disease isolated to the left neck. Laboratory studies are notable for an erythrocyte sedimentation rate (ESR) 5 mm/h (reference range, 0–20 mm/h). Which of the following is the most appropriate treatment strategy?
   A. ABVD × 2 cycles plus 20 Gy of IFRT
   B. AVD × 2 cycles plus 20 Gy involved-field radiation therapy
   C. Escalated BEACOPPesc × 2 cycles plus 30 Gy of IFRT
   D. Six cycles of brentuximab vedotin
   E. ABVD × 3 cycles plus 30 Gy of IFRT

11. A 30-year-old woman presents to establish ongoing care. She feels well and enjoys long-distance running. 10 years earlier she was treated with 4 cycles of ABVD plus involved-field radiation therapy for stage IIA classical Hodgkin lymphoma involving the left neck, left axilla, and mediastinum. She is feeling well and has not seen a physician for 7 years. What do you recommend for the patient?
   A. CBC and ESR
   B. Breast imaging
   C. Pulmonary function tests
   D. Surveillance CT of the chest, abdomen, and pelvis
   E. Stress echocardiography

12. A 40-year-old woman presents with drenching night sweats and fevers and is found to have diffuse lymphadenopathy in the bilateral neck and axilla. Excisional lymph node biopsy of a right neck node reveals classical HL, mixed cellularity subtype. PET-CT reveals FDG-avid disease in the bilateral neck, axilla, mediastinum, upper abdomen, and spleen. She has stage IIIB disease with risk factors of hypoalbuminemia (albumin 3.2 g/dL), anemia (hemoglobin of 10 g/dL), and lymphopenia (absolute lymphocyte count of 500/mm^3). Her oncologist recommends therapy with ABVD. ABVD is associated with all the following toxicities except:
   A. Risk of cardiac dysfunction
   B. Pulmonary toxicity
   C. Neutropenia
   D. Ileus
   E. Infertility

ANSWERS

1. C
A surgical biopsy is critical to establish the diagnosis of HL. Given that the RS cells constitute approximately 1% of the cells in an involved lymph node, a specimen derived from a needle biopsy may not include the diagnostic cells and lacks the architecture necessary to subclassify the lymphoma. A PET scan is required as part of the staging evaluation, but it is not necessary to identifying a site to biopsy given the appearance of her CT scans. Bone marrow biopsy is not required given the sensitivity of PET to identifying bone marrow or bony sites of disease. An echocardiogram is typically obtained prior to the administration of anthracycline containing therapy but is not helpful in establishing the diagnosis.

2. C
The diagnosis is NLPHL. Patients typically present with asymptomatic lymphadenopathy that frequently spares the mediastinum. The RS cells, referred to as "popcorn cells" or lymphocytic and histiocytic (L&H) cells, express CD20 and are typically negative for CD15 and CD30, which are typically found on the RS cells of classical HL. Gray zone lymphoma shares features of classical HL and primary mediastinal large B-cell lymphoma.

3. A
Patients with HIV are at increased risk for the development of HL and frequently develop an advanced-stage disease that is associated with Epstein-Barr virus.

ABVD is the standard of care in patients with HIV-associated HL, and outcomes in patient on antiretrovirals are similar to HIV-negative patients. This patient has no contraindication to the inclusion of bleomycin, but the patient requires careful monitoring for the development of respiratory symptoms. Although escalated BEACOPP is associated with improved progression-free survival compared to ABVD without overall survival benefit, it is associated with significantly higher myelosuppression and risk of infection. Brentuximab vedotin is a CD30 directed antibody drug conjugate approved for use in the relapsed setting but not for upfront use. Nivolumab, an antibody against PD-1 (programmed cell death protein-1), is currently being studied in relapsed/refractory HL.

4. D

Long-term follow-up of patients treated with IFRT shows that approximately 90% of patients with stage I disease have long-term disease-free survival. The addition of chemotherapy does not improve outcomes, and there are no data to support the use of chemotherapy alone in patients with stage I NLPHL. Mantle radiation is not associated with improved disease control and has a high risk of late cardiovascular disease and increased risk of second malignancies. Although rituximab has high response rates in NLPHL, the durability is inferior compared to radiotherapy in stage I patients.

5. D

The malignant cell in HL is the RS cell is a multinucleated cell derived from a germinal center B-cell in the vast majority of cases. RS cells comprise approximately 1% of the cells in the involved site and are surrounded by mixed inflammatory cells. The RS cells in classical HL typically express CD30 and CD15. PAX-5 expression is weak. Genetic analysis of RS cells shows near uniform amplification of 9p24.1, leading to the expression of PDL-1 and PDL-2 (programmed cell death-ligands 1 and 2). PD-1 (programmed cell death 1) is expressed on a subset of surrounding immune cells.

6. A

The ESR is an important component of risk stratification for patients with early-stage HL. Both the German Hodgkin Study Group and the European Organization for Research and Treatment of Cancer classification identify an ESR ≥50 mm/h without symptoms or ≥30 mm/h with B symptoms as an adverse prognostic indicator. The serum lactate dehydrogenase level is typically normal in early-stage HL (although it may be elevated in patients with bulky mediastinal disease) and is not prognostic in early-stage HL. Patients without underlying pulmonary disease are unlikely to have abnormal baseline pulmonary function testing, and this does not necessarily predict the development of bleomycin-related pulmonary toxicity. Patients presenting with stage I/II classical HL without B symptoms have a low risk of bone marrow involvement, and PET scan has a higher sensitivity for detecting occult marrow involvement than bone marrow biopsy.

7. D

More than half of patients who develop recurrent HL that remains sensitive to chemotherapy have long-term disease control with autologous stem cell transplantation. Patients are treated with second-line chemotherapy, with regimens such as ifosfamide, carboplatin, and etoposide. Responding patients then undergo stem cell collection followed by high-dose chemotherapy and autologous stem-cell transplants. No comparative data exist to evaluate the possibility of curative therapy with radiation alone in the relapsed setting. Given the patient has recurred following prior ABVD chemotherapy, an alternative second-line regimen is used. Although gemcitabine is an active drug, combination therapy is associated with higher overall and complete remission rates.

8. B

Nodular lymphocyte predominate HL is associated with a risk of transformation to diffuse large B-cell lymphoma of approximately 10%, and patients typically present with abdominal disease, often involving the spleen. B symptoms are more likely seen in patients with aggressive lymphoma than NLPHL. Although radiotherapy is associated with a risk of secondary malignancies, the patient received treatment only to the neck. The pattern of disease involvement is atypical for HL or sarcoid.

9. C

Per the HD6 Canadian/US Intergroup study, patients with early-stage disease were randomly assigned to ABVD chemotherapy alone or to subtotal radiation to the nodes alone or with 2 cycles of ABVD for favorable and unfavorable risk disease, respectively. Patients in the chemotherapy-only group who had a complete response (according to CT images) after 2 cycles of ABVD received a total of 4 cycles of chemotherapy. The remainder of patients received 6 cycles. At 12 years, the overall survival was superior for patients who only received chemotherapy. Patients who achieved a CR after 4 cycles of ABVD had a 92% freedom from disease progression at 12 years. The patient in this clinical scenario has stage IIA disease with three sites of involvement (bilateral cervical/supraclavicular, and mediastinum). She therefore has unfavorable disease according to the German Hodgkin Study Group and does not fit criteria for the HD10 study with 2 cycles of ABVD plus 20 Gy of IFRT. Given the patient is younger than 30 years, she is at high risk for the subsequent development of radiation-induced breast cancer, with the disease involvement in the mediastinum and axilla.

10. A

This patient has stage IIA favorable disease with two sites of disease involvement without any other risk factors, (bulky disease, B symptoms, an ESR ≥50 mm/h, or extranodal disease). In the HD10 trial, patients were randomized in a factorial design to four versus 2 cycles of ABVD chemotherapy and 30 Gy versus 20 Gy of IRFT. There was no difference in freedom from treatment failure in any of the treatment arms, and 2 cycles of ABVD followed by 20 Gy of radiotherapy was associated with less toxicity. In the HD13 GHSG trial, patients were assigned to one of four chemotherapy regimens (ABVD, AVD, ABV, and AV) followed by 30 Gy of IFRT. The omission of dacarbazine and bleomycin was associated with inferior rates of freedom from treatment failure. Escalated bleomycin, etoposide, doxorubicin, cyclophosphamide, vincristine, procarbazine, and prednisone (BEACOPPesc) has not been studied in early, favorable disease, and it is not recommended for patients over 60 given its toxicity. Brentuximab vedotin is approved for relapsed HL.

11. B

Patients under the age of 30 treated with radiotherapy to the chest are at a significantly increased risk of breast cancer. Patients should initiate screening 8 years after radiation or at the age of 40, whichever occurs first. Given the patient is asymptomatic and 10 years out from therapy, the likelihood of disease recurrence is extremely low and there is no role for surveillance imaging or an ESR. She has no cardiac or respiratory symptoms, and pulmonary function testing or stress echocardiogram is not routinely recommended.

12. E

ABVD is not associated with an increased risk of infertility. Adriamycin can rarely cause cardiac dysfunction. The risk is dose related, and patients receiving 6 cycles of ABVD receive a cumulative dose of 300 mg/m^2, which is below 450 mg/m^2, above which the incidence of cardiomyopathy rises significantly. Bleomycin is associated with pulmonary toxicity, and patients must be followed carefully for the development of cough, dyspnea, or crackles on chest exam. Neutropenia occurs commonly in patients receiving ABVD, although the risk of febrile neutropenia is very low and most patients do not require white blood cell growth factors. Vinblastine commonly causes peripheral neuropathy and constipation that can be severe and result in ileus.

REFERENCES

Question 1

1. Cheson BD, Fisher RI, Barrington SF, et al. Recommendations for initial evaluation, staging, and response assessment of Hodgkin and non-Hodgkin lymphoma: the Lugano classification. *J Clin Oncol.* 2014;32:3059–3068.

Question 4

1. Montoto S, Shaw K, Okosun J, et al. HIV status does not influence outcome in patients with classical Hodgkin lymphoma treated with chemotherapy using doxorubicin, bleomycin, vinblastine, and dacarbazine in the highly active antiretroviral therapy era. *J Clin Oncol.* 2012;30:4111–4116.
2. Merli F, Luminari S, Gobbi PG, et al. Long-term results of the HD2000 trial comparing ABVD versus BEACOPP versus COPP-EBV-CAD in untreated patients with advanced Hodgkin lymphoma: a study by Fondazione Italiana Linfomi. *J Clin Oncol.* 2016;34:1175–1181.
3. Eichenauer DA, Plutschow A, Fuchs M, et al. Long-term course of patients with stage IA nodular lymphocyte-predominant Hodgkin lymphoma: a report from the German Hodgkin Study Group. *J Clin Oncol.* 2015;33:2857–2862.

Question 5

1. Ansell SM, Lesokhin AM, Borrello I, et al. PD-1 blockade with nivolumab in relapsed or refractory Hodgkin's lymphoma. *N Engl J Med.* 2015;372:311–319.

Question 6

1. Cheson BD, Fisher RI, Barrington SF, et al. Recommendations for initial evaluation, staging, and response assessment of Hodgkin and non-Hodgkin lymphoma: the Lugano classification. *J Clin Oncol.* 2014;32:3059–3068.

Question 7

1. Zelenetz AD, Hamlin P, Kewalramani T, Yahalom J, Nimer S, Moskowitz CH. Ifosfamide, carboplatin, etoposide (ICE)-based second-line chemotherapy for the management of relapsed and refractory aggressive non-Hodgkin's lymphoma. *Ann Oncol.* 2003;14(suppl 1):i5–i10.

Question 8

1. Biasoli I, Stamatoullas A, Meignin V, et al. Nodular, lymphocyte-predominant Hodgkin lymphoma: a long-term study and analysis of transformation to diffuse large B-cell lymphoma in a cohort of 164 patients from the Adult Lymphoma Study Group. *Cancer.* 2010;116:631–639.

Question 9

1. Meyer RM, Gospodarowicz MK, Connors JM, et al. ABVD alone versus radiation-based therapy in limited-stage Hodgkin's lymphoma. *N Engl J Med.* 2012;366:399–408.
2. Engert A, Plutschow A, Eich HT, et al. Reduced treatment intensity in patients with early-stage Hodgkin's lymphoma. *N Engl J Med.* 2010;363:640–652.

Question 10

1. Engert A, Plutschow A, Eich HT, et al. Reduced treatment intensity in patients with early-stage Hodgkin's lymphoma. *N Engl J Med.* 2010;363:640–652.
2. Behringer K, Goergen H, Hitz F, et al. Omission of dacarbazine or bleomycin, or both, from the ABVD regimen in treatment of early-stage favourable Hodgkin's lymphoma (GHSG HD13): an open-label, randomised, non-inferiority trial. *Lancet.* 2015;385:1418–1427.

Question 11

1. Yahalom J. Evidence-based breast cancer screening guidelines for women who received chest irradiation at a young age. *J Clin Oncol.* 2013;31:2240–2242.

Question 12

1. Hodgson DC, Pintilie M, Gitterman L, et al. Fertility among female Hodgkin lymphoma survivors attempting pregnancy following ABVD chemotherapy. *Hematol Oncol.* 2007;25:11–15.

CHAPTER 9

Non-Hodgkin Lymphoma

Nathan Fowler

QUESTIONS

1. A 62-year-old woman presents to your office with relapsed mantle cell lymphoma. Her prior therapy includes rituximab plus cyclophosphamide, Adriamycin, vincristine, and prednisone (R-CHOP), and localized radiation to a node in the axilla on relapse. She now has evidence of progressive disease and inquires about ibrutinib. She would like to discuss potential adverse events associated with the drug. You inform her that ibrutinib is associated with an increased risk of:
   A. Atrial fibrillation
   B. Colitis
   C. Myelosuppression
   D. Infection
   E. Pneumonitis

2. A 45-year-old male presented to his primary care physician complaining of headache and diplopia. MRI of the brain shows a 3-cm mass in the occipital lobe. Brain biopsy demonstrates a CD20+, CD5– population of large B cells. Staging does not show evidence of disease outside of the brain, and the patient is HIV negative. A lumbar puncture is positive for a small population of large cells, which are positive for CD20, CD19, and CD10 by flow cytometry. Which of the following agents is most likely to be active in his disease?
   A. Cyclophosphamide
   B. Vincristine
   C. High-dose methotrexate
   D. Cisplatin
   E. Oxaliplatin

3. A 70-year-old male with recently diagnosed follicular lymphoma presents to your office. He complains of a 10-pound weight loss, but denies fever or night sweats. PET imaging shows evidence of nonbulky disease limited to three nodal sites above the diaphragm. His CBC shows a hemoglobin of 14.2, a WBC of 4.5, and a platelet count of 240. His LDH is normal, and his albumin is 3.0. Bone marrow is hypocellular, but without evidence of lymphoma. Based upon the follicular lymphoma international prognostic index (FLIPI) scoring system, his expected 10-year survival is:
   A. 5%
   B. 10%
   C. 30%
   D. 50%
   E. 70%

4. A 64-year-old male with a history of hypothyroidism, controlled congestive heart failure, and osteoarthritis was recently found to have night sweats and an enlarged node in the right groin. He underwent excisional biopsy, which showed a CD20+, CD10+, grade 2 follicular lymphoma. He noted a 15-pound weight loss over the past 3 months.

PET-CT scans demonstrate disease both above and below the diaphragm, with the largest node in the right groin measuring 5 cm. A bone marrow biopsy shows 20% involvement by a low-grade process consistent with follicular lymphoma. What is your recommended first-line treatment option?
   A. Observation
   B. Bendamustine plus rituximab
   C. Cyclophosphamide, Adriamycin, vincristine, and prednisone (CHOP) + rituximab
   D. Fludarabine, mitoxantrone, and decadron (FND) + rituximab
   E. Cyclophosphamide, Adriamycin, vincristine, and prednisone (CHOP)

5. A 60-year-old male with follicular lymphoma is diagnosed with stage III bulky disease. He is initially treated with rituximab, cyclophosphamide, Adriamycin, vincristine, and prednisone (R-CHOP) and achieves a complete remission. Three years later, he progresses and is treated with bendamustine and rituximab and achieves a partial remission by CT imaging. He is started on maintenance rituximab, given every 2 months. Six months into maintenance dosing, he is found to have a new axillary node (3 cm). Biopsy confirms recurrent grade 1–2 follicular lymphoma. You would now recommend:
   A. R-CHOP
   B. Re-dose with bendamustine
   C. Continue rituximab maintenance
   D. Radiation to axillary bed
   E. Idelalisib

6. A 42-year-old Caucasian woman with a history of relapsed follicular lymphoma is interested in starting idelalisib. She asks about potential side effects of the study drug. Which of the following adverse events are not associated with idelalisib?
   A. Diarrhea
   B. Cardiac dysfunction
   C. Transient transaminitis
   D. Pneumonitis
   E. Infection

7. A 54-year-old male presents with a new diagnosis of diffuse large B-cell lymphoma. He is HIV negative and hepatitis C negative. After staging, he is found to have nonbulky disease limited to nodal areas both above and below the diaphragm. He is slightly anemic (hemoglobin 12.2), and his lactate dehydrogenase (LDH) is normal. What is his risk of central nervous system involvement by lymphoma?
   A. 0%
   B. 5%
   C. 13%
   D. 20%
   E. 30%

8. A 68-year-old female was recently diagnosed with mantle cell lymphoma. PET imaging shows evidence of lymphadenopathy in the neck, axilla, and retroperitoneum. Her bone marrow biopsy shows 5% involvement by mantle cell lymphoma. There is no evidence of blastoid transformation in her nodal biopsy or on bone marrow. Which of the following is the most common site of extranodal involvement of her mantle cell lymphoma?
   A. Skin
   B. Brain
   C. GI tract
   D. Spleen
   E. Liver

9. You are called during a patient's first cycle of rituximab plus bendamustine for treatment of follicular lymphoma. During escalation of the rituximab infusion, and prior to starting bendamustine, the patient experiences hives and shortness of breath. His nurse reports a temperature of 101.3, blood pressure of 124/78, and pulse of 100. The patient denies dizziness, nausea, or chest pain. The patient has no prior history of cardiac disease, pulmonary disease, or infectious exposures. Thirty minutes after stopping the infusion, the patient's symptoms resolve. You instruct the nurse to:
   A. Discontinue rituximab and ask the patient to return to your clinic
   B. Reduce the rituximab dose by 20%
   C. Restart the rituximab at a slower rate
   D. Restart the rituximab at the same rate
   E. Discontinue rituximab, order EKG and blood cultures

10. Which of the following treatments are associated with an increased risk of cardiotoxicity?
   A. Adriamycin total dose greater than 450 mg/m^2
   B. Adriamycin total dose greater than 300 mg/m^2
   C. Lenalidomide dose greater than 20 mg
   D. Vincristine dose greater than 2 mg/m^2
   E. Vincristine dose greater than 3 mg/m^2

11. A 62-year-old female is being treated for newly diagnosed diffuse large B-cell lymphoma. She has a history of well-controlled diabetes, hypertension, and anxiety. Following her third course of R-CHOP chemotherapy, she complains of difficulty with handwriting as well as difficulty buttoning up her shirt. You plan to make the following adjustments to her chemotherapy course:
   A. Decrease her vincristine dose by 50%
   B. Decrease her rituximab dose by 20%
   C. Hold prednisone on next cycle of therapy
   D. Make no change in her chemotherapy
   E. Decrease cyclophosphamide dose by 20%

12. A 25-year-old female presented with swelling in the neck, shortness of breath, and facial edema. She was found to have a large mediastinal mass measuring 12 cm in maximum diameter. She underwent a mediastinal biopsy, which showed evidence of a diffuse large B-cell lymphoma. PET-CT scan showed disease limited to the mediastinum. She was started on a course of rituximab, cyclophosphamide, Adriamycin, vincristine, and prednisone (R-CHOP). She tolerated 6 cycles of therapy, and the imaging studies at the completion of treatment demonstrate complete remission. What is your next step in management?
   A. Autologous stem cell transplant
   B. Radiotherapy

C. Begin maintenance rituximab × 24 months
D. Begin maintenance rituximab × 12 months
E. Give 2 more cycles of R-CHOP as consolidation

13. A 45-year-old male recently presented with night sweats, fever, weight loss, and enlarged bilateral axillary adenopathy. Excisional biopsy shows a population of large cells positive for CD20 and CD19, and negative for CD5 and CD10. Cytogenetics demonstrate BCL 2 and C-MYC mutations. PET scan shows evidence of adenopathy in the axilla and groin. Bone marrow biopsy is negative for involvement by disease. The patient is given 6 cycles of rituximab, cyclophosphamide, Adriamycin, vincristine, and prednisone (R-CHOP) chemotherapy. This patient's 3-year progression-free survival is approximately:
   A. 0%
   B. 20%
   C. 60%
   D. 75%
   E. 90%

14. A 72-year-old female is receiving her second cycle of bendamustine and rituximab for a grade 2, stage III follicular lymphoma. Prior to initiating therapy, she inquires about the common toxicities associated with bendamustine. You inform her of the following:
   A. Alopecia
   B. Nausea
   C. Peripheral neuropathy
   D. Cardiac dysfunction
   E. Transient hepatitis

15. A 52-year-old female with a history of previously treated follicular lymphoma presents to your office. Her prior therapy includes bendamustine plus rituximab followed by 2 years of rituximab maintenance. She completed therapy 4 years ago. Two weeks ago she developed intermittent dizziness and diplopia. MRI of the brain shows diffuse white matter changes with no evidence of leptomeningeal enhancement or mass effect. A lumbar puncture shows no malignant cells. Your next step in diagnostic workup should include:
   A. Lumbar puncture with viral studies
   B. EEG
   C. Blood cultures
   D. MRI of the cervical spine
   E. Brain biopsy

16. A 62-year-old presents to his primary care physician complaining of 7-month history of slowly enlarging nodes in his neck, bilaterally. He eventually consents to an excisional biopsy of a left-sided cervical lymph node. Pathology shows a population of small cells, which are positive for CD20, CD10, and CD19, but negative for CD5 and cyclin D1. The most common cytogenetic abnormality associated with this diagnosis is:
   A. t(14;18)(q32;q21)
   B. t(8;14)(q24;q32)
   C. t(2;8)(p12;q24)
   D. t(8;22)(q24;q11)
   E. t(11;14)(q13;q32)

17. A 45-year-old male presents to his physician complaining of stomach upset for the past 3 months. He was given proton pump inhibitor (PPI) with minimal effect. Upper endoscopy demonstrates several nodular lesions within the stomach and the proximal duodenum. Stomach biopsy shows evidence of a population of intermediate-sized

cells, which are CD20+ and CD10, CD5, and CD138 negative. Staging studies fail to show evidence of local or distant adenopathy. The infection most associated with this diagnosis is:
A. HIV
B. *H. pylori*
C. Hepatitis C
D. *B. burgdorferi*
E. *C. psittaci*

18. A 65-year-old male has evidence of lymphocytosis, 30% bone marrow involvement by marginal zone lymphoma, and splenomegaly. No significant adenopathy is noted on CT imaging. The patient received four doses of single agent rituximab with partial remission. One year later, he is found to have recurrent splenomegaly and anemia. A bone marrow biopsy confirms persistent marginal zone lymphoma. He receives 6 cycles of ibrutinib, but again only achieves partial remission, and has persistent anemia and splenomegaly 4 months after completing therapy. Your next step in management includes:
A. Switch to R-CHOP chemotherapy
B. Start rituximab maintenance
C. Splenectomy
D. Give two more doses of bendamustine
E. Allogeneic stem cell transplant

19. A 63-year-old male presents to his primary care physician complaining of diarrhea, abdominal cramping, and a 15-pound weight loss. Colonoscopy with biopsy is positive for mantle cell lymphoma. Staging studies show low-volume adenopathy both above and below the diaphragm. The diagnosis is associated with which cytogenetic abnormality?
A. t(14;18)(q32;q21)
B. t(8;14)(q24;q32)
C. t(2;8)(p12;q24)
D. t(8;22)(q24;q11)
E. t(11;14)(q13;q32)

20. A 48-year-old male was recently diagnosed with stage III, bulky diffuse large B-cell lymphoma. He received 4 cycles of rituximab, cyclophosphamide, Adriamycin, vincristine, and prednisone (R-CHOP) and achieves a partial remission. Following his sixth cycle of therapy, he is found to have progression of disease. He then received 2 cycles of rituximab, ifosfamide, carboplatin, and etoposide (R-ICE) chemotherapy. PET imaging following his second cycle of R-ICE shows a complete metabolic response. What is the next step in management?
A. Refer the patient for autologous stem cell transplant
B. Give two more cycles of R-ICE chemotherapy as consolidation
C. Begin rituximab maintenance
D. Give 4 more cycles of R-ICE as consolidation
E. Begin observation and repeat staging studies in 3 months

21. A 52-year-old female with relapsed mantle cell lymphoma is started on a course of lenalidomide. On the 15th day of her first cycle of therapy, she presents to your clinic with a raised erythematous rash covering her back, bilateral arms, and torso (>50% of her body surface area). She denies blistering, fever, pruritus, or recent toxic exposures. She has no mucosal lesions and denies recent bleeding events.
What is your next step in management?
A. Order skin biopsy
B. Start antibiotics

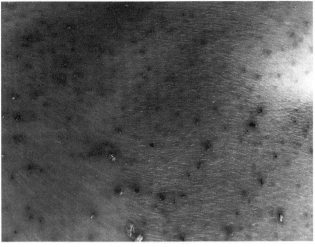

FIG. 9.1 Dorsal rash.

C. Stop lenalidomide
D. Start allopurinol
E. Start topical steroids

22. A 66-year-old male was recently diagnosed with stage III, diffuse large B-cell lymphoma. Staging studies show evidence of nonbulky disease both above and below the diaphragm, splenomegaly, and bone marrow involvement. He is started on rituximab, cyclophosphamide, Adriamycin, vincristine, and prednisone (R-CHOP) chemotherapy and receives growth factor support with pegfilgrastim 24 hours after completing his first cycle. On day 14, he presents to the emergency room with an absolute neutrophil count of 0.3 and fever. A chest x-ray shows a new opacity in the right middle lobe. The patient is admitted to the hospital and improves after 3 days of IV antibiotics. How would you manage his next cycle of therapy?
A. Decrease his dose of rituximab by 50%
B. Change pegfilgrastim to filgrastim
C. Decrease cyclophosphamide and Adriamycin by 20%
D. Switch R-CHOP to rituximab plus bendamustine
E. Hold prednisone on next cycle

23. A 62-year-old male was recently diagnosed with stage III, diffuse large B-cell lymphoma. He has evidence of nodal disease above and below the diaphragm without bone marrow involvement. He complains of abdominal bloating, but otherwise feels well and is out of bed the entire day. His platelet count is 98 and hemoglobin is 13.4. His erythrocyte sedimentation rate is normal. According the international prognostic index (IPI), which of the following are not adverse prognostic factors?
A. Elevated LDH
B. Poor performance status
C. Low hemoglobin
D. Extranodal sites of involvement
E. Elevated erythrocyte sedimentation rate

24. A 52-year-old female is diagnosed with a bulky stage III, grade 2 follicular lymphoma. She received 6 cycles of bendamustine and rituximab and achieved a complete remission. She is followed with routine surveillance imaging as well as physical exams. Three years after completing treatment, she develops an enlarging nontender node in the left axilla. A CT scan shows several nodes above and below the

diaphragm, including a 4-cm node in the left retroperitoneum. Your next step in management includes:
A. Biopsy
B. Start R-CHOP chemotherapy
C. Rechallenge with bendamustine
D. Stem cell transplant consult
E. Rituximab as a single agent

25. A 64-year-old male with a history of well-controlled diabetes is diagnosed with ALK(−) anaplastic large cell lymphoma (ALCL). Staging studies show evidence of nonbulky disease both above and below the diaphragm. He receives 6 cycles of cyclophosphamide, Adriamycin, vincristine, and prednisone (CHOP) chemotherapy and achieves a partial remission. Eighteen months later, repeat imaging shows progressive disease in the retroperitoneum and mediastinum. You are considering brentuximab vedotin as his next line of therapy. Which of the following side effects are commonly associated with brentuximab vedotin?
A. Cardiac toxicity
B. Anemia
C. Peripheral neuropathy
D. Renal toxicity
E. Cystitis

26. A 32-year-old man was recently diagnosed with diffuse large B-cell lymphoma. He is found to have stage III disease with enlarged nodes above and below the diaphragm. On day 17 of cycle 1 of chemotherapy, he is found to have elevated liver enzymes. His aspartate aminotransferase (AST) and alanine aminotransferase (ALT) are 225 and 430, respectively. He is found to have a positive hepatitis B surface antigen (HBsAg). Which of the following agents is most associated with an increased risk of hepatitis B reactivation?
A. Cyclophosphamide
B. Etoposide
C. Rituximab
D. Prednisone
E. Adriamycin

27. On day 6 of cycle 1 of rituximab, ifosfamide, carboplatin, and etoposide (R-ICE) chemotherapy, a 64-year-old male with a history of chronic renal insufficiency develops an acute episode of confusion, lethargy, and dysarthria. He is afebrile, and no acute abnormalities are seen on brain MRI. Urinalysis is normal, and there is no clear evidence of infection. What is the next appropriate step in the management of this patient?
A. Obtain EEG
B. Administer methylene blue
C. Blood culture
D. Start high-dose dexamethasone
E. Start empiric ceftriaxone and vancomycin

28. A recent mammogram in a woman with a history of bilateral breast implants shows a 2.5-cm lesion at the periphery of the right breast. Ultrasound of the right breast confirms a solid mass at the 3 o'clock position. Excluding a benign lesion, which of the following diagnosis is most common?
A. ALCL, ALK(−)
B. Peripheral T-cell lymphoma not otherwise specified (PTCL-NOS)
C. Follicular lymphoma
D. Posttransplant lymphoproliferative disorder (PTLD)
E. Mycosis fungoides

29. A male patient is recently found to be anemic with abdominal bloating. A CT scan of the abdomen shows a spleen measuring 21 cm in maximum diameter. A bone marrow biopsy shows an intrasinusoidal infiltration of medium-sized cells, which are positive for CD20 and CD19, and negative for CD5 and CD10. B cells express immunoglobulin M (IgM) and are negative for cyclin D1. Which of the following infections are associated with this diagnosis?
A. Hepatitis C
B. Epstein-Barr virus (EBV)
C. *H. pylori*
D. *B. burgdorferi*
E. Human herpes virus-8

30. A 42-year-old female with HIV recently presented to her infectious disease physician complaining of night sweats, fever, and abdominal pain. A PET scan showed enlarged nodes in the abdomen, chest, and pelvis. An excisional biopsy of an inguinal lymph node shows diffuse large B-cell lymphoma. Bone marrow biopsy is positive for involvement with B-cell lymphoma. He has been compliant with his antiretroviral therapy and has a CD4 count of 220. Which of the following approaches is most appropriate to managing his HIV during treatment?
A. Hold antiretroviral therapy during chemotherapy
B. Hold rituximab during chemotherapy to minimize infectious risk
C. Hold vincristine during chemotherapy to minimize neuropathy
D. Reduce his cytotoxic therapy dose by 20% to minimize infectious risk
E. Continue retroviral therapy and full-dose chemotherapy

31. A 59-year-old male was recently diagnosed with a stage III follicular lymphoma. Histology from an excisional biopsy shows 5–10 centroblasts per high-powered field. Bone marrow biopsy demonstrates 10% involvement with a population of small CD10+ and CD 20+ B cells. This patient's 10-year risk of aggressive transformation is approximately:
A. 10%
B. 30%
C. 50%
D. 70%
E. 90%

32. A 54-year-old male was recently diagnosed with a grade 2 follicular lymphoma. Imaging studies show evidence of diffuse adenopathy both above and below the diaphragm. The patient complains of night sweats and fevers, along with abdominal bloating. He received 6 cycles of rituximab, cyclophosphamide, Adriamycin, vincristine, and prednisone (R-CHOP). PET imaging at the end of treatment shows a complete metabolic response. Two months after finishing chemotherapy, he is started on rituximab maintenance given every 2 months. Rituximab maintenance in this setting is associated with which of the following benefits?
A. Prolonged progression-free survival
B. Decreased infection
C. Improved overall survival
D. Decreased transformation risk
E. Decreased cost

33. A 43-year-old male presents to his primary care physician complaining of a painless unilateral testicular mass. Orchiectomy demonstrates a population of CD20+ large B cells abutting the removed testicle. A PET-CT scan shows evidence of a 3-cm node in the left inguinal area with no evidence of FDG avid adenopathy in the contralateral testis or above the diaphragm. The patient received 6 cycles of rituximab, cyclophosphamide, Adriamycin, vincristine, and

prednisone (R-CHOP) with intrathecal chemoprophylaxis. What is your next step in management of the patient?
A. Consult stem cell transplant
B. Total nodal irradiation
C. Radiation to the contralateral testis
D. Removal of the contralateral testis
E. Low-dose radiotherapy to the craniospinal axis

ANSWERS

1. A

Ibrutinib irreversibility inhibits Bruton's tyrosine kinase, a critical component of the pro-survival B-cell receptor pathway. Ibrutinib is administered once daily and is active in mantle cell lymphoma and chronic lymphocytic leukemia. Clinical studies have shown the drug to be associated with atrial fibrillation, increased risk of bleeding, and hypertension, but rarely infection or myelosuppression.

2. C

Primary brain lymphoma is an aggressive extranodal non-Hodgkin lymphoma. The majority of cases are diffuse large B cell lymphoma (DLBCL) subtype. Methotrexate is an antimetabolite that competes with folic acid leading to cell death. Intravenous high-dose (>3.5 g/m^2) methotrexate is effective in primary central nervous system (CNS) lymphoma due to its ability to cross the blood-brain barrier at higher concentrations (>3 gm/m^2). Although cyclophosphamide, cisplatin, oxaliplatin, and vincristine are active in B-cell malignancies, their CNS penetration is poor.

3. E

The follicular lymphoma international prognostic index (FLIPI) was developed after studying the clinical characteristics of newly diagnosed patients with follicular lymphoma. Several clinical parameters were identified that strongly predict a poor clinical outcome. These factors include age greater than 60, stage III–IV, hemoglobin level less than 12 g/dL, lactate dehydrogenase (LDH) level greater than the upper limit of normal, and greater than three nodal sites. Patients are grouped into low-, intermediate-, or high-risk disease, and each group has dramatically different 10-year outcomes.

4. B

Observation is not recommended in follicular lymphoma patients who have evidence of a high tumor burden. This includes patients who have "B" symptoms, such as night sweats, fever, or significant weight loss. Treatment is also indicated in patients who have bulky disease, threatened organ function, or cytopenias secondary to lymphoma. Excellent response rates have been observed with combination chemotherapy regimens and rituximab. With this combined approach, overall response rates are over 80% in several studies. Recently, two randomized studies comparing bendamustine and rituximab to either R-CHOP or rituximab plus CVP showed equivalent overall response and complete response rates.[1,2] Anthracycline-containing regimens have been associated with a low but consistent rate of cardiotoxicity, and their use is not recommended in patients who have alternate treatment options. Fludarabine has also been associated with an increased risk of secondary late malignancies, including myelodysplasia and secondary acute leukemia.

5. E

Although overall response rates are high with induction therapy in follicular lymphoma, the majority of patients still relapse following traditional chemoimmunotherapy regimens. Maintenance rituximab has been shown to extend progression-free survival in both the frontline and relapsed setting following rituximab-containing combinations. When patients relapse, multiple salvage combinations are effective. Generally, it is recommended to use alternative chemotherapy regimens in patients who progress within 1 year of the last regimen. Rituximab as a single agent is not recommended in patients who progress within 6 months of a rituximab-containing regimen. This patient has previously received 300 mg/m^2 of Adriamycin with 6 cycles of R-CHOP chemotherapy. Subsequent dosing of an anthracycline above 450 mg/m^2 has been associated with a significant increase in the incidence of congestive heart failure. Localized radiotherapy can be palliative and is associated with local control, but is not generally associated with prolonged systemic control of relapsed lymphoma. Idelalisib is approved for relapsed follicular lymphoma following two lines of prior therapy.

6. B

Idelalisib inhibits phosphoinositide 3-kinase (PI3K) and is used to treat relapsed chronic lymphocytic leukemia (CLL) as well as relapsed follicular lymphoma. Adverse events associated with idelalisib include transient but sometimes severe hepatotoxicity, diarrhea, colitis, pneumonitis, and infection. Diarrhea and colitis can occur after several months of therapy. Patients with suspected colitis or pneumonitis should interrupt dosing until the resolution of symptoms. Steroids have been shown to be effective in some cases.

7. B

Diffuse large B-cell lymphoma can present with both systemic and central nervous system involvement. Although the risk in most patients is low (5%), known clinical factors can increase the risk of central nervous system involvement at initial presentation or at relapse. Known risk factors include HIV positivity, multiple extranodal sites (notably renal, adrenal, and testicular), as well as Burkitt or Burkitt-like histology. Many patients with increased risk factors are given prophylactic therapy with intrathecal (IT) methotrexate.

8. C

Mantle cell lymphoma is an aggressive B-cell malignancy comprising approximately 3%–7% of all new diagnosed lymphomas. The disease is characterized by translocation t(11;14)(q13;q32) and the overexpression of CCND1. Although mantle cell lymphoma can occur in multiple extranodal sites the gastrointestinal (GI) tract is the most common extranodal site and can be involved in up to 80% of patients. Endoscopy as part of initial staging is especially recommended in patients who have GI symptoms, such as diarrhea, cramping, or bloating.

9. C

Rituximab is an anti-CD20 chimeric monoclonal antibody. Infusions are associated with reactions including hypotension, shortness of breath, rash, fever, and chills. Infusion reactions are most common during the first exposure to the drug, and patients are often premedicated with antihistamines and acetaminophen prior to dosing. In the event of a reaction, the infusion is held. If symptoms are not severe and do resolve, the infusion can generally be safely restarted at a minimum 50% reduction in the rate.

10. **A**

The anthracycline Adriamycin is associated with rare but potential life-threating cardiotoxicity. If congestive heart failure occurs, mortality approaches 50%. Symptoms can occur within 2 weeks of initial treatment or potentially up to 6–10 years following exposure. The risk increases substantially at total lifetime dose exposures of more than 450 mg/m^2.

11. **A**

Vinca alkaloids, such as vincristine, produce a dose-related sensorimotor neuropathy. Peripheral neuropathy can affect sensory, motor, and autonomic function. Patients who develop significant neuropathic symptoms that do not recover between cycles require dose reduction or interruption of vinca alkaloid therapy.

12. **B**

Primary mediastinal lymphoma often occurs as stage II disease only. Presenting symptoms include chest pain, shortness of breath, and occasionally superior vena cava (SVC) syndrome. R-EPOCH as well as R-CHOP chemotherapy is associated with excellent outcomes, including overall response rates over 80%. Consolidative radiotherapy is recommended in patients with limited stage disease who receive R-CHOP chemotherapy.

13. **B**

"Double hit" lymphomas are characterized by a C-MYC plus BCL2 translocation. Morphologically, these aggressive lymphomas resemble diffuse large B-cell lymphoma. They can occur de novo or as transformation from underlying follicular lymphoma. The subtype occurs in 3%–10% of all newly diagnosed diffuse large B-cell lymphomas, and is associated with a long-term survival of less than 30% following standard R-CHOP chemotherapy.

14. **B**

The bifunctional alkylator bendamustine is approved for the treatment of follicular lymphoma. Bendamustine is associated with nausea, lymphopenia, increased risk of infection, and rash. Alopecia, cardiotoxicity, and hepatotoxicity are rare.

15. **E**

Progressive multifocal leukoencephalopathy (PML), caused by the John Cunningham (JC) virus, is a rare but devastating complication of treatment with monoclonal antibodies, including rituximab. The disease should be suspected in patients with a prior history of rituximab exposure, new neurological dysfunction, abnormal findings on MRI, and a negative malignancy workup. In this patient, occult recurrence of lymphoma cannot be excluded. A brain biopsy is required to confirm a diagnosis.

16. **A**

Follicular lymphoma is an indolent B-cell non-Hodgkin lymphoma that often presents with a slowly progressive adenopathy. Cells are typically positive for CD20 and CD19, and negative for CD5 and cyclin D1. A total of 85% of follicular lymphomas are associated with a t(14;18)

(q32;q21)(BCL-2) translocation. BCL-2 translocation is associated with a survival phenotype.

17. **B**

Marginal zone lymphoma occurring in the mucosa has been associated with several infections. Mucosal associated lymphoid tissue (MALT) of the stomach is associated with *Helicobacter pylori* (*H. pylori*) infection. Eradication of the infection results in remission in over 60% of patients with localized disease. *Chlamydia psittaci* (*C. psittaci*) has been associated with orbital/conjunctival MALT, and *Borrelia burgdorferi* (*B. burgdorferi*) has been associated with cutaneous marginal zone lymphoma.

18. **C**

Splenic marginal zone lymphoma (SMZL) is an uncommon low-grade lymphoma that often presents with lymphocytosis, bone marrow involvement, and splenomegaly. Excellent response rates are associated with rituximab as a single agent, as well as splenectomy. Splenectomy is associated with prolonged disease control and improvements in cytopenias and is considered in patients who fail or cannot tolerate systemic therapy.

19. **E**

Mantle cell lymphoma is an aggressive but uncommon B-cell lymphoma. The disease occurs in elderly patients and commonly involves the GI tract. Mantle cell lymphoma is characterized by the translocation t(11;14)(q13;q32) leading to the constitutive overexpression of cyclin D1. Long-term outcomes have dramatically improved due to the introduction of small molecule inhibitors that block the B-cell receptor signaling pathway.

20. **A**

High-dose chemotherapy followed by autologous stem cell transplant is considered standard for patients with diffuse large B-cell lymphoma who progress following frontline chemotherapy. In the landmark PARMA study, autologous stem cell transplant was associated with improved event-free survival and overall survival when compared with observation in chemosensitive patients.[3]

21. **C**

The immunomodulatory drug (IMID), lenalidomide, is associated with a cutaneous rash in up to 30% of patients. The rash is generally self-limited and resolves without treatment. In patients where rash occurs in over 50% of the body surface area, lenalidomide should be held until the resolution of the rash. In most cases, the drug can be restarted without incident. In patients who develop significant mucosal ulcerations or blisters, the drug is permanently discontinued.

22. **C**

R-CHOP chemotherapy is associated with significant neutropenia in over 40% of patients. Prophylaxis with granulocyte-colony stimulating factor (GCSF) should be considered in elderly patients, patients with comorbidities, or when there is bone marrow involvement. If neutropenic fever occurs despite growth factor prophylaxis, dose reduction of myelosuppressive agents, such as cyclophosphamide and Adriamycin, is recommended.

23. **E**

The international non-Hodgkin lymphoma prognostic index is a model that predicts relapse-free survival and overall survival in patients with aggressive non-Hodgkin lymphoma based upon pretreatment clinical characteristics. Patients are grouped into low, low-intermediate, high-intermediate, and high-risk groups based on the number of risk factors. Factors include advanced age, poor performance status, stage III–IV, elevated LDH, and the presence of more than one extranodal site of disease.

24. A

Several salvage treatment options exist for patients who relapse following frontline therapy for follicular lymphoma. However, prior to initiating therapy, aggressive transformation must be ruled out. Aggressive transformation occurs in approximately 3% of follicular lymphoma patients annually, with a lifetime risk of over 30%. Biopsy is required in all patients who relapse after attaining initial remission, especially patients who attain initial remission greater than 24 months.

25. C

The antibody-drug conjugate brentuximab vedotin targets CD30 and is approved for the treatment of relapsed ACLC and relapsed Hodgkin lymphoma. Brentuximab vedotin is associated with peripheral neuropathy, hepatotoxicity, rash, nausea, and neutropenia. The drug should never be used with bleomycin, as serious and fatal pulmonary events can occur.

26. C

Hepatitis B reactivation is a serious complication of rituximab treatment. Rituximab can suppress both T cell and B cells, and accelerates HBV replication. Screening for hepatitis B is always indicated prior to rituximab exposure. During treatment, the monitoring of HBV-DNA levels of at-risk patients is recommended, and antiviral prophylaxis with nucleoside analogs should be considered.

27. B

Ifosfamide has been associated with dose-dependent encephalopathy. The mechanism is unknown but may be associated with the accumulation of toxic metabolites. Risk factors for encephalopathy include preexisting renal conditions, hyponatremia, low abdomen, and patients over 60. The majority of cases are reversible. Treatment includes discontinuation of the drug, neurological monitoring, and the administration of methylene blue.

28. A

The development of ALCL has been associated with silicone breast implants. The disease often presents as a localized mass or persistent seroma adjacent to the implant site. Most patients have an excellent prognosis after surgical resection of the implant, capsule, and associated mass. A worse prognosis is associated in patients who develop extracapsular extension or have bilateral disease.

29. A

SMZL often presents with splenomegaly, cytopenias, and elevated peripheral white blood cell count. Tumor B cells typically express surface immunoglobulin (e.g., IgM+, IgD+), CD19, CD20 and BCL-2, but are negative for CD5 and CD10. The disease is associated with advanced age (>65) and cooccurrence of hepatitis C virus (HCV) infection or Kaposi's sarcoma-associated herpes virus.

30. E

Patients with HIV and diffuse large B-cell lymphoma should continue antiretroviral therapy during chemotherapy. Antiretroviral therapy has been shown to improve clinical outcomes. Dose reduction of chemotherapy or holding rituximab during treatment has not been shown to improve outcomes.

31. B

Histological transformation of follicular lymphoma is a biological event that occurs at a fairly a constant (2%–4%) annual rate. The risk is additive, and a patient's 10-year risk is approximately 30%. Biopsy is generally required to confirm the diagnosis.

32. A

In the landmark PRIMA study, rituximab maintenance following a rituximab-containing induction regimen was associated with improvement in progression-free survival. This study did not show an improvement in overall survival, and maintenance therapy was associated with a small increase in infectious risk.[4]

33. C

Testicular lymphoma has a propensity to recur in the contralateral testes and central nervous system (CNS). Prophylactic CNS therapy with high-dose methotrexate or intrathecal therapy is indicated. The blood-testes barrier prevents the passage of cytotoxic agents into the seminiferous tubules and can limit the efficacy of chemotherapy. Irradiation to the contralateral testes in patients who have prior orchiectomy is indicated.

REFERENCES

Question 4
1. Rummell M, Niederle N, Maschmeyer G, et al. Bendamustine plus rituximab versus CHOP plus rituximab as first-line treatment for patients with indolent and mantle-cell lymphomas: an open-label, multicentre, randomised, phase 3 non-inferiority trial. *Lancet.* 2013;381(9873):1203–1210.
2. Flinn IW, van der Jagt R, Kahl BS, et al. Randomized trial of bendamustine-rituximab or R-CHOP/R-CVP in first-line treatment of indolent NHL or MCL: the BRIGHT study. *Blood.* 2014;123(19):2944–2952.

Question 20
1. Philip T, Guglielmi C, Hagenbeek A, et al. Autologous bone marrow transplantation as compared with salvage chemotherapy in relapses of chemotherapy-sensitive non-Hodgkin's lymphoma. *N Engl J Med.* 1995;333(23):1540–1545.

Question 32
1. Salles G, Seymour JF, Offner F, et al. Rituximab maintenance for 2 years in patients with high tumour burden follicular lymphoma responding to rituximab plus chemotherapy (PRIMt): a phase 3, randomised controlled trial. *Lancet.* 2010;377(9759):42–51.

10

Multiple Myeloma and Other Plasma Cell Dyscrasias

David H. Vesole

QUESTIONS

1. A 56-year-old male is found to have an elevated total protein at 8.6 g/dL by his primary care doctor. There are no other laboratory abnormalities (normal calcium, hemoglobin, creatinine, and random urine for protein). A serum protein electrophoresis showed a polyclonal gammopathy with a serum immunofixation electrophoresis showing oligoclonal banding. On further history, the patient informs you that his grandmother died of myeloma 16 years ago. He wants to know which epidemiological features have been associated with myeloma:
   A. Obesity
   B. 9/11 exposure
   C. Agent orange
   D. Immediate family member with monoclonal gammopathy of undetermined significance (MGUS)
   E. All of the above

2. The criteria for the revised International Staging System includes the following parameters:
   A. Beta-2 microglobulin, albumin, M component, skeletal survey
   B. Beta-2 microglobulin, albumin, LDH, M component
   C. Beta-2 microglobulin, albumin, metaphase karyotype, LDH
   D. Beta-2 microglobulin, albumin, LDH, FISH
   E. Beta-2 microglobulin, albumin, FISH, serum creatinine

3. In 2016, there were approximately 30,280 new cases of myeloma diagnosed with a prevalence projected at 118,000 cases. Based upon the most recent SEER data, a newly diagnosed patient with multiple myeloma, across all age groups, will have a 5-year estimated survival of the following:
   A. 33%
   B. 50%
   C. 66%
   D. 74%
   E. 81%

4. A 52-year-old healthy male presents with bone pain in the left leg; the MRI shows marrow infiltration, but no bone disease. An extensive workup reveals: no M protein spike; normal renal and other blood chemistry profile; hemoglobin 11.3 g/dL, β_2-M 2.2 mg/L, albumin 3.9 mg/dL; free light chain ratio of greater than 100; PET and MRI show no lytic disease; bone marrow biopsy of 65% plasma cell involvement, with normal cytogenetics and a negative FISH panel. What is your diagnosis for this patient?

   A. MGUS
   B. Smoldering myeloma (low risk)
   C. Smoldering myeloma (high risk)
   D. Multiple myeloma
   E. AL amyloidosis

5. A 43-year-old male with standard-risk, stage I immunoglobulin (Ig)G kappa multiple myeloma with SPEP 4.87 g/dL, serum free kappa light chain 862 mg/L, serum free lambda light chain 17.2 mg/L with a free light chain ratio of 50.12, 24-hour total urine protein 1.25 g with urine protein electrophoresis (UPEP) negative, but urine immunofixation electrophoresis showing an IgG kappa plus kappa monoclonal protein. He received lenalidomide/bortezomib/dexamethasone induction × 3 cycles and achieved a very good partial remission. He then received melphalan 200 mg/m² and autologous stem cell transplantation (ASCT) and, by day 60, had fully recovered. He was also treated with zoledronic acid to minimize bone complications. Repeat myeloma parameters reveal a negative serum protein electrophoresis (SPEP) and UPEP; negative serum and urine immunofixation, bone marrow with no clonal plasma cells by immunohistochemistry and flow cytometry; and a free light chain ratio of 2.85. The patient inquires about how well the transplant worked. You inform him that he has achieved what depth of response?
   A. Very good partial response
   B. Near complete response
   C. Complete response
   D. Stringent complete response
   E. Minimal residual disease

6. An 80-year-old male with a history of type 2 diabetes, hypertension, and compensated congestive heart failure presents with back pain and increasing fatigue. His daughter is concerned that he is depressed. A workup of his back pain and fatigue included the following: x-ray of lumbar spine reveals L4 compression fracture, lytic disease in L2 and L5. Blood work shows Hb 9.5 mg/L, plt 178 k/mm³, creatinine 1.5 mg/dL (CrCl: 35 mL/min), albumin 3.5 mg/dL, β_2-M 3.1 mg/L, Ca 9.8 mg/dL. SPEP M-protein 4.5 g/dL, IgG lambda, IgG 5200 mg/dL, IgA 35 g/L, IgM 25 g/L. Bone marrow: 40% plasma cells, cytogenetics normal; FISH: no adverse features. In addition to zoledronic acid administration monthly, you plan to initiate the following double:
   A. Lenalidomide 25 mg/day on days 1–21, dexamethasone 40 mg/day on days 1, 8, 15, 22
   B. Lenalidomide 25 mg/day on days 1–21, dexamethasone 20 mg/day on days 1, 8, 15, 22

C. Lenalidomide 10 mg/day on days 1–21, dexamethasone 40 mg/day on days 1, 8, 15, 22

D. Lenalidomide 10 mg/day on days 1–21, dexamethasone 20 mg/day on days 1, 8, 15, 22

E. Lenalidomide 10 mg/day on days 1–21, dexamethasone 20 mg/day on days 1, 8, 15

7. A 63-year-old woman with IgA kappa multiple myeloma, ISS 2, presented with rib pain and fatigue. Initial studies showing 85% plasma cells in the bone marrow, hyperdiploidy, IgAκ 5 g/L, multiple lytic lesions, hemoglobin 9.7 g/dL, calculated creatinine clearance 68 mL/min, beta-2 microglobulin 3.3 mg, albumin 3.1 g/dL. She was treated initially with lenalidomide/bortezomib/dexamethasone × 4 cycles with monthly zoledronic acid. Her course was complicated by streptococcal pneumonia and grade 2 sensory neuropathy. She went on to high-dose therapy with ASCT and achieved a stringent complete remission. She was not placed on maintenance therapy. Her neuropathy improved to grade 1 numbness in her feet. Four years later, her M protein reappears and she has a 1.5 g drop in her hemoglobin from her baseline. Which of the following would not be an approved treatment option for first relapse?
   A. Elotuzumab/lenalidomide/dexamethasone
   B. Lenalidomide/bortezomib/dexamethasone
   C. Pomalidomide and dexamethasone
   D. Carfilzomib/lenalidomide/dexamethasone
   E. Ixazomib/lenalidomide/dexamethasone

8. Which of the following monoclonal antibodies targets SLAMF7 and activates NK activity?
   A. Daratumumab
   B. Elotuzumab
   C. Indatuximab ravtansine
   D. Isatuximab
   E. Pembrolizumab

9. A 74-year-old female presents with relapsed IgG lambda myeloma. Her history includes initial FISH studies: t(4;14) translocation. Two years ago, she received induction therapy with bortezomib/cyclophosphamide/dexamethasone followed by autologous transplant. She then received maintenance SQ bortezomib every 2 weeks for 1 year, but relapsed. She was switched to lenalidomide plus low-dose dexamethasone but progressed after 9 months. A 2-month course of lenalidomide/ixazomib/dexamethasone resulted in progressive disease. Given her high-risk disease, you recommend the following regimen:
   A. Elotuzumab/lenalidomide/dexamethasone
   B. Daratumumab
   C. Carfilzomib/lenalidomide/dexamethasone
   D. Carfilzomib/pomalidomide/dexamethasone
   E. Bortezomib/panobinostat/dexamethasone

10. In the revised International Staging System, high-risk cytogenetic features include the following:
   A. t(11;14), t(4;14), −13
   B. t(4;14; t(14;20), −17p
   C. t(4;14), t(14;16), −17p
   D. t(8;14), t(11;14), −13
   E. t(4;14), t(14;16), t(14;20)

11. The mainstays of myeloma therapy are immunomodulatory agents and proteasome inhibitors in combination with corticosteroids (dexamethasone). The proteasome inhibitors are reversible or irreversible, boron-based or epoxyketone-based. One of the main pathways of inhibition is through which of following?

   A. Bcl-2
   B. C-myc
   C. Nf-kappa B
   D. CTLA 4
   E. PD-1

12. A 63-year-old woman with newly diagnosed multiple myeloma begins induction therapy with lenalidomide/bortezomib/dexamethasone with the bortezomib administered as an SQ injection on days 1, 4, 8, and 11; lenalidomide 25 mg days 1–14 and dexamethasone 40 mg on days 1, 2, 8, 9, 11, and 12. After 3 cycles of therapy, the patient began to complain of loss of feeling and numbness in her feet that has gotten worse and is now painful. You explain to the patient that the neuropathy is from bortezomib and discuss the following options with her:
   A. "We need to adjust the dose of bortezomib; the pain will resolve after we do."
   B. "Since the neuropathy is causing you pain, we should halt bortezomib until the pain improves and then we can resume the drug with a reduced dose and/or use SC administration."
   C. "Since the neuropathy is causing you pain, we should stop the bortezomib permanently and consider other treatment options."
   D. "We can continue the bortezomib at the current dose; the pain will decrease over time and we can treat the pain."
   E. "We can continue the current dose but change the schedule to once weekly."

13. Which of the following is true of ASCT for myeloma?
   A. It is curative in 10% of patients.
   B. It is not curative but prolongs event-free survival and overall survival.
   C. Typically patients receive 4–6 cycles of melphalan-based induction therapy prior to transplantation.
   D. Response to induction therapy is not important prior to transplantation.
   E. Graft versus host disease occurs in 25% of patients.

14. A 45-year-old patient has newly diagnosed myeloma and is treated with 4 cycles of lenalidomide and dexamethasone (Rd) chemotherapy. He achieves a very good response and is now in good performance status. Cytogenetics are normal. Which of the following would be an ideal therapeutic choice for this patient?
   A. Stop therapy and observe closely for evidence of progression
   B. Collect stem cells and proceed with ASCT
   C. Stop Rd chemotherapy and switch to bortezomib therapy for 4 cycles
   D. Continue Rd chemotherapy until disease progression
   E. Add bortezomib to the regimen to improve the complete response rate

15. Which of the following is not a risk factor for progression in MGUS?
   A. Size of the M protein
   B. Type of the M protein
   C. Age of the patient
   D. Abnormal free light chain ratio
   E. Years since diagnosis

16. A 55-year-old male with newly diagnosed IgGκ multiple myeloma is referred to you to discuss therapeutic options. He has previously been in good health and has a normal renal function, and an ECOG performance status of 1. Serum

β2-microglobulin is 3.9 mg/dL. He has multiple lytic lesions, but none are at significant risk for fracture. You suggest starting him on treatment with lenalidomide, bortezomib, and dexamethasone, as well as a bisphosphonate. In addition, as part of his initial treatment plan, you suggest that the patient should:

A. Receive a reduced-intensity allogeneic stem cell transplant from his HLA-matched sister

B. Receive a fully myeloablative allogeneic stem cell transplant from his HLA-matched sister

C. Have autologous blood stem cells collected for an ASCT in the event his disease does not respond to lenalidomide, bortezomib, and dexamethasone

D. Have an ASCT to consolidate his response to lenalidomide, bortezomib, and dexamethasone followed by lenalidomide maintenance

E. Receive 4–6 cycles of lenalidomide, bortezomib, and dexamethasone, then proceed to bortezomib maintenance due to his high-risk cytogenetics

ANSWERS

1. E

Although the etiology of myeloma remains uncertain, there are associated risk factors, including obesity, workers extensively exposed post 9/11, and Vietnam veterans exposed to agent orange. There are a database studies (Sweden) that have studied familial association and found there is a slight risk increase in lymphoproliferative disorders (CLL, NHL, amyloid) in family members of individuals with monoclonal gammopathy, such as multiple myeloma application.

2. D

The initial international staging system did not have sufficient cytogenetic data to include cytogenetic risk stratification in the ISS. Subsequently, Palumbo et al. have published the revised-ISS, which includes cytogenetics and LDH.

3. B

The number of newly diagnosed myeloma patients is increasing yearly, mainly due to an increase in the population aged 65–75 (Baby Boomers) resulting in approximately a 118,000 prevalence. With the incorporation of immunomodulatory agents and proteasome inhibitors into standard treatment algorithms, the 5-year survival has essentially doubled over the past 5 years to 50%.

4. D

Based upon the increased risk of developing symptomatic organ compromise, approximately 60%–80% within 2 years, the International Myeloma Working Group has revised the definition of active myeloma to include patients with ≥1 lesion on MRI, a free light chain ratio greater than 100, or bone marrow plasma cell concentration of greater than 60%.

5. C

The International Myeloma Working Group response criteria would categorize this depth of response as a complete remission (negative SPEP/UPEP, sIFE/uIFE and negative bone marrow by immunohistochemistry). The free light chain has not yet normalized (0.25–1.65), so a stringent complete response has not been achieved. There are now criteria for minimal residual disease by flow cytometry, by next-generation sequencing, and by MRI/PET/CT.

6. D

Per insert prescribing guidelines for lenalidomide, the lenalidomide should be dose-reduced for a creatinine clearance of less than 60 mL/min. The dexamethasone is recommended to be dose-reduced to 20 mg from 40 mg weekly for individuals older than 75 years of age.

7. C

Only pomalidomide and dexamethasone would not be indicated in this patient who is in first relapse. There are a wide range of available regimens that are FDA approved for individuals with one to three prior therapies, all of which are effective, although the mode of administration (IV/SQ/PO) and toxicity profiles differ. Pomalidomide is approved for patients with at least two prior therapies (including lenalidomide and bortezomib) who have demonstrated progressive disease within 60 days of the last therapy.

8. B

Elotuzumab targets signaling lymphocyte activation molecule family member 7 (SLAMF7) whereas daratumumab/isatuximab target CD38, indatuximab ravtansine CD138. Pembrolizumab is a programmed death-1 (PD-1) monoclonal antibody.

9. B or D

The initial FDA approval for daratumumab, an anti-CD38 monoclonal antibody, was for patients with three or more prior lines of therapy. Subsequently, daratumumab has been approved with either bortezomib or lenalidomide for one to three lines of prior therapy. Elotuzumab/lenalidomide/dexamethasone would not be indicated; there are no data combining elotuzumab in lenalidomide refractory patients. Similarly, there are no data to support carfilzomib/lenalidomide/dexamethasone in lenalidomide-refractory patients. Bortezomib/panobinostat/dexamethasone is an FDA-approved regimen, but this patient has progressed on bortezomib maintenance and became refractory to the oral boron-based proteasome inhibitor, ixazomib. Answer D is a very attractive option: the patient has not been treated with either pomalidomide or carfilzomib; pomalidomide is active in lenalidomide-refractory patients, and carfilzomib is active in bortezomib-refractory patients.

10. C

In the revised International Staging System, high-risk cytogenetics by FISH includes t(4;14), t(14;16), and 17p. There are other cytogenetic risks that are not included in the Mayo Stratification for Myeloma and Risk-Adapted Therapy (mSMART).

11. C

Although a number of pathways for proteasome inhibition may contribute to clinical activity, the most well studied is through Nf-kappa B.

12. B

Peripheral neuropathy can be a devastating treatment-related complication in multiple myeloma. Treatment choices are limited and variably effective. The clinician must be proactive in dose reduction or discontinuation in the setting of emergent neuropathy in an attempt to prevent long-term symptoms.

13. B

Approximately 15% of patients achieve long, durable remission exceeding 10 years following transplantation. However, there is not yet a plateau on survival curves with current treatment approaches. Patients with chemotherapy-sensitive disease have better outcomes posttransplant. The typical induction regimen consists of an immunomodulatory agent, a proteasome inhibitor, and corticosteroids. Melphalan, an alkylating agent, should be avoided as it can compromise stem cell mobilization and may increase the risk of myelodysplasia/acute leukemia.

14. B

There are now four randomized clinical trials that have been completed (two published, two presented in abstract) comparing either transplant versus no transplant, or early versus late transplant. All four show definite improvement in progression-free survival in the patients who receive an early transplant. Therefore, early transplant continues to be the recommended treatment. In addition, if the patient was considered ineligible for transplant, the current recommendations are to continue the induction therapy indefinitely.

15. C

The risk of MGUS evolving into active myeloma is approximately 1%/year (cumulative). This can be further stratified based upon the size of the M protein (>1.5 g/dL), the type of M protein (IgA or IgM), and an abnormal free light chain ratio (>8). Since this is cumulative, the risk of evolution increases over time.

16. D

The standard of care for newly diagnosed myeloma patients is for induction therapy, usually with a triplet (immunomodulatory agent, proteasome inhibitor, and corticosteroids) followed by a consolidative high-dose therapy with ASCT. Lenalidomide is now FDA approved as maintenance therapy post-autologous transplant with improvement in progressive-free survival and, in some trials, overall survival.

REFERENCES

Question 1
1. Frank C, Fallah M, Chen T, et al. Search for familial clustering of multiple myeloma with any cancer. *Leukemia.* 2016;30:627–632.

Question 2
1. Greipp, et al. 2005. International staging system for multiple myeloma. *J Clin Oncol.* 2005;23:3412–3420.

2. Palumbo A, Avet-Loiseau H, Oliva S, et al. Revised international staging system for multiple myeloma: a report from International Myeloma Working Group. *J Clin Oncol.* 2015;33(26): 2863–2869.

Question 3
1. Cancer Stat Facts. Myeloma. https://seer.cancer.gov/statfacts/html/mulmy.html; Accessed 01.06.17.

Question 4
1. Rajkumar SV, Dimopoulos MA, Palumbo A, et al. International Myeloma Working Group updated criteria for the diagnosis of multiple myeloma. *Lancet Oncol.* 2014;15(12):e538–e548.

Question 5
1. Kumar S, Paiva B, Anderson KC, et al. International Myeloma Working Group consensus criteria for response and minimal residual disease assessment in multiple myeloma. *Lancet Oncol.* 2016;17(8):e328–e346.

Question 6
1. Highlights of Prescribing Information. https://www.accessdata.fda.gov/drugsatfda_docs/label/2013/021880s034lbl.pdf; Accessed 01.06.17.

Question 7
1. Highlights of Prescribing Information. https://www.accessdata.fda.gov/drugsatfda_docs/label/2013/204026lbl.pdf; Accessed 01.06.17.

Question 10
1. Palumbo A, Avet-Loiseau H, Oliva S, et al. Revised international staging system for multiple myeloma: a report from International Myeloma Working Group. *J Clin Oncol.* 2015;33(26):2863.
2. mSMART. Mayo Stratification for Myeloma and Risk-Adapted Therapy. Newly Diagnosed Myeloma. https://nebula.wsimg.com/e1520dd2009dae7c8ea5ca513775b8fa?AccessKeyId=A0994494BBBCBE4A0363&disposition=0&alloworigin=1; Accessed 01.06.17.

Questions 12
1. Richardson PG, Delforge M, Beksac M, et al. Management of treatment-emergent peripheral neuropathy in multiple myeloma. *Leukemia.* 2012;26(4):595–608.

Question 14
1. Benbouker L, Dimopoulos MA, Dispenzieri A, et al. Lenalidomide and dexamethasone in transplant-ineligible patients with myeloma. *N Engl J Med.* 2014;371(10):906–917.

Question 15
1. Kyle RA, Durie BG, Rajkumar SV, et al. Monoclonal gammopathy of undetermined significance (MGUS) and smoldering (asymptomatic) multiple myeloma: IMWG consensus perspectives risk factors for progression and guidelines for monitoring and management. *Leukemia.* 2010;24(6):1121–1127.

T-Cell and Natural Killer Cell Neoplasms and Other Lymphoid Malignancies

Steven Horwitz

QUESTION

1. A 76-year-old woman presents with rapid onset of "bruises" as shown below. She is otherwise healthy except for hypertension and hyperlipidemia. She does not take any anticoagulants and does not recall any trauma. A physical exam shows the lesion (below), but there is an absence of lymphadenopathy. A complete blood count shows a normal WBC, a platelet count of 120,000 K/μL, and an hgb of 9.9 g/dL. PT and PTT are normal. A metabolic panel is normal, and lactate dehydrogenase is normal. A skin biopsy shows an infiltrate of medium-sized cells involving the dermis and subcutaneous fat. Immunohistochemistry shows that the abnormal cells express CD4 and CD56.

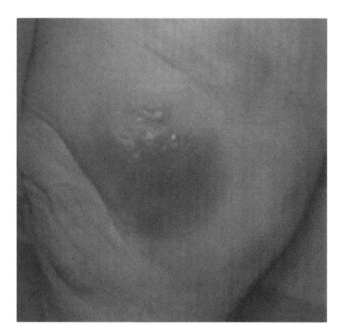

CD20 and CD30 are negative, and EBER is negative. The most likely diagnosis is:
A. Primary cutaneous anaplastic large cell lymphoma
B. Subcutaneous panniculitis–like T-cell lymphoma
C. Extranodal natural killer (NK)/T-cell lymphoma
D. Blastic plasmacytoid dendritic cell neoplasm

2. What do you tell her regarding her prognosis and recommended management?

A. This is usually an indolent process that can be expectantly monitored in most patients.
B. This is an often rapidly progressive malignancy that is usually treated with combination chemotherapy regimens typically used for aggressive lymphomas or acute lymphoid leukemias.
C. Topical mechlorethamine gel is often a first-line treatment.
D. Tyrosine kinase inhibitors, such as imatinib, are effective for the majority of patients.

3. A 45-year-old man, who is 5 years s/p a kidney transplant for end-stage renal disease, is maintained on cyclosporine. He has not had any episodes of rejection in the last 4 years. He reports to his primary care physician with 3 months of increasing crampy abdominal pain. He denies fevers, sweats, or weight loss. On physical exam, he is noted to have mild tenderness in the left lower quadrant of his abdomen, a nontender palpable graft on the right abdomen, and a 2 cm left inguinal node. Hemeoccult positive stools are noted on rectal exam. The rest of the physical exam is unremarkable. Laboratory work-up shows a baseline creatinine of 1.4 mg/dL, an hgb of 10.2 g/dL (baseline 11.8 g/dL), a WBC of 4.7 K/μL, with a normal differential, and platelets of 188,000/μL. A colonoscopy is performed showing a 3 cm mass in the sigmoid colon. The biopsy shows an infiltrate of mostly small- and medium-sized lymphocytes with occasional larger cells. In the background are eosinophils, histiocytes, and plasma cells. The larger cells express CD20 and lack CD2, CD3, CD30, and CD56. These larger cells, as well as some of the small- and medium-sized lymphocytes, also express EBER. Kappa and lambda light chains appear to be expressed in equal amounts. The most likely diagnosis is:
A. Hodgkin lymphoma
B. Posttransplant lymphoproliferative disorder
C. Extranodal NK/T-cell lymphoma
D. Diffuse large B-cell lymphoma

4. This patient is referred to you. Positron emission tomography/computed tomography (PET-CT) shows multifocal FDG-avid areas in the large bowel as well as the left inguinal lymph nodes. For initial therapy you recommend:
A. Halving his dose of cyclosporine and rituximab at 375 mg/m^2 weekly for 4 weeks
B. Holding cyclosporine for 2 months and then repeating the PET-CT scan
C. R-CHOP
D. R-Hyper CVAD

5. A 29-year-old woman is now 9 months post a matched-related donor allogeneic stem cell transplantation from her brother for refractory diffuse large B-cell lymphoma. She recently had a flare of graft versus host disease (GVHD) with a rash and moderate elevation of her liver function tests about 1 month ago. Her tacrolimus was increased, and she was placed on prednisone with resolution of all symptoms of GVH. She now presents with 3 days of low-grade fever and small, tender, cervical lymph nodes. On exam you note cervical, axillary, and inguinal lymphadenopathy up to 2 cm in size. WBC is 5.2 K/μL and her LDH is elevated at 462 U/L (ULN 248 U/L). Quantitative assessment of serum EBV is 42,000 IU/mL. A core needle biopsy of one of the larger cervical nodes shows a diffuse infiltrate of large CD20 positive B-cells. The cells express EBER and kappa light chain restriction. The most critical next step in terms of evaluating the biopsy specimen for diagnosis would be:

A. FISH to evaluate for c-myc and bcl-2 translocations
B. Immunohistochemistry to determine the cell of origin, and the germinal center versus the activated B-cell
C. Karyotype for XY chromosomes
D. Quantify CD30 expression to see if brentuximab vedotin is an option

6. The karyotype comes back as XY showing a donor origin for the lymphoma. Your initial therapy recommendation is:
A. Hold the tacrolimus and reduce the prednisone by half
B. Rituximab 375 mg/m^2 for four doses
C. Collect additional cells from her brother for a donor lymphocyte infusion
D. Start R-CHOP

ANSWERS

1. **D**
Blastic plasmacytoid dendritic cell neoplasm is a malignancy that usually presents in the skin. The cells express CD4 and CD56. Primary cutaneous anaplastic large cell lymphoma is always universally CD30 expressing. Subcutaneous panniculitis–like T-cell lymphoma expresses CD8 and not NK markers, such as CD56. Extranodal NK/T cell lymphoma always expresses markers of EBV such as EBER.

2. **B**
In children, induction regimens, such as ALL or for aggressive non-Hodgkin lymphomas, are usually effective. In adults, these regimens can induce remissions, but better results seem to be obtained with consolidation with allogeneic stem cell transplant. Topical mechlorethamine and imatinib are not known to be active treatments.

3. **B**
The development of and EBV+ lymphoproliferation in a patient with a history of previous organ transplant with ongoing immunosuppression is indicative of PTLD. In this case, it is a polymorphic subtype. Absence of CD30 and CD56 argue against Hodgkin lymphoma and extranodal NK T-cell lymphoma. The mixed inflammatory background and lack of light chain restriction argue against diffuse large B-cell lymphoma.

4. **A**
This patient has what is best characterized as polymorphic PTLD. In these cases, some patients will respond to a reduction in immunosuppression alone. However, given the multifocal and symptomatic disease, it is most prudent to treat rather than to wait for a slow response. Many patients will respond to rituximab with a reduction in immunosuppression with rituximab. For those with early lesions or polymorphic PTLD, combination chemo-immunotherapy, such as R-CHOP, is generally reserved for those not responding completely to a reduction in immunosuppression and rituximab.

5. **C**
This is suspicious for monomorphic PTLD. However, given that the original diagnosis was DLBCL, this also could be a recurrence after the patient had an increase in her immunosuppressive regimen. Since she had a male donor, evaluating the biopsy for XY chromosomes will quickly tell you whether it is the donor or the host. If it is the donor, this is PTLD and can be treated accordingly. However, if it is the host, this is a recurrence of her lymphoma and represents a failure of the transplant.

6. **B**
Rituximab. Reducing immunosuppression is not likely to help when the PTLD is of donor origin. The donor's immune system will be unlikely to recognize the PTLD even if there is less immunosuppression. In addition, with the recent flare of GVHD, this could precipitate further GVHD. For similar reasons, DLI would not be helpful and would carry significant risk. Many patients with PTLD post-allogeneic SCT respond to rituximab. R-CHOP is likely not ideal here as it carries more toxicity than the single agent rituximab, and it is likely that this patient has had full doses of anthracycline in the past.

REFERENCE

Question 1
1. Swerdlow SH, Campo E, Harris NL, et al., eds. *WHO Classification of Tumors of Haematopoietic and Lymphoid Tissues.* Lyon: IARC; 2008.

Hematopoietic Cell Transplantation

Pashna N. Munshi and Corey Cutler

QUESTIONS

1. What is the objective of using a conditioning regimen for hematopoietic stem cell (HSC) transplantation?
   A. To reduce the bulk of malignant cells
   B. To decrease the risk of graft rejection via general host immune suppression
   C. To improve the engraftment of donor HSCs by providing profound immunosuppression of the host
   D. All the above

2. What is the main mechanism of graft-versus-leukemia effect using donor lymphocyte infusion?
   A. Increase in CD8+ cells that recognize target antigens on tumor cells
   B. CD8+/CD4+T cells recognize target antigens on tumor cells
   C. Enhancing the presence of killer inhibitory receptors (KIRs) recognized by donor NK cells
   D. Increase in TCR repertoire diversity
   E. Release of cytokine mediators generated by the graft versus host disease (GVHD) reaction initiated by DLI

3. Which of the following increases the risk of relapse after an allogeneic and/or autologous stem cell transplant (ASCT)?
   A. Human leukocyte antigen (HLA) mismatched transplant
   B. CD34+ cell dose less than 2 × 10e6/kg
   C. Presence of acute or chronic GVHD
   D. Disease burden prior to stem cell transplantation

4. Risk factors for increased acute and/or chronic GVHD are all the following except—
   A. Recipient HLA mismatching
   B. Use of unrelated donors versus related donors
   C. Use of female donors for male recipients
   D. Use of total body irradiation (TBI) as part of the conditioning regimen
   E. Use of T-cell depleted graft

5. A 45-year-old cytomegalovirus (CMV) IgG negative man with Philadelphia chromosome positive B-cell acute lymphoblastic leukemia underwent an allogeneic stem cell transplant from his CMV IgG negative, 10/10 HLA matched brother using a myeloablative conditioning regimen. He returns for follow-up 45 days following the transplant. He is on tacrolimus for GVHD prevention. He is compliant with all other medications following transplant. He denies any nausea, anorexia, diarrhea, or rash. He notices a painful sore in his mouth that started 2 days ago. On examination, you find a shallow ulcer over the palate. His blood work reveals white blood cell (WBC) count of 4300 cells/μL, hemoglobin 9.7 g/dL, platelets 90,000/μL, tacrolimus level 7 ng/mL, S. sodium 142 mEq/L, S. potassium 3.7 mEq/L, S. creatinine 0.87 mg/dL, total bilirubin 0.5 mg/dL.
   What is the likely cause of his oral symptoms?
   A. Acute graft versus host disease
   B. Chronic graft versus host disease
   C. Herpes simplex virus (HSV) reactivation
   D. Tacrolimus-induced aphthous ulcer
   E. CMV reactivation

6. A 35-year-old woman with acute myeloid leukemia (AML) is in complete remission after induction therapy with cytarabine and idarubicin (7+3 regimen). She received cyclophosphamide and 12 Gy TBI as conditioning regimen followed by a transplant from her 10/10 HLA matched brother. Her admission weight is 58 kg. She is receiving tacrolimus and methotrexate for immunosuppression. Six days later, her weight is 67 kg. On physical examination, she has pitting pedal edema above her ankles, her abdomen is distended, and there is tenderness to palpation in her right upper quadrant. The patient is afebrile. Pretransplant laboratory values were within the normal range. Today, her laboratory values show ALT 161 U/L, AST 142 U/L, creatinine 2.7 mg/dL, total bilirubin 4.8 mg/dL, WBC 1200 cells/μL. She has no known preexisting liver conditions. What is the likely diagnosis?
   A. Acute cholangitis
   B. Relapsed AML
   C. Acute GVHD of the liver
   D. Methotrexate toxicity
   E. Hepatic sinusoidal obstruction syndrome (SOS)

7. Following HSC transplantation, what is the correct order of immune reconstitution?
   A. Neutrophils > NK cells > B lymphocytes > CD8+ T-cells > plasma cells, dendritic cells > CD4+ T-cells
   B. NK cells > B lymphocytes > neutrophils > CD8+ T cells > CD4+ T-cells > plasma cells, dendritic cells
   C. Plasma cells, dendritic cells > neutrophils > NK cells > CD8+ T-cells > B lymphocytes > CD4+ T-cells
   D. Neutrophils > NK cells > CD8+ T-cells > plasma cells, dendritic cells > B lymphocytes > CD4+ T-cells
   E. NK cells > B lymphocytes > CD8+ T-cells > neutrophils > plasma cells, dendritic cells > CD4+ T cells

8. A 67-year-old man returns for his follow-up visit. Sixty-five days ago he underwent an allogeneic stem cell transplant AML. Over the past 3 weeks, you notice his platelet counts have shown a steady decline from 120,000 to 43,000/μL. His hemoglobin is 9.8 g/dL, previously 11 g/dL. His creatinine is slowly rising from 0.7 to 2.2 mg/dL. A direct antiglobulin

test returns negative. He is otherwise asymptomatic. He is taking tacrolimus and sirolimus for prevention of GVHD. Tacrolimus levels have been within 7–9 ng/mL range. A bone marrow biopsy is without any leukemic blasts but shows a slightly hypocellular marrow with increased megakaryocytes and erythroblasts. What is the most likely cause of his abnormal studies?

A. Acute GVHD
B. Immune thrombocytopenic purpura (ITP)
C. Tacrolimus toxicity
D. Thrombotic microangiopathy (TMA)
E. Relapsed AML

9. A 46-year-old man has IPSS Intermediate-2 risk MDS and has an HLA-matched sibling available to be a stem cell donor. Which of the following transplantation strategies is the most appropriate recommendation for him?

A. Immediate myeloablative transplantation
B. Defer myeloablative transplantation until IPSS risk score is high
C. Immediate reduced intensity transplantation
D. Nontransplant therapy with a DNA hypomethylating agent alone

10. A 56-year-old otherwise healthy woman with AML presents for evaluation for transplantation. She had a monosomal karyotype at presentation and is in remission after one induction course and a course of consolidation chemotherapy. A suitably matched unrelated donor has been identified from the Bone Marrow Donor Registry. Which of the following transplantation strategies is the most appropriate recommendation for her?

A. Reduced intensity transplantation
B. Myeloablative transplantation
C. Consolidation therapy for 2 additional cycles followed by transplantation
D. Consolidation therapy alone, reserving allogeneic transplantation in the event of AML relapse

11. Which of these statements is true?

A. Antibacterial prophylaxis is generally started at the time of stem cell infusion and continued until recovery from neutropenia or initiation of empirical antibacterial therapy for fever during neutropenia.
B. The prophylaxis should not be continued after recovery from neutropenia.
C. Fluoroquinolone prophylaxis is preferred.
D. Emergence of resistance in bacterial pathogens should be monitored closely because of increasing quinolone resistance worldwide among gram-negative bacteria (e.g., *Escherichia coli*, *Klebsiella pneumoniae*, and *Pseudomonas aeruginosa*).
E. All of the above.

12. A 47-year-old man underwent matched unrelated donor allogeneic stem cell transplant for T-cell ALL in first remission. He has no CNS involvement of disease. He is now 14 days into his treatment course. His systolic blood pressure over the past 2 days has been between 140 and 160 mm Hg. He is now reporting headaches, which are worsening over 24 hours, and blurry vision. The nurse calls you to report that the patient is now confused and is unable to tell her where he is. He is currently taking tacrolimus and methotrexate for immunosuppression. He receives prochlorperazine and lorazepam for nausea alternatingly. He is taking fluconazole and valaciclovir for prophylaxis. He is afebrile. He has ongoing pancytopenia as expected from his conditioning chemotherapy. His creatinine is 1.9

mg/dL. He received a platelet transfusion yesterday for platelet count of 9000 cells/μL. What is the likely cause of this patient's symptoms?

A. Central nervous system leukemia
B. HSV encephalitis
C. Tacrolimus toxicity
D. Methotrexate toxicity
E. Intracranial hemorrhage

13. A 19-year-old woman is a stem cell donor for her 25-year-old sister with AML. She suddenly develops left upper quadrant abdominal pain and has a near syncopal episode. Her BP is 98/64 mm Hg with a heart rate of 118 beats/minute. She is on the third day of taking high dose filgrastim. She denies any abdominal pain prior to this. She is otherwise healthy and has normal menses. Her last menstrual cycle was 2 weeks ago. What is the reason for her abdominal pain?

A. Nephrolithiasis that was previously undiscovered
B. Ectopic pregnancy
C. Splenic rupture
D. Pain caused by bone marrow expansion
E. Pancreatitis

14. Your patient is a 57-year-old man with AML. He is CMV IgG negative. His ABO blood type is O Rh+. You recommend that he undergoes an allogeneic stem cell transplant. He has two sisters and one brother. His sisters are 45 and 63 years old. His sisters have no children, but his younger sister has had one miscarriage in the past. His brother is 52 years old with mild hypertension. Who would you choose as a donor?

A. 10/10 HLA matched 63-year-old sister who is CMV IgG negative
B. One haplotype HLA matched 45-year-old sister, B Rh positive
C. 10/10 HLA matched brother, CMV IgG positive
D. None of the above

15. A patient with the following HLA type is scheduled to undergo allogeneic stem cell transplantation for MDS:
A*02:01 B*27:02 C*02:02 DRβ1*04:01 DQβ1*03:02 DPβ1*01:01
A*25:01 B*18:01 C*12:03 DRβ1*14:54 DQβ1*05:03 DPβ1*02:02
Which of the following donors should be selected to reduce the risk of GVHD (HLA disparities indicated in bold)?

A. A*02:01 **B*08:01** C*02:02 DRβ1*04:01 DQβ1*03:02 DPβ1*01:01
A*25:01 B*18:01 C*12:03 DRβ1*14:54 DQβ1*05:03 DPβ1*02:02
B. A*02:01 B*27:02 C*02:02 DRβ1*04:01 DQβ1*03:02 DPβ1*01:01
A*25:01 B*18:01 **C*12:07** DRβ1*14:54 DQβ1*05:03 DPβ1*02:02
C. A*02:01 B*27:02 C*02:02 **DRβ1*04:02** DQβ1*03:02 DPβ1*01:01
A*25:01 B*18:01 C*12:03 DRβ1*14:54 DQβ1*05:03 DPβ1*02:02
D. A*02:01 B*27:02 C*02:02 DRβ1*04:01 DQβ1*03:02 DPβ1*01:01
A*25:01 B*18:01 C*12:03 DRβ1*14:54 **DQβ1*08:03** DPβ1*02:02

16. Concerning the following two donor recipient pairs, which is the true statement (HLA disparities indicated in bold)?
Pair 1:
Recipient
A*02:01 B*27:02 C*02:02 DRβ1*04:01 DQβ1*03:02 DPβ1*01:01
A*25:01 B*27:02 C*12:03 DRβ1*14:54 DQβ1*05:03 DPβ1*02:02
Donor
A*02:01 B*27:02 C*02:02 DRβ1*04:01 DQβ1*03:02 DPβ1*01:01
A*25:01 **B*18:01** C*12:03 DRβ1*14:54 DQβ1*05:03 DPβ1*02:02
Pair 2:
Recipient
A*02:01 B*27:02 C*02:02 DRβ1*04:01 DQβ1*03:02 DPβ1*01:01
A*25:01 B*18:01 C*12:03 DRβ1*14:54 DQβ1*05:03 DPβ1*02:02

Donor

A*02:01 B*27:02 C*02:02 DRβ1*04:01 DQβ1*03:02 DPβ1*01:01
A*02:01 B*18:01 C*12:03 DRβ1*14:54 DQβ1*05:03 DPβ1*02:02

- **A.** Recipient 1 is more likely to have GVHD and graft rejection.
- **B.** Recipient 2 is more likely to have GVHD and graft rejection.
- **C.** Recipient 1 is more likely to have GVHD.
- **D.** Recipient 2 is more likely to have GVHD.

17. A 32-year-old man with adverse risk AML is scheduled to undergo allogeneic transplantation. He has three biological siblings and two half-siblings. Which of the following statements regarding the likelihood of finding a family member for donation is true?
    - **A.** All siblings should be typed to determine if he has a suitable, fully matched donor.
    - **B.** Only siblings who share the same mother should be typed.
    - **C.** The likelihood of finding a donor in his family is greater than 50%.
    - **D.** A search of the NMDP registry should occur immediately as the chance of a sibling match is low.

18. A 64-year-old man is 35 days following allogeneic stem cell transplant from his fully matched sibling. He feels well overall and is without any skin rash, nausea, vomiting, anorexia, or diarrhea. Immunosuppression is with tacrolimus and methotrexate. His laboratory tests are significant for mild anemia hemoglobin 10.4 g/dL and mild thrombocytopenia 90,000 cells/μL. He is reporting discomfort during urination with increasing frequency. He feels he is not being able to void completely. He notices his urine is slightly dark and thinks he might have seen some blood. What is your diagnosis?
    - **A.** Bladder cancer
    - **B.** Benign prostatic hypertrophy (BPH)
    - **C.** BK virus cystitis
    - **D.** Bladder stone
    - **E.** Hemoglobinuria

19. A 54-year-old man is complaining of urinary bleeding 45 days following allogeneic stem cell transplant. BK virus in the urine is 40,000,000 gEq/mL. He is on tacrolimus with levels between 6 and 9 ng/μL. He has mild skin GVHD, which is controlled with topical triamcinolone cream. He has had rising creatinine over the past 1 week and gradually declining platelet counts. He is started on low dose cidofovir 1 mg/kg intravenously three times a week. After 4 weeks of treatment, his hematuria has resolved and his BK viral loads are 90,000 gEq/mL. He now reports right eye tearing and pain that started 2 days ago. He denies any fevers, cough, or cold symptoms. His right eye appears inflamed with erythematous conjunctiva. His left eye shows mild erythema. His vision in the right eye is blurry. The light bothers him, and he prefers to remain in a dark room. His 2-year-old grandchild recently recovered from conjunctivitis. What is the likely cause of his symptoms?
    - **A.** Acute angle glaucoma
    - **B.** Bacterial conjunctivitis
    - **C.** Viral conjunctivitis
    - **D.** Optic neuritis
    - **E.** Cidofovir toxicity

20. What is routinely checked in an asymptomatic patient following a full matched allogeneic hematopoietic stem cell transplant (HSCT)?
    - **A.** BK virus
    - **B.** CMV
    - **C.** Epstein-Barr virus (EBV)
    - **D.** HSV
    - **E.** Hepatitis B virus

21. What category of patients should receive antibiotic prophylaxis against pneumococcal infection?
    - **A.** A 45-year-old man who underwent allogeneic HCT 40 days ago
    - **B.** A 23-year-old woman with chronic skin GVHD on oral prednisone and sirolimus
    - **C.** A 38-year-old woman with IgG levels of 250 mg/dL who underwent reduced intensity conditioning for Hodgkin lymphoma 6 months ago
    - **D.** A 52-year-old man with recurrent sinopulmonary infections, dry eyes, difficulty swallowing, weight loss, and skin rash 250 days following mismatched unrelated donor transplant
    - **E.** All of the above

22. On day+4 after mismatched myeloablative allogeneic stem cell transplantation, a 36-year-old develops profuse watery diarrhea, totaling 1.75 L over a 24-hour period. Appropriate diagnostic and therapeutic maneuvers in this patient include:
    - **A.** Endoscopy with biopsy to diagnose acute GI GVHD before administration of corticosteroids
    - **B.** Empiric corticosteroids with methylprednisolone at 2 mg/kg to treat acute grade III GI GVHD with endoscopy to confirm diagnosis
    - **C.** Empiric corticosteroids with methylprednisolone at 1 mg/kg to treat acute grade III GI GVHD with endoscopy to confirm diagnosis
    - **D.** Stool culture and infectious disease investigation

23. A 42-year-old woman develops a generalized skin rash over her face, torso, abdomen, arms, and legs 30 days after allogeneic HCT for AML. The rash started out on her chest and neck after she took a walk in her neighborhood around midday. In 48 hours, the rash spread to her entire body. She reports itching. She is taking tacrolimus and sirolimus, the levels of which are therapeutic on recent laboratory check. On examination, she has an erythematous macular popular rash involving her forehead, chin, anterior neck, chest, abdomen, back, arms, and legs along with excoriation marks over her thighs. What is the next step in management for this patient's clinical symptoms?
    - **A.** Take a skin biopsy
    - **B.** Start oral prednisone 1 mg/kg body weight daily
    - **C.** Apply topical triamcinolone cream 0.1%
    - **D.** Increase the dose of sirolimus
    - **E.** Change tacrolimus to mycophenolate mofetil (MMF)

24. A 49-year-old man with AML underwent a matched related donor transplant 60 days ago. He remains on tacrolimus and sirolimus for immunosuppression. One week ago, CMV DNA PCR in the blood was undetectable. Today CMV PCR is 1886 copies/μL. The patient is on valacyclovir 500 mg by mouth twice daily. Laboratory testing today also reveals WBC 2.7×10^9/L, hemoglobin 9.8 g/dL, platelets 78,000/μL, creatinine 0.6 mg/dL. What is the next best step in the management of CMV reactivation?
    - **A.** Stop valacyclovir and start valganciclovir 900 mg by mouth twice daily
    - **B.** Continue valacyclovir and start foscarnet 90 mg/kg intravenously twice daily
    - **C.** Stop valacyclovir and start foscarnet 90 mg/kg intravenously twice daily
    - **D.** Stop valacyclovir and start intravenous ganciclovir
    - **E.** None of the above

25. A 52-year-old woman with AML is undergoing treatment with foscarnet infusions daily for CMV reactivation since 2 weeks. She has ongoing leucopenia and anemia. She is taking tacrolimus and MMF for immunosuppression. She feels well and denies any nausea, vomiting, diarrhea, anorexia, or skin rash. Yesterday she noted burning during urination. Today she reports itching after urination. On examination, you notice erythema in the inner labial folds. There is no vaginal discharge and no ulceration. What is the cause of her current complaint?
    A. HSV sores
    B. Bacterial vaginosis
    C. Candida
    D. Foscarnet toxicity
    E. Graft versus host disease

26. A 27-year-old woman is undergoing a myeloablative double umbilical cord blood transplant for AML. She has poor appetite lingering from the side effects of her conditioning regimen. She is currently in complete remission. What is the best choice of agent for prophylaxis against mold infections?
    A. Itraconazole
    B. Posaconazole
    C. Voriconazole
    D. Fluconazole
    E. Caspofungin

27. A previously healthy 50-year old man with a 10 year history of alcohol use, diagnosed with Philadelphia chromosome positive ALL is being considered for allogeneic stem cell transplantation. Which of the following myeloablative regimens is the most appropriate for use as conditioning?
    A. Cyclophosphamide total dose 120mg/kg IV, plus total body irradiation 12 Gy fractionated
    B. Busulfan total dose 16mg/kg IV, plus cyclophosphamide total dose 120mg/kg IV
    C. Fludarabine total dose 120mg/m2 IV, plus Busulfan 12.8 mg/kg IV over 4 days
    D. Fludarabine total dose 150mg/m2 IV, plus Busulfan 8-10mg/kg orally over 2 days

28. Uncommon but serious side effects of myeloablative doses of cyclophosphamide include:
    A. Hemorrhagic cystitis and seizures
    B. Nephrotoxicity and avascular bone necrosis
    C. Hemorrhagic cystitis and cardiotoxicity
    D. Seizure and nephrotoxicity

29. A 46-year-old man is undergoing high dose chemotherapy with BEAM and ASCT for high-risk relapsed Hodgkin lymphoma. Which of the following antiinfective prophylaxis would you NOT give to this patient?
    A. Levofloxacin 500 mg daily until resolution of neutropenia
    B. Fluconazole 400 mg daily until 30 days following ASCT
    C. Trimethoprim-sulfamethoxazole (TMP-SMX) one double strength tablet daily for up to 6 months after ASCT
    D. Valacyclovir 500 mg daily for up to 3 months following ASCT
    E. Fluconazole 400 mg daily until resolution of neutropenia

30. A 48-year-old man who is 20 days from myeloablative transplantation now has a bilirubin of 3.6 with hepatic tenderness and leg edema on examination. The most appropriate initial investigation of his liver dysfunction is which of the following?
    A. 2-D ultrasound of the right upper quadrant
    B. Duplex ultrasound of the right upper quadrant
    C. CT scan without contrast of the abdomen
    D. Liver biopsy

31. A 58-year-old man underwent a myeloablative allogeneic HCT from an unrelated donor 18 months ago with fludarabine and busulfan. He is currently on sirolimus and extracorporeal photophoresis for chronic GVHD of the skin. He reports a nonproductive cough and mild dyspnea on exertion after climbing two flights of stairs that started 1 month ago. Infectious workup has been negative. Pulmonary function testing (PFT) 6 months following allogeneic HCT revealed FEV1 80% predicted, FEV1/FVC ratio 1.2. His PFTs today reveal FEV1 65%, FEV1/FVC ratio 0.6. A high-resolution CT scan of the chest shows bronchiectasis, bronchial wall thickening, centrilobular opacities, and air trapping. A trial of bronchodilator therapy failed. What is your diagnosis?
    A. Chronic obstructive pulmonary disease (COPD)
    B. Bronchiolitis obliterans syndrome (BOS)
    C. Cryptogenic organizing pneumonia (COP)
    D. Sirolimus toxicity
    E. Viral pneumonia

32. What is the proposed treatment for BOS?
    A. Nebulization therapy
    B. Oral prednisone 1 mg/kg per day
    C. Inhaled fluticasone, oral azithromycin, oral montelukast sodium (FAM)
    D. Both A and B
    E. Inhaled ipratropium/albuterol

33. A 26-year-old woman with relapsed Hodgkin lymphoma underwent high-dose chemotherapy with cyclophosphamide, carmustine, and etoposide followed by ASCT 7 months ago. She reports a nonproductive cough over the past two weeks. She is an active soccer player and is now unable to participate on the field. Her physical exam is notable for bilateral basilar crackles and normal jugular venous pressure. There is no evidence of pedal edema, cardiac rub, murmur, or gallop. Her vital signs show a heart rate of 78 bpm, blood pressure of 125/80 mm Hg, temperature 98.9°F, respiratory rate 22 breaths/min, and oxygen saturation of 90% on room air. The patient recently stopped TMP-SMX and valacyclovir prophylaxis 1 month ago. A restaging positron emission tomography (PET)-CT scan performed 4 weeks ago revealed subtle bilateral interstitial infiltrate but no evidence of disease recurrence. What is the likely diagnosis?
    A. Pulmonary embolism (PE)
    B. Carmustine induced pulmonary toxicity
    C. *Pneumocystis jiroveci* pneumonia
    D. Relapsed Hodgkin lymphoma
    E. COPD

34. Which of the following vaccines will you **NOT** provide to a patient within 1 year of a stem cell transplant?
    A. Pneumococcal conjugate (PCV)
    B. Tetanus, diphtheria, acellular pertussis
    C. *Haemophilus influenzae* conjugate
    D. Measles-mumps-rubella
    E. Inactivated polio

35. A 67-year-old man returns for his annual follow-up visit. He underwent a matched related donor stem cell transplant 1 year ago. He feels well and wants to travel to Orlando, Florida, with his grandchildren. He is off all immunosuppressant therapy and is without evidence of GVHD. What is the current vaccination advised to this patient?
    A. Chickenpox (Varivax)
    B. Shingles vaccine (Zostavax)
    C. *Hemophilus influenzae* type b (Hib)
    D. Measles-mumps-rubella
    E. Oral polio vaccine

36. On routine monitoring of a 60-year-old man 30 days after a matched related allogeneic HCT, CMV reactivation is noted at 1457 copies/μL. Intravenous ganciclovir is begun and bi-weekly levels are followed. After 2 weeks of therapy, CMV PCR shows 2760 copies/μL. What is the next step in management?
    A. Increase dose of ganciclovir
    B. Stop ganciclovir and start valganciclovir
    C. Stop ganciclovir and start foscarnet
    D. Add foscarnet therapy to ganciclovir
    E. Add valganciclovir

37. A 42-year-old man reports mild nausea, appetite changes, loss of 2 lbs weight, and loose stools over the past 2 weeks. He underwent a matched related donor transplant for AML 45 days ago. He is taking tacrolimus 1 mg twice daily and MMF 1000 mg 3 times daily. His tacrolimus blood levels are 7 ng/mL. He has undetectable viral loads as of last week. His physical exam shows a mild erythematous macular popular rash. He is applying hydrocortisone cream to the rash. He underwent an esophagogastroduodenoscopy (EGD)/sigmoidoscopy, which was unremarkable. Pathology from gastric and sigmoid colon biopsies show single cell apoptosis with crypt epithelium in the gastric fundus and destruction of single crypts and glands with apoptotic crypt abscesses in the sigmoid colon.
    What is the lead cause of his GI symptoms?
    A. Acute GVHD
    B. MMF side effect
    C. Viral gastroenteritis
    D. CMV reactivation
    E. Tacrolimus toxicity

38. A 49-year-old man comes for a follow-up visit 40 days after ASCT. His past medical history is significant for CD15+, CD30+ nodular sclerosing Hodgkin lymphoma. He undergoes 4 cycles of chemotherapy with ABVD. Restaging PET-CT show complete resolution of disease. Two months later he reports new-onset chest tightness, cough, night sweats, and fever 101°F. A repeat CT scan of the chest, abdomen, and pelvis reveal bulky mediastinal adenopathy and enlarged inguinal lymph nodes. A biopsy of the right inguinal lymph node is consistent with nodular sclerosing Hodgkin disease. He receives 3 cycles of brentuximab vedotin and achieves a complete response. One month later, he receives high-dose chemotherapy with BEAM followed by ASCT. What is the next best treatment approach for this patient?
    A. Brentuximab vedotin therapy for total 16 cycles as tolerated
    B. Consolidation radiation therapy to the mediastinum
    C. Observation
    D. Single agent Rituxan therapy for 6 months
    E. Allogeneic stem cell transplant

39. A 57-year-old man with new onset runny nose and rhinovirus should delay his upcoming allogeneic HCT until symptoms resolve.
    Which of the following statements is true?
    A. All patients undergoing autologous and allogeneic HCT should receive the annual inactivated influenza vaccine.
    B. HCT recipients less than 6 months after HCT should receive chemoprophylaxis with neuraminidase inhibitors during community influenza outbreaks that lead to nosocomial outbreaks.
    C. There is no evidence to support routine testing of HCT recipients or donors for the presence of BKV-specific or JCV-specific antibodies.
    D. All of the above.

ANSWERS

1. **D**
    The pretransplant regimen is intended to accomplish two goals: ablate the tumor (autologous and allogeneic transplantation) and achieve adequate immunosuppression to allow donor engraftment (allogeneic transplantation, only). Cancers treatable by HCT are usually those that exhibit a strong dose-sensitivity, justifying the treatment of patients with dose-intense regimens. Bone marrow is also exquisitely sensitive to many of the agents used in the pretransplant conditioning regimens, which is the basis for infusion of HCT. Conditioning regimens range from fully myeloablative (which destroy the inherent hematopoietic function of the bone marrow) and nonmyeloablative or reduced intensity conditioning, which are chosen to be used in the elderly population or for transplant of nonmalignant conditions, such as severe aplastic anemia.

2. **B**
    Relapse is the main cause of failure after allogeneic HCT. The effect of graft versus tumor response depends on factors that improve the activity of cytotoxic T lymphocytes that recognize tumor-specific antigens presented by major histocompatibility complex (MHC) class I or class II molecules. Many tumors evade recognition by the immune system by downregulating surface MHC, which is one reason for relapses after allogeneic HSCT. Other factors that contribute are secretion by tumor cells of inhibitory cytokines, such as TGF-beta.

3. **D**
    The inability to achieve a complete remission with prior chemotherapy is predictive of higher risk of relapse after autologous or allogeneic HCT. Aggressiveness of the tumor is judged by disease responsiveness to induction regimens as well as the duration of the response. Transplants may not be appropriate when the expected benefit is slim, such as in the setting of a large disease burden or rapid kinetics of tumor growth in the period preceding HCT.

4. **E**
    GVHD occurs after all allogeneic HSCTs. The likelihood of GVHD may vary based on the degree of HLA matching; for example, higher risk of GVHD in a mismatched unrelated HSCT compared with a matched unrelated HSCT and matched related HSCT. This is due to several factors not limited to major HLA matching. Mismatch at minor histocompatibility antigens also play a role in initiating GVHD. The more myeloablative the regimen, the higher the chance of acute GVHD as a result of tissue injury from the conditioning regimen. Researchers found that using peripheral blood stem cells, compared with bone marrow stem cells, results in a higher incidence of chronic GVHD. Ultimately, the higher the cytotoxic T-cell to the regulatory T-cell ratio, the greater the GVHD. In addition, any insults in the form of infections, surgeries, or phototoxicity can trigger GVHD.

5. **C**
    Acute GVHD presents with three-organ involvement; GI resulting in nausea, vomiting, anorexia, and diarrhea;

skin resulting is varying degrees of rash; and liver resulting is rising total bilirubin. This patient has none of these. Chronic GVHD involves multiple organs. This patient does not seem to have any organ involvement of symptoms of GVHD. Tacrolimus toxicity occurs most commonly if blood levels are greater than 15 ng/mL. While some patients can be sensitive to tacrolimus even at lower levels, oral ulcers are very rare side effects of tacrolimus and do not typically occur at levels below 10 ng/mL. CMV reactivation is a possibility following allogeneic HCT. However, both patient and donor are CMV negative, with very low risk of reactivation. In the post-engraftment phase (30–100 days after hematopoietic cell transplant) infections relate primarily to impaired cell-mediated immunity. The depth of this defect is determined by the extent of GVHD and immunosuppressive therapy in use. HSV, particularly CMV, are common infectious agents during this period. HSV typically causes painful oral sores, and a testing with viral cultures/PCRs is warranted.

6. **E**

Hepatic SOS or, as it was previously known, venoocclusive disease (VOD) occurs after an injury to the hepatic venous endothelium. Preexisting liver disease, use of busulfan, cyclophosphamide, high doses of TBI, and female gender are all considered risk factors for SOS. The triad of clinical signs is weight gain, increased abdominal girth with tender hepatomegaly, and rise in total bilirubin. Serial Doppler ultrasounds of the liver will reveal reversal of portal vein flow indicative of sinusoidal obstruction. Thrombocytopenia eventually ensues. Depending on the severity of the disease, it can be fatal. Immediate clinical diagnosis is necessary and treatment involves prompt institution of recently approved defibrotide along with aggressive supportive care.

7. **A**

The recovery of the innate immune system (e.g., neutrophils, monocytes, and NK cells) is influenced by the graft type and is fastest with filgrastim-mobilized blood stem cells, is intermediate with bone marrow, and is slowest with umbilical cord blood. This is followed by recovery of CD8+ T-cells and B-cells, whose counts may become supranormal transiently. B-cell recovery is influenced by graft type (fastest after cord blood transplant) and is delayed by GVHD and/or its treatment. Subsequently, plasma cells, and tissue macrophages/microglia, which are relatively resistant to chemo/radiotherapy, recover. The nadir of these cells may be lower in the presence of acute GVHD due to the graft versus host plasma cell effect. Finally, the recovery of CD4+ T-cells is influenced by the T-cell content of the graft and patient age (faster in children than adults). Therefore close monitoring of the patient's immune reconstitution markers (e.g., IgG levels and CD4+ counts) assists in guiding physicians about discontinuing prophylactic antiinfective therapy.

8. **D**

The Blood and Marrow Transplant Clinical Trials Network (BMT-CTN) operational definition of TMA requires the following: microangiopathic hemolysis (red blood cell fragmentation and ≥2 schistocytes per high-power field on a peripheral blood smear), concurrent increased serum LDH above institutional baseline, concurrent renal (defined as doubling of serum creatinine from baseline or 50% decrease in creatinine clearance from baseline) and/or neurologic dysfunction without other explanations, and negative direct and indirect Coombs tests results. TMA

may occur after allogeneic hematopoietic stem cell transplantation and is related, in part, to calcineurin inhibitor toxicity particularly in combination with sirolimus even when tacrolimus levels are within normal range (nanograms per milliliter). Acute GVHD affects the liver with rising total bilirubin and can suppress the bone marrow function; however, the patient has no clinical evidence of involvement of skin, gut, or hepatic systems. ITP can result in declining platelets and similar bone marrow biopsy findings, but it does not explain the rising creatinine. Relapsed AML is unlikely in a bone marrow biopsy that is unrevealing of disease.

9. **A**

Immediate transplantation from an HLA matched sibling is most appropriate. Given his age, a reduced toxicity approach is not recommended, and the decision to delay transplantation or not to undergo transplantation at all are both associated with a loss of total life years.

10. **B**

Myeloablative transplantation should be offered. This woman has adverse risk AML by virtue of her monosomal karyotype; therefore, transplantation in first remission is indicated. There is no advantage to pursuing further courses of consolidation chemotherapy prior to transplantation, and myeloablative transplantation is preferred over reduced intensity transplantation on the basis of a large randomized trial, prematurely halted, that demonstrated improved outcomes in leukemic patients offered myeloablative transplantation over reduced intensity transplantation.

11. **E**

The consensus recommendations from the CDC, IDSA, CIBMTR, ASBMT, EBMT, NMDP, and SHEA jointly suggest using fluoroquinolones as primary prophylaxis to prevent bacterial infections for the period of neutropenia. In case of drug allergy or other reasons, azithromycin 250 mg daily can be used instead. Due to lack of data, there are currently no antimicrobial prophylactic regimens that can be recommended for children. Some experts use levofloxacin for pediatric antibacterial prophylaxis.

12. **C**

Tacrolimus is a calcineurin inhibitor developed from a fungus. It reduced inflammation by decreasing cytokine release and subsequently interleukin-2. It is metabolized through the cytochrome p450 pathway in the liver and interacts with several drugs, such as like antiemetics and antibiotics. Such interactions can result in increased tacrolimus levels and signs of toxicity, including uncontrolled hypertension, headache, confusion, and renal insufficiency. Another concerning complication of tacrolimus toxicity is posterior reversal encephalopathy syndrome (PRES), which is usually reversible on drug discontinuation. Therefore, this patient should get magnetic resonance imaging of the brain to rule out any flare or hyperintensity in the T2-weighted diffusion images. CNS leukemia can result in headaches and vision changes, but is unlikely to cause renal insufficiency. HSV encephalitis is unlikely in a patient taking antiviral prophylaxis. Methotrexate toxicity, while causing renal injury, does not cause headaches and confusion. Intracranial bleeds will result in stroke like symptoms rather than renal injury and confusion.

13. **C**

Splenic rupture is a very rare yet potentially fatal complication of granulocyte-colony stimulating factor (G-CSF) such as filgrastim. Ectopic pregnancy is unlikely since female donors are screened for pregnancy prior to the collection of stem cells. She also just had her menstrual cycle recently. G-CSF-induced bone pain is more gradual in onset and is generalized and dull in nature. Pancreatitis typically causes pain radiating to the midback and is associated with nausea and vomiting. G-CSF is not known to promote kidney stones.

14. C

The choice of a donor is of great importance because it can predict the outcome of the transplant based on HLA typing, age, gender, CMV status, and ABO compatibility of the donor. Matching donor and recipient for HLA class I (-A, -B, and -C) and class II (-DRB1 and -DQB1) haplotypes is a key part of successful allogeneic HCT. A 12 of 12 HLA match refers to donor-recipient pairs matched for HLA-A, HLA-B, HLA-C, HLA-DRB1, HLA-DQB1, and HLA-DP1 at the allele level. A full HLA matched donor is preferred over a mismatched or an unrelated donor. Many transplant centers are now performing half-matched (haploidentical) donor transplants with the advent of posttransplant cyclophosphamide and the low risk of graft failure. However, the transplant community is yet to reach a consensus on favoring these transplants over a full HLA-matched donor. When available, a matched sibling donor is preferred over other donor sources due to improved clinical outcomes following transplant (e.g., less GVHD) and the speed and cost-effectiveness of the search. As such, the initial search should center on molecular HLA typing of the patient's full biological siblings. The next important screen is the donor's age. A younger donor is always preferred over an older donor. The effect of donor age was best demonstrated in a retrospective analysis from the Center for International Blood and Marrow Transplant Research of over 11,000 unrelated transplants performed from 1988 to 2011 that evaluated the effects of various donor characteristics (e.g., age, sex, CMV serologic status, ABO compatibility, race, and parity) on recipient outcome. For every 10-year increment in donor age, there was a 5.5% increase in the hazard ratio (HR) for mortality. Older donor age was also associated with an increase in acute GVHD but not chronic GVHD. Recipients with female donors who had undergone multiple pregnancies have a higher rate of chronic GVHD than recipients with male donors or nulliparous female donors. Therefore, this patient's 45-year-old sister would not be an ideal candidate. The CMV serostatus impacts transplant-related morbidity and mortality in some studies (Schmidt-Hieber M. et al, Blood 2013). CMV reactivation is a challenging problem following allogeneic stem cell transplants, hence a CMV-negative donor is favored for a CMV-negative recipient. In choosing a donor, the physician must remember that the above-mentioned factors only come into effect when there are multiple donor choices available. An unrelated donor search can be time consuming, and delays might result in disease relapse in the interim.

15. D

An HLA-DQβ1 mismatched donor is the best option presented here. HLA-A, -B, -C, and -DRβ1 are more important considerations over HLA-DQβ1, which only minimally impacts on the rate of GVHD. Also note that allelic mismatches carry the same risk of antigenic mismatches.

16. D

Recipient 2 is more likely to experience GVHD. Recipient 1 is homozygous at HLA-B and is more likely to experience graft rejection due to the recognition of foreign HLA-B. The risk of GVHD is not increased in the scenario. Donor 2 is homozygous at HLA-A and is more likely to induce GVHD due to the recognition of foreign HLA-A in the recipient. There is no increased risk of graft rejection in Recipient 2.

17. C

The likelihood of finding a match exceeds 50%. The likelihood of finding a donor among biological siblings can be estimated by the formula:

$$\text{Likelihood of Match} = 1 - (0.75)^n$$

where n represents the number of biological siblings. In this case, with three siblings, the likelihood of match is approximately 58%. Note that only full biological siblings should be typed when a full HLA match is sought. At most, half siblings can be haploidentical to their half sibling.

18. C

The BK virus is a member of the polyoma virus. It can cause significant morbidity in an immunocompromised patient. Any urinary urgency, discomfort, or hematuria in a patient following allogeneic stem cell transplant should alert the physician for testing BK virus in the urine and subsequently blood. BK viruria is often asymptomatic, but warrants treatment if symptoms of pain, frequency, or bleeding occur. If left untreated, the BK virus can invade the kidneys and cause BK-virus-associated nephropathy (BKVAN), which can quickly become irreversible. Treatment is with cidofovir and aggressive hydration with close follow-up for BK virus clearing and renal dysfunction. Bladder cancer does not cause painful urination. Bladder stone is possible; therefore, a complete workup including renal ultrasound should be performed, although a bladder stone will not cause increased frequency. BPH does not result in hematuria or painful urination.

19. E

Cidofovir demonstrates in vitro activity against a number of DNA viruses, including the herpesviruses, adenovirus, polyomavirus, papillomavirus, and poxvirus. The most important toxicity of the drug is renal; this can be reduced by co-administration with saline and probenecid, which blocks active renal tubular secretion. Acute iritis and ocular hypotony have also been associated with intravenous cidofovir and are usually dose dependent. Patients with ocular symptoms while on cidofovir need immediate evaluation by a retina specialist. Cidofovir should be permanently discontinued in these patients. Resolution of symptoms typically occurs with prompt diagnosis and aggressive therapy with ocular steroids and supportive care. Acute angle glaucoma is unlikely in a patient without any history of glaucoma. Bacterial and viral conjunctivitis typically do not cause vision changes. Optic neuritis is a possibility, but typical symptoms are painful eye movements, which this patient does not have.

20. B

CMV is a common cause of morbidity and mortality following HCT. CMV PCR testing is routinely done since serologic testing is not adequate for monitoring reactivation in an immunocompromised host who cannot mount an effective antibody response. The risk of CMV reactivation is highest when either donor or recipient is CMV positive. Preemptive treatment reduces CMV infections and mortality. The BK virus is only tested if patients have urinary frequency, pain, or hematuria. Some centers perform EBV testing as an early marker for posttransplant lymphoproliferative disease (PTLD), but this is not routine. HSV reactivation is common, but less so if patients are on antiviral prophylaxis. Hepatitis B testing is only done on patients who are known to be positive prior to transplant. Posttransplant risk of acquiring hepatitis B is practically zero due to stringent blood bank quality measures.

21. **E**

Invasive pneumococcal infection (IPI) is a life-threatening complication that can occur at any time point following allogeneic HCT, particularly in patients with chronic GVHD or patients with low IgG levels. Antibiotic prophylaxis should be administered even to patients who have received pneumococcal vaccination (1) because not all strains are included in the vaccines, so the immunogenicity of vaccines against the vaccine strains in HCT patients is only about 80%; and (2) because of the theoretic concern that strains not included in the vaccine will replace vaccine strains. Oral penicillin remains the preferred choice, but antibiotic selection depends on the local pattern of pneumococcal resistance to penicillin and other antibiotics (i.e., second-generation cephalosporins, macrolides, and quinolones).

22. **D**

Day 4 is in general too early for severe acute GI GVHD, and an infectious etiology or the effects of conditioning chemotherapy should be considered. In the absence of a skin rash, the diagnosis of hyperacute GVHD is very unlikely.

23. **B**

This patient has acute GVHD of the skin. Based on the body surface area involved, she has greater than 50% involvement of the skin constituting stage 3 skin GVHD (generalized erythroderma) by Glucksberg criteria. While a skin biopsy should be done to confirm the diagnosis, the first step is to start the patient on high-dose steroids. Additionally, topical steroids may be added for additional supportive care, particularly for hypersensitivity and itching symptoms. Flare of acute GVHD is common following allogeneic HCT, and the incidence is higher in matched unrelated donor (MUD) transplants, increasing parity of the donor (female donors), and female donors to male recipients. Acute GVHD is also triggered on direct exposure to the sun; therefore, patients should be instructed to wear sunscreen and protective clothing and to avoid the midday sun. Increasing sirolimus will lead to added toxicity without additional benefit. Changing to another calcineurin inhibitor will not be sufficient in this instance.

24. **C**

CMV reactivation increases morbidity and mortality following allogeneic HCT. Prompt preemptive treatment is needed to prevent organ involvement and damage by CMV. Valacyclovir is used for prophylaxis only, but once viral reactivation occurs, induction treatment is warranted. The threshold of starting therapy after viral reactivation varies in different transplant centers. In a patient with ongoing pancytopenia, ganciclovir or valganciclovir can worsen cytopenias. In a patient with normal creatinine clearance, foscarnet is a good treatment option and requires supportive care with fluid and electrolyte infusions.

25. **D**

Foscarnet is excreted in the urine and can cause genital ulcers. Prevention of ulcers can be done with maintaining thorough hygiene after urination. Steroid cream can be used to relieve the symptoms of itching and burning. HSV can also cause genital ulcers. Sending of cultures from the sore is a definitive diagnosis; however, since this patient has been on foscarnet at least 2 weeks, the most likely cause of her symptoms is drug induced. GVHD does not affect a limited genital area. The patient does not have any vaginal discharge, thereby ruling out bacterial vaginosis and yeast infection.

26. **C**

Invasive mold infections have a trimodal incidence distribution among allogeneic HCT recipients. Before engraftment (i.e., during phase I), the main risk factor is prolonged neutropenia; therefore, the risk is higher with bone marrow and umbilical cord blood transplants, and lower with peripheral blood and nonmyeloablative transplants. In addition, the risk is higher among patients with prolonged low-level neutropenia prior to transplant, such as aplastic anemia patients. In phases II and III (peri- and postengraftment), the main risk factor is severe cell-mediated immunodeficiency caused by GVHD and its treatment. Therefore, recipients of transplants with higher risks for severe GVHD (unrelated donor, mismatched transplant, haploidentical) are at greater risk of mold infections. Patients at high risk for mold infections should be considered for prophylaxis with mold-active drugs during periods of risk.

Absorption of itraconazole and posaconazole is poor in patients who are not eating, so it is not a good choice for this patient. Also, posaconazole has not been studied in the pre-engraftment phase of transplant. Voriconazole blood levels of at least $1\ \mu g/mL$ are thought to be required for efficacy. Low voriconazole levels have been reported in patients with documented breakthrough infections. Breakthrough mold infections have been recorded in patients taking caspofungin. Fluconazole has no activity against mold.

27. **A**

A standard conventional myeloablative regimen for patients with ALL is cyclophosphamide 120mg/kg total dose and TBI 12Gy in fractionated dosing. With this regimen, the 3 year overall survival or disease free survival of 50% is obtained if transplanted in CR. TBI is the most common preparative regimen used for allogeneic HCT for ALL. Myeloablative regimens using fludarabine and busulfan combinations can be considered if patients are deemed ineligible for TBI. Further, patients with prior liver insult/injury can have increased busulfan toxicity like sinusoidal obstruction syndrome. Use of fractionated TBI regimens have less toxicity to normal cells while the larger doses provide more effective kill of resistant tumor cells. Overall, the choice of myeloablative regimens is considered based on patient tolerance and presence of other co-morbidities that can influence outcomes.

References: (1) Sebban C, et al. J Clin Oncol 1994;12:2580-7. (2) Thomas X, et al. J Clin Oncol. 2004;2:4075-86. (3) Copelan EA, et al. J Clin Oncol. 1992;10(2):237.

28. **C**

In high doses, cyclophosphamide is associated with hemorrhagic cystitis and cardiotoxicity. Hemorrhagic cystitis can be prevented with forced saline diureses and the use of MESNA, while there are no specific preventative measures for the cardiotoxicity. Supportive care, bladder irrigation, and topical analgesia are indicated for the treatment of hemorrhagic cystitis, while cardiac care is based on the manifestations of the cardiotoxicity (pericardial, myocardial, or arrhythmogenic).

29. B

Antifungal prophylaxis extension is only needed if prolonged degree of neutropenia is expected, which is not the case here. Antibiotic prophylaxis with a fluoroquinolone is standard practice in most transplant centers (alternately cephalosporin) and is typically continued until neutropenia resolves, or it is changed to broader coverage if patients experience a neutropenic fever. Antiviral prophylaxis is recommended for at least 3 months following ASCT or longer if patients are getting more chemotherapy. TMP-SMX is the preferred drug of choice for *Pneumocystis jiroveci* pneumonia (PCP) treatment and prevention. TMP-SMX can delay engraftment and thus is not usually administered before engraftment occurs. TMP-SMX is variably tolerated, and toxicities include myelosuppression, hypersensitivity, hyperkalemia, nephritis, hepatitis, and pancreatitis. The optimal dosage has not been defined in HCT patients. Many HCT programs use once- or twice-daily regimens (single-strength or double-strength tablets) 2–7 days/week, and all appear efficacious. PCP prophylaxis should be considered for ASCT recipients whose immunosuppression is substantial, either from an underlying condition or its treatment. Such patients include those with underlying lymphoma, leukemia, or myeloma, especially when intensive treatment or conditioning regimens have included purine analogues (fludarabine, cladribine [2CdA]) or high-dose corticosteroids.

30. B

VOD of the liver is clinically suspected, so a duplex (Doppler) ultrasound of the liver is the best initial test. In comparison to traditional 2D ultrasound, duplex ultrasound can measure portal blood flow and document reduced portal vein flow velocity, the absence of flow, and the reversal of flow in the portal system. A CT scan is useful to exclude other intraabdominal pathology, but is not as useful as ultrasound for evaluation of the right upper quadrant. Liver biopsy is reserved for equivocal cases on ultrasound and should be performed in conjunction with intrahepatic venous pressure measurements to document VOD.

31. B

BOS, a form of irreversible airflow obstruction (AFO), is the most common long-term, noninfectious pulmonary complication of allogeneic HCT. The current definition of BOS includes (1) FEV1 less than 75% predicted and an irreversible ≥10% decline in less than 2 years; (2) FEV1-to-vital capacity ratio less than 0.7 or the lower limit of the 90% confidence interval of the ratio; (3) absence of infection; and (4) either (a) preexisting diagnosis of chronic GVHD, (b) air trapping by expiratory CT, or (c) air trapping on PFTs by residual volume (RV) greater than 120% or RV/total lung capacity (TLC) exceeding the 90% confidence interval. It is very important to exclude other diagnoses, including idiopathic pneumonia syndrome, COP, pulmonary fibrosis, and late radiation effects, infection, asthma, or COPD, and rare disorders such as tracheomegaly, tracheobronchomalacia, or α-1-antitrypsin deficiency. COP produces a restrictive pattern on PFTs. The patient here has an obstructive pattern with evidence of air trapping and the presence of chronic GVHD, which all identify the diagnosis of BOS.

32. D

This patient has already developed symptoms of cough and dyspnea related to BOS, and therefore it is likely not enough that only an FAM regimen would prevent progression. High-dose steroids, particularly in the setting of chronic active GVHD, is the preferred option in combination with pulmonary directed therapy. PFT testing should be repeated every 3 months to assess for the FEV1 curve.

33. B

Pulmonary toxicity has historically been a frequent complication of high-dose therapy with ASCT, particularly with conditioning regimens containing 1,3-bis[2-chloroethyl]-1-nitrosurea (BCNU, or carmustine). Numerous studies in lymphomas, malignant gliomas, and breast cancer have established a strong correlation between BCNU dose and pulmonary toxicity. This can occur weeks to years after carmustine exposure. The incidence of pulmonary toxicity is less than 10% when cumulative BCNU doses are less than 800 mg/m^2 as a single agent, but in combination with other cytotoxic drugs, particularly cyclophosphamide, the tolerated dose is lower. Patients are usually treated with steroids. This condition can be severe and fatal at times. The patient has a normal heart rate making PE unlikely. She received appropriate prophylaxis against PCP for 6 months, and her PET-CT does not show any suspicion of pneumonia or relapsed disease. COPD is unlikely in this young, otherwise healthy, patient.

34. D

Antibody titers to vaccine-preventable diseases (e.g., tetanus, polio, measles, mumps, rubella) decline during the 1–10 years after allogeneic or autologous HCT if the recipient is not revaccinated. Evidence exists that certain vaccine-preventable diseases, such as pneumococcal infection, *Haemophilus influenzae* type b (Hib infection, measles, varicella, and influenza) can pose increased risk for HCT recipients. Therefore, HCT recipients should be routinely revaccinated after HCT so that they can experience immunity to the same vaccine-preventable diseases as others. In order for a vaccine to mount a clinically relevant response (e.g., a fourfold rise in specific antibody levels or a rise to a level considered protective), adaptive (T- and B-cell) immunity post-transplant must have been at least partially reconstituted. B-cell counts, which are typically zero or near-zero in the first 1–3 months after HCT, return to normal by 3–12 months post-transplant. MMR is a live vaccine and should only be offered 24 months following autologous and/or allogeneic HCT if the patient is without any active GVHD.

35. C

The patient is 1 year following allogeneic HCT. The CDC and ASBMT guidelines do not recommend administration of live vaccines to patients until 2 years following HCT or until they are free of an active flare of GVHD. Varivax can be given when patients fulfill the criteria to receive live vaccines. Shingles vaccine is not recommended in this subgroup of patients. MMR and oral polio vaccine are both live vaccines and therefore not recommended. Hib is a common encapsulated pathogen and patients should be vaccinated following autologous and/or allogeneic HCT.

36. C

After 2 weeks of therapy for CMV reactivation, if viral loads continue to increase, resistant strains should be considered and therapy should be switched. The addition of other therapies just increases the risk of toxicity without the benefit of the drug in case of CMV resistance. Valganciclovir is a prodrug of ganciclovir and cross-resistance is likely. When possible, blood samples should be sent to a laboratory capable of documenting antiviral resistance.

37. **A**

The patient has grade I GVHD findings in the stomach and grade II GVHD in the colon. Grading is a pathology criteria, which is different from the clinical stage of acute GVHD. MMF can also cause neutrophilic cryptitis and mimic GVHD on biopsy; however, since this patient has other signs and symptoms of GVHD, that is the likely diagnosis. CMV reactivation is unlikely if PCR in the blood was recently negative. However, immunohistology should be done to rule out CMV inclusion bodies. Tacrolimus toxicity does not cause this type of pathology.

38. **A**

Posttransplant consolidation treatment with brentuximab vedotin (Bv) for patients with high risk of relapse of Hodgkin disease is recommended based on the landmark phase III AETHERA trial. In this trial, 329 HL patients at high risk of relapse (defined as failure to achieve a complete remission with initial chemotherapy, evidence of disease progression within the first year after initial treatment, or the presence of extranodal involvement at the time of disease progression even if the period was longer than 1 year) following ASCT, achieved its primary endpoint and demonstrated a significant increase in PFS per independent review facility, with a hazard ratio of 0.57 and a P-value of 0.001. Median PFS was 43 months for patients who received Bv versus 24 months for patients who received placebo. The 2-year PFS rate was 63% in the Bv arm compared with 51% in the placebo arm. Bv is an antibody-drug conjugate (ADC) for intravenous injection comprising of an anti-CD30 monoclonal antibody attached by a protease-cleavable linker to a microtubule disrupting agent, monomethyl auristatin E (MMAE). The antibody-drug conjugate employs a linker system that is designed to be stable in the bloodstream but releases MMAE upon internalization into CD30-expressing tumor cells. This patient is at increased risk of relapse following ASCT due to a relapse within 12 months of frontline therapy as well as the presence of bulky disease. Single agent Rituxan has no role to play in this patient. Consolidation radiation therapy following ASCT is highly controversial and not practiced routinely. Observation would not be in the best interest of this patient. Allogeneic stem cell transplant would only be considered if the patient failed ASCT.

39. **D**

All statements are true. Then how can the correct answer be E? HCT candidates with URI symptoms at the time conditioning therapy is scheduled to start should postpone their conditioning regimen until the URI resolves, if possible, because certain URIs might progress to LRI during immunosuppression. BK virus testing is performed on patients with urinary symptoms of dysuria, hematuria, and frequency.

REFERENCES

Question 11

1. Tomblyn M, Chiller T, Einsele H, et al. Guidelines for preventing infectious complications among hematopoietic cell transplantation recipients: a global perspective. *Biol Blood Marrow Transplant.* 2009;15:1143–1238.

Question 21

1. Tauro S, et al. *Bone Marrow Transplant.* 2000.

Question 23

1. Rowlings PA, et al. *Br J Haematol.* 1997.

Question 26

1. Baddley JW, et al. *Clin Infect Dis.* 2001.

Question 32

1. Williams KM. *Blood;* 2017.

Question 35

1. Tomblyn M, et al. *Biol Blood Marrow Transplant.* 2011.

CHAPTER
13

Breast Cancer

Erica Mayer, Beth Overmoyer, Antoinette Tan, Paula R. Pohlmann, and Filipa Lynce

Early-Stage Breast Cancer

QUESTIONS

1. You meet a new consult patient and together are reviewing the pathology report from her recent surgery. Which of the following profiles is least consistent with HER2-positive breast cancer?
   A. HER2 IHC 2+, HER2 FISH ratio, 1.5, HER2 copy number >6
   B. HER2 IHC 2+, HER2 FISH ratio 1.1, HER2 copy number 5
   C. HER2 IHC 2+, HER2 FISH ratio 3.5, HER2 copy number 4
   D. HER2 IHC 3+, HER2 FISH ratio 1.9, HER2 copy number 3

2. A 50-year-old woman has a stage 2 HER2-positive breast cancer and will receive a trastuzumab-based regimen. She asks you about the toxicity profile. You reply that trastuzumab is generally safe, but rare adverse effects can include:
   A. Rash, diarrhea, stomatitis
   B. Renal impairment, lowering of cardiac ejection fraction, infusion reaction
   C. Lower seizure threshold, rash, long QT interval
   D. Infusion reaction, lowering of cardiac ejection fraction, interstitial pneumonitis
   E. Hypertension, vomiting, renal impairment

3. A 51-year-old woman is found to have an asymmetry on screening mammography, with ultrasound showing a 1.2-cm hypoechoic mass. A biopsy is performed, showing invasive ductal carcinoma, grade 2, ER 80%, PR 20%, HER3 IHC 2+, FISH ratio 4.5, HER2 copy number 7. She undergoes breast-conserving surgery and a sentinel lymph node procedure, finding a 1.4-cm invasive cancer, grade 2, without lymphovascular invasion and with clear margins. A single sentinel lymph node was negative. She comes in for a medical oncology opinion on management. What is the preferred systemic recommendation?
   A. Docetaxel, carboplatin, trastuzumab for six cycles, then completion of 1 year of trastuzumab
   B. Docetaxel, trastuzumab, pertuzumab for three cycles, then completion of 1 year of trastuzumab
   C. Weekly paclitaxel and trastuzumab × 12 weeks, then completion of 1 year of trastuzumab
   D. Doxorubicin and cyclophosphamide for 4 cycles, weekly paclitaxel and trastuzumab × 12 weeks, followed by completion of 1 year of trastuzumab
   E. TDM1 every 3 weeks for a year

4. A 61-year-old woman has routine screening mammography which demonstrates new microcalcifications in the upper outer quadrant of her right breast. A stereotactic biopsy is performed, finding ductal carcinoma in situ. She undergoes localized excision, and pathology reveals a 1.8 cm ductal carcinoma in situ. Immunohistochemistry shows the tumor to be ER >95%, PR 50%, HER2 3+. Adjuvant radiotherapy is planned. What is the best systemic management plan?
   A. No systemic therapy
   B. Weekly paclitaxel and trastuzumab x 12 weeks, then completion of 1 year of trastuzumab
   C. Either tamoxifen or aromatase inhibitor for 5 years
   D. Perform a sentinel lymph node biopsy before making a treatment decision
   E. Tamoxifen with concurrent trastuzumab for 1 year, then completion of 4 more years of trastuzumab

5. A 53-year-old woman presents with a palpable mass in the upper outer quadrant of her left breast. Breast imaging confirms the presence of a 2.0-cm mass, and a core needle biopsy finds invasive ductal carcinoma, grade 3, ER < 5%, PR < 5%, HER2 IHC 0. She proceeded with breast-conserving surgery and a sentinel lymph node biopsy. Pathology showed a 2.2-cm invasive cancer with negative margins. A total of two sentinel lymph nodes were recovered, one of which contained a 0.8-cm macrometastasis. Adjuvant chemotherapy and radiotherapy are planned. What is the preferred next step in locoregional management?

A. Ultrasound of the axilla to evaluate for residual disease
B. Completion axillary lymph node dissection
C. No further axillary surgery
D. Completion mastectomy
E. Completion mastectomy with axillary lymph node dissection

6. A 71-year-old woman presents with a 6-month history of a slowly evolving central breast mass. On radiologic evaluation, the mass is 3.2 cm in size. A biopsy is performed, showing invasive ductal carcinoma, grade 1, ER >95%, PR >95%, HER2 0. She proceeds with breast-conserving surgery and a sentinel lymph node biopsy. Pathology confirms a 3.0-cm invasive cancer, with one of three axillary lymph nodes with a macrometastasis and $\frac{1}{3}$ with a micrometastasis. A 21-gene recurrence score assay is sent and returns with a low recurrence score of 10. What is best systemic management for this patient?
   A. Dose-dense Adriamycin, Cytoxan, and paclitaxel for eight cycles followed by at least 5 years of aromatase inhibitor therapy
   B. Docetaxel cyclophosphamide for four cycles, followed by 10 years of tamoxifen therapy
   C. Cyclophosphamide, methotrexate, and fluorouracil (CMF) for six cycles, followed by at least 5 years of aromatase inhibitor therapy
   D. 10 years of tamoxifen therapy
   E. At least 5 years of aromatase inhibitor therapy

7. A 34-year-old woman presented last year with a 3.7-cm invasive ductal carcinoma, grade 3, with extensive lymphovascular invasion and three involved axillary lymph nodes. She received adjuvant chemotherapy as well as radiotherapy. She was then started on adjuvant tamoxifen. Although her periods stopped during chemotherapy, within 4 months she has had resolution of hot flashes and resumption of menses. What is the optimal adjuvant endocrine therapy plan?
   A. Continue tamoxifen × 5 years
   B. Continue tamoxifen × 10 years
   C. Oophorectomy and no further endocrine therapy
   D. Initiation of luteinizing hormone-releasing hormone (LHRH) agonist with tamoxifen or aromatase inhibitor for at least 5 years
   E. Change to aromatase inhibitor for 5 years

8. A 34-year-old woman presented with a palpable right breast mass. A biopsy found high-grade invasive ductal carcinoma, negative for ER/PR and HER2, with lymphovascular invasion. She underwent a lumpectomy and sentinel lymph node biopsy, finding a 1.9-cm tumor with negative resection margins, and 0/2 sentinel lymph nodes involved. She comes to your clinic for systemic therapy recommendations. Which option is least acceptable for her?
   A. Adriamycin/cyclophosphamide every 3 weeks for four cycles
   B. Adriamycin/cyclophosphamide every 2 weeks for four cycles followed by weekly paclitaxel × 12 weeks
   C. Docetaxel/cyclophosphamide every 3 weeks for four cycles
   D. Carboplatin/paclitaxel every 3 weeks for six cycles
   E. Adriamycin/cyclophosphamide every 2 weeks for four cycles followed by paclitaxel every 2 weeks for four cycles

9. A 48-year-old woman was diagnosed with a right-sided T1cN2 breast cancer, negative for ER and PR and positive for HER2. She underwent upfront lumpectomy and axillary lymph node dissection followed by adjuvant systemic therapy consisting of Adriamycin, cyclophosphamide, paclitaxel, and trastuzumab, as well as radiation therapy completed 1 year ago. She has done very well and returns to the clinic for a follow-up visit. She asks how she should be monitored, and you reply:
   A. Annual visit with physical exam, annual mammogram, and annual PET-CT
   B. Visit every 6 months with a physical exam, every 6 month tumor markers every 6 months, and an annual PET-CT
   C. Annual mammogram, a visit every 6 months with a physical exam, and a routine pap smear
   D. PET-CT every 6 months, annual brain MRI, and an annual visit with a physical exam
   E. Mammogram every 6 months, annual tumor markers, and an annual echocardiogram

10. A 68-year-old woman with a history of a T1cN0 ER-positive, PR-positive, HER2-negative breast cancer has been maintained on aromatase inhibitor for the past 2 years. She is 5′5″ and weighs 185 pounds. She comes for routine follow-up and asks what she can best be doing to optimize her breast cancer care. You tell her:
    A. Try to lose weight, increase dietary fiber, and avoid all alcohol
    B. Perform weight-bearing exercise, eat organic whenever possible, and try to lose weight
    C. Try to lose weight, perform weight-bearing exercise, and take calcium and vitamin D
    D. Take calcium and vitamin D, try to lose weight, and avoid aluminum deodorants
    E. Avoid all alcohol, perform weight-bearing exercise, and eat organic whenever possible

11. A premenopausal 45-year-old woman is found to have a screen-detected T1bN0 breast cancer, ER+/PR+, HER2 negative. She elects to have a bilateral mastectomy with ipsilateral sentinel lymph node biopsy, which identifies a 6-mm grade 1 invasive ductal carcinoma and a negative sentinel lymph node. Which of the following is the preferred treatment option?
    A. Adjuvant aromatase inhibitor and ovarian suppression × 5 years
    B. Adjuvant raloxifene × 5 years
    C. Observation only
    D. Adjuvant tamoxifen × 5 years
    E. Adjuvant fulvestrant × 5 years

12. A 39-year-old premenopausal woman presents with a left-sided breast cancer. She undergoes surgical resection finding a 2.4-cm grade 2, ER-positive, PR-positive, HER2-negative invasive ductal carcinoma with lymphovascular invasion, and a negative sentinel lymph node. A 21-gene recurrence score test is sent, returning with a high score of 31. What is the best systemic management for this patient?
    A. Ovarian suppression and tamoxifen × 5 years
    B. Ovarian suppression and aromatase inhibitor × 5 years
    C. 10 years of tamoxifen therapy
    D. Adriamycin/cyclophosphamide × 4 cycles + paclitaxel × 4 cycles, followed by at least 5 years of aromatase inhibitor therapy alone
    E. Docetaxel/cyclophosphamide × 4 cycles, followed by up to 10 years of adjuvant endocrine therapy

13. A 32-year-old woman presented with a superficial palpable left breast lesion. On examination the mass was 4 cm, and a biopsy showed a high-grade breast cancer, that was ER and PR negative and HER2 1+, FISH 1.3. She proceeded

with preoperative chemotherapy and received Adriamycin/cyclophosphamide for four cycles and paclitaxel for four cycles, followed by a mastectomy and sentinel lymph node biopsy. Pathology shows a pathologic complete response. She received postmastectomy radiotherapy and has been in observation. Her menses stopped during treatment but resumed about 6 months after chemotherapy. She comes in for a follow-up visit 2 years after completion of chemotherapy. She is interested in trying to get pregnant. How do you advise her?

A. Due to her history of chemotherapy exposure, she should proceed with a cycle of IVF and preimplantation genetic analysis of fertilized embryos.

B. Pregnancy after a breast cancer diagnosis is not safe at any time and is discouraged.

C. She should not become pregnant as that will require an unacceptable stoppage in adjuvant endocrine therapy.

D. She can attempt pregnancy at any time.

E. It is suggested that she wait 5 years after completion of chemotherapy before attempting pregnancy.

14. A 28-year-old woman presented to her primary care doctor with a right breast mass that persisted through three menstrual cycles. A mammogram was not interpretable due to dense breast tissue, and an ultrasound showed a 2.5-cm breast mass with associated left axillary lymphadenopathy. A core biopsy of the breast mass was obtained, showing invasive ductal carcinoma, grade 3, ER/PR negative, HER2 2+ by immunohistochemistry, with a FISH ratio of 4.3 and a HER2 copy number of 9.5. She reports a family history of breast cancer in a paternal aunt at age 35, a history of a brain tumor in that aunt's child at age 10, and a history of a bone cancer in a paternal grandmother. She is referred for genetic testing. What is the most likely genetic abnormality identified?

A. BRCA1 mutation

B. BRCA2 mutation

C. APC mutation

D. p53 mutation

E. PALB2 mutation

15. A 63-year-old woman presented with a left breast mass, which on biopsy was found to be a high-grade invasive ductal carcinoma, negative for ER/PR and HER2 0. She completed upfront surgery, finding a 5.3-cm high-grade cancer with extensive lymphovascular invasion and two involved axillary lymph nodes. Systemic staging is negative for distant metastatic disease. Anthracycline-containing adjuvant chemotherapy is planned (cumulating dose 240 mg/m^2). She has a history of hypertension, but is very active and exercises 3 times a week at the gym. Which prechemotherapy cardiac evaluation is preferred?

A. Baseline cardiac MRI with baseline troponin and brain natriuretic peptide levels

B. Baseline cardiac stress test with cardiac catheterization if abnormal

C. Baseline echocardiogram with cardiooncology consultation if ejection fraction is less than 55%

D. No baseline cardiac evaluation needed

E. Initiation of dexrazoxane prior to anthracycline exposure

16. A 52-year-old woman presents with right axillary discomfort. On examination there are multiple enlarged right axillary lymph nodes and a 5-cm palpable right breast mass. A biopsy of the breast mass shows high-grade invasive breast cancer, negative for ER/PR, and HER2 3+. A fine needle aspiration of an axillary node is positive as well. Systemic staging is negative for evidence of metastatic disease. What are the preferred approaches for this patient?

A. Upfront surgical resection and axillary lymph node dissection, followed by adjuvant Adriamycin/cyclophosphamide for four cycles and weekly paclitaxel and trastuzumab/pertuzumab × 12 weeks, with completion of 1 year of adjuvant trastuzumab

B. Preoperative dose dense Adriamycin/cyclophosphamide for four cycles + paclitaxel for four cycles, followed by surgery, with 1 year of adjuvant trastuzumab

C. Preoperative radiotherapy, followed by surgery, then adjuvant Adriamycin/cyclophosphamide for four cycles + weekly paclitaxel and trastuzumab × 12 weeks, with completion of 1 year of adjuvant trastuzumab

D. Preoperative weekly paclitaxel with trastuzumab and pertuzumab for 12 weeks, followed by surgery, then adjuvant Adriamycin/cyclophosphamide for four cycles, followed by completion of a year of trastuzumab

E. Preoperative docetaxel/carboplatin/trastuzumab/pertuzumab for six cycles, followed by surgery, then completion of 1 year of trastuzumab

17. A 32-year-old woman presents for a prenatal evaluation at 14 weeks gestation. She mentions breast asymmetry; on examination, a mass is noted in the right breast, which is fixed to the chest wall and confirmed as a 4-cm solid lesion on a subsequent ultrasound. A biopsy is performed showing invasive ductal carcinoma that is high grade and negative for ER/PR and HER2. Her axilla is clinically negative, and a chest x-ray and right upper quadrant ultrasound are negative for metastatic involvement. What is the preferred next step?

A. Complete a modified radical mastectomy, defer on further anticancer therapy until completion of the pregnancy, then initiate adjuvant Adriamycin/cyclophosphamide for four cycles + weekly paclitaxel × 12 weeks

B. Terminate the pregnancy, then initiate preoperative Adriamycin/cyclophosphamide for four cycles + weekly paclitaxel, followed by surgical resection

C. Initiate preoperative Adriamycin/cyclophosphamide for four cycles, induce delivery early to facilitate continuation of anticancer therapy with weekly paclitaxel, followed by surgical resection

D. Initiate preoperative Adriamycin/cyclophosphamide for four cycles + weekly paclitaxel × 12 weeks, holding chemotherapy at 36 weeks gestation to await delivery, followed by surgical resection

E. Complete a modified radical mastectomy, then initiate adjuvant Adriamycin/cyclophosphamide for four cycles + weekly paclitaxel, holding chemotherapy at 36 weeks to await delivery, then completing 12 weeks after delivery

18. A 58-year-old woman with no family history of breast cancer presents to her primary care doctor with a left breast mass. On examination, the mass is 4 cm in size, and there are no skin changes or clinically apparent regional lymphadenopathy. A core biopsy is performed, showing invasive ductal carcinoma, grade 3, and negative for ER/PR and HER2. Staging studies including CT scans of the chest, abdomen, and pelvis show no definitive evidence of metastatic breast cancer. An upfront mastectomy is suggested by surgical oncology; however, the patient expresses a preference for breast conservation if possible, and neoadjuvant therapy is discussed. What preoperative systemic therapy regimen do you recommend for this patient to maximize her survival?

A. Carboplatin and paclitaxel × 12 weeks, followed by Adriamycin/cyclophosphamide every 2 weeks for four cycles, followed by surgical resection

B. Adriamycin/cyclophosphamide for four cycles, followed by weekly paclitaxel × 12 weeks, followed by surgical resection

C. Preoperative weekly paclitaxel with trastuzumab and pertuzumab for 12 weeks, followed by surgery, then adjuvant Adriamycin/cyclophosphamide every 3 weeks for four cycles, followed by completion of 1 year of trastuzumab

D. Cisplatin every 3 weeks for four cycles, followed by surgical resection, followed by Adriamycin/cyclophosphamide every 2 weeks for four cycles

E. Adriamycin/cyclophosphamide for four cycles, followed by weekly paclitaxel × 12 weeks, followed by surgical resection, followed by 12 weeks of weekly carboplatin in combination with poly (adenosine diphosphate [ADP]-ribose) polymerase (PARP) inhibitor in a setting of residual disease

19. A 78-year-old woman presents after her daughter noted a left breast mass while shopping with her mother. On examination, an 8-cm mass was noted with skin dimpling and nipple inversion, as well as slight skin erythema over the lesion. The ipsilateral axilla was clinically negative. The woman said she had noticed breast heaviness several months ago, but had not yet sought out care. A biopsy was performed, confirming invasive ductal cancer, grade 1, strongly positive for ER and PR and negative for HER2. The preferred treatment option for this patient is:

A. Upfront mastectomy and sentinel lymph node biopsy

B. Preoperative CMF for six cycles, then surgical resection

C. Preoperative aromatase inhibitor for at least 6 months, then determine surgical resectability

D. Preoperative Adriamycin/cyclophosphamide followed by weekly paclitaxel prior to surgery

E. Preoperative radiotherapy, then attempt at surgical resection

20. A 48-year-old man presents to his primary care doctor with a chest wall mass noted while showering at the gym. Further imaging showed a 4-cm mass adherent to the pectoralis muscle, and regional enlarged lymph nodes. A biopsy is obtained showing invasive ductal carcinoma, grade 2, positive for ER and PR, and negative for HER2. A fine needle aspiration of an ipsilateral axillary lymph node confirms involvement with carcinoma; systemic staging studies are negative. He proceeds with preoperative Adriamycin/cyclophosphamide followed by paclitaxel, and then undergoes a mastectomy and axillary lymph node dissection. Pathology shows residual invasive disease with 60% tumor regression, 2 of 14 axillary nodes involved, and 2 additional nodes with evidence of fibrosis. Adjuvant postmastectomy radiotherapy is planned. What is the preferred adjuvant therapy plan?

A. Tamoxifen for 5–10 years

B. Two years of palbociclib in combination with tamoxifen, then continuation of tamoxifen up to 10 years

C. Capecitabine × 18 weeks, followed by tamoxifen for up to 10 years

D. Cisplatin every 3 weeks for four cycles, followed by tamoxifen for up to 10 years

E. Observation only

21. A 62-year-old woman was treated 3 years ago for a stage 2 triple negative (ER/PR−, HER2−) breast cancer. She underwent a lumpectomy and sentinel lymph node biopsy, followed by adjuvant anthracycline/cyclophosphamide (Adriamycin 60 mg/m², cyclophosphamide 600 mg/m²) × 4 and taxane-containing chemotherapy, as well as adjuvant radiotherapy. She now presents for routine follow-up after her annual mammogram found an ipsilateral breast mass. A biopsy is obtained showing triple negative breast cancer, morphologically similar to her disease 3 years ago. She undergoes a mastectomy and axillary lymph node dissection that finds 2.7-cm invasive disease at the prior surgical site with a negative deep margin and no involved axillary lymph nodes. Systemic staging is negative for metastatic disease. What is the next best step for her?

A. Observation

B. Adriamycin/cyclophosphamide for four cycles

C. Epirubicin/5-FU/cyclophosphamide for four cycles

D. Docetaxel/cyclophosphamide for four cycles

E. Trial of aromatase inhibitor

22. A 72-year-old woman with a history of stage 3 ER+/HER2 negative invasive ductal breast cancer presented to your office with a complaint of a new chest wall lesion. She had been originally diagnosed 4 years prior and, after a mastectomy and completion of adjuvant anthracycline-based chemotherapy and radiotherapy, she recovered well and had been maintained on adjuvant anastrozole. On examination a hard fixed nodule was present near the mastectomy scar. A biopsy confirmed recurrent ER/PR+ HER2 negative grade 1 invasive breast cancer.

Best options for her:

A. Upfront surgical resection to achieve negative margins with skin grafting as necessary, followed by adjuvant capecitabine x 4 months, followed by adjuvant exemestane

B. Preoperative endocrine therapy with tamoxifen for 4-6 months, followed by surgical resection to negative margins, followed by continuation of adjuvant endocrine therapy

C. Preoperative CMF chemotherapy x 6 months, followed by surgical resection to negative margins, followed by continuation of endocrine therapy

D. Preoperative capecitabine x 4 months, followed by surgical resection to negative margins, followed by adjuvant tamoxifen

E. Upfront surgical resection to achieve negative margins with skin grafting as necessary, followed by adjuvant exemestane

23. The following patients present with a breast cancer diagnosis, and are without systemic complaints. In which settings is systemic staging recommended?

A. A 32-year-old woman with a diagnosis of resected 5-cm unilateral ductal carcinoma in situ, HER2 positive, with comedonecrosis

B. A 41-year-old woman with a diagnosis of bilateral breast cancer: on the right, 1.5-cm grade 3 with extensive lymphovascular invasion, N0, ER−/PR−/HER2−; on the left, 2.0-cm grade 2 disease, ER+/PR+/HER2 negative, with a micrometastatic deposit in 1 of 1 sentinel lymph nodes

C. A 55-year-old woman found to have a mammographic density, biopsy-proven grade 3 invasive ductal carcinoma, ER, PR, and HER2 positive, confirmed as 2.3 cm in size on MRI, surrounded by an additional 4 cm of non-mass-like enhancement, and with at least two abnormal appearing ipsilateral axillary lymph nodes

D. A 44-year-old woman who undergoes a mastectomy finding a 3-cm encapsulated papillary carcinoma, ER+/PR+/HER2−, without nodal sampling

E. A 52-year-old woman with a history of a stage 1 grade 2 breast cancer, with a 21-gene recurrence score of 20, in her right breast treated with breast-conserving surgery, adjuvant radiotherapy, and adjuvant tamoxifen, now with a new 3.0-cm mass in the ipsilateral breast 3 years later, biopsy proven to be recurrent grade 2 disease, ER+/PR+/HER2−

24. A 32-year-old premenopausal woman palpated a right breast mass that was determined to be a grade 3 invasive ductal carcinoma. Estrogen receptors were positive, progesterone receptors were negative, and HER2 was negative. On examination, the mass was located at the upper outer quadrant of the left breast, was mobile, and the right axilla did not contain palpable lymph nodes. The patient would like to undergo breast conservation surgery, but was told that the primary tumor size, 3.8 cm, was too large to obtain an adequate cosmetic outcome, given the small size of her breast. What is her best therapeutic option?
   A. Receive neoadjuvant chemotherapy with four cycles of doxorubicin and cyclophosphamide followed by four cycles of paclitaxel
   B. Receive neoadjuvant endocrine therapy with anastrozole for 6 months
   C. Receive neoadjuvant endocrine therapy with tamoxifen for 6 months
   D. Receive neoadjuvant radiation followed by breast-conserving surgery
   E. Mastectomy with axillary lymph node dissection

25. A 43-year-old premenopausal woman palpated a mass in the left breast prior to initiating screening mammography. A diagnostic mammogram showed a 2.5-cm spiculated mass with extensive calcifications over a 5-cm area. An ultrasound of the left breast demonstrated a 3.5-cm hypoechoic mass with prominent left axillary adenopathy. A core biopsy of the left breast mass demonstrated an invasive ductal carcinoma, grade 3, which was ER positive, PR negative, and HER2 positive by FISH with a ratio of 3.4. An FNA of the left axillary lymph node was positive for carcinoma. Staging studies including a CT scan of the chest, abdomen, and pelvis and bone scan were negative for distant disease but confirmed left axillary adenopathy and a left breast mass. Which of the following is the most appropriate treatment option?
   A. Preoperative therapy with trastuzumab, pertuzumab, and a taxane-containing regimen
   B. Breast conservation surgery with sentinel lymph node sampling
   C. Preoperative therapy with an anthracycline and cyclophosphamide combination
   D. Preoperative therapy with tamoxifen
   E. Preoperative therapy with tamoxifen and trastuzumab

26. A 60-year-old woman was found to have a 2.2-cm, grade 3, invasive ductal carcinoma after undergoing her routine mammographic screening exam, which she has been diligent in obtaining because of a family history of breast cancer. She wishes to undergo breast-conserving therapy and therefore underwent an excisional biopsy and sentinel lymph node sampling, which found two of three axillary lymph nodes involved with disease and the medial margin was involved with ductal carcinoma in situ. The maximum dimension of involvement in the nodes was 3 mm, and there was no extracapsular extension. The invasive ductal carcinoma was estrogen receptor negative, progesterone receptor negative, and HER2 negative. What is the next best step in the management of her disease?
   A. Genetic testing to determine whether she carries the BRCA 1 mutation
   B. A completion axillary lymph node dissection
   C. Adjuvant chemotherapy with paclitaxel and carboplatin for four cycles

   D. Oncotype DX analysis to determine whether she would benefit from adjuvant chemotherapy
   E. Surgical re-excision of the biopsy cavity to obtain negative margins

27. A 51-year-old postmenopausal woman underwent a screening mammogram that showed architectural distortion within the right breast. Same-day targeted ultrasound showed two areas of hypoechoic density, one at the 11 o'clock position measuring 8 × 7 × 4 mm, the other at the 4 o'clock position measuring 1.0 × 0.9 cm. She underwent a core needle biopsy of both areas with the pathology revealing invasive lobular carcinoma, well differentiated, with no lymphatic vascular invasion. Estrogen receptors were positive, progesterone receptors were positive, and HER2 was negative. Which of the following is the most appropriate next step in her management?
   A. Separate wire localized excisions of the sites of invasive carcinoma with sentinel lymph node sampling
   B. Preoperative endocrine therapy with an aromatase inhibitor for 6 months
   C. Preoperative radiation therapy to the breast followed by breast-conserving surgery
   D. Mastectomy with sentinel lymph node sampling
   E. Preoperative chemotherapy with doxorubicin and cyclophosphamide

28. A 53-year-old postmenopausal woman underwent a screening mammogram demonstrating a spiculated density within the right breast. Diagnostic mammogram confirmed the spiculated density at the 1 o'clock position and a targeted ultrasound demonstrated a 1.5-cm hypoechoic mass corresponding to the mammographic change. An ultrasound of the right axilla was negative for lymph node enlargement. A core biopsy of the mass confirmed invasive ductal carcinoma, grade 3, ER positive, PR negative, and HER2 negative. She opted to undergo breast-conserving surgery, removing a 2.0-cm, grade 3, invasive ductal carcinoma with focal lymphovascular invasion. Estrogen receptors were positive, progesterone receptors were negative, and HER2/neu was negative. Zero of 3 sentinel lymph nodes were involved with disease. An evaluation of the overlying skin demonstrated dermal lymphatic involvement with cancer. The invasive carcinoma was within 3 mm of the surgical margins, and ductal carcinoma in situ was within 2 mm of the surgical margins. Which of the following is true regarding the local therapy of this condition?
   A. This stage of this disease is T4d, N0.
   B. A complete axillary lymph node dissection is now indicated.
   C. A completion mastectomy with an axillary lymph node dissection is now indicated.
   D. Radiation to the breast is now indicated.
   E. An immediate reconstruction at the time of mastectomy is contraindicated.

29. A 38-year-old premenopausal woman palpated a left breast mass, which was demonstrated by mammogram to be a 2.5-cm spiculated density in the upper outer quadrant. She underwent breast-conservation surgery that revealed a 3.0-cm, grade 2, invasive ductal carcinoma, which involved 1 of 3 sentinel lymph nodes. The invasive carcinoma was estrogen receptor positive, progesterone receptor positive, and HER2 positive. She received adjuvant carboplatin, docetaxel, and trastuzumab for six cycles, and continued with maintenance trastuzumab to complete 1 year of trastuzumab therapy. Although she was menstruating regularly prior to chemotherapy,

her menses stopped after her first cycle of treatment. It is now 1 month after completing her chemotherapy and she has not resumed her menses. Which of the following statements is correct?

A. She is now postmenopausal due to the effects of chemotherapy.
B. Endocrine therapy is not beneficial as long as she is receiving trastuzumab.
C. Endocrine therapy with tamoxifen therapy is not beneficial because she is not menstruating.
D. Her menstrual function may return up to 1 year following discontinuation of chemotherapy.
E. She should begin endocrine therapy with an aromatase inhibitor.

30. A 64-year-old postmenopausal woman was interested in breast augmentation and consulted a plastic surgeon who palpated an abnormality within the left breast. She had a diagnostic mammogram that was unremarkable, but an ultrasound confirmed the presence of a hypoechoic nodule at the 6:00 position measuring 1.9 cm. An ultrasound-guided biopsy revealed an invasive ductal carcinoma, grade I, associated with DCIS. She subsequently underwent an MRI of the breast that demonstrated the abnormality within the left breast with a normal right breast. The patient opted for a left mastectomy and implant reconstruction, which revealed an invasive ductal carcinoma, grade I, measuring 1.1 centimeters. Lymphovascular invasion was present, and 1 of 3 sentinel lymph nodes were involved. The estrogen receptors were positive, progesterone receptors were positive, and HER2 was negative. An Oncotype DX analysis was requested, and the results showed a recurrence score of 15. She began anastrozole endocrine therapy and has tolerated this treatment for the past 5 years. What is the next best step in management?

A. Discontinue anastrozole and begin tamoxifen for 5 years
B. Discontinue anastrozole because she has completed 5 years of treatment
C. Continue anastrozole to complete 10 years of treatment.
D. Bilateral salpingo-oophorectomy now followed by tamoxifen for 5 years
E. Fulvestrant for 5 years

31. A 49-year-old postmenopausal woman felt a right breast mass for 2–3 months prior to seeking the attention of her primary care physician. Breast imaging was performed with the following results: a mammogram showed a spiculated mass and calcifications in the area of palpable density within the right breast, and a right breast ultrasound confirmed a solid mass measuring 1.7 cm. A core biopsy of the mass showed invasive ductal carcinoma, ER positive, PR positive, and HER2 2+, but negative by FISH with a ratio of 1.8. She underwent breast-conserving surgery, and the pathology revealed a 2.6-cm, grade 3, invasive ductal carcinoma, with isolated lymphovascular invasion, and metastatic involvement in 2 of 6 axillary lymph nodes. Repeat markers on the invasive carcinoma confirmed ER positive, PR positive, and HER2 2+, but the FISH was positive with a ratio of 9.35. Which of the following is the most appropriate treatment option for adjuvant chemotherapy?

A. Doxorubicin and cyclophosphamide for four cycles followed by trastuzumab, lapatinib, and paclitaxel for 12 weeks, followed by trastuzumab and lapatinib to complete 1 year
B. Doxorubicin and cyclophosphamide for four cycles followed by trastuzumab, pertuzumab, and paclitaxel for 12 weeks, followed by trastuzumab and pertuzumab to complete 1 year

C. Doxorubicin and cyclophosphamide for four cycles followed by trastuzumab and paclitaxel for 12 weeks, followed by trastuzumab to complete 1 year
D. Doxorubicin and cyclophosphamide for four cycles followed by paclitaxel for 12 weeks
E. Doxorubicin and cyclophosphamide for four cycles followed by weekly paclitaxel and carboplatin for 12 weeks

32. A 48-year-old premenopausal woman presented for her routine screening mammogram, which demonstrated microcalcifications in the upper central left breast without a suspicious mass. Diagnostic imaging confirmed suspicious calcifications, prompting a stereotactic biopsy that revealed invasive ductal carcinoma, grade 2, with a focus suspicious for lymphovascular invasion. She underwent a left wire localized excisional biopsy and sentinel lymph node sampling, which revealed a grade 3 invasive ductal carcinoma measuring 0.9 cm without lymphovascular invasion. The carcinoma was estrogen receptor positive and progesterone receptor positive as well as HER2 +3+ by IHC. Both of the two left axillary sentinel lymph nodes were negative. In addition to radiation therapy to the left breast, which of the following is the most appropriate next treatment option?

A. Ovarian suppression with goserelin and tamoxifen for 10 years
B. Doxorubicin and cyclophosphamide for four cycles followed by weekly paclitaxel for 12 weeks with trastuzumab followed by maintenance trastuzumab to complete 1 year
C. Weekly paclitaxel for 12 weeks with trastuzumab followed by maintenance trastuzumab to complete 1 year
D. Trastuzumab given concurrent with doxorubicin and cyclophosphamide for four cycles followed by weekly paclitaxel for 12 weeks followed by continued trastuzumab to complete 1 year
E. Trastuzumab for 1 year given concurrent with ovarian suppression with goserelin and tamoxifen for 10 years

33. A 52-year-old premenopausal woman palpated a mass within the left breast and brought this to the attention of her primary care provider. A diagnostic mammogram demonstrated a new density measuring 1.5 cm at the 6 o'clock position in the right breast. A same-day targeted ultrasound confirmed the 6 o'clock density as well as a separate satellite lesion approximately 4 cm away from the 1.5-cm mass. She underwent a biopsy of both lesions, and the pathology revealed an invasive ductal carcinoma, grade 2, with lymphovascular invasion. She subsequently underwent a right completion mastectomy and axillary lymph node dissection showing multifocal invasive ductal carcinoma, one focus measuring 1.5 cm and the second focus measuring 1.2 cm. Both were estrogen receptor positive, progesterone receptor positive, and HER2 negative. One of 16 lymph nodes was positive for disease, which measured 0.9 cm. She received adjuvant chemotherapy with doxorubicin and cyclophosphamide for four cycles followed by paclitaxel for four cycles, and then began tamoxifen. She has now been on tamoxifen for 5 years and has been amenorrheic since initiating chemotherapy. What is the next best step in management?

A. Discontinue tamoxifen, having completed 5 years of adjuvant endocrine therapy
B. Discontinue tamoxifen and begin extended endocrine therapy with letrozole for 5 years
C. Continue tamoxifen to complete 10 years of adjuvant endocrine therapy

D. Undergo bilateral salpingo-oophorectomy, and begin letrozole for 5 years

E. Continue tamoxifen and add letrozole for 5 years to complete 10 years of endocrine therapy

34. A 66-year-old postmenopausal woman underwent a screening mammogram demonstrating heterogeneously dense parenchyma with an area of architectural distortion in the lower inner quadrant of the right breast. Diagnostic imaging confirmed this area of distortion, and a targeted ultrasound of this area revealed a 1.0-cm hypoechoic density. She underwent an ultrasound-guided biopsy of the right breast revealing invasive ductal carcinoma. The patient subsequently underwent breast-conserving surgery, and the pathology contained a 1.6-cm invasive carcinoma with ductal and lobular features, grade 2, with focal lymphovascular invasion. Estrogen receptors were positive, progesterone receptors positive, and HER2 was negative. One of three sentinel lymph nodes was involved with micrometastatic disease measuring 0.6 mm. What is the most appropriate next step in management?

A. Initiate adjuvant chemotherapy with doxorubicin and cyclophosphamide for four cycles

B. Initiate adjuvant endocrine therapy with anastrozole for 5 years

C. Request an Oncotype DX analysis on the primary tumor

D. Initiate radiation to the breast followed by adjuvant endocrine therapy with anastrozole for 5 years

E. Initiate adjuvant chemotherapy with weekly paclitaxel for 12 weeks

35. A 51-year-old premenopausal woman felt a thickening within the right breast for approximately 1 year prior to palpating a discrete mass at the 1 o'clock position. She contacted her primary care physician who arranged for a diagnostic mammogram, which was unremarkable. She had undergone routine mammography since the age of 40 because of a family history of breast cancer including her mother diagnosed with breast cancer at age 37, her maternal grandmother diagnosed with breast cancer at age 40, and her maternal aunt diagnosed with breast cancer at age 41. A targeted ultrasound of the right breast confirmed a solid density corresponding to the palpable mass, prompting a biopsy that revealed a grade 1 invasive lobular carcinoma. A magnetic resonance imaging (MRI) scan of the breasts showed a 7-cm area of nonmass-like enhancement corresponding to the biopsy site. She subsequently underwent a right mastectomy and sentinel lymph node sampling revealing multifocal, grade 2, invasive lobular carcinoma, ranging in size from 1.0 to 2.5 cm, over a 9-cm area, without lymphovascular invasion. Estrogen receptors were positive, progesterone receptors were positive, HER-2 was negative, and six axillary lymph nodes were removed without evidence of disease. Which of the following is the most appropriate intervention?

A. Perform a left prophylactic mastectomy

B. Administer radiation therapy to the right chest wall and regional lymph nodes

C. Administer adjuvant chemotherapy with Adriamycin and cyclophosphamide ×4 cycles followed by paclitaxel for four cycles

D. Obtain an Oncotype DX analysis on the largest focus of cancer

E. Perform a bilateral salpingo-oophorectomy

36. A 43-year-old premenopausal woman presented with an 8-week history of right breast pain associated with nipple inversion. Bilateral mammogram showed dense breast parenchyma and nipple inversion associated with

an ill-defined mass measuring 3.4 cm at the 9 o'clock position of the right breast. She underwent a biopsy of the right breast, which revealed a grade 2, invasive ductal carcinoma with lobular features, which was estrogen receptor positive, progesterone receptor positive, and HER2 negative. She underwent a right mastectomy which contained a 4.1-cm, grade 2, invasive carcinoma with ductal and lobular features, involving 1 of 6 axillary lymph nodes. She received adjuvant chemotherapy with dose-dense doxorubicin and cyclophosphamide for four cycles followed by dose-dense paclitaxel for four cycles, and is now anticipating postmastectomy radiation therapy. Her last menstrual period was on the day of her surgery; however, a recent estradiol level was 86 pmol/L. Which of the following is the most appropriate treatment option?

A. Tamoxifen for 2 years followed by an aromatase inhibitor for 3 years

B. Ovarian suppression with exemestane for 5 years

C. An aromatase inhibitor for 5 years

D. An aromatase inhibitor for 5 years with zoledronic acid given twice annually

E. Tamoxifen for 5 years with zoledronic acid given twice annually

37. A 52-year-old premenopausal woman was recently diagnosed with a 1.3-cm, grade 1, invasive lobular carcinoma of the right breast. She had breast-conserving surgery and sentinel lymph node sampling that revealed 0 of 3 sentinel lymph nodes involved. An Oncotype DX Recurrence Score was 5, and she therefore opted to receive adjuvant tamoxifen. Her last menses was during her surgery, and she is now seeing you at her 6-month follow-up after completing radiation therapy. The purpose of her office visit is to discuss her treatment plan and long-term follow-up. You discuss performing a physical exam every 6 months for 3 years, followed by annual visits. Which of the following statements is correct concerning her scheduled follow-up screening?

A. She will have annual CT and bone scans.

B. She will have annual bilateral mammograms.

C. She will have annual bilateral mammograms and bone density evaluation every 2 years.

D. She will have annual bilateral mammograms and transvaginal ultrasound every 6 months.

E. She will have transvaginal ultrasounds, CBC, differential, liver function tests, and a basic metabolic panel every 6 months.

38. A 55-year-old postmenopausal woman was recently diagnosed with a 1.7-cm, grade 1, invasive lobular carcinoma of the left breast. Zero of three sentinel lymph nodes were involved with the disease, and the cancer was estrogen receptor positive, progesterone receptor positive, and HER2 negative. She underwent breast-conserving surgery, and an Oncotype DX analysis was sent, which revealed a recurrence score of 10. She has now completed radiation therapy to the right breast and is about to initiate adjuvant endocrine therapy with anastrozole. Which of the following statements is correct?

A. Aromatase inhibitors are associated with an increased risk of thrombosis.

B. Aromatase inhibitors increase bone density.

C. Aromatase inhibitors may cause vaginal dryness and loss of sexual desire.

D. Low-dose estrogens can be given with aromatase inhibitors to alleviate hot flashes.

E. Aromatase inhibitors are associated with weight gain.

39. A 37-year-old premenopausal woman recently delivered a baby and breastfed for 1 year. She noted that after discontinuing breastfeeding, the left breast returned to its baseline size and consistency but the right breast remained engorged and slightly pink. She discussed these changes with her Ob/Gyn who recommended breast imaging and performed a mammogram. The mammogram demonstrated heterogeneous dense breast tissue with skin thickening but no discrete mass. A right breast ultrasound performed on the same day confirmed a 1.9-cm mass at the 6 o'clock position with surrounding edematous tissue and right axillary adenopathy, the largest lymph node measuring 4.5 cm. An ultrasound-guided biopsy of the right breast contained a grade 3, invasive ductal carcinoma that was ER negative, PR negative, and HER2 negative. Which of the following statements is true regarding this condition?

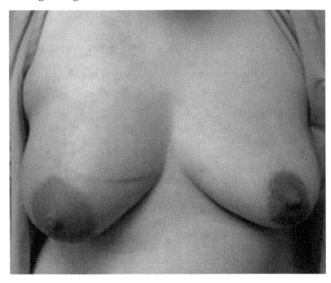

A. Chemotherapy is administered prior to surgery.
B. An adequate disease response to preoperative chemotherapy allows for breast-conserving surgery.
C. A skin biopsy is necessary to confirm the diagnosis of this disease.
D. This subtype of breast cancer is often associated with a PALB2 mutation.
E. This subtype of breast cancer is never seen in male patients.

40. An 83-year-old woman was found to have enlargement of the left breast with a patch of erythema and nipple inversion during a massage therapy session. This prompted a visit to her primary care physician who had been treating her for hypertension, diabetes, and congestive heart failure. The patient states that she noted changes within the left breast over the past 6–9 months; however, her last mammogram was 5 years ago. A diagnostic mammogram demonstrated marked nipple inversion with a diffuse pattern of distortion within the center and

a nodular density in the lower outer quadrant of the left breast. A targeted ultrasound confirmed a poorly defined hypoechoic area with associated skin thickening. She denied any pain, nipple discharge, or other symptoms. An ultrasound-guided core biopsy of the breast mass confirmed invasive lobular carcinoma, ER positive, PR positive, HER2 negative. The patient had been living with her daughter because of worsening hearing loss and early dementia. Which is the following is the most appropriate treatment option?

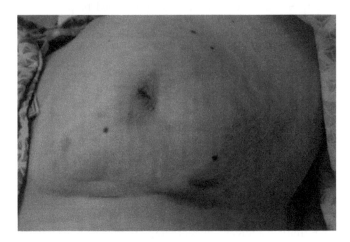

A. A complete right mastectomy with an axillary lymph node dissection
B. Radiation therapy to the right breast and regional lymph nodes
C. Chemotherapy with cyclophosphamide, methotrexate, and 5-fluorouracil for six cycles
D. Chemotherapy with doxorubicin and cyclophosphamide for four cycles
E. An aromatase inhibitor for at least 6 months

41. One month prior to undergoing her routine screening mammogram, a 70-year-old postmenopausal woman noted intermittent erythema and swelling of the right breast. She denied any palpable mass but developed pain within the right breast after her dog jumped on her chest and struck the right breast. Her subsequent routine screening mammogram showed microcalcifications within the right breast but no other abnormality. A stereotactic biopsy was performed and revealed invasive poorly differentiated carcinoma with mixed lobular and ductal features, which was estrogen receptor positive, progesterone receptor negative, and HER2 positive 3+ by IHC. MRI imaging of the breasts showed markedly thickened skin of the right breast associated with a 1.7-cm density with biopsy clip in place and multiple enlarged right axillary lymph nodes, right internal mammary lymph nodes, and subpectoral lymph nodes. There was extensive non-mass-like enhancement extending from the nipple to the chest wall measuring more than 9 cm diffusely. What is the most likely diagnosis?

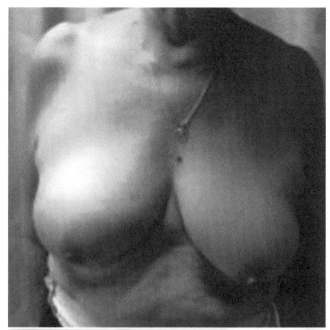

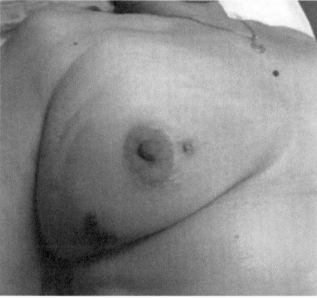

A. Neglected locally advanced breast cancer
B. Mastitis with concurrent diagnosis of invasive breast cancer
C. Inflammatory breast cancer
D. Stage II operable breast cancer
E. Trauma-associated invasive breast cancer

42. A 68-year-old postmenopausal woman noted a left breast mass for 1 year prior to discussing this with her primary care physician. She found that the mass waxed and waned in size and was otherwise asymptomatic. Breast imaging included a mammogram that demonstrated a spiculated density corresponding to the area of the palpable mass, with associated extensive calcifications measuring up to 7 cm. An ultrasound confirmed the density to be solid and 4.0 cm in size. Because of her family history of breast cancer, the patient's primary physician requested an MRI of the breast, which showed a 5.5-cm mass within the right breast with enhancement of the pectoralis muscle, with multiple enlarged right axillary lymph nodes.

A core biopsy of the mass confirmed an invasive ductal carcinoma grade 2, which was estrogen receptor positive, progesterone receptor positive, and HER2 negative by FISH (ratio = 1.4). An FNA of the right axillary lymph node confirmed carcinoma. Which option is true regarding this condition?
A. Preoperative chemotherapy is more likely to achieve breast conservation compared with endocrine therapy.
B. Preoperative chemotherapy improves survival compared with preoperative endocrine therapy.
C. Following preoperative treatment, mastectomy with radiation therapy is indicated.
D. Preoperative aromatase inhibitor can be used to achieve breast conservation.
E. Preoperative tamoxifen is more likely to downstage her cancer compared with an aromatase inhibitor.

43. A 66-year-old woman presented to her primary care physician with an upper respiratory infection and palpable right supraclavicular lymphadenopathy. A supraclavicular lymph node was subsequently biopsied and revealed a metastatic poorly differentiated carcinoma with squamous features. Estrogen receptors were negative, progesterone receptors negative, and HER2 was negative by FISH with a ratio of 1.2. A CT scan of the chest, abdomen, and pelvis demonstrated a large right breast mass measuring 6.1 cm, right axillary adenopathy, with the largest lymph node measuring 3.0 cm, and right subpectoral lymphadenopathy. There was no sign of distant metastases. A diagnostic mammogram and targeted ultrasound of the right breast localized the mass in the tail of the right breast, extending into the right axilla, which was associated with bulky right axillary adenopathy. A core biopsy of the right breast mass demonstrated a metaplastic carcinoma. During the workup of her disease, the patient developed significant right-arm lymphedema and needle-like pain with movement of the arm, extending into her right hand. What is the most appropriate next step in management?
A. Chemotherapy with doxorubicin and cyclophosphamide
B. Lymphedema therapy to the right arm
C. Radiation therapy to the right breast and regional lymph nodes
D. Radical mastectomy with axillary lymph node dissection
E. Endocrine therapy with anastrozole

44. A 48-year-old premenopausal woman palpated a mass within the left breast. This prompted a diagnostic mammogram, which showed asymmetry at the 2 o'clock position associated with a 9-mm hypoechoic mass demonstrated by ultrasound. An ultrasound-guided core biopsy of the mass revealed a grade 1 invasive ductal carcinoma that was estrogen receptor positive and progesterone receptor positive but HER2/neu negative. Because of the presence of breast augmentation and small breast size, she decided to undergo a mastectomy with implant reconstruction. The final pathology revealed a grade 1 invasive ductal carcinoma, measuring 1 cm, estrogen receptor and progesterone receptor positive, with HER2 negative, with 0 of 1 sentinel lymph node involved. She began tamoxifen but quickly discontinued it after 3 months because of emotional intolerance. Three years later, her oncologist palpated a small subcentimeter density along the lateral aspect of her implant and a subsequent biopsy confirmed adenocarcinoma, which was estrogen receptor positive, progesterone receptor positive, and HER2 negative. A CT of the chest,

abdomen, and pelvis and bone scan were both negative for systemic disease. Which of the following is the most appropriate intervention?
A. Surgical excision of the chest wall recurrence followed by radiation therapy
B. Radiation therapy to the chest wall followed by surgical excision of the chest wall recurrence
C. Ovarian suppression followed by tamoxifen
D. Doxorubicin and cyclophosphamide for four cycles followed by paclitaxel for four cycles followed by surgical excision of the chest wall recurrence
E. Paclitaxel weekly for 12 weeks followed by surgical excision of the chest wall recurrence

45. A 39-year-old premenopausal woman noted a mass within the right breast with some changes in the overlying skin prompting an evaluation by her gynecologist. Breast imaging was recommended, and a mammogram revealed calcifications over a 5-cm area associated with an irregular mass measuring 1.4 cm within the right breast. An ultrasound-guided biopsy of the mass revealed an invasive ductal carcinoma, grade 2, with positive estrogen and progesterone receptors, and negative for HER2. A second stereotactic biopsy of calcifications confirmed ductal carcinoma in situ. This prompted a right mastectomy with sentinel lymph node biopsy revealing a 2.5-cm invasive ductal carcinoma, grade 3, with an extensive intraductal component and lymphovascular invasion. One of two sentinel lymph nodes contained isolated tumor cells. An Oncotype DX Recurrence Score was 20. She opted to receive adjuvant ovarian suppression using goserelin and tamoxifen. Three years later she was found to have a right axillary mass, which was biopsied and confirmed to be a recurrence within an axillary lymph node. She underwent a completion axillary lymph node dissection, which revealed a 1.5-cm lymph node completely replaced by a poorly differentiated carcinoma that was ER and PR positive and HER2 negative. Staging studies including a CT scan of the chest, abdomen, and pelvis and bone scan were completely negative for distant disease. Which of the following is the most appropriate treatment option?
A. Discontinue goserelin and begin anastrozole for 5 years
B. Doxorubicin and cyclophosphamide for four cycles followed by paclitaxel for four cycles
C. Continue goserelin and tamoxifen to complete 10 years of treatment
D. Discontinue goserelin and begin monthly zoledronic acid with tamoxifen to complete 10 years of treatment
E. Doxorubicin and cyclophosphamide for four cycles

46. A 64-year-old postmenopausal woman was originally diagnosed with a 1.2-cm invasive ductal carcinoma, grade 1, involving the left breast in 1998. The carcinoma was estrogen receptor positive, progesterone receptor positive, and involved 0 of 24 axillary lymph nodes. She had undergone breast conservation surgery and axillary lymph node dissection and then received adjuvant CMF chemotherapy for 6 months followed by radiation to the left breast and tamoxifen for 5 years, which was completed in 2005. Her most recent screening mammogram, in 2016, revealed a spiculated density within the left breast confirmed by ultrasound to be a 1-cm hypoechoic mass. She underwent an ultrasound-guided core biopsy of the left breast revealing an invasive ductal carcinoma, grade 2, without lymphovascular invasion. Estrogen receptors were positive, progesterone receptors were positive, and

HER2 was negative. What is the next best step in management?
A. Continue with an additional 5 years of tamoxifen
B. Perform a completion mastectomy
C. Preoperative chemotherapy with doxorubicin and cyclophosphamide for four cycles
D. Breast conservation with an excision of the primary tumor
E. Radiation therapy to the breast

47. A 65-year-old male comes to see you to discuss adjuvant therapy for his recent diagnosis of breast cancer. He was diagnosed with a stage IIIC (pT2pN3a) left breast cancer that is ER 95%, PR 60%, and HER2 negative (ratio 1.0). He has no significant family history. He underwent a left modified radical mastectomy. This showed a 3-cm invasive ductal carcinoma, negative margins, and 19/19 positive axillary lymph nodes with the largest metastatic deposit of 2.5 cm and extracapsular extension. Staging studies with a CT scan of the chest, abdomen, and pelvis and bone scan did not reveal any site of distant metastasis. He has a history of hypercholesterolemia. His ECOG PS is 0. He works part time. He plays tennis twice a week. He is motivated to receive chemotherapy. What is the most appropriate treatment option?
A. Anthracycline- and taxane-based chemotherapy, followed by postmastectomy radiation and tamoxifen
B. Anthracycline- and taxane-based chemotherapy followed by tamoxifen
C. Taxane-based chemotherapy followed by postmastectomy radiation and tamoxifen
D. No chemotherapy, but recommend tamoxifen
E. No additional therapy

48. A 49-year-old male was diagnosed with a stage IIA (pT2N0) left breast cancer. He underwent a lumpectomy and sentinel lymph node biopsy. Per the pathology report, he has a 2.5-cm tumor, grade 3, ER5%, PR1%, and HER2:CEP17 ratio was 0.8 (nonamplified), negative margins, and 0/3 involved sentinel lymph nodes. He was treated with adjuvant docetaxel and cyclophosphamide for four cycles. He is asking you what happens next with regard to his treatment. Which of the following is the next most appropriate course of action?
A. Additional chemotherapy with anthracycline followed by radiation therapy
B. Radiation therapy alone
C. Radiation therapy followed by tamoxifen
D. Tamoxifen alone
E. No additional therapy

49. A 45-year-old premenopausal woman presents to your clinic for a second opinion. Three weeks ago, she felt a painless lump in her left breast, and she said it was enlarging over that time period. A mammogram and ultrasound described a 3.5-cm lobulated circumscribed mass and no axillary adenopathy. A core needle biopsy revealed a cellular biphasic neoplasm, suspicious for a phyllodes tumor. She then underwent an excisional biopsy, and this showed a 3.0-cm cellular fibroepithelial lesion with a circumscribed border, consistent with a benign phyllodes tumor. The surgical specimen revealed that the lesion abutted the margin of excision. She then underwent a wide local excision and there was a residual 1.0-cm phyllodes tumor that was greater than 1 cm from the margins. She presents to you for a consultation. Which of the following statements is true?

A. Surgical axillary staging and axillary dissection is indicated because the frequency of nodal disease in phyllodes tumor is high.

B. Adjuvant radiation therapy should be offered to this patient.

C. Patients with Li-Fraumeni syndrome (germline *TP53* mutation) experience an increased risk of developing phyllodes tumors.

D. There is evidence that adjuvant chemotherapy provides benefit in terms of reducing the risk of a recurrent phyllodes tumor.

50. An 80-year-old woman has a history of stage IA(pT1cN0) invasive ductal carcinoma of the breast diagnosed 8 years ago; it was ER positive, PR positive, and HER2 negative. She underwent a left lumpectomy and sentinel lymph node biopsy, and received adjuvant whole breast external beam radiation with a standard dose of 4680 cGy, followed by a boost of 1400 cGy to the lumpectomy cavity. She took tamoxifen for 5 years. She presents to your office describing a "new knot" in her left breast.

On physical exam, there is a well-healed lumpectomy scar in the upper outer quadrant. Inferolateral to the scar there is a 5-mm patch of erythema present. There is a 3-cm purple nodule lateral to the incision. There is no axillary adenopathy. A mammogram 6 months ago showed stable postoperative changes in the left breast. A punch biopsy was performed, and sections of skin demonstrated involvement of the dermis by high-grade neoplasm. Immunohistochemical stains demonstrate the tumor cells to be strongly positive for CD31 and negative for cytokeratin, ER, PR, and HER2.

Which of the following is the next most appropriate step for this patient?

A. Order CT scans of the chest, abdomen, and pelvis prior to surgical resection

B. Perform chemotherapy followed by surgery

C. Perform radiation therapy followed by surgery

D. Proceed with surgery

E. No additional action needed

51. A 55-year-old postmenopausal woman presents to your office for evaluation of her newly diagnosed left breast cancer. A mammogram and ultrasound showed a 3.0-cm irregularly shaped mass with spiculated margins in the left breast. A core biopsy showed a tubular carcinoma of the breast, ER 99%, PR 100%, and HER2 negative by FISH (HER2:CEP17 ratio 1.4). She underwent a lumpectomy and sentinel lymph node biopsy. The surgical specimen revealed a 3.0-cm tubular carcinoma, grade 1, no lymphovascular space invasion. The margins were free of tumor, and three sentinel lymph nodes were negative for cancer. Which option is the next best step to manage this patient?

A. Combination chemotherapy followed by radiation therapy and anastrozole

B. Anastrozole alone

C. Radiation therapy alone

D. Radiation therapy followed by anastrozole

E. No additional therapy

52. A 62-year-old female is referred to you by a dermatologist. She describes a red, pruritic area on her left nipple and areola associated with burning. She also noted some flaking and scaling of the nipple skin of the left breast. She applied some skin creams as she thought she had a contact dermatitis. The dermatologist performed a shave biopsy, and it showed that the epidermis was invaded by large round cells with clear cytoplasm and hyperchromatic nuclei, arranged in groups. On physical exam, the left nipple was erythematous and slightly retracted. The left nipple-areolar complex had some mild ulceration. There was no palpable mass in the left breast. The right breast had no skin changes or palpable masses. What is the next best step in management?

A. Refer her back to the dermatologist for treatment of eczema

B. Order a mammogram and if negative, follow with a breast MRI

C. Perform a skin punch biopsy

D. Refer her for excision of the nipple-areolar complex

E. No additional therapy

53. A 65-year-old woman underwent a screening mammogram, and an abnormality was noted in her left breast. Additional imaging with ultrasound revealed a circumscribed mass in the left breast measuring 7 mm. There was no axillary adenopathy. A core needle biopsy showed detached papillary fragments, suggestive of part of an intraductal papilloma and ductal hyperplasia. Which of the following is true regarding this condition?

A. No further treatment needed

B. Order a breast MRI

C. Refer her for an excision

D. Redo a core biopsy of the mass

ANSWERS

1. B

Identification of HER2 positivity can be challenging, but is of great importance in knowing when to recommend the addition of HER2-directed therapy for a patient. Based on the American Society of Clinical Oncology/College of American Pathologists (ASCO CAP) 2013 guidelines, HER2 positivity can be defined by at least one of the following parameters: immunohistochemistry score of 3+, a HER2/CEP17 ratio greater than 2.0, and/or a HER2 copy number greater than 6.

2. D

Trastuzumab is a monoclonal antibody that precisely targets the HER2 receptor. Although generally extremely well tolerated, one of the rare toxicities that can occur with trastuzumab exposure is cardiac toxicity, which manifests as a drop in left ventricular ejection fraction. Rates of cardiac toxicity appear to be higher when trastuzumab is used concurrently or sequentially with anthracycline-based therapy, and is typically reversible by withholding the drug and treating with cardiac medication. Other rare toxicities of trastuzumab include infusion reaction and interstitial pneumonitis.

3. C

Several database analyses have shown that small HER2-positive cancers carry increased risk of recurrence compared with HER2-negative cancers of the same size. Longer duration trastuzumab-based regimens provide efficacy, but may exposure a patient to excessive risk. The APT trial treated patients with predominantly stage 1 HER2+ cancer with a regimen of 12 weeks of weekly paclitaxel and trastuzumab, followed by trastuzumab for a year. Therapy was extremely well tolerated and the rate of recurrence was extremely low, supporting the "TH + H" regimen as the standard of care for small HER2+ cancers.

4. C

DCIS is preinvasive breast cancer, requiring complete local therapy and consideration of systemic methods to reduce the risk of local recurrence as well as the risk of new breast primary. NSABP B-24, which enrolled patients who had completed lumpectomy and radiotherapy for DCIS and randomized to 5 years of tamoxifen versus placebo, showed a significantly reduced risk of ipsilateral recurrent disease and contralateral new disease with the use of tamoxifen. More recently, NSABP B-35, a similarly structured trial, confirmed a similar benefit for aromatase inhibitors. In a healthy woman who had excision of ER+ DCIS, it would be appropriate to offer a 5-year course of endocrine therapy with either agent. While brief duration of HER2-directed therapy is being investigated in a clinical trial, there is no role for HER2-directed therapy for HER2+ DCIS outside of a clinical trial. Additionally, a sentinel lymph node biopsy is not necessary in the setting of non-invasive disease.

5. C

ACOSOG Z-011 randomized patients who had a lumpectomy and a positive sentinel lymph node biopsy and for whom adjuvant radiotherapy was planned to either completion dissection or no further axillary surgery. Importantly, eligible patients were clinical node negative at baseline, had no more than three positive sentinel nodes, and had not received preoperative systemic therapy. No survival difference was seen between the two groups, including at 10-year follow-up. Additionally, patients who avoided axillary lymph node dissection had less perioperative complications and morbidity from the procedure. This finding has led to a change in the standard of care for a patient with a positive sentinel lymph node from completion axillary dissection to no further axillary surgery.

6. E

The 21-gene recurrence score assay has been retrospectively validated in both node-negative as well as postmenopausal patients with 1–3 positive nodes. Low scores less than 18 suggest a favorable cancer biology not responsive to adjuvant chemotherapy. Additionally, recent studies in node-negative breast cancer patients with recurrence scores <11 and in those with 0–3 positive nodes with recurrence scores < 11 indicated that these patients had excellent disease-free survivals with endocrine therapy alone. Thus, particularly in this older patient with a history of a slow growing tumor, a score of 10 supports no role for chemotherapy and a focus on adjuvant endocrine therapy exclusively. For a postmenopausal woman with a node-positive cancer, including an aromatase inhibitor is a fundamental part of adjuvant endocrine therapy.

7. D

At minimum, adjuvant endocrine therapy for a premenopausal woman with a hormone receptor–positive breast cancer consists of at least 5 years adjuvant tamoxifen. The SOFT trial explored the role of the addition of ovarian suppression in combination with 5 years of either tamoxifen or aromatase inhibitor (AI) in premenopausal women with hormone receptor–positive breast cancer. The study enrolled patients with heterogeneous risk, and overall

results of the study did not show superiority with addition of ovarian suppression over tamoxifen alone. However, in the subgroup of women younger than 35 years who regained menses after adjuvant chemotherapy, the addition of ovarian suppression to endocrine therapy significantly improved survival outcomes compared with tamoxifen alone, with the ovarian suppression and AI regimen producing the most favorable outcomes. Although 10 years of adjuvant endocrine therapy could also be considered, for a very young woman, addition of ovarian suppression is a preferred strategy.

8. D

Anthracycline and taxane-based chemotherapy remains the standard of care for higher-risk triple negative breast cancer. Shorter-duration regimens, including AC × 4 and the nonanthracycline-containing TC × 4, are acceptable for a T1cN0 triple negative breast cancer. There is considerable interest in the role of platinum chemotherapy as part of neo/adjuvant management of triple negative breast cancer; however, a survival benefit from the addition of platinum chemotherapy has not been confirmed. Therefore, substituting a proven regimen for a carboplatin-containing regimen would be the least acceptable option compared with the other more standard options.

9. C

Follow-up care for breast cancer survivors is well described by evidence-based guidelines and consists of annual breast imaging, provider visits every 6 months with clinical examination for several years after diagnosis, and routine health maintenance. There is no role for other routine imaging or serologic testing in an asymptomatic patient, and further investigations are driven by emergent symptoms.

10. C

Emerging data have helped define target health behaviors in breast cancer survivors. Patients can be counseled to pursue regular exercise, preferably weight bearing to support bone health, maintain body weight, or lose weight if desired, and consume no more than one or two glasses of alcohol per day on average. Taking calcium and vitamin D can be encouraged to maintain bone health, especially for patients receiving aromatase inhibitors.

11. D

This patient has been diagnosed with a low-risk breast cancer. Because she is premenopausal, tamoxifen is the preferred agent for adjuvant endocrine therapy, recommended for a 5-year course. The addition of ovarian suppression to oral endocrine therapy in premenopausal women with hormone receptor–positive breast cancer was evaluated in the SOFT trial (Francis et al, NEJM 2014). In this trial, patients with lower-risk cancer for which chemotherapy was not indicated did not benefit from the addition of ovarian suppression, and so ovarian suppression would not be indicated in this situation. Additionally, the selective estrogen receptor degrader fulvestrant is an approved agent for postmenopausal metastatic breast cancer, but would not be indicated in the care of a premenopausal woman with early-stage breast cancer.

12. E

A 21-gene recurrence score of 31 is a high-risk score, suggesting not only a higher risk of recurrence, but also suggesting benefit from adjuvant chemotherapy. Therefore, adjuvant chemotherapy is indicated, and either an anthracycline-based or nonanthracycline-based regimen could be considered. Because the cancer is hormone receptor positive, adjuvant endocrine therapy is also indicated. She may experience a loss of ovarian function during chemotherapy, but is likely to regain menses afterward. Therefore, treatment with aromatase inhibitor alone is dangerous because the agent is ineffective in the setting of functioning ovaries. Data from ATLAS, ATTOM, and Ma.17 have all supported benefits of 10 years rather than 5 years of adjuvant endocrine therapy for premenopausal patients, and this strategy is recommended to reduce the risk of late recurrence.

13. D

Cohort analyses of women who choose to get pregnant after a breast cancer diagnosis have not demonstrated an increased risk of breast cancer recurrence. In fact, the population appears to have improved outcomes compared with matched controls, an observation that has been referred to as the "healthy mother bias," and may reflect subtle differences in tumor biology and expectations. Conventional wisdom tends to recommend waiting at least 2 years after initial diagnosis and treatment to confirm no early recurrence. This patient, with a history of triple negative breast cancer 2 years out from diagnosis, can be encouraged to pursue pregnancy if so desired.

14. D

All listed mutations can increase the risk of development of breast cancer and can be assessed on multigene panel testing. Of these, mutations in p53 (Li-Fraumeni syndrome) are associated with development of cancer in very young women (<30 years old) and are more likely to be HER2 positive. Li-Fraumeni is also associated with development of primary brain tumors, sarcomas, adrenocortical malignancies, and leukemia. Additionally, there is an elevated risk of second malignancy in radiated fields, so radiation therapy should be avoided if possible.

15. C

The risks of cardiac toxicity with anthracycline-based chemotherapy increase with older age, preexisting cardiovascular disease such as hypertension, concurrent exposure to other cardiotoxic medications, and cumulative dose. In a standard to higher-risk patient, baseline cardiac evaluation is necessary prior to initiation of therapy. At minimum, an echocardiogram (preferred) or a multigated acquisition (MUGA) to confirm normal ejection fraction is recommended, although in this patient, cardiooncology consultation should be considered if there are any abnormalities seen on echo. Advanced imaging by MRI and/or cardiac markers are under study and are not recommended as part of routine care. There is no role for dexrazoxane in the adjuvant setting for less than 240 mg/m^2 anthracycline.

16. D and E

The anti-HER2 and HER3 antibody pertuzumab was approved to be used in the preoperative setting for locally advanced HER2+ breast cancer. The approval was based on data from the NeoSPHERE and TYPHAENA studies showing improved pathologic complete response when pertuzumab was added to taxane and trastuzumab-based therapy. For a locally advanced HER2+ cancer, initiation of preoperative therapy with HER-directed agents is preferable to starting with an anthracycline to avoid the risk of upfront cardiac toxicity that could complicate subsequent use of HER2-directed therapy.

17. D

Treatment of breast cancer during pregnancy requires balancing risks and benefits for the woman with breast cancer as well as the developing fetus. Evolving cohort studies have demonstrated that use during pregnancy of several traditional modalities for breast cancer treatment, including administration of standard chemotherapeutics during the 2nd and 3rd trimester as well as surgical procedures, do not appear to increase complications of pregnancy or fetal malformation above population baselines. Preterm delivery (<37 weeks), however, is a well-described risk for newborn complication. Therefore, in the setting of locally advanced disease requiring preoperative therapy, it is acceptable to pursue an anthracycline and taxane-based chemotherapy regimen to optimize surgical outcomes, and early delivery or even termination of the pregnancy are discouraged.

18. B

Standard therapy for higher-risk triple negative breast cancer is anthracycline and taxane-based chemotherapy, which can be given before or after surgery. Because this patient desires breast conservation, preoperative chemotherapy is indicated. There is significant interest in the role of platinum chemotherapy for triple negative breast cancer due to the DNA-damaging method of action. Studies of preoperative cisplatin chemotherapy for triple negative breast cancer have demonstrated robust response rates, especially for BRCA1/2 associated breast cancer. Trials evaluating the addition of carboplatin to anthracycline and taxane-based chemotherapy have demonstrated an increase in pathologic response rate with the addition of platinum therapy; however, they also report conflicting information on whether this translates into improvements in survival. Therefore, for this patient with clinical T2N0 disease, preoperative anthracycline and taxane would be indicated, reserving platinum-based preoperative therapy for a research setting preferably.

19. C

A grade 1 hormone receptor–positive, HER2-negative breast cancer in an elderly patient will exhibit greater sensitivity to endocrine therapy over chemotherapy. Preoperative chemotherapy not only may increase the risk of toxicity in this patient but also may result in less than 10% pathologic complete response rate. Preoperative endocrine therapy is preferred in this situation and is recommended for at least a 6-month course before surgery for optimal cytoreduction.

20. A

The annual incidence of male breast cancer in the United States is about 2000 cases. Treatment paradigms for male breast mirror those in women, because randomized trials in male populations are limited by the low incidence of the disease. Tamoxifen has been demonstrated to be safe and effective in men and is a preferred endocrine approach, as aromatase inhibitors are not well studied. In an individual with hormone receptor–positive breast cancer who has completed preoperative anthracycline and taxane-based therapy yet has residual disease at surgery, there are no recommended standard adjuvant chemotherapy or targeted therapy programs that will decrease the risk of recurrence beyond endocrine therapy. Multiple ongoing trials are underway to improve outcomes in this higher-risk population.

21. D

Local recurrence after initial breast cancer therapy suggests elevated risk of distant recurrence. The CALOR study asked if further systemic chemotherapy could reduce this risk, randomizing patients with resected recurrent disease to further chemotherapy or not. Despite accruing a heterogeneous population, the study was positive showing additional therapy was beneficial, especially in hormone receptor–negative populations. In a patient who is at least 1 year out from adjuvant chemotherapy with locally recurrent triple negative breast cancer, further chemotherapy is warranted. Because this patient has received 240 mg/m^2 cumulative dose of anthracycline, a further anthracycline-based comprehensive regimen would push too close to lifetime limits in the curative setting. A nonanthracycline-based regimen, for example docetaxel/cyclophosphamide, would be suggested.

22. B

Given the presentation with a fixed chest wall lesion, this patient is not a candidate for upfront surgical resection and would benefit from preoperative systemic therapy. A low-grade hormone receptor positive cancer in an older patient with a 4-year disease-free interval suggests a tumor biology best treated with endocrine therapy. As disease recurrence occurred while on aromatase inhibitor, a change to tamoxifen would be indicated. If chemotherapy is pursued, CMF would be a reasonable option, although not preferred over endocrine therapy. Neo/adjuvant capecitabine does not have a role in the curative management of older women with breast cancer.

23. C and E

Although helpful in detecting evidence of distant metastatic disease, systemic staging carries the risk of findings that may lead to unnecessary further evaluation in an otherwise nonmetastatic patient. NCCN guidelines recommend staging for clinical stage IIB patients, patients with symptoms worrisome for distant spread of disease, and given the high risks associated, for those with locoregional recurrence. Staging is not needed for patients with lower stage or noninvasive disease.

24. A

Although this patient has operable breast cancer and can undergo a mastectomy for her clinical stage II disease, she wishes to preserve her breast; therefore the optimal therapeutic option for her is to receive neoadjuvant chemotherapy with doxorubicin and cyclophosphamide followed by paclitaxel, which is a standard adjuvant therapy regimen. Neoadjuvant chemotherapy has been shown to result in a greater proportion of patients undergoing breast conservation, with a comparable disease-free survival and overall survival when standard adjuvant therapy regimens are administered preoperatively. Neoadjuvant endocrine therapy has only been studied in postmenopausal women; therefore the option of using tamoxifen as preoperative therapy is not standard, and anastrozole, an aromatase inhibitor, is not effective in premenopausal women. Radiation therapy as primary treatment of breast cancer is only used for palliation.

25. A

Although this patient has operable disease, her large tumor size and palpable axillary adenopathy is best treated with preoperative systemic therapy to downstage her cancer and allow breast conservation. The large tumor size and palpable axillary adenopathy would not be optimally treated with breast-conserving surgery but would require a mastectomy and lymph node dissection. In the case of HER2-positive disease, dual HER2-directed therapy with trastuzumab and pertuzumab administered with chemotherapy, results in a greater pathologic complete response rate compared with chemotherapy administered with trastuzumab or pertuzumab alone. The NeoSphere study demonstrated a 39.3% pathologic complete response rate when pertuzumab, trastuzumab, and docetaxel was administered preoperatively compared with a 21.5% and 17.7% PCR rate when docetaxel was given with trastuzumab or pertuzumab as single HER2-directed therapy, respectively. In North America, a regimen commonly administered in this setting is docetaxel, carboplatin, pertuzumab, and trastuzumab. In addition, pertuzumab is currently only FDA approved in early-stage disease when administered preoperatively with trastuzumab and a taxane. Preoperative therapy with tamoxifen is not effective in premenopausal women.

26. E

There is comparable survival outcome between mastectomy and breast conservation surgery with radiation. The optimal characteristics for breast conservation include the ability to resect the entire tumor with negative surgical margins, because there is an estimated twofold higher risk of an in-breast recurrence with positive surgical margins. The definition of negative margins is no evidence of invasive or noninvasive cancer seen at the inked surgical margins; therefore the next step in the management of this patient is a re-excision of the biopsy cavity to obtain negative margins. ACOSOG trial Z0011 found no difference in axillary recurrence rate, disease-free survival, or overall survival among patients with one to two positive axillary lymph nodes treated with sentinel lymph node sampling compared with completion axillary lymph node dissection when breast conservation surgery is followed by whole breast radiation therapy. Germ-line mutations do not influence systemic adjuvant therapy recommendations, though in younger women, it may prompt a discussion about prophylactic mastectomy. The Oncotype Dx analysis applies only to estrogen receptor–positive breast cancer. Combination paclitaxel and carboplatin is not considered a standard of care adjuvant regimen for breast cancer. The addition of platinum agents to adjuvant therapy in triple negative disease is still being investigated, and if pursued, should be given in addition to Adriamycin and cytoxan chemotherapy.

27. D

Multicentric disease, defined as carcinoma in more than one quadrant of the breast, is associated with a significant risk of in-breast recurrence when breast conservation and radiation therapy are used.[1] A separate excision of distinct foci of breast cancer followed by radiation is being investigated and is not the standard of care at this time. Preoperative systemic therapy with either endocrine therapy or chemotherapy will not change the ultimate surgical procedure, which is mastectomy. The sizes of the foci of cancer are very small, and preoperative therapy will not change the ability of the patient to undergo surgery, nor will it allow for breast conservation. Radiation is only used as initial therapy for breast cancer, that is, prior to systemic therapy or surgery, when palliation is indicated.

28. D

Breast-conserving surgery is appropriate when negative surgical margins can be obtained following resection of the primary breast cancer and the cosmetic outcome of the breast is acceptable. Whole breast radiation therapy is given following breast-conserving surgery, which results in a comparable overall survival compared with mastectomy. This patient meets the criteria for breast conservation. The presence of dermal lymphatic involvement seen on a skin biopsy can be seen at any stage breast cancer and does not denote T4 disease. Therefore, a completion mastectomy is not indicated, but if mastectomy is chosen, an immediate reconstruction can be performed. Sentinel lymph node dissection is associated with less upper extremity lymphedema and other complications and is the procedure of choice for surgical evaluation of the clinically negative axilla. The false-negative rate of sentinel lymph node dissection is approximately 8%, and therefore a completion axillary lymph node dissection is not indicated in this patient.

29. D

Adjuvant endocrine therapy reduces the risk of disease recurrence and improves overall survival, and therefore should be offered to all patients with hormone receptor–positive breast cancer (estrogen receptor positive and/or progesterone receptor positive). Trastuzumab only targets HER2 and does not replace the need for endocrine therapy. Options for endocrine therapy include AIs, which target aromatase, an enzyme that converts androgens to estrogens, and tamoxifen, which is a partial antagonist of the estrogen receptor. AIs are only effective in postmenopausal women, and although this patient has experienced chemotherapy amenorrhea, she is young enough that her menstrual function may return within 1–2 years after completing chemotherapy. An AI should not be used in this setting because a return of ovarian function would render the treatment ineffective. Tamoxifen is effective endocrine therapy regardless of menopausal status; therefore it is the treatment of choice for this patient. If the patient's menstrual function resumes within 8 months of completing chemotherapy, then she may benefit from the addition of ovarian suppression to endocrine therapy.

30. C

Multiple studies comparing the efficacy of AIs with tamoxifen as adjuvant therapy demonstrate superiority in the use of AI in postmenopausal women. A metaanalysis of these studies showed a 29% proportional reduction in risk of recurrence with primary treatment using an AI compared with tamoxifen. The ATLAS trial demonstrated a 2.8% absolute reduction in death at 15 years when 10 years of tamoxifen was compared with 5 years of tamoxifen. Recently, the MA 17R study supported the benefit of prolonged AI use beyond 5 years. The majority of the patients in the study received 4–6 years of tamoxifen prior to beginning extended endocrine therapy with AI. This patient is at high enough risk to warrant extended endocrine therapy. The use of tamoxifen following 5 years of an AI has not been studied, and fulvestrant is only used for advanced disease. Bilateral salpingo-oophorectomy is not beneficial in a postmenopausal woman.

31. C

Adjuvant therapy recommendations should be based upon the final pathology determined at the time of surgery. For this reason, although the original core biopsy contained HER2-negative disease, the final specimen was HER2 positive, and anti-HER2 therapy should be offered. The ALLTO trial did not find a benefit when lapatinib, a small molecule tyrosine kinase inhibitor of HER2, was added to trastuzumab (humanized monoclonal antibody to HER2) for adjuvant therapy. Although the addition of pertuzumab (humanized monoclonal antibody to HER2) to trastuzumab is beneficial for neoadjuvant therapy, this combination anti-HER2 therapy is still being investigated in the adjuvant setting. The optimal adjuvant treatment for this patient is supported by the NCCTG N9831 study, which found that the addition of trastuzumab to standard adjuvant therapy using four cycles of doxorubicin and cyclophosphamide, followed by weekly paclitaxel with trastuzumab, followed by trastuzumab to complete 1 year of anti-HER2 therapy, resulted in a 48% improvement in disease-free survival and a 39% improvement in overall survival.

32. C

This patient has a T1b, N0, HER2-positive breast cancer which would not meet the criteria for enrollment on any of the initial HER2-positive adjuvant therapy trials and yet, retrospective data suggest that T1b HER2-positive breast cancer may have up to a 30% risk of systemic recurrence. For this reason, HER2 directed therapy using trastuzumab is indicated in addition to endocrine therapy. In the adjuvant setting, trastuzumab is given concurrently with chemotherapy and continues for a total of 1-year duration. The risk of cardiac toxicity is elevated when trastuzumab is given concurrently with an anthracycline; therefore that combination is avoided. One of the standard chemotherapy regimens for high-risk HER2-positive disease includes doxorubicin and cyclophosphamide followed by weekly paclitaxel with trastuzumab for 12 weeks followed by maintenance trastuzumab to complete 1 year. Recent data suggest that patients with T1b, N0 HER2-positive disease have a low enough risk of recurrence to allow them to avoid anthracyclines. In these cancers, adjuvant therapy includes weekly paclitaxel with trastuzumab for 12 weeks followed by maintenance trastuzumab to complete 1 year. Recurrence rates are low, less than 2%, and cardiac toxicity is less than 0.5%. Endocrine therapy is initiated during trastuzumab maintenance therapy.

33. B

Extended endocrine therapy with 10 years of tamoxifen compared with 5 years of tamoxifen has been shown to reduce the absolute mortality associated with breast cancer by approximately 2.8%. However, the ATLAS trial demonstrated a higher risk of endometrial cancer among postmenopausal women taking tamoxifen for greater than 5 years. Clinical trial MA-17 demonstrated a comparable improvement in overall survival with extended endocrine therapy using 5 years of tamoxifen followed by 5 years of letrozole, without the added risk of endometrial cancer. The benefit of extended endocrine therapy appears to be more advantageous for high-risk disease such as node-positive breast cancer. The combination of tamoxifen and an aromatase inhibitor has not been shown to be superior to tamoxifen or an aromatase inhibitor given alone. Ovarian suppression with bilateral stopping oophorectomy is not beneficial in postmenopausal women.

34. C

An Oncotype DX analysis on breast cancer specimens obtained from early-stage disease provides both prognostic data and predictive information about the benefit of adding chemotherapy to adjuvant endocrine therapy. This analysis was first used in estrogen receptor–positive, lymph node–negative early-stage breast cancer, but has subsequently been found to be beneficial in identifying postmenopausal patients with lymph node–positive disease who would not benefit from adjuvant chemotherapy in addition to endocrine therapy. An Oncotype DX analysis helps guide adjuvant therapy decisions in patients with 0–3 positive axillary lymph nodes and estrogen receptor–positive, HER2-negative breast cancer. Oncotype DX Recurrence Scores of less than 18 are not associated with an additional benefit from adjuvant chemotherapy, whereas scores greater than 30 predict an added efficacy when adjuvant chemotherapy is given in addition to endocrine therapy.

35. D

Although one could consider prophylactic contralateral mastectomy given her maternal family history, this would not be the next most appropriate step. Genetic testing would first be recommended; in addition, prophylactic contralateral mastectomy has not been shown to improve overall survival in the absence of a documented germline mutation. Postmastectomy radiation therapy has not been shown to be of benefit in lymph node–negative disease. An Oncotype DX Recurrence Score analysis would provide predictive information on whether adjuvant chemotherapy, in addition to endocrine therapy, would result in an improvement in disease-free survival compared with endocrine therapy alone. This is shown to be helpful in determining adjuvant therapy recommendations in stage II, node-negative, ER-positive, HER2-negative breast cancer. The SOFT trial determined that ovarian suppression, in addition to endocrine therapy, is of benefit to women who are 35 years or younger, and/or who have high-risk disease requiring adjuvant chemotherapy.

36. B

Although this patient has a high-risk breast cancer that required adjuvant chemotherapy, endocrine therapy is still an important component of her treatment. Chemotherapy often suppresses menstrual cycling, but it does not completely suppress ovarian function as is demonstrated in this patient who has a premenopausal estradiol level. Aromatase inhibitors are not effective in premenopausal women, and therefore tamoxifen is the endocrine therapy of choice. However, the SOFT trial demonstrated a 10%–15% improvement in the 5-year breast-cancer-free interval when ovarian suppression was combined with exemestane, compared with ovarian suppression and tamoxifen or tamoxifen alone. This was seen among the high-risk patients who required adjuvant chemotherapy, such as this patient. As a number of patients do not tolerate ovarian suppression with exemestane, one can also consider ovarian suppression with tamoxifen.

37. C

Metastatic breast cancer presents with systemic symptoms, unlike early-stage disease, which is curable. Routine imaging to detect systemic recurrence has not been shown to improve long-term survival, and therefore CT scans and bone scans should only be performed when symptoms warrant an evaluation. Annual breast imaging with mammograms are indicated because the detection of a new primary in the breast favorably impacts breast cancer survival. Premenopausal women on tamoxifen have a higher risk of developing osteoporosis, and therefore a bone density should be performed every 2 years. Transvaginal ultrasounds are associated with a high false-positive rate among patients taking tamoxifen because tamoxifen causes benign thickening of the endometrium and are therefore not recommended. Additionally, transvaginal ultrasounds have not been shown to detect ovarian cancer at an earlier stage.

38. C

Aromatase inhibitors have more musculoskeletal toxicity, such as myalgias, arthralgias, and increased risk of osteoporosis, compared with tamoxifen, whereas tamoxifen is associated with more endocrine-related toxicities such as increased risk of thrombosis and increased risk of endometrial cancer. Because of the reduction of estrogen associated with aromatase inhibitors, they are associated with vaginal dryness and decreased libido. Neither of the endocrine therapies is independently associated with increased weight gain. We do not have safety data for the administration of oral estrogens among breast cancer patients receiving aromatase inhibitors, but randomized trials have suggested an increased risk of recurrence in breast cancer survivors who took hormone replacement therapy.

39. A

The rapid onset of changes within the breast such as erythema, edema, and breast swelling, which occur in the setting of documented invasive breast carcinoma, are consistent with a diagnosis of inflammatory breast cancer. Confirmation of dermal lymphatic involvement with breast cancer is not required for this diagnosis and can be present in earlier-stage breast cancer. Although this cancer is rare, accounting for 2%–5% of all breast cancers diagnosed in the United States, it can occur in men and is not associated with a specific inherited gene mutation. At the time of diagnosis, this disease is not operable, and therefore preoperative chemotherapy is indicated. Because the disease is extensive within the breast at the time of diagnosis, stage III, a modified radical mastectomy is performed following preoperative chemotherapy, and breast-conserving surgery remains investigational.

40. E

This patient presents with a locally advanced breast cancer with direct extension to the skin. Based on her history and clinical findings, that is, her compromised mental status, lack of screening breast imaging over many years, and hormone receptor–positive invasive lobular carcinoma, it is most likely that she has indolent disease. Given her comorbidities and the indolent nature of her disease, systemic therapy is preferred compared with the potential toxicities of local therapy with surgery or primary radiation. In addition, given the extent of her disease, primary systemic therapy is preferred. Hormone receptor–positive invasive lobular cancer is less responsive to chemotherapy, but endocrine therapy is very effective. Therefore, the optimal treatment for this patient is primary therapy with an aromatase inhibitor. In postmenopausal women, preoperative therapy using an aromatase inhibitor is superior to tamoxifen and is associated with a clinical response of 55% versus 36%, respectively.

41. C

This patient experienced a rapid onset (1-month duration) of erythema and swelling of the breast associated with a diagnosis of invasive breast cancer. The breast imaging confirmed extensive disease involving the skin, parenchyma, and regional lymph nodes. This constellation of signs and symptoms is consistent with inflammatory breast cancer, which is not operable at the time of diagnosis. The rapid onset of signs and symptoms does not support a neglected, indolent, locally advanced breast cancer. Trauma is not associated with the development of invasive breast cancer, but rather brings attention to changes within the breast.

42. C

This scenario describes a locally advanced breast cancer that involves the pectoralis muscle, is classified as T4c, and is not considered operable. Preoperative therapy is indicated; however, the extent of disease warrants local control with a mastectomy and axillary lymph node dissection regardless of disease response to preoperative therapy. Preoperative tamoxifen is not as effective as aromatase inhibitors in the treatment of locally advanced disease in postmenopausal women. Although neoadjuvant endocrine therapy is associated with a low PCR rate (1%–8%), neoadjuvant chemotherapy is not associated with a superior overall survival.

43. A

This patient has extensive locally advanced triple negative breast cancer that involves the right axillary lymph nodes and appears to be causing symptoms of a brachial plexopathy, that is, neuropathic pain within the right arm. Surgical resection of the cancer is unlikely to result in negative surgical margins and has potential to cause nerve damage during dissection of the axilla, given the extensive adenopathy. Because of effective preoperative chemotherapy, radical mastectomies are rarely performed. Primary radiation to a bulky tumor is unlikely to be effective and is associated with significant toxicity because of the higher doses of radiation required. Metaplastic breast cancer is a rare subtype of triple negative breast cancer that responds to standard breast cancer treatment, such as doxorubicin and cyclophosphamide. The optimal treatment for this patient is to administer preoperative doxorubicin and cyclophosphamide, with the goal of reducing the bulk of the tumor and reverse injury to the brachial plexus caused by tumor invasion. Endocrine therapy is not effective in ER-negative, PR-negative disease.

44. A

To determine whether this breast cancer recurrence is a new primary that arose within residual breast tissue left at the time of mastectomy, or a chest wall recurrence, the nodule needs to be completely excised. This recurrence occurred within the first 5 years after diagnosis, and so it is less likely to be a second primary breast cancer. Because there is no evidence of disease elsewhere, radiation therapy is indicated to control the local regional disease following a chest wall recurrence. Although endocrine therapy would be offered following surgery, and ovarian suppression is indicated in this premenopausal woman, endocrine therapy is recommended as an adjuvant treatment rather than primary therapy, that is, surgery. The lesion is very small by physical exam, and therefore presurgical systemic therapy, such as chemotherapy, is not necessary to achieve an adequate surgical resection.

45. B

An axillary lymph node recurrence without evidence of distant metastases suggests a failure of local regional disease control. This clinical situation should be treated with curable intent. Endocrine therapy will remain the mainstay of treatment given the fact that her recurrent lymph node involvement remains estrogen receptor and progesterone receptor positive. However, this patient's disease has a component of endocrine resistance because it grew on tamoxifen; therefore switching endocrine therapy alone would not maximize her adjuvant treatment. The CALOR trial demonstrated a benefit in 5-year disease-free survival with chemotherapy compared with no chemotherapy (69% vs. 57%) when administered after an isolated local disease recurrence. The benefit was primarily seen in triple negative breast cancer. Given evidence of axillary lymph node disease that grew on endocrine therapy, the optimal treatment would include standard adjuvant chemotherapy with doxorubicin and cyclophosphamide followed by

paclitaxel. In hormone receptor–positive breast cancer, the addition of taxanes to an anthracycline regimen, such as doxorubicin and cyclophosphamide, has been shown to reduce the risk of recurrence by an additional 26% and reduces the risk of death by additional 23%.

46. B

An in-breast recurrence following breast-conserving surgery and radiation is associated with a two- to threefold increase in the risk of metastasis; however, the majority of these "recurrences" are actually second cancers that occur more than 5 years after the completion of radiation therapy. This cancer occurred 18 years after the initial diagnosis and is most likely a second primary breast cancer with a curative goal of treatment. Local regional disease control with surgical removal of the tumor is of greater benefit compared with systemic therapy alone (chemotherapy or endocrine therapy), which is used for palliation. Because the breast has been irradiated previously, a completion mastectomy is indicated and an attempt at a second course of breast-conserving surgery and/or re-radiation remains investigational.

47. A

This patient has a node-positive breast cancer and an excellent performance status. Male breast cancer is uncommon, accounting for less than 1% of all breast cancer cases.

The most common surgical operation for male breast cancer is a modified radical mastectomy. The axillary node involvement is the strongest predictor of local recurrence and distant recurrence. The indications for adjuvant chemotherapy and postmastectomy radiation therapy should follow the treatment recommendations used to treat women with a node-positive breast cancer. Patients with lymph node–positive disease are candidates for chemotherapy. Given that the tumor is hormone receptor–positive, endocrine therapy is also indicated. For high-risk patients, which this patient would be, given the involved nodes, an anthracycline- plus taxane-containing regimen is preferred and can be given, presuming he has no contraindication to being treated with an anthracycline. In this particular case, the indication for radiation therapy postmastectomy is that he has four or more nodes that are pathologically involved. There is limited data regarding the indications for postmastectomy radiation in men, but the management of male breast cancer follows the recommendations for women with breast cancer. Tamoxifen is the most extensively studied endocrine therapy in male breast cancer.

48. C

The indications for radiation therapy for women with breast cancer apply also to men with breast cancer. After breast-conserving surgery, whole breast radiation reduces the risk of local recurrence and improves survival. An additional point to this question is that breast cancers that have at least 1% of cells staining positive for ER should be considered ER-positive cancers. Endocrine therapy should be discussed. For men with hormone receptor–positive breast cancer, endocrine therapy is recommended. Tamoxifen is the most extensively studied endocrine therapy in male breast cancer.

49. C

Phyllodes tumors of the breast, also known as cystosarcoma phyllodes, are rare tumors composed of stromal and epithelial elements. They are characterized into benign, borderline, or malignant categories. Patients with a diagnosis of Li-Fraumeni syndrome are described as having an increased risk of phyllodes tumors. The treatment is complete surgical excision. This should include a wide local excision and histologic margins negative for tumor. Recurrence rates are high after local excision or enuclea- tion without negative margins. Axillary dissection is not required due to the infrequency of nodal disease, and in the absence of clinically palpable nodes. Adjuvant radia- tion therapy is not necessary for widely excised benign phyllodes tumors. There have been no randomized studies of adjuvant therapy that have been conducted specifically in phyllodes tumors; patients with benign or borderline phyllodes tumors should not be offered chemotherapy.

50. A

Angiosarcoma of the breast is a rare disease. It comprises about 0.04% of malignant breast neoplasms. Angiosar- comas are a subtype of soft tissue sarcomas that have a vascular or endothelial origin. There are two forms of this disease. Primary angiosarcoma occurs in younger patients and is more likely to present as a palpable mass. Second- ary angiosarcoma may occur after local radiation or in the setting of chronic postoperative lymphedema (Stewart– Treves syndrome). It is commonly referred to as cutaneous angiosarcoma and involves the subcutaneous tissues of the breast, while sparing the underlying breast parenchy- ma. It most commonly presents as a violaceous or erythe- matous lesion. It may be accompanied by a palpable mass. This patient has a diagnosis of secondary angiosarcoma or radiation-associated angiosarcoma. Metastases from angiosarcoma are thought to primarily be hematogenous, and CT scanning should be considered prior to surgical resection. Due to the rarity of this tumor, there are no rand- omized trials comparing wide local excision or completion mastectomy. Total mastectomy with or without an axillary node dissection is the preferred treatment. Administration of radiation is limited for secondary angiosarcoma as the area has likely received a maximum dosage. There is no definitive role for adjuvant chemotherapy.

51. D

Tubular carcinoma is a rare, subtype of invasive breast can- cer with a prevalence of 1%–4%. It has an excellent long- term prognosis. The analysis by Rakha et al. compared the biological behavior and outcomes of tubular carcinomas compared with low-grade ductal or mixed tubular car- cinomas and confirmed that patients with tubular carci- nomas have a very favorable prognosis and an excellent outcome. The favorable histology of tubular carcinomas supports recommendations that adjuvant chemotherapy can be avoided. Adjuvant endocrine therapy is considered because most tumors are hormone receptor–positive.

52. B

This patient has a diagnosis of Paget disease, which is uncommon. Paget disease of the breast presents with a pruritic eczema-like rash involving the nipple-areolar complex. There can be flaking and scaling of the nipple skin, and nipple retraction. Associated symptoms include tingling, burning, or pain. In advanced stages, there can be ulceration, crusting, skin erosion, and a discharge. It is typ- ically associated with underlying invasive or noninvasive breast cancer. Paget disease involves the nipple-areolar complex. If the symptoms are bilateral or confined to the areola with sparing of the nipple, eczema is the more likely diagnosis. Histologically, Paget disease is characterized by large round cells with clear cytoplasm and hyperchromatic nuclei, arranged in groups or singly, involving the epider- mis of the skin. In this case a shave biopsy was obtained

to confirm the diagnosis of Paget disease. A skin punch biopsy is sometimes performed. Further imaging with mammogram and/or breast MRI should be performed be- cause in the majority of cases, there is an associated breast cancer. The presence of a concurrent breast cancer drives the type of surgery (lumpectomy or mastectomy), axillary nodal evaluation, and adjuvant therapy. For patients with localized Paget disease, breast-conserving therapy with excision of the nipple-areolar complex is recommended followed by adjuvant radiation therapy.

53. C

Intraductal papilloma is a type of papillary breast lesion and is a benign finding. Papillary breast lesions comprise a range of benign and malignant entities including intra- ductal papilloma, atypical papilloma, papillary ductal carcinoma in situ, encapsulated papillary carcinoma, and invasive papillary carcinoma. These lesions can be diffi- cult to differentiate based on the tissue fragments obtained from a biopsy. Because papillary lesions are heterogeneous, full histologic evaluation is necessary to rule out cancer or atypical hyperplasia. It has been reported that when a pap- illary lesion is diagnosed by core biopsy, and then followed by surgical excision, the rate of the lesion being upgraded to a cancer ranges from 10% to 35% across several series.

REFERENCES

Question 1
1. Wolff AC, Hammond ME, Hicks DG, et al. Recommendations for human epidermal growth factor receptor 2 testing in breast can- cer: American Society of Clinical Oncology/College of Ameri- can Pathologists clinical practice guideline update. *J Clin Oncol.* 2013;31:3997–4013.

Question 2
1. Romond EH, Jeong JH, Rastogi P, et al. Seven-year follow-up assessment of cardiac func- tion in NSABP B-31, a randomized trial comparing doxorubicin and cyclophosphamide followed by paclitaxel (ACP) with ACP plus trastuzumab as adjuvant therapy for patients with node-positive, human epidermal growth factor receptor 2-positive breast cancer. *J Clin Oncol.* 2012;30:3792–3799.

Question 3
1. Tolaney SM, Barry WT, Dang CT, et al. Adjuvant paclitaxel and trastuzumab for node-negative, HER2-positive breast cancer. *N Engl J Med.* 2015;372:134–141.
2. Curigliano G, Viale G, Bagnardi V, et al. Clinical relevance of HER2 overexpression/amplification in patients with small tumor size and node-negative breast cancer. *J Clin Oncol.* 2009;27:5693–5699.
3. Gonzalez-Angulo AM, Litton JK, Broglio KR, et al. High risk of recurrence for patients with breast cancer who have human epider- mal growth factor receptor 2-positive, node-negative tumors 1 cm or smaller. *J Clin Oncol.* 2009;27:5700–5706.

Question 4
1. Fisher B, Dignam N, Wolmark N, et al. Tamoxifen in treatment of intraductal breast cancer: National Surgical Adjuvant Breast and Bowel Project B-24 randomised controlled trial. *Lancet.* 1999;353:1993–2000.
2. Margolese RG, Cecchini RS, Julian TB, et al. Anastrozole versus ta- moxifen in postmenopausal women with ductal carcinoma in situ undergoing lumpectomy plus radiotherapy (NSABP B-35): a ran- domised, double-blind, phase 3 clinical trial. *Lancet.* 2015.

Question 5
1. Giuliano AE, Hawes D, Ballman KV, et al. Association of occult metastases in sentinel lymph nodes and bone marrow with surviv- al among women with early-stage invasive breast cancer. *JAMA.* 2011;306:385–393.

2. Lucci A, McCall LM, Beitsch PD, et al. American College of Surgeons Oncology Group. Surgical complications associated with sentinel lymph node dissection (SLND) plus axillary lymph node dissection com- pared with SLND alone in the American College of Surgeons Oncology Group trial Z0011. *J Clin Oncol.* 2007;25(24):3657–3663.

Question 6

1. Paik S, Tang G, Shak S, et al. Gene expression and benefit of chemotherapy in women with node-negative, estrogen receptor-positive breast cancer. *J Clin Oncol.* 2006;24:3726–3734.
2. Albain KS, Barlow WE, Shak S, et al. Prognostic and predictive value of the 21-gene recurrence score assay in postmenopausal women with node-positive, oestrogen-receptor-positive breast cancer on chemotherapy: a retrospective analysis of a randomised trial. *Lancet Oncol.* 2010;11:55–65.
3. Gluz O, Nitz UA, Christgen M, et al. West German Study Group Phase III Plan B Trial: First Prospective Outcome Data for the 21-Gene Recurrence Score Assay and Concordance of Prognostic Markers by Central and Local Pathology Assessment. *J Clin Oncol.* 2016;34(20):2341–2349.

Question 7

1. Francis PA, Regan MM, Fleming GF, et al. Adjuvant ovarian suppression in premenopausal breast cancer. *N Engl J Med.* 2015;372:436–446.

Question 9

1. Runowicz CD, Leach CR, Henry NL, et al. American Cancer Society/American Society of Clinical Oncology Breast Cancer Survivorship Care Guideline. *J Clin Oncol.* 2016;34:611–635.

Question 10

1. Runowicz CD, Leach CR, Henry NL, et al. American Cancer Society/American Society of Clinical Oncology Breast Cancer Survivorship Care Guideline. *J Clin Oncol.* 2016;34:611–635.

Question 11

1. Francis PA, Regan MM, Fleming GF, et al. Adjuvant ovarian suppression in premenopausal breast cancer. *N Engl J Med.* 2015;372:436–446.

Question 12

1. Davies C, Pan H, Godwin J, et al. Long-term effects of continuing adjuvant tamoxifen to 10 years versus stopping at 5 years after diagnosis of oestrogen receptor-positive breast cancer: ATLAS, a randomised trial. *Lancet.* 2013;381:805–816.
2. Gray RG, Rea DW, Handley K, et al. ATTom: randomized trial of 10 versus 5 years of adjuvant tamoxifen among 6,934 women with estrogen receptor-positive (ER+) or ER untested breast cancer—preliminary results. *Proc Am J Clin Oncol.* 2008;26(suppl 10). abstr 513.
3. Goss PE, Ingle JN, Pritchard KI, et al. Extending aromatase-inhibitor adjuvant therapy to 10 years. *N Engl J Med.* 2016;375:209–219.

Question 16

1. Schneeweiss A, Chia S, Hickish T, et al. Pertuzumab plus trastuzumab in combination with standard neoadjuvant anthracycline-containing and anthracycline-free chemotherapy regimens in patients with HER2-positive early breast cancer: a randomized phase II cardiac safety study (TRYPHAENA). *Ann Oncol.* 2013;24:2278–2284.
2. Gianni L, Pienkowski T, Im YH, et al. Efficacy and safety of neoadjuvant pertuzumab and trastuzumab in women with locally advanced, inflammatory, or early HER2-positive breast cancer (NeoSphere): a randomised multicentre, open-label, phase 2 trial. *Lancet Oncol.* 2012;13:25–32.

Question 17

1. Loibl S, Schmidt A, Gentilini O, et al. Breast cancer diagnosed during pregnancy adapting recent advances in breast cancer care for pregnant patients. *JAMA Oncol.* 2015;1(8):1145–1153.
2. Hance KW, Anderson WF, Devesa SS, Young HA, Levine PH. Trends in inflammatory breast carcinoma incidence and survival: the surveillance, epidemiology, and end results program at the National Cancer Institute. *J Natl Cancer Inst.* 2005;97:966–975.

3. Dawood S, Merajver SD, Viens P, et al. International expert panel on inflammatory breast cancer: consensus statement for standardized diagnosis and treatment. *Ann Oncol.* 2011;22:515–523.

Question 18

1. Sikov WM, Berry DA, Perou CM, et al. Impact of the addition of carboplatin and/or bevacizumab to neoadjuvant once-per-week paclitaxel followed by dose-dense doxorubicin and cyclophosphamide on pathologic complete response rates in stage II to III triple-negative breast cancer: CALGB 40603 (Alliance). *J Clin Oncol.* 2015;33:13–21.

Question 21

1. Aebi S, Gelber S, Anderson SJ, et al. Chemotherapy for isolated locoregional recurrence of breast cancer (CALOR): a randomised trial. *Lancet Oncol.* 2014;15:156–163.

Question 22

1. Muss HB, Berry DA, Cirrincione CT, et al. Adjuvant Chemotherapy in Older Women with Early-Stage Breast Cancer. *N Engl J Med.* 2009;360:2055–2065.

Question 24

1. Mauri D, Pavlidis N, Ioannidis JP. Neoadjuvant versus adjuvant systemic treatment in breast cancer: a meta-analysis. *J Natl Cancer Inst.* 2005;97:188–194.
2. Kaufmann M, Hortobagyi GN, Goldhirsch A, et al. Recommendations from an international expert panel on the use of neoadjuvant (primary) systemic treatment of operable breast cancer: an update. *J Clin Oncol.* 2006;24:1940–1949.

Question 25

1. Schneeweiss A, Chia S, Hickish T, et al. Pertuzumab plus trastuzumab in combination with standard neoadjuvant anthracycline-containing and anthracycline-free chemotherapy regimens in patients with HER2-positive early breast cancer: a randomized phase II cardiac safety study (TRYPHAENA). *Ann Oncol.* 2013;24:2278–2284.
2. Gianni L, Pienkowski T, Im YH, et al. Efficacy and safety of neoadjuvant pertuzumab and trastuzumab in women with locally advanced, inflammatory, or early HER2-positive breast cancer (NeoSphere): a randomised multicentre, open-label, phase 2 trial. *Lancet Oncol.* 2012;13:25–32.

Question 26

1. Buchholz TA, Somerfield MR, Griggs JJ, et al. Margins for breast-conserving surgery with whole-breast irradiation in stage I and II invasive breast cancer: American Society of Clinical Oncology endorsement of the Society of Surgical Oncology/American Society for Radiation Oncology consensus guideline. *J Clin Oncol.* 2014;32:1502–1506.
2. Giuliano AE, Hunt KK, Ballman KV, et al. Axillary dissection vs no axillary dissection in women with invasive breast cancer and sentinel node metastasis: a randomized clinical trial. *JAMA.* 2011;305:569–575.
3. Sikov WM, Berry DA, Perou CM, et al. Impact of the addition of carboplatin and/or bevacizumab to neoadjuvant once-per-week paclitaxel followed by dose-dense doxorubicin and cyclophosphamide on pathologic complete response rates in stage II to III triple-negative breast cancer: CALGB 40603 (Alliance). *J Clin Oncol.* 2015;33:13–21.

Question 27

1. Vera-Badillo FE, Napoleone M, Ocana A, et al. Effect of multifocality and multicentricity on outcome in early stage breast cancer: a systematic review and meta-analysis. *Breast Cancer Res Treat.* 2014;146:235–244.

Question 28

1. Fisher B, Anderson S, Bryant J, et al. Twenty-year follow-up of a randomized trial comparing total mastectomy, lumpectomy, and lumpectomy plus irradiation for the treatment of invasive breast cancer. *N Engl J Med.* 2002;347:1233–1241.

2. Lyman GH, Giuliano AE, Somerfield MR, et al. American Society of Clinical Oncology guideline recommendations for sentinel lymph node biopsy in early-stage breast cancer. *J Clin Oncol.* 2005;23:7703–7720.

Question 29

1. Early Breast Cancer Trialists' Collaborative Group (EBCTCG). Effects of chemotherapy and hormonal therapy for early breast cancer on recurrence and 15-year survival: an overview of the randomised trials. *Lancet.* 2005;365:1687–1717.
2. Burstein HJ, Lacchetti C, Anderson H, et al. Adjuvant endocrine therapy for women with hormone receptor-positive breast cancer: American Society of Clinical Oncology Clinical Practice Guideline Update on Ovarian Suppression. *J Clin Oncol.* 2016;12(4):390–393.
3. Smith IE, Dowsett M, Yap YS, et al. Adjuvant aromatase inhibitors for early breast cancer after chemotherapy-induced amenorrhoea: caution and suggested guidelines. *J Clin Oncol.* 2006;24:2444–2447.
4. Regan MM, Francis PA, Pagani O, et al. absolute benefit of adjuvant endocrine therapies for premenopausal women with hormone receptor-positive, human epidermal growth factor receptor 2-negative early breast cancer: TEXT and SOFT trials. *J Clin Oncol.* 2016;34(19):2221–2231.

Question 30

1. Dowsett M, Cuzick J, Ingle J, et al. Meta-analysis of breast cancer outcomes in adjuvant trials of aromatase inhibitors versus tamoxifen. *J Clin Oncol.* 2010;28:509–518.
2. Davies C, Pan H, Godwin J, et al. Long-term effects of continuing adjuvant tamoxifen to 10 years versus stopping at 5 years after diagnosis of oestrogen receptor-positive breast cancer: ATLAS, a randomised trial. *Lancet.* 2013;381:805–816.
3. Goss PE, Ingle JN, Pritchard KI, et al. Extending aromatase-inhibitor adjuvant therapy to 10 years. *N Engl J Med.* 2016;375:209–219.

Question 31

1. Piccart-Gebhart M, Holmes E, Baselga J, et al. Adjuvant lapatinib and trastuzumab for early human epidermal growth factor receptor 2-positive breast cancer: results from the randomized phase III adjuvant lapatinib and/or trastuzumab treatment optimization trial. *J Clin Oncol.* 2016;34:1034–1042.
2. Perez EA, Romond EH, Suman VJ, et al. Four-year follow-up of trastuzumab plus adjuvant chemotherapy for operable human epidermal growth factor receptor 2-positive breast cancer: joint analysis of data from NCCTG N9831 and NSABP B-31. *J Clin Oncol.* 2011;29:3366–3373.

Question 32

1. Perez EA, Romond EH, Suman VJ, et al. Four-year follow-up of trastuzumab plus adjuvant chemotherapy for operable human epidermal growth factor receptor 2-positive breast cancer: joint analysis of data from NCCTG N9831 and NSABP B-31. *J Clin Oncol.* 2011;29:3366–3373.
2. Gonzalez-Angulo AM, Litton JK, Broglio KR, et al. High risk of recurrence for patients with breast cancer who have human epidermal growth factor receptor 2-positive, node-negative tumors 1 cm or smaller. *J Clin Oncol.* 2009;27:5700–5706.
3. Tolaney SM, Barry WT, Dang CT, et al. Adjuvant paclitaxel and trastuzumab for node-negative, HER2-positive breast cancer. *N Engl J Med.* 2015;372:134–141.

Question 33

1. Davies C, Pan H, Godwin J, et al. Long-term effects of continuing adjuvant tamoxifen to 10 years versus stopping at 5 years after diagnosis of oestrogen receptor-positive breast cancer: ATLAS, a randomised trial. *Lancet.* 2013;381:805–816.
2. Jin H, Tu D, Zhao N, Shepherd LE, Goss PE. Longer-term outcomes of letrozole versus placebo after 5 years of tamoxifen in the NCIC CTG MA.17 trial: analyses adjusting for treatment crossover. *J Clin Oncol.* 2012;30:718–721.

Question 34

1. Paik S, Tang G, Shak S, et al. Gene expression and benefit of chemotherapy in women with node-negative, estrogen receptor-positive breast cancer. *J Clin Oncol.* 2006;24:3726–3734.

2. Albain KS, Barlow WE, Shak S, et al. Prognostic and predictive value of the 21-gene recurrence score assay in postmenopausal women with node-positive, oestrogen receptor–positive breast cancer on chemotherapy: a retrospective analysis of a randomised trial. *Lancet Oncol.* 2010;11:55–65.

Question 35

1. Wong SM, Freedman RA, Sagara Y, Aydogan F, Barry WT, Golshan M. Growing use of contralateral prophylactic mastectomy despite no improvement in long-term survival for invasive breast cancer. *Ann Surg.* 2016. [Epub ahead of print.].
2. Paik S, Tang G, Shak S, et al. Gene expression and benefit of chemotherapy in women with node-negative, estrogen receptor-positive breast cancer. *J Clin Oncol.* 2006;24:3726–3734.
3. Regan MM, Francis PA, Pagani O, et al. Absolute benefit of adjuvant endocrine therapies for premenopausal women with hormone receptor-positive, human epidermal growth factor receptor 2-negative early breast cancer: TEXT and SOFT trials. *J Clin Oncol.* 2016;34(19):2221–2231.

Question 36

1. Regan MM, Francis PA, Pagani O, et al. absolute benefit of adjuvant endocrine therapies for premenopausal women with hormone-receptor-positive, human epidermal growth factor receptor 2-negative early breast cancer: TEXT and SOFT trials. *J Clin Oncol.* 2016;34(19):2221–2231.

Question 37

1. Hayes DF. Clinical practice. Follow-up of patients with early breast cancer. *N Engl J Med.* 2007;356:2505–2513.
2. Runowicz CD, Leach CR, Henry NL, et al. American Cancer Society/American Society of Clinical Oncology Breast Cancer Survivorship Care Guideline. *J Clin Oncol.* 2016;34:611–635.

Question 38

1. Runowicz CD, Leach CR, Henry NL, et al. American Cancer Society/American Society of Clinical Oncology Breast Cancer Survivorship Care Guideline. *J Clin Oncol.* 2016;34:611–635.
2. Holmberg L, Iversen OE, Rudenstam CM, et al. Increased risk of recurrence after hormone replacement therapy in breast cancer survivors. *J Natl Cancer Inst.* 2008;100:475–482.

Question 40

1. Barnadas A, Gil M, Sanchez-Rovira P, et al. Neoadjuvant endocrine therapy for breast cancer: past, present and future. *Anticancer Drugs.* 2008;19:339–347.
2. Eiermann W, Paepke S, Appfelstaedt J, et al. Preoperative treatment of postmenopausal breast cancer patients with letrozole: a randomized double-blind multicenter study. *Ann Oncol.* 2001;12:1527–1532.

Question 41

1. Dawood S, Merajver SD, Viens P, et al. International expert panel on inflammatory breast cancer: consensus statement for standardized diagnosis and treatment. *Ann Oncol.* 2011;22:515–523.

Question 42

1. Kaufmann M, Hortobagyi GN, Goldhirsch A, et al. Recommendations from an international expert panel on the use of neoadjuvant (primary) systemic treatment of operable breast cancer: an update. *J Clin Oncol.* 2006;24:1940–1949.
2. Barnadas A, Gil M, Sanchez-Rovira P, et al. Neoadjuvant endocrine therapy for breast cancer: past, present and future. *Anticancer Drugs.* 2008;19:339–347.

Question 43

1. McKinnon E, Xiao P. Metaplastic carcinoma of the breast. *Arch Pathol Lab Med.* 2015;139:819–822.

Question 44

1. Harms W, Geretschlager A, Cescato C, Buess M, Koberle D, Asadpour B. Current treatment of isolated locoregional breast cancer recurrences. *Breast Care (Basel).* 2015;10:265–271.

Question 45

1. Aebi S, Gelber S, Anderson SJ, et al. Chemotherapy for isolated locoregional recurrence of breast cancer (CALOR): a randomised trial. *Lancet Oncol.* 2014;15:156–163.
2. Berry DA, Cirrincione C, Henderson IC, et al. Estrogen-receptor status and outcomes of modern chemotherapy for patients with node-positive breast cancer. *JAMA.* 2006;295:1658–1667.

Question 46

1. Wapnir IL, Anderson SJ, Mamounas EP, et al. Prognosis after ipsilateral breast tumor recurrence and locoregional recurrences in five National Surgical Adjuvant Breast and Bowel Project node-positive adjuvant breast cancer trials. *J Clin Oncol.* 2006;24:2028–2037.

Question 47

1. Korde LA, Zujewski JA, Kamin L, et al. Multidisciplinary meeting on male breast cancer: summary and research recommendations. *J Clin Oncol.* 2010;28:2114–2122.
2. Early Breast Cancer Trialists' Collaborative Group (EBCTCG), Peto R, et al. Comparisons between different polychemotherapy regimens for early breast cancer: meta-analyses of long-term outcome among 100,000 women in 123 randomised trials. *Lancet.* 2012;379:432–444.

Question 48

1. Korde LA, Zujewski JA, Kamin L, et al. Multidisciplinary meeting on male breast cancer: summary and research recommendations. *J Clin Oncol.* 2010;28:2114–2122.
2. Eggemann H, Ignatov A, Smith BJ, et al. Adjuvant therapy with tamoxifen compared to aromatase inhibitors for 257 male breast cancer patients. *Breast Can Res Treat.* 2013;127:465–470.
3. Early Breast Cancer Trialists' Collaborative Group, Darby S, McGale P, et al. Effect of radiotherapy after breast-conserving surgery on 10-year recurrence and 15-year breast cancer death: meta-analysis of individual patient data for 10,801 women in 17 randomised trials. *Lancet.* 2011;378:1707–1716.

Question 49

1. Tan BY, Acs G, Apple SK, et al. Phyllodes tumours of the breast: a consensus review. *Histopathology.* 2016;68:5–21.

2. Birch JM, Alston RD, McNally RJ, et al. Relative frequency and morphology of cancers in carriers of germline TP53 mutations. *Oncogene.* 2001;20:4621–4628.

Question 50

1. Arora TK, Terracina KP, Soong J, Idowu MO, Takabe K. Primary and secondary angiosarcoma of the breast. *Gland Surg.* 2014;3:28–34.
2. Abbott R, Styring E, Verstappen V, et al. Angiosarcoma of the breast following surgery and radiotherapy for breast cancer. *Nat Clin Pract Oncol.* 2008;12:727–736.

Question 51

1. Diab SG, Clark GM, Osborne CK, Libby A, Allred DC, Elledge RM. Tumor characteristics and clinical outcome of tubular and mucinous breast carcinomas. *J Clin Oncol.* 1999;17:1442–1448.
2. Liu GF, Yang Q, Haffty BG, Moran MS. Clinical-pathologic features and long-term outcomes of tubular carcinoma of the breast compared with invasive ductal carcinoma treated with breast conservation therapy. *Int J Radiat Oncol Biol Phys.* 2009;75:1304–1308.
3. Rakha EA, Lee AH, Evans AJ, et al. Tubular carcinoma of the breast: further evidence to supports its excellent prognosis. *J Clin Oncol.* 2010;28:99–104.

Question 52

1. Trebska-McGowan K, Terracina KP, Takabe K. Update on the surgical management of Paget's disease. *Gland Surg.* 2013;2:137–142.

Question 53

1. Valdes EK, Feldman SM, Boolbol SK. Papillary lesions: a review of the literature. *Ann Surg Oncol.* 2007;14:1009–1013.
2. Rizzo M, Linebarger J, Lowe MC, et al. Management of papillary breast lesions diagnosed on core-needle biopsy: clinical pathologic and radiologic analysis of 276 cases with surgical follow-up. *J Am Coll Surg.* 2012;214:280–287.
3. Degnim AC, King TA. Surgical management of high-risk breast lesions. *Surg Clin North Am.* 2013;93:329–340.

Metastatic Breast Cancer

QUESTIONS

1. A 68-year-old woman was referred to your office for evaluation of a newly diagnosed left breast cancer. A mammogram showed a 2.5-cm invasive left breast cancer with enlarged left axillary nodes. A core biopsy of the left breast showed invasive ductal carcinoma, grade 3, ER90%, PR0%, HER2 by IHC2+, and the HER2 FISH was positive for amplification with a HER2:CEP17 ratio of 3.2. A core biopsy of the left axilla also showed involvement by invasive ductal carcinoma. She reports experiencing fatigue, anorexia, and abdominal pain in the epigastric area. Her complete blood count and comprehensive metabolic panel are normal. A CT scan of her chest, abdomen, and pelvis shows several hepatic lesions. She undergoes a biopsy of one of the liver lesions, and it is consistent with her breast primary. ER95%, PR0%, and HER2 FISH was positive for amplification with a HER2:CEP17 ratio of 3.6. Her ECOG performance status is 1. Which of the following is the most appropriate treatment option?

   A. Docetaxel, trastuzumab, and pertuzumab
   B. Paclitaxel and trastuzumab
   C. Anastrozole and trastuzumab
   D. Letrozole and lapatinib
   E. Ado-trastuzumab emtansine

2. A 38-year old woman with a medical history significant for hypertension and beta-thalassemia intermedia was treated with mastectomy and adjuvant dose-dense doxorubicin and cyclophosphamide, followed by paclitaxel for a stage IIIA triple negative breast cancer (TNBC). The patient was due to begin radiation therapy next week, but her primary oncologist has canceled this treatment after obtaining a PET-CT scan that revealed two new bilateral 5.0 cm FDG-avid bilateral paraspinal soft-tissue masses from T8 to T10, without associated bone invasion/erosion. He recommended palliative chemotherapy, starting tomorrow. She presents at your office for a second opinion. She is tearful and very anxious. The best next step would be:

   A. Agree with your colleague, reassure the patient she needs treatment, and proceed immediately with palliative chemotherapy
   B. MRI of the thoracic spine
   C. Palliative radiation to T8–T10 region first, followed by palliative systemic chemotherapy

D. Screen patient for clinical trials evaluating new treatment strategies such as immunotherapy for patients with metastatic TNBC

E. Obtain tissue for diagnosis

3. A 49-year-old woman with metastatic breast cancer is referred to you for a second opinion. Four years ago, she was found to have a 2.0-cm, ER negative, PR negative, and HER2-negative, node negative left breast cancer. She underwent lumpectomy, sentinel lymph node biopsy, and received radiation therapy to the breast and four cycles of adjuvant chemotherapy with docetaxel and cyclophosphamide. Eighteen months ago, she was diagnosed with biopsy-proven metastatic disease involving the lungs and liver. She received weekly paclitaxel and experienced a partial response lasting 12 months. Then her disease progressed, and she began treatment with liposomal doxorubicin. Restaging studies after four cycles of liposomal doxorubicin chemotherapy showed stable disease. She then received an additional two cycles of liposomal doxorubicin. During her consultation with you, she reports no trouble doing most of her daily activities. She denies any peripheral neuropathy. She is anicteric. Physical examination findings are notable for a left breast incision. No pulmonary abnormalities are detected, and the lymph nodes and liver are not enlarged. Results of liver function tests and serum creatinine level are normal. Follow-up computed tomography shows tumor progression, with an increase in the size and number of liver metastases and pulmonary nodules. Which of the following is the most appropriate treatment option?

A. Ixabepilone and capecitabine

B. Eribulin

C. Doxorubicin

D. Docetaxel

E. Capecitabine

4. A 66-year-old woman with hormone receptor positive, HER2 negative, metastatic breast cancer on anastrozole and denosumab, as first-line therapy presents with right hip pain after a vacation to Hawaii. Scans reveal progression of disease in the lungs and sclerotic lesions in the bones without evidence of fracture. She denies dyspnea. Oxygen saturation in room air is 99%. What is the best course of action?

A. Switch endocrine therapy to fulvestrant and add palbociclib

B. Continue anastrozole, add everolimus, and switch zoledronate for denosumab

C. Start palbociclib at the same time as radiation to the hip, and switch letrozole for anastrozole

D. Start eribulin

E. Stop denosumab

5. A 52-year-old woman presents to you with a history of metastatic breast cancer initially diagnosed 5 years ago. When she presented at that time, she had a mass in the right breast, right axillary lymph node, and pulmonary nodules. A core biopsy of the right breast mass showed invasive ductal carcinoma, ER0%, PR0%, and HER2-FISH was amplified (HER2:CEP17 ratio 5.5). Core biopsy of a lung nodule confirmed metastatic breast cancer that was ER-negative, PR-negative, and HER2-amplified. She received initial therapy with docetaxel, pertuzumab, and trastuzumab for six cycles and achieved a partial response. She was then maintained on therapy with trastuzumab and pertuzumab for 6 months. She then developed progressive disease with development of liver metastases.

She was then treated with ado-trastuzumab emtansine (T-DM1). After 6 months, she develops headaches associated with mild nausea and vomiting. An MRI of the brain reveals she has developed five new brain metastases. She received whole brain radiotherapy. Restaging of her extracranial disease shows an increase in the size of the pulmonary and liver lesions. Her ECOG performance status is a 1. She is very motivated to continue with additional therapy.

A. Restart ado-trastuzumab emtansine (T-DM1)

B. Initiate lapatinib and capecitabine

C. Start pertuzumab

D. Start lapatinib

E. No further therapy is available

6. A 46-year-old woman is status post multiple lines of therapy for metastatic HER2+ breast cancer. She is currently receiving navelbine 25 mg/m^2 and trastuzumab 2 mg/kg IV weekly. After completing 6 weeks of therapy, she traveled to visit her family in another state. She presents today after returning from her trip to resume her systemic therapy. She missed a total of 3 weeks of therapy. Laboratory tests are acceptable for treatment. The last ECHO completed 10 weeks ago had normal ejection fraction. The patient is doing very well, and in great spirits, with a performance status of 1. What do you order?

A. Trastuzumab maintenance, 2 mg/kg IV weekly

B. Navelbine loading dose 50 mg/m^2 and trastuzumab loading dose 4 mg/kg followed by 2 mg/kg weekly thereafter

C. Navelbine alone until a new ECHO is performed

D. Navelbine 25 mg/m^2 and trastuzumab at 2 mg/kg IV weekly

E. Navelbine 25 mg/m^2 and trastuzumab loading dose 4 mg/kg followed by 2 mg/kg weekly thereafter

7. A healthy 40-year-old female presents with a 1-week history of headaches, nausea, and dizziness. Two years ago, she was diagnosed with a stage II (T2N1), ER-negative, PR-negative, and HER2-negative left breast cancer. She underwent lumpectomy, sentinel lymph node biopsy, radiation, and anthracycline/taxane-based adjuvant chemotherapy. On an MRI brain with contrast, she is found to have a 2-cm enhancing mass in the right occipital region, with some surrounding vasogenic edema. There are no other metastatic lesions. A CT scan of the chest, abdomen, pelvis, and bone scan does not show evidence of metastatic disease. She is started on oral steroids. She has an ECOG performance status of 1. Which of the following is the most appropriate intervention?

A. Refer to radiation oncology for whole brain radiation

B. Start anticonvulsants

C. Refer to a neurosurgeon for consideration of resection of the brain lesion to then be followed by irradiation

D. Start capecitabine

E. Start weekly paclitaxel

8. A 52-year-old woman with a history of hypertension, high cholesterol, and seasonal allergies is receiving exemestane and everolimus for treatment of hormone receptor positive, HER2 negative metastatic breast cancer. She has bone-only disease. She developed a skin rash and stomatitis, which has persisted since the second month of therapy. She presents today for scheduled follow-up at month 5 of therapy. She describes a new progressive dry cough associated with increasing shortness of breath when going upstairs at home. This first manifested 10 days ago, and she tells you she has not been upstairs for the past 3 days. She

also noticed increasing fatigue after work and a few days of temperature between 99.5°F and 100.6°F. She denies sick contacts. What are the best next steps?

A. Prescribe a course of amoxicillin and clavulanate; continue treatment with exemestane and everolimus

B. Refer the patient to immunologist for seasonal allergies treatment optimization

C. Stop exemestane and send labs containing complete blood count and blood cultures

D. Order an US Doppler of lower extremities

E. Order a high-resolution computed tomography scan of the chest; draw labs including complete blood count and blood cultures; send pulmonary consultation and hold everolimus

9. A 52-year-old postmenopausal woman is being treated with palbociclib and letrozole for metastatic breast cancer to the lungs and lymph nodes. You are seeing her in your office for consideration for her next cycle of therapy. Her complete blood count today reveals hematocrit 32%, hemoglobin 10 g/dL, WBC 2000/mm^3, absolute neutrophil count 800/mm^3, and platelets 130,000/mm^3. She is afebrile. The patient has been compliant with her treatment. She gives you a diary of her medicines. She completed 21 days of palbociclib 48 hours ago. What is the best next step?

A. Discontinue treatment with palbociclib due to hematologic toxicity

B. Repeat blood counts in 5 days and consider next cycle initiation at the same dose level

C. Hold palbociclib and repeat labs in 7 days; if counts recovered, resume palbociclib at lower dose level

D. Hold letrozole

E. Change abemaciclib for palbociclib

10. A postmenopausal woman presents for a second opinion regarding therapy for metastatic breast cancer. She describes new bone pain and right upper quadrant discomfort while on paclitaxel, trastuzumab, and pertuzumab. CT scans of chest, abdomen, and pelvis with IV contrast, as well as bone scan, reveal multiple new metastatic lesions in the bones and liver, and an increase in size of the previous hepatic masses. Her left ventricular ejection fraction measured by ECHO is unchanged at 55%. A liver biopsy performed 4 months ago confirmed ER+50%, PR+20%, and HER2 positive metastatic breast cancer. What would be the best treatment approach?

A. Continue paclitaxel, trastuzumab and pertuzumab, and add fulvestrant and zoledronate

B. Switch treatment to trastuzumab emtansine and zoledronate

C. Switch her treatment to lapatinib and capecitabine

D. Stop anti-HER2 therapy, and start letrozole and palbociclib

E. Transarterial chemoembolization (TACE) for liver metastases and radiation to affected bones

11. A 42-year-old woman was just diagnosed with metastatic triple negative breast cancer last week following a biopsy of a mediastinal node. She presents for a consultation and is requesting treatment on a clinical trial involving immunotherapy. Her symptoms are fatigue, right upper quadrant discomfort, and upper back pain. Over the past week, she has noticed urinary hesitancy and constipation. She is afebrile. She also describes residual numbness and tingling from adjuvant taxane-based chemotherapy that was completed 4 months ago. She takes lisinopril for hypertension and paracetamol as needed for pain. You get

STAT scans and diagnose metastases to right lower lobe of the lung, mediastinum, and thoracic spine. There is T8 vertebral body lesions with soft tissue component, causing narrowing of spinal canal. The most appropriate next steps are:

A. Enroll the patient in the trial and start immunotherapy with checkpoint inhibitors immediately

B. Schedule outpatient systemic chemotherapy with carboplatin/gemcitabine doublet starting during the next few days

C. Admit the patient to the hospital, and obtain neurosurgery and radiation oncology urgent consultations

D. Order MRI to be done as an outpatient, with follow-up appointment in clinic next week to wrap up the plan

E. Give her antibiotics, including community acquired pneumonia coverage, starting immediately

12. A 62-year-old female was diagnosed with a stage II (T1N1M0) ER-positive, PR-positive, and HER2-unknown breast cancer 15 years ago. She underwent lumpectomy, adjuvant chemotherapy, and radiation therapy. She declined adjuvant endocrine therapy. Then, 2 years ago, she presented with flank pain. A bone scan showed a moderately intense focus involving much of the right side of L1, consistent with metastatic focus. A CT scan did not show any visceral disease. An FNA of this region confirmed malignant tumor cells consistent with metastatic mammary carcinoma, ER greater than 90%, PR0%, and HER2:CEP17 ratio of 1.1. She was treated with radiation therapy to L1. She also was treated with anastrozole and denosumab and experienced stable disease for 18 months. She now has progression of disease in the bones, specifically in the left superior acetabulum, left pedicle of L4, and right iliac crest in addition to mediastinal lymphadenopathy. She was then treated with fulvestrant and palbociclib. Nine months later, restaging studies show progressive disease with new foci in the cervical and thoracic vertebrae. She still has minimal symptoms and denies any back pain. Which of the following is the most appropriate treatment option?

A. Combination chemotherapy

B. Fulvestrant and everolimus

C. Anastrozole and everolimus

D. Exemestane and everolimus

E. Letrozole and palbociclib

13. A 57-year-old postmenopausal woman with a history of a stage I (pT1N0) right breast cancer, ER65%, PR25%, and HER2 1+ diagnosed about 13 years ago underwent a lumpectomy, radiation therapy, and adjuvant chemotherapy with doxorubicin and cyclophosphamide for four cycles. She was on tamoxifen for 5 years. She then presented to her primary care physician with a complaint of midback pain. Her past medical history is also significant for paroxysmal atrial fibrillation and glaucoma. An MRI of her thoracic spine showed extensive osseous metastatic disease. There was also an enhancing epidural metastatic tumor extending from T3 through T6, exerting mild mass effect on the spinal cord, and enhancing epidural tumor extending into both neural foramina at the T4–T5 level. A CT scan did not show any visceral disease. A bone scan was positive in several areas including the cervical, thoracic, and lumbar spine as well as the pelvis. A core biopsy of the left ileum confirmed metastatic carcinoma, favoring breast origin, ER70%, PR 50%, and HER2 negative score was 0. Which of the following is the most appropriate therapy?

A. Combination chemotherapy and denosumab

B. Radiation therapy, aromatase inhibitor, palbociclib, and denosumab

C. Radiation therapy, tamoxifen, palbociclib, and denosumab
D. Aromatase inhibitor and denosumab
E. Radiation therapy alone

14. A 42-year-old woman with hormone receptor positive, HER2 negative metastatic breast cancer, comes for a consultation for a second opinion. She was initially diagnosed with breast cancer 6 years ago. She is status postbilateral mastectomies, reconstruction, adjuvant chemotherapy, radiation, and adjuvant endocrine therapy. After biopsy proven metastatic disease was diagnosed 4 years ago, she has gone on to receive multiple therapies, including bilateral oophorectomies, radiation to spine, aromatase inhibitor, mTOR inhibitor, CDK 4/6 inhibitor, fulvestrant, capecitabine, weekly taxol, carboplatin, gemcitabine, eribulin, vinorelbine, and ixabepilone. She has also been treated with a PI3K inhibitor as part of a trial. Six weeks ago, she underwent whole brain radiation for metastatic disease to the brain. Dexamethasone has now been completely tapered. She has experienced a significant and progressive clinical decline in the past 3 months. She was recently admitted to her local hospital for failure to thrive. She has bone pain, today 3/10, on narcotics. She is hungry but can only take small amounts of food at a time. She spends most of her time in bed or reclining on the couch and requires assistance to bathe, dress, and eat. She is able to walk in her house but no longer goes outside, except for medical appointments. The patient demands participation in an immunotherapy trial that you have open at your institution, or off-label use of pembrolizumab. Her sister is the caregiver. She looks exhausted while requesting help. What are the appropriate recommendations?
    A. Discuss goals of care, advance directives, and hospice care options; consider fractionated diet and nutritional supplement drinks
    B. Change the pain treatment regimen because uncontrolled pain may be the cause for clinical decline
    C. Consent the patient for the immunotherapy trial of a PD-1 checkpoint inhibitor and start the screening process
    D. MRI of the brain and CT scans of chest, abdomen, and pelvis, to evaluate for recent disease progression
    E. Order medical marijuana

15. An active 65-year-old woman was diagnosed 3 years ago with a stage III (T3N2) invasive left breast cancer, ER-positive, PR-positive, and HER-negative. Her only significant past medical history is bradyarrhythmias. She was treated with neoadjuvant doxorubicin and cyclophosphamide, followed by paclitaxel chemotherapy, mastectomy, postmastectomy radiation therapy, and then 5 years of anastrozole. She then recurred 12 months later with predominant osseous metastasis that was biopsy-proven to be consistent with her primary breast cancer with the same biomarkers. She then was initiated on fulvestrant and had improvement of disease that lasted 6 months. Her disease progressed, and she was treated with weekly paclitaxel, with clinical improvement lasting 12 months. Restaging studies reveal lung metastases. She began treatment with capecitabine. She developed hand-foot syndrome requiring a dose reduction after two cycles.
She received an additional four cycles of capecitabine to date. On follow-up evaluation today, she reports no trouble performing most of her daily activities. She denies any shortness of breath or peripheral neuropathy. Physical examination findings are notable for a left breast incision. No pulmonary abnormalities are detected, and the lymph

nodes and liver are not enlarged. Results of liver function tests and serum creatinine level are normal. Follow-up computed tomography shows tumor progression, with an increase in the size and number of pulmonary nodules and new bone lesions. You are considering treatment with eribulin. Which of the following is the most appropriate intervention?
    A. Obtain a baseline echocardiogram
    B. Obtain baseline pulmonary function tests
    C. Obtain a baseline ECG
    D. Check a urinalysis for protein
    E. Give prophylactic growth colony stimulating factors with the first cycle of treatment

16. A 62-year-old woman presents to your office to establish care. Four years ago, she was diagnosed with stage II (T2N1aM0) ER-negative, PR-negative, and HER2-positive right breast cancer. She presented with a 4.7 cm mass in the right breast. She underwent neoadjuvant chemotherapy with doxorubicin and cyclophosphamide for four cycles, followed by paclitaxel and trastuzumab for 12 weeks. She underwent a mastectomy and had residual disease of 2.3 cm in the breast with negative nodes and negative margins. Her pathologic stage was ypT2ypN0. She received postmastectomy radiation therapy. She completed adjuvant trastuzumab therapy. One year ago, she was diagnosed with metastatic disease. A CT scan of the chest, abdomen, and pelvis showed presumed metastatic bone lesions of the pelvis with a large destructive left sacral mass measuring 5.7×4.6 cm^2. A subsequent CT-guided pelvic biopsy was performed and described metastatic carcinoma, features consistent with metastatic breast carcinoma, ER-negative, PR-negative, and HER IHC 3+. She received palliative radiation to the left sacroiliac area and was started on zoledronic acid. She was treated with docetaxel, trastuzumab, and pertuzumab for six cycles. She underwent restaging studies of her spine, which showed an increase in the size and number of metastatic foci throughout the thoracic vertebral bodies, and findings consistent with progression of disease. An MRI of the brain was significant for an 8-mm focus of increased contrast enhancement in the left parietal lobe. She underwent radiosurgery to the left parietal lobe. Due to side effects from treatment, she elects not to receive additional systemic therapy. She sees you for the first time and reports symptoms of progressive fatigue, anorexia, headaches, and blurred vision. An ophthalmologic exam confirms she has bitemporal hemianopia. An MRI of the brain with contrast shows new abnormal thickening and enhancement of the pituitary stalk.
Laboratory studies:
Sodium 129 [136–145 mEq/L]
Chloride 97 [98–106 mEq/L]
Potassium 3.7 [3.5–5 mEq/L]
Carbon dioxide 20 [23–28 mEq/L]
Serum osmolality 301 [275–295 mOsm/kg]
What are the next best steps in the management? Choose all the correct answers.
    A. Convince her to start systemic therapy with ado-trastuzumab emtansine
    B. Order a specialized MRI of the brain with attention to the pituitary gland
    C. Order a prolactin level, thyroid function tests, and cortisol stimulation test
    D. Refer her to radiation oncology for evaluation
    E. Refer to neurosurgery for evaluation

17. A 63-year-old woman with metastatic triple negative breast cancer to the liver and spine was started on nab-paclitaxel

and denosumab. She presents after three cycles, with restaging CT scans for consideration of continuation of therapy. She feels better than she has in a very long time, except for grade 1 peripheral neuropathy related to the treatment. She is no longer taking narcotics. You review the current images, and the following findings are present:

- There is an approximately 40% decrease in the size of liver lesions.
- There are two vertebral lesions measuring 2.5 and 2.1 cm in T11 and L2, respectively (previously 2.5 and 2.2 cm), with a more prominent density pattern than baseline (at baseline they were osteolytic and now osteoblastic).
- There are three new satellite osteoblastic lesions in the vertebral body of L2, measuring approximately 2 mm each (not seen at baseline scans).

At baseline, T11 and L2 were positive on the bone scan. What is the most appropriate approach?

A. Stop nab-paclitaxel and obtain MRI of spine
B. Obtain serum protein electrophoresis
C. Stop denosumab
D. Continue treatment as planned, with nab-paclitaxel and denosumab
E. Obtain a PET-CT scan

18. A 52-year-old female is hospitalized because of abdominal pain. She was well until about 1 week ago when she presented with pain in the right upper quadrant, fatigue, and anorexia. On physical exam, she has a 5-cm mass in the right breast at 3 o'clock, and there is right axillary adenopathy. There is also tenderness in the right upper abdominal area, and the liver edge is palpable about 2 cm below the right costal margin.

Laboratory studies:

Serum total bilirubin	1.0 mg/dL [0.3–1.0]
Serum total alkaline phosphatase	302 IU/mL [30–120]
Serum aspartate transaminase	201 U/L [10–40]
Serum alanine transaminase	78 U/L [10–40]
Serum albumin	3.3 g/dL [3.5–5.5]

A core biopsy of the right breast tumor confirms infiltrating ductal carcinoma, ER0%, PR0%, with a HER2:CEP17 ratio of 3.4. CT scan showing multiple liver lesions. A core needle biopsy of one of the liver lesions confirms metastatic breast cancer, ER0%, PR0%, and a HER2:CEP17 ratio of 3.7. Which of the following would you recommend?

A. Docetaxel, trastuzumab, and pertuzumab
B. Paclitaxel, trastuzumab, and pertuzumab
C. Trastuzumab and pertuzumab
D. Trastuzumab and capecitabine
E. Surgically resect the right breast tumor and start a trastuzumab-based regimen

19. A 54-year-old female was treated with curative intent for her breast cancer with left lumpectomy, left sentinel lymph node biopsy, adjuvant docetaxel, cyclophosphamide and trastuzumab for six cycles, radiation therapy, trastuzumab to complete 1 year (completed 20 months ago), and adjuvant endocrine therapy with anastrozole (currently ongoing). As part of the investigation of her recent symptoms, scans revealed new nodules in the lungs and liver. A CT-guided biopsy of the liver confirmed recurrent breast cancer, ER negative, PR negative, HER2 3+ by immunohistochemistry. What is the best treatment option?

A. Lapatinib and capecitabine
B. Trastuzumab emtansine, single agent

C. Trastuzumab emtansine and zoledronate
D. A taxane combined with trastuzumab and pertuzumab
E. Exemestane and everolimus

20. A 67-year-old woman who was diagnosed with an early-stage hormone receptor-positive, HER2-negative left breast cancer in 2000 and was treated with adjuvant tamoxifen for 5 years presents to your office with increasing back pain. Her only significant past medical history is hyperlipidemia. A bone scan showed multiple abnormal foci of increased uptake suggesting metastatic disease, including the skull, pelvis, lumbosacral spine, and left femur. CT scans did not show any visceral disease. Biopsy of a metastatic bone lesion confirmed bone involved by carcinoma consistent with metastasis from a mammary primary, ER70%, PR20%, and HER2-negative (score = 0). You initiate therapy with letrozole and palbociclib and denosumab. Treatment with palbociclib has been associated with which of the following adverse effects?

A. Cardiomyopathy
B. Neutropenia
C. Interstitial pneumonitis
D. Hand-foot syndrome
E. Neuropathy

21. A 53-year-old woman with stage IV HER2+ breast cancer received her first cycle of taxotere, trastuzumab, and pertuzumab. On day 3 postinfusion, she developed grade 3 diarrhea (had 10 episodes of diarrhea in 24 hours, limiting self-care) and became dehydrated requiring hospitalization. In the hospital, blood counts were normal and chemistry was remarkable for a creatinine of 1.3 mg/dL and a BUN of 22 mg/dL. The patient was afebrile and clinically dehydrated. Stool studies were negative for fecal leukocytes, *Clostridium difficile*, or blood. Cultures were negative. She received IV fluids, loperamide, lomotil, and octreotide with improvement. At discharge from the hospital, you recommend:

A. Colonoscopy as outpatient after consultation with gastroenterologist
B. Ciprofloxacin PO course
C. Dietary changes
D. Scheduled loperamide and PO hydration after hospitalization until the next visit for treatment cycle 2, with lomotil as needed for resistant diarrhea
E. Vancomycin PO

22. You have been caring for a 58-year-old woman who has metastatic breast cancer. She was found to have a 1.5-cm estrogen receptor–negative, progesterone receptor–negative, HER2-negative, node-positive (2 out of 12) infiltrating ductal carcinoma. She underwent lumpectomy and four cycles of adjuvant chemotherapy with dose-dense doxorubicin and cyclophosphamide, followed by 12 weekly treatments of paclitaxel. She received radiation therapy to the breast. She underwent genetic testing, and this did not reveal a BRCA1 or BRCA2 mutation. Five months after her last paclitaxel chemotherapy, she presents to you with abdominal pain. She is diagnosed with biopsy-proven metastatic disease to the liver. The liver lesion is ER-negative, PR-negative, and HER2-negative. Imaging also reveals lung metastases. She states she does not want to go back on IV chemotherapy. You treat her with capecitabine. After 6 weeks of therapy, she has progressive disease in the liver and lungs, but is still asymptomatic. She is now willing to take IV chemotherapy. Which of the following is the most appropriate course of action at this point?

A. Paclitaxel
B. Paclitaxel and gemcitabine
C. Ixabepilone
D. Nab-paclitaxel
E. Docetaxel and capecitabine

23. A 59-year-old woman is receiving capecitabine for metastatic hormone receptor positive, HER2 negative breast cancer that became endocrine therapy resistant. She is also on denosumab due to the diagnosis of bone metastases. Her treatment is complicated, with grade 1 stomatitis and erythrodysesthesia, and grade 2 diarrhea, all clinically managed. She presents for consideration of another cycle of therapy, with new complaints of discomfort close to her left mandibular second molar. She describes a hard rough white area in the gum just below the tooth crown, which started after eating crunchy chips. On exam, you identify a 8 × 4 mm² ulceration with bone exposure in that area. There is no associated erythema or bleeding. Submandibular and cervical lymph nodes are unremarkable on exam. The patient is afebrile. What is the next most appropriate step?
    A. Start fluconazole
    B. Start acyclovir
    C. Change capecitabine to weekly paclitaxel
    D. Obtain ear, nose, and throat specialist consultation, and consider stopping denosumab
    E. Switch zoledronate for denosumab

24. A 55-year-old woman who has metastatic breast cancer presents to you for a second opinion regarding her treatment options. Two years ago, she was evaluated for a palpable mass in the right breast. Ultrasonography-guided core needle biopsy revealed a poorly differentiated, estrogen receptor–negative, progesterone receptor–negative, HER2-positive invasive ductal cancer. Staging studies showed a left pleural effusion, bone, and liver lesions that were consistent with metastatic disease. At that time, she had been experiencing increasing dyspnea with exertion. She underwent a left-sided thoracentesis, and 800 mL of serosanguineous fluid was removed. Cytology of the fluid was positive for adenocarcinoma; immunohistochemistry staining was negative for ER, negative for PR, and positive (3+) for HER2. She was treated with paclitaxel, trastuzumab, pertuzumab, and denosumab. She received six cycles of paclitaxel, trastuzumab, and pertuzumab, and then remained on trastuzumab, pertuzumab, and denosumab. She had an excellent initial response both clinically and radiographically, with resolution of the left pleural effusion. On follow-up evaluation today, however, repeat staging studies show an increase in the size and number of the liver and bone lesions, and reoccurrence of the left pleural effusion, consistent with tumor progression. Which of the following is the most appropriate therapy?
    A. Lapatinib and capecitabine
    B. Docetaxel, carboplatin, and trastuzumab
    C. Ado-trastuzumab emtansine (T-DM1)
    D. Trastuzumab
    E. Trastuzumab and capecitabine

25. A 44-year-old woman with metastatic triple negative breast cancer to liver and lungs is status postadjuvant chemotherapy and two lines of chemotherapy in the metastatic setting. She presented for her second cycle of eribulin. After the first cycle of this therapy, the right upper quadrant pain resolved. Unfortunately, she experienced severe nausea and vomiting, requiring escalation of antiemetics at home and at the infusion center. She was at the infusion center for cycle 2 day 1 of eribulin, receiving the initial premedication with ondansetron, when she complained of odd dizziness with epigastric discomfort. Vital signs were normal. Within minutes of checking the vital signs, the nurse noted that the patient had a motionless stare, followed by automatic and cyclic movements of her mouth. Lorazepam 1 mg IV was administered, and the rapid response team was called. No tonic/clonic activity was noted. The event subsided after lorazepam, and the patient remained somnolent and aphasic for approximately 20 minutes. After that, she was able to talk and respond to questions appropriately. On your exam, she is oriented to person, place, and time. There are no neurologic findings; however, she does not recall the event. What are the next steps?
    A. Reassure the patient and her husband that this was a side effect from ondansetron, and that this drug will no longer be used.
    B. Initiate cognitive and behavioral therapies, and prescribe selective serotonin reuptake inhibitors (SSRIs).
    C. You bring the patient to emergency room with the rapid response team, and order a noncontrast CT scan of the head. If normal, you recommend a brain MRI with contrast.
    D. Give NS 0.9% 500 cc IV at infusion center. If stable, continue eribulin treatment as planned.
    E. Check magnesium levels. If normal, proceed with eribulin as planned.

26. Twelve years ago, a 76-year-old woman was found to have a 1.6-cm left breast cancer without lymph node involvement. The tumor was ER-negative, PR-positive, and HER2-negative. After breast conservation surgery, she received four cycles of chemotherapy with doxorubicin and cyclophosphamide, and radiation therapy to the breast. She completed 5 years of anastrozole. Recently, a lymph node in the right supraclavicular fossa was noted. Fine-needle aspiration confirmed carcinoma consistent with the primary breast cancer. There was not enough material to perform ER, PR, or HER2. On evaluation in your office, she reports no symptoms. Vital signs are normal. A 2.5-cm lymph node is palpable in the right supraclavicular fossa. No other lymph node enlargement is apparent. Other findings of the physical examination, including breast examination findings, are unremarkable. Complete blood count is normal, results of liver function tests are normal, and serum CA 27–29 is elevated at 313.0 U/mL (<38.0). Bilateral mammography and breast magnetic resonance imaging show no evidence of recurrence or new breast abnormality. Contrast-enhanced computed tomography of the chest, abdomen, and pelvis shows several bilateral less than 1 cm pulmonary nodules. The liver is normal. Multiple foci of osteoblastic metastasis are noted in the spine and pelvis. A bone scan shows abnormal uptake in the calvarium, thoracic and lumbar spine, and right iliac wing. She is asymptomatic. What is the next best step in her management?
    A. PET-CT scan
    B. Excision of the supraclavicular lymph node for assessment of ER, PR, and HER2 status
    C. Initiate radiation therapy to all areas of the bone that are abnormal on bone scan
    D. Start fulvestrant
    E. Start weekly paclitaxel

27. A 36-year-old woman with a history of a stage IIB (T2N1) right breast cancer who underwent a right mastectomy and axillary lymph node dissection for a 3.4-cm ER81%,

PR33%, and HER2-negative tumor with 1/18 positive lymph nodes, and completed adjuvant chemotherapy with dose-dense doxorubicin and cyclophosphamide, and weekly paclitaxel, and has been on adjuvant tamoxifen for the last 2 years. She presented to the ER with flank pain and a CT scan of the abdomen revealed a kidney stone, in addition to four liver lesions. An US-guided core biopsy of one of these liver lesions confirmed it to be an ER-positive, PR-positive, and HER2-negative breast cancer. She receives therapy with ovarian suppression and letrozole. Ten months later, restaging studies show bone metastases in her ribs with stable liver lesions. She continues to be asymptomatic with an ECOG performance status of 0. Which of the following is the most appropriate therapy?
  A. Anastrozole
  B. Continue ovarian suppression and letrozole
  C. Progestins
  D. Ovarian suppression, fulvestrant, and palbociclib
  E. Liposomal doxorubicin

28. A 72-year-old woman presented with shortness of breath to the emergency department. She had a history of hormone receptor positive breast cancer treated with surgery alone in 1986. She had been on raloxifene for osteoporosis from 2001 to 2016. Investigation at the ED revealed a left-sided pleural effusion. Thoracentesis was performed with cytology and cellblock revealing ER+100%, PR+80%, HER2 negative, and metastatic breast cancer. Breast mammogram and MRI were negative for new suspicious lesions. Systemic staging revealed bone lesions in the ribs and hip, without immediate risk for fracture. She had an indwelling pleural catheter (Pleurx) placed with resolution of her dyspnea. At the time she was discharged from the hospital, she was referred to you for further treatment planning. She has been draining the pleural fluid twice a week. At your office, her ECOG PS is 1. Saturation of oxygen at rest and exertion is 100% and 97%, respectively. She denies supplemental oxygen use. There is no evidence of infection on exam. The best treatment option at this point is:
  A. Letrozole and denosumab
  B. Anastrozole and zoledronate
  C. Letrozole, palbociclib, and denosumab
  D. Carboplatin and gemcitabine
  E. Trastuzumab, pertuzumab, and paclitaxel

ANSWERS

1. A

This patient has a HER2-positive breast cancer with symptomatic visceral metastases. The best treatment option is dual HER2 blockade in combination with chemotherapy. The phase III CLEOPATRA trial was designed to evaluate dual HER2 inhibition through the addition of pertuzumab, a HER2-directed antibody, to trastuzumab and docetaxel for HER2-positive metastatic breast cancer (MBC). Results showed that the median overall survival was 56.5 months (95% confidence interval [CI], 49.3 to not reached) in the group receiving the pertuzumab combination, as compared with 40.8 months (95% CI, 35.8–48.3) in the group receiving the placebo combination (hazard ratio favoring the pertuzumab group, 0.68; 95% CI, 0.56–0.84; $P < .001$), a difference of 15.7 months. Median progression-free survival as assessed by investigators improved by 6.3 months in the pertuzumab group (hazard ratio, 0.68; 95% CI, 0.58–0.80). The toxicity profiles of the two treatment groups were similar. As a result of this trial, pertuzumab plus trastuzumab plus docetaxel was approved by the US Food and Drug Administration, and pertuzumab plus trastuzumab plus taxane has been recommended by the National Comprehensive Cancer Network as a preferred regimen for the first-line treatment of HER2-positive MBC. The patient is symptomatic, and anastrozole or letrozole with a HER2-targeted agent are not good choices for this patient. Ado-trastuzumab emtansine is not approved as a single-agent in the first-line setting. Given the substantial survival associated with docetaxel plus trastuzumab and pertuzumab of over 56 months, there would be no reason to give only trastuzumab and paclitaxel as a first-line regimen.

2. E

Differential diagnosis of soft tissue mass in patients with a history of breast cancer treated with curative intent. The recommendation is for biopsy of metastatic disease as part of the workup of suspicious lesions in patients who present with metastatic disease, or at first disease recurrence after curative treatment. This is performed in order to confirm diagnosis of metastasis, and to determine the receptor status. This recommendation is endorsed by the NCCN Panel. Patients with beta-thalassemia may develop extramedullary hematopoiesis, which may present as paraspinal masses. Recent use of chemotherapy may cause FDG avidity in any tissue with marrow activity, including the extramedullary hematopoietic sites; placing it in the differential diagnosis with recurring/metastatic breast cancer. Answer A is not acceptable before tissue diagnosis of metastatic disease. Answer B would evaluate the anatomy of lesion, but would not provide definitive diagnosis. Spinal MRI would potentially be useful if there were concerns for bone involvement or spinal cord compromise. Answers C and D could represent a valid options, after histologic confirmation of metastatic disease.

3. B

The approval of eribulin was based on phase III data showing eribulin to be the first monotherapy to prolong survival in women with heavily pretreated metastatic breast cancer.

Eribulin is a microtubule inhibitor indicated for the treatment of patients with metastatic breast cancer who have previously received at least two chemotherapeutic regimens for the treatment of metastatic disease. Prior therapy should have included an anthracycline and a taxane in either the adjuvant or metastatic setting. This was based on the results of Eisai Metastatic Breast Cancer Study Assessing Physician's Choice Versus E7389 (EMBRACE), a phase III study in pretreated metastatic breast cancer patients (previously treated with ≥2 prior chemotherapies, including an anthracycline and a taxane, unless contraindicated) to compare overall survival with eribulin compared with treatment of choice. Patients were randomized (2:1) to receive eribulin 1.4 mg/m^2 in 2–5 minutes intravenous bolus on days 1 and 8 of a 21-day cycle or treatment of physician's choice (TPC). TPC included any single-agent chemotherapy, hormonal, or biological treatment approved for the treatment of cancer, radiotherapy, or symptomatic treatment alone. The primary endpoint of the trial was OS. A total of 762 patients were randomized as follows: 508

patients to eribulin and 254 patients to TPC. The study met its primary endpoint. Overall survival was longer for patients who received eribulin than for those who received treatment of physician's choice (13.1 months vs. 10.6 months; HR, 0.81; $P = .04$). Overall response rates (12% with eribulin versus 5% with TPC [$P = .002$] and progression-free survival also favored patients who received eribulin [PFS was 3.7 months with eribulin and 2.2 months with TPC [HR 0.87; 95% CI 0.71–1.05; $P = .137$]). The majority of patients received chemotherapy (96%), which included vinorelbine (25%), gemcitabine (19%), and capecitabine (18%). The remaining 4% of patients received endocrine therapy, and no patient was treated with supportive care alone. Median number of prior chemotherapy regimens was four, and 73% of them had received prior capecitabine. Ixabepilone and capecitabine is not necessary for this patient. Although combination chemotherapy provides higher rates of response and longer time to progression, compared with single-agent chemotherapy, combination chemotherapy is associated with increase in toxicity, and studies have not demonstrated a survival benefit. Single-agent chemotherapy is preferred to minimize the side effects. Combination cytotoxic regimens are usually given to those who are very symptomatic and have rapidly progressive disease. This patient is asymptomatic and has a volume of visceral disease that does not appear to be fast growing or appears to have any imminent threat of organ compromise. Doxorubicin and docetaxel are not good choices for this patient, given prior treatment with liposomal doxorubicin and docetaxel, respectively.

4. A

Second-line therapy for patients with metastatic disease that is HR+HER2−. The phase III trial PALOMA-3 randomized patients with hormone receptor positive, HER2 negative metastatic breast cancer that had progressed during endocrine therapy to receive fulvestrant or fulvestrant combined with palbociclib. The median progression-free survival with combined treatment was 9.2 months, and with fulvestrant alone 3.8 months. This study led to FDA approval of palbociclib/fulvestrant as second-line therapy for patients with hormone-receptor positive metastatic breast cancer that had progressed on endocrine therapy. The mTOR inhibitor everolimus is an option combined with exemestane, not with anastrozole (answer B). There are no data on safety of palbociclib concomitant with radiation. Upon progression on the aromatase inhibitor anastrozole, it is preferred to use palbociclib in combination with fulvestrant, rather than with letrozole (answer C). Chemotherapy could be an option in the case of visceral crisis; however, the presented clinical history does not suggest lung compromise is severe (answer D). Stopping denosumab will not address the problem of resistance to first-line endocrine therapy (answer E).

5. B

Lapatinib is an oral small molecule that targets the intracellular kinase domain of HER1 and HER2. Lapatinib binds to intracellular ATP binding site of EGFR and HER2 preventing phosphorylation and activation. It causes reversible inhibition of HER1 and HER2 homodimer and heterodimer formation. A phase III trial was conducted that compared lapatinib and capecitabine versus capecitabine alone in women with HER2-positive metastatic breast cancer. All participants had been previously treated with an anthracycline, taxane, and trastuzumab. None had prior capecitabine. Patients were randomized to receive either 1250 mg of lapatinib daily plus 2000 mg/m²/day of

capecitabine days 1–14 every 3 weeks or capecitabine 2500 mg/m²/day on days 1–14 every 3 weeks. Treatment continued until disease progression or unacceptable toxicity. The benefit of combining lapatinib with capecitabine was demonstrated. The median time to progression was 8.4 months in the combination arm, as compared with 4.4 months in the capecitabine arm (HR = 0.49, $P < .001$). These results led to the FDA approval of lapatinib in combination with capecitabine, in the treatment of patients with MBC that progress after receiving trastuzumab, anthracycline, and taxanes. The overall response rate was 22% (95% CI, 16–29) and 14% in the monotherapy group (95% CI, 9–21; $P = .09$), but this was not statistically significant, primarily due to the fact that fewer patients were enrolled than originally planned, and the study was noted adequately powered to evaluate this difference. The corresponding clinical benefit-benefit rates were 27% for the combination and 18% for the monotherapy group. In the phase III trial evaluating capecitabine with or without lapatinib in patients with HER2-positive metastatic breast cancer, fewer women in the lapatinib-containing arm developed central nervous system metastases compared with the capecitabine alone arm (13 vs. 4 patients, respectively; $P = .045$). Thus in a patient like this with HER2-positive disease with brain metastases who has received prior therapy with chemotherapy, pertuzumab and trastuzumab, and TDM-1, lapatinib, and capecitabine is the most reasonable combination to administer, given lapatinib's potential for better penetration of the blood-brain barrier compared with trastuzumab.

6. E

When does trastuzumab need to be reloaded? According to a package insert of trastuzumab, if a patient who is on weekly schedule has missed a dose of trastuzumab by more than 1 week, a reloading dose of trastuzumab should be administered over approximately 90 minutes (weekly schedule: 4 mg/kg) as soon as possible. Subsequent trastuzumab maintenance doses (weekly schedule: 2 mg/kg) should then be resumed every 7 days according to the weekly schedule. Based on FDA recommendations, ECHO is typically repeated every 3 months while the patient is receiving trastuzumab (every 12 weeks). Navelbine does not require loading dose.

7. C

Surgical excision should be considered for patients with minimal or no evidence of extracranial disease, good performance status, and a surgically accessible single brain metastasis that is amenable to complete excision. To reduce the risk of recurrence in patients who have undergone resection of a single brain metastasis, postoperative radiotherapy should be considered. In 1998 Patchell and colleagues investigated the benefit of using whole brain radiation (WBRT) as an adjunctive therapy following surgical tumor removal in these patients. The study randomized 95 patients to surgery alone or surgery plus (WBRT). Progression of intracranial disease was fourfold greater in the surgery-alone group, and local recurrence was also higher in this group. Patients treated with surgery alone received WBRT at the time of CNS disease progression, and so survival data did not reflect the initial randomization of the groups. There was comparable survival between the groups: surgery plus WBRT, median survival 12.0 months; and surgery alone, median survival 10.8 months. These data support the use of WBRT with surgery for improvement in recurrence and local control. Seizures are another problem affecting patients with brain metastases. However, this does not justify the prophylactic use of anticonvulsants, especially given that typical anticonvulsants have side effects that include cognitive impairment, liver dysfunction, myelosuppression, and skin reactions. Systemic therapy does not need to be initiated in the absence of any extracranial disease.

8. E

Noninfectious pneumonitis as a complication of anticancer therapies in the metastatic setting. Noninfectious pneumonitis (NIP) is a well-recognized potential adverse event of everolimus. Its incidence is approximately 10%, with grade 3/4 incidence rates of 0.8%–5.0% in reports from BOLERO-2 and BALLET trials, with higher reported incidences within the older population. In the BALLET trial, NIP caused two out of four deaths attributed to treatment toxicity. Patients may present with nonproductive cough, dyspnea, with or without systemic symptoms of fever and fatigue. Many patients are asymptomatic, with signs detected on high-resolution CT (HRCT) scan of the chest. The most common findings of HRCT are ground-glass opacities, lobular septal linear thickening, and multifocal areas of lung consolidation more commonly seen at bases. For NIP interfering with ADL, fiberoptic bronchoscopy and BAL are strongly recommended after HRCT rules out other causes/confirms initial suspicion. A respiratory infection would potentially be in the differential diagnosis, and amoxicillin and clavulanate could be an option to treat this; however, everolimus should be on hold until HRCT is done (answer A). Referral to the allergist may be useful after HRCT rules out NIP (answer B). Exemestane is not associated with NIP (answer C). If a pulmonary embolism is suspected, a CT angiogram of the chest should be ordered, instead of US Doppler of lower extremities (answer D). The BOLERO-2 trial was a randomized phase III trial comparing exemestane plus or minus everolimus as treatment for ER positive HER2 negative metastatic breast cancer patients. Median progression-free survival was 10.6 months with the combination and 4.1 months with exemestane alone. The BALLET trial was a phase IIIb expanded access safety study of everolimus and exemestane for patients with metastatic hormone receptor positive, HER2 negative advanced breast cancer. In this trial, 81.8% of patients experienced adverse events, with 27.2% being of grade 3/4 severity.

9. B

Palbociclib pharmacology. In the phase I clinical trial defining the palbociclib dose of 125 mg daily for 21 days followed by 7-day rest, there was a 12% incidence of neutropenia, which was considered a dose limiting toxicity (DLT). That study showed the neutropenia occurs gradually during the 21 days of treatment, with nadir at day 21. During the following 7 days off palbociclib, counts recover, allowing reinitiating treatment, typically at day 28 of the cycle. Therefore, labs on day 23 of cycle, as in this case, would be premature for assessment of hematologic toxicity that would lead to treatment changes.

10. B

Second-line therapy for patients with metastatic disease that is HER2 positive. The strongest evidence supporting the use of the antibody-drug conjugate trastuzumab emtansine (T-DM1, Kadcyla) in this setting comes from the EMILIA trial, in which patients with metastatic HER2 positive breast cancer were randomized to receive treatment with capecitabine/lapatinib or with trastuzumab emtansine. In this study, most enrolled patients had not previously been exposed to pertuzumab. Patients treated with trastuzumab emtansine had significant longer disease-free

and overall survival, and less toxicity than patients receiving lapatinib/capecitabine. The median overall survival at second interim analysis was 25.1 months with lapatinib/capecitabine and 30.9 months with trastuzumab emtansine. The results of the EMILIA trial led to FDA approval of trastuzumab emtansine as second-line treatment for patients with metastatic HER2+ breast cancer. A retrospective study of 78 patients treated with trastuzumab emtansine after being exposed to pertuzumab reported approximately 30% of the patients remained on therapy for 6 months or longer, with a tumor response rate of 18%. With the diagnosis of metastatic disease to bone, antiresorptive therapy would be recommended. There are no clinical data to support answer A or D as appropriate second-line therapy options for patients with HER2+ disease after progression to taxane/trastuzumab/pertuzumab combination. The experience with TACE in patients with breast cancer is limited. Furthermore, local therapy for liver metastases would not be a consideration in patients with multiple liver and bone lesions (answer E).

11. C

Spinal cord compression. Spinal cord compression is an emergency and should be treated immediately. The presence of spinal cord compression caused by cancer is typically a contraindication for immunotherapy treatments such as checkpoint inhibitors, due to the potential risk of pseudoprogression with worsening of neurologic symptoms/compromise (answer A). Chemotherapy will be likely necessary at a later time point; however, neurosurgery and/or radiation strategies should be implemented prior to systemic chemotherapy initiation (answer B). MRI of the spine should be done as inpatient, while being evaluated and followed by neurosurgeon and radiation oncologist, so that prompt intervention can be done (answer D). The clinical scenario does not suggest pneumonia (answer E).

12. D

This patient has hormone receptor positive, HER2 negative disease (HER2:CEP17 ratio of >2 is considered positive). Postmenopausal women with hormone-responsive metastatic breast cancer (MBC) benefit from sequential use of endocrine therapies at disease progression. Women who respond to one endocrine approach with reduction in tumor volume or long-term disease stabilization should receive additional endocrine therapies at disease progression. Results of the phase III randomized controlled trial Breast Cancer Trials of Oral Everolimus-2 (BOLERO-2) showed that postmenopausal women refractory to letrozole or anastrozole, which are nonsteroidal aromatase inhibitors, treated with a combination of everolimus, an mTOR inhibitor, and exemestane, a nonsteroidal aromatase inhibitor, had an improved PFS of 10.6 months compared with 4.1 months in women treated with exemestane alone. This combination is a reasonable next treatment regimen for this patient. Combination chemotherapy is not indicated for hormone receptor-positive, HER2-negative MBC that is limited to bone or soft tissue, or both. There are no data to use letrozole and palbociclib beyond the first-line setting. Everolimus is only FDA approved in combination with exemestane and not anastrozole or fulvestrant.

13. B

For spinal cord compression, radiation therapy is directed at vertebral metastatic sites that are associated with significant epidural involvement. Women who have recurrent hormone receptor-positive HER2-negative disease are appropriate candidates for initial endocrine therapy.

Postmenopausal women should be offered an aromatase inhibitor as first-line therapy for their metastatic disease. The usual upfront choices are a nonsteroidal aromatase inhibitor such as anastrozole or letrozole. Two large randomized trials in which postmenopausal women who were endocrine therapy-naïve in the metastatic setting showed that anastrozole was at least equivalent to tamoxifen in the first-line setting; unplanned subgroup analysis restricted to patients with known positive hormone receptors demonstrated a superior TTP for anastrozole. Letrozole has also been directly compared with tamoxifen in the first-line setting among women with MBC, and similarly increased the TTP. Anastrozole and letrozole, which are nonsteroidal AIs, are appropriate first-line endocrine options in postmenopausal MBC. Based on the recent results of the PALOMA-1/TRIO-18 trial and FDA approval of the combination of letrozole and palbociclib, an oral small-molecule inhibitor of cyclin-dependent kinases 4 and 6, addition of palbociclib to letrozole should be considered. The combination resulted in significant improvement in progression-free survival as first-line treatment for advanced disease in postmenopausal women with estrogen receptor–positive and HER2-negative breast cancer. Women with metastatic breast cancer to the bones may be considered for treatment with a bisphosphonate or denosumab, a fully human monoclonal antibody directed against RANK ligand, a mediator of osteoclast function. These agents are used in patients with metastatic breast cancer to the bones and have been shown to prevent bone fractures, decrease bone pain, and prevention of skeletal-related events (SRE). With regard to denosumab, a randomized study showed equivalency and superiority of time to occurrence of an SRE with denosumab. Since this patient has hormone receptor-positive MBC limited to bone, cytotoxic chemotherapy does not have to be utilized as first-line, and endocrine therapy is preferred.

14. A

Palliative care in patients with metastatic breast cancer. A discussion about goals of care would be appropriate in this case. Hospice provides care including pain management, and emotional and spiritual support tailored to the patient's needs and wishes, while also providing support to patients' families. It is very unlikely that any additional anticancer therapy could change the outcome for this patient, and it could cause toxicity and additional suffering. Answer B is not appropriate, because the pain seems to be well controlled. Answer C: Most immunotherapy clinical trials would not enroll patients with ECOG performance status (PS) 2–4. This patient's current PS is 3. Immunotherapy is emerging as a potential anticancer strategy earlier rather than later in the treatment history of a patient, since the number of previous treatment lines may negatively affect the impact of immunotherapy against the disease. There are no approved immunotherapies for patients with ER/PR+, HER2 negative metastatic breast cancer. Answer D is not appropriate because the listed tests will not change the medical recommendations. In some highly selected cases, though, scans confirming progression of disease may be required to enable a patient and/or family members to make progress in the discussion of goals of care. This would be done after the failure of the approach described in answer A. Answer E is not appropriate because patient is not experiencing nausea from chemotherapy or poor appetite.

15. C

A baseline ECG is recommended to obtain in a patient with a history of bradyarrhythmias who is to be treated with eribulin. In an uncontrolled ECG study in 26 patients, QT prolongation was observed on day 8, independent of eribulin concentration, with no prolongation on day 1. ECG monitoring is recommended for patients with congestive heart failure, bradyarrhythmias, concomitant use of drugs that prolong QT interval, including Class Ia and III antiarrhythmics, and electrolyte abnormalities. Correction of hypokalemia or hypomagnesemia prior to initiating eribulin and electrolytes should be monitored periodically during therapy. Eribulin does not cause cardiac dysfunction, proteinuria, or pneumonitis, so there would be no reason to obtain a baseline echocardiogram, pulmonary function tests, or a urinalysis. Growth colony-stimulating factors are not indicated with the first cycle of therapy with eribulin.

16. B, C, D, and **E**

This patient's symptoms and laboratory findings are suspicious for metastatic involvement of the pituitary. Pituitary metastases are uncommon, in the range of 1%–5%. About 10%–30% of pituitary lesions cause symptoms and can result in diabetes insipidus, visual field defects, or cranial nerve palsy. MRI scans performed with standard techniques may miss abnormalities of the pituitary and stalk, and therefore MRI with contrast and thin cuts with specific attention to the pituitary must be performed when disease is suspected. Whether or not the imaging is positive, initial laboratory should include ACTH, cortisol, thyroid function studies, gonadal hormones, gonadotropins, and prolactin for clues as to the extent of involvement. Serum and urine electrolytes and osmolality should be done to assess both for hyponatremia associated with adrenal insufficiency due to lack of ACTH, as well as the possibility of diabetes insipidus in these patients. Treatment should be initiated with steroids immediately after drawing blood tests, along with education regarding adrenal insufficiency while awaiting the results of studies. Pituitary metastases are uncommon, but more often present with symptoms of posterior pituitary involvement (diabetes insipidus) than anterior involvement (hypopituitarism). There are many management considerations in these patients, and a multidisciplinary team is optimal, including endocrinology to address diagnosis of hypopituitarism and manage hormone replacement needs, and neurosurgery and radiation oncology to address local disease control. When surgery cannot be considered, an alternative option is radiation therapy, either traditional or stereotactic.

17. D

Evaluation of response to therapy. The presence of "new" osteoblastic/sclerotic bone lesions may represent healing lytic lesions upon treatment with effective agents. Typically, a lytic lesion becomes blastic. Occasionally, smaller lytic lesions that were not appreciated at baseline scan may be detected after treatment because of changes to its characteristics due to healing. Therefore with clinical improvement and no critical location for lesions, it would be acceptable to continue treatment and repeat scans in 8 weeks to ensure stability. Nothing on restaging CT or clinical history suggests spinal cord compression (answer A) or multiple myeloma (answer B). Findings are not compatible with denosumab toxicity (answer C). For accurate comparison among scans obtained at different time points, it is recommended that the same modality be used for comparison. In addition, the number of documented sites of disease being followed for effect will not change the treatment recommendation in the metastatic setting. Therefore PET-CT has little to add in this case (answer E).

18. B

This patient needs systemic chemotherapy combined with HER2-targeted agents. There is no role for surgical resection, given the extensive liver metastases. Pertuzumab plus trastuzumab and docetaxel was approved by the US Food and Drug Administration, and pertuzumab plus trastuzumab plus taxane has been recommended by the National Comprehensive Cancer Network as a preferred regimen for the first-line treatment of HER2-positive MBC. Dual HER2 blockade is considered the standard of care for first-line treatment of HER2-positive metastatic breast cancer. However, docetaxel should not be given if AST and/or ALT is greater than 1.5 × ULN concomitant with alkaline phosphatase greater than 2.5 × ULN. LFT elevations increase the risk of severe and life-threatening complications. A reasonable alternative is to treat with weekly paclitaxel, trastuzumab, and pertuzumab in this situation. There is a phase II trial of weekly paclitaxel, trastuzumab, and pertuzumab given in HER2-positive metastatic breast cancer patients that received zero to one prior regimens, which showed an 86% PFS rate at 6 months and a favorable safety profile. The median PFS was 19.5 months (95% CI, 14–26 months) overall.

19. D

First-line therapy for patients with metastatic disease that is HER2 positive. The strongest evidence to support the use of a taxane with double anti-HER2 Mab-based therapy comes from the CLEOPATRA trial. This trial randomized patients with metastatic HER2-positive breast cancer treated in the first-line setting to pertuzumab, docetaxel, and trastuzumab versus docetaxel and trastuzumab (control), and demonstrated a statistically significant 16 months increase in median overall survival in those receiving pertuzumab (56 months vs. 40 months, respectively). Previous use of trastuzumab and taxanes was recorded in 11% and 23% of participants, respectively. An interval of at least 12 months since completion of the adjuvant or neoadjuvant therapy was required for eligibility. Answers A, B, and C are not appropriate in first-line therapy for metastatic HER2+ disease. Answer E would be potentially appropriate for hormone receptor positive, HER2 negative metastatic breast cancer

20. B

Based on the recent results of the PALOMA-1/TRIO-18 trial, the combination of letrozole and palbociclib, an oral small-molecule inhibitor of cyclin-dependent kinases 4 and 6, was approved by the FDA in 2015 as first-line therapy for metastatic hormone receptor-positive, HER2-negative breast cancer. The addition of palbociclib to letrozole resulted in significant improvement in progression-free survival as first-line treatment for advanced disease in postmenopausal women with hormone receptor–positive, HER2-negative breast cancer. The trial enrolled 165 patients randomly allocated to receive either palbociclib (125 mg orally daily for 21 consecutive days, followed by 7 days off treatment), plus letrozole (2.5 mg daily continuously throughout the 28-day cycle) or letrozole alone. Median progression-free survival was 20.2 months in the palbociclib/letrozole group versus 10.2 months in the letrozole group (hazard ratio [HR] = 0.488, P = .0004). Response rates were 43% versus 33% (including complete response in 1% of both groups), respectively, and median duration of response was 20.3 versus 11.1 months. Median overall survival, assessed at the same time as progression-free survival, was 37.5 versus 33.3 months (HR = 0.813, P = .42). The most common adverse events in the palbociclib/letrozole group were neutropenia, leukopenia, and fatigue. Grade 3–4 neutropenia was reported in 45 (54%) of 83 patients in the palbociclib plus letrozole group versus one (1%) of 77 patients in the letrozole group, leukopenia in 16 (19%) versus none, and fatigue in four (4%) versus one (1%).

21. D

Dual anti-HER2 therapy-related severe diarrhea. Chemotherapy-induced diarrhea (CID) occurs in 40%–80% of breast cancer patients who receive HER2 directed therapy with trastuzumab, pertuzumab, lapatinib, or neratinib. The risk of severe diarrhea with double anti-HER2 treatment is approximately 8%. In the luminal side of the colon, chloride efflux is mediated via apical chloride channels, which may be affected by these therapies and cause excess chloride secretion, resulting in impaired gut absorption and producing secretory diarrhea. Since therapeutic monoclonal antibodies have long half-lives measured in weeks, it is common for the diarrhea to continue until the next treatment cycle, and beyond, justifying the scheduled use of antidiarrheal treatment. Answer A would be appropriate in the setting of inflammation or bleeding. Answer B would be appropriate in the setting of infectious gastroenteritis. Answer C would be appropriate with food poisoning or food allergies. Answer E would be appropriate treatment for *C. difficile* colitis.

22. C

The best choice is ixabepilone. This patient demonstrates that she has a tumor that is resistant to anthracycline, taxane, and capecitabine, given the short time to relapse and the shortened duration on capecitabine. Ixabepilone (Ixempra, Bristol-Myers Squibb) is the first epothilone to be approved by the Food and Drug Administration (FDA). Ixabepilone as a single agent is indicated for the treatment of metastatic breast cancer as monotherapy in patients whose tumors are resistant to anthracyclines, taxanes, and capecitabine. The basis for FDA approval of ixabepilone as a single agent was an international, multicenter phase II trial conducted in 126 metastatic breast cancer patients whose disease was resistant to anthracyclines, taxanes, and capecitabine. Resistance to each agent was defined as progressive disease within 8 weeks of the last dose of the drug in the metastatic setting, or recurrence within 6 months of adjuvant or neoadjuvant anthracycline or taxane therapy. Approximately 88% of patients had received two or more prior chemotherapy regimens for metastatic disease. Ixabepilone was administered at 40 mg/m^2 as a 3-hour infusion every 3 weeks. The ORR based on independent radiologic review was 11.5% [95% CI, 6.3%–18.9%], and 13 out of 113 patients had a partial response. In addition, 13% experienced stable disease for ≥6 months. Eribulin is not indicated, as she has not previously received at least two chemotherapeutic regimens for treatment of metastatic disease. Although combination chemotherapy provides higher rates of response and longer time to progression, compared with single-agent chemotherapy, combination chemotherapy is associated with increase in toxicity and is of little survival benefit. Single-agent chemotherapy is preferred to minimize the side effects. Combination cytotoxic regimens are usually given to those who are very symptomatic and have rapidly progressive disease. This patient is asymptomatic and has a volume of visceral disease that does not appear to be fast growing or appears to have any imminent threat of organ compromise. Therefore the combinations of paclitaxel/gemcitabine and docetaxel/capecitabine are not necessary for this patient. Paclitaxel is not a good choice for this patient, given prior treatment with it less than 6 months prior to relapse.

23. D

Management of antiresorptive therapy toxicity in patients with metastatic breast cancer. Antiresorptive therapy with bisphosphonates or denosumab is an approved treatment to prevent skeletal events in patients with breast cancer metastatic to the bones. Osteonecrosis of the jaw (ONJ) is a potential serious complication of this treatment. Based on data from clinical trials evaluating these agents, the incidence of ONJ with zoledronate or denosumab was between 1% and 2% at 3 years follow-up. Although there are no prospective data evaluating the potential beneficial effects of discontinuing antiresorptive therapy versus continuing it, discontinuation of the agent is thought to allow recovery of the ONJ site while reducing the risk of new ONJ lesions. The therapy is typically discontinued at least temporarily, as was done in the registration trials of these agents. Conservative management is recommended, consisting of topical mouth rinses, antibiotic therapy to control secondary infection when present, and limited débridement to prevent injury from rough bone surface to tongue. The clinical description is not compatible with yeast (answer A) or viral (answer B) infections, or with disease progression and worsening of osteoblastic mandibular metastases (answer C). There are no data supportive of the switch from one to the other antiresorptive agent as management of ONJ (answer E).

24. C

Ado-trastuzumab emtansine (T-DM1) is an antibody-drug conjugate that incorporates the HER2-targeted antitumor properties of trastuzumab with the cytotoxic activity of the microtubule-inhibitory agent DM1 (derivative of maytansine); the antibody and the cytotoxic agent are conjugated by means of a stable linker. T-DM1 allows intracellular drug delivery specifically to HER2-overexpressing cells, thereby improving the therapeutic index and minimizing exposure of normal tissue. Ado-trastuzumab emtansine as a single-agent is indicated, for the treatment of patients with HER2-positive metastatic breast cancer, who previously received trastuzumab and a taxane, separately or in combination. Patients should have either received prior therapy for metastatic disease or developed disease recurrence during or within 6 months of completing adjuvant therapy. The drug was approved based on the results of the EMILIA study, which was a randomized, phase III international trial of patients with unresectable locally advanced or metastatic HER2-positive breast cancer, previously treated with trastuzumab and a taxane, to demonstrate the utility of ado-trastuzumab emtansine. In this study, 991 patients were randomly assigned in a 1:1 ratio to TDM-1 or lapatinib plus capecitabine. Treatment with TDM-1 significantly improved progression-free survival as assessed by independent review, and median survival was 9.6 months versus 6.4 months with lapatinib and capecitabine. At the second interim analysis of overall survival (331 deaths), TDM-1 significantly improved increased median overall survival, 30.9 months versus 25.15 months with lapatinib and capecitabine.

The ASCO Clinical Practice Guideline Update of Systemic Therapy for Patients With Advanced HER2-Positive Breast Cancer strongly recommends that if a patient's HER2-positive advanced breast cancer has progressed during or after first-line HER2-targeted therapy, clinicians should recommend trastuzumab emtansine (T-DM1) as second-line treatment.

25. C

CNS disease. Epilepsy may be the first sign of central nervous system (CNS) metastatic disease. This patient presented with a complex partial seizure, characterized by impaired consciousness, automatisms, and possibly autonomic aura. Brain imaging, including MRI of the brain with contrast, can detect brain metastasis and has greater sensitivity than CT scan with contrast. Answer A attributes the seizure event to ondansetron. Ondansetron has been described as a potential cause for seizures. However, this would be a diagnosis of exclusion for this patient. Answer B describes a potential approach to panic attack. Although this is still in the differential, in this patient, CNS disease must be ruled out first. Answer D treats dehydration; however, there is nothing in the clinical picture suggesting this diagnosis. Answer E addresses the issue that electrolyte abnormalities should be evaluated, and that the routine complete metabolic profile does not include magnesium levels. Certainly part of differential diagnosis; however, normal or abnormal magnesium levels will not exclude other important causes for seizures, such as brain metastatic disease.

26. B

Metastatic disease at first recurrence or at presentation should be biopsied as part of the workup for the patients with stage IV or recurrent disease. This ensures adequate determination of recurrent or metastatic disease and tumor histology, and allows for determination of biomarkers for selection of appropriate treatment. In addition, given the potential for discordance between the receptor status of the primary cancer and metachronous metastases, biopsy of metastatic disease at the time of recurrence should be performed if it can be safely done to confirm the diagnosis, but also to guide therapies. Reported rates of discordance range from 10% to 40% and may reflect a true change in tumor biology, sampling error, or assay error. Since the FNA did not yield enough material for biomarker assessment, the next step is to surgically remove the lymph node to obtain enough tissue to assess ER, PR, and HER2. Starting therapy with fulvestrant or weekly paclitaxel are not correct. Therapy should not be started until an attempt is made to confirm the ER, PR, and HER2 status of the recurrence. A PET-CT scan will not add additional information. The pleural effusion is small and still may not yield enough tissue to run the receptors.

27. D

Endocrine therapy remains an important approach in the treatment of hormone receptor-positive metastatic breast cancer and is reasonable to treat with this, given her low volume of disease and lack of symptoms. In premenopausal woman with previous antiestrogen therapy who are within 1 year of antiestrogen exposure, preferred therapy is oophorectomy, ovarian radiation, or LHRH agonists with endocrine therapy, such as aromatase inhibitors. Since she had prior antiestrogen exposure in the adjuvant setting with tamoxifen, it was reasonable to then treat her with ovarian suppression and an aromatase inhibitor. Switching her to fulvestrant and palbociclib, a cyclin-dependent kinase (CDK) 4/6 inhibitor, based on the PALOMA-3 study, is a reasonable next step. This combination was approved in the treatment of hormone-receptor positive, HER2-negative metastatic breast cancer patients, who have had prior endocrine therapy. This is a trial that randomized postmenopausal women who had prior aromatase inhibitor therapy, to fulvestrant versus fulvestrant and palbociclib. Premenopausal or perimenopausal women also received ovarian suppression via a luteinizing hormone-releasing hormone agonist during the treatment period. The median progression-free survival was 9.5 months in the fulvestrant plus palbociclib group, compared with 5.4 months in the fulvestrant plus placebo group, which was statistically significant [HR 0.46; 95% CI: 0.36–0.59; *P* < .0001]. Therefore, this would be a reasonable appropriate regimen to go to next in this patient who has had prior aromatase inhibitor and no prior palbociclib. There would be no reason to start off with liposomal doxorubicin, given she has minimal symptoms. Anastrozole cannot be used alone safely in premenopausal females without concurrent ovarian suppression or ablation, since inhibition of the aromatase enzyme in the setting of functional ovaries will lead to ovarian hyperstimulation. Progestins, such as megestrol acetate, indirectly decrease serum estrogen levels by reducing androgen levels, and are usually utilized as a third- and fourth-line therapy.

28. C

First-line therapy for patients with metastatic breast cancer that is HR+HER2–. The ideal sample for first diagnosis of metastatic disease is soft tissue. Such samples have higher yield for histological diagnosis and receptor testing. In the absence of a soft tissue site to biopsy, this patient's recurrence information is coming from pleural fluid cytology and cellblock. Based on the PALOMA-1/TRIO-18 (phase II) and PALOMA-2 (phase III) trials, in first-line metastatic hormone receptor positive, HER2 negative breast cancer, the recommendation would be for palbociclib and letrozole, instead of the aromatase inhibitor alone. In the PALOMA-1 trial, the median progression-free survival was 20.2 months for the group of patients treated with palbociclib and letrozole, and 10.2 months for the group treated with letrozole alone (HR 0.488). The use of antiresorptive agent such as denosumab to reduce the incidence of skeletal events (pathological fracture, radiotherapy to bone, surgery to bone, or spinal cord compression) is also indicated. When compared with zoledronate, denosumab reduced the risk of first on-study skeletal event by 17% (the median of first skeletal event with denosumab was 27.6 months and with zoledronate, 19.4 months), although zoledronate would also be an appropriate option. Systemic chemotherapy, single agent, or doublets could be considered and option in case of visceral crisis (answer D); however, the pleural effusion is now controlled with the use of an indwelling catheter. Anti-HER2 therapy would be indicated only with proven HER2 positive disease (answer E).

REFERENCES

Question 1
1. Swain SM, Baselga J, Kim SB, et al. Pertuzumab, trastuzumab, and docetaxel in HER2-positive metastatic breast Cancer. *N Engl J Med.* 2015;372:724–734.

Question 3
1. Cortes J, O'Shaughnessy J, Loesch D, et al. Eribulin monotherapy versus treatment of physician's choice in patients with metastatic breast cancer (EMBRACE): a phase 3 open-label randomised study. *Lancet.* 2011;377:914–923.
2. Carrick S, Parker S, Wilcken N, Ghersi D, Marzo M, Simes J. Single agent versus combination chemotherapy for metastatic breast cancer. *Cochrane Database Syst Rev.* 2005;(2):CD003372.

Question 6
1. Trastuzumab package insert (Revised 03/2016): http://www.gene.com/download/pdf/herceptin_prescribing.pdf.

Question 7
1. Patchell RA, Tibbs PA, Walsh JW, et al. A randomized trial of surgery in the treatment of single metastases to the brain. *N Engl J Med.* 1990;322:494–500.
2. Patchell RA, Tibbs PA, Regine WF, et al. Postoperative radiotherapy on the treatment of single metastases to the brain: a randomized trial. *JAMA.* 1998;280:1485–1489.
3. Glantz MJ, Cole BF, Forsyth PA, et al. Practice parameter: anticonvulsant prophylaxis in patients with newly diagnosed brain tumors. Report of the Quality Standards Subcommittee of the American Academy of Neurology. *Neurology.* 2000;54:1886–1893.

Question 12
1. Baselga J, Campone M, Piccart M, et al. Everolimus in postmenopausal hormone-receptor-positive advanced breast cancer. *N Engl J Med.* 2012;366:520–529.

Question 13
1. Bonneterre J, Buzdar A, Nabholtz JM, et al. Anastrozole is superior to tamoxifen as first-line therapy in hormone receptor positive advanced breast carcinoma. *Cancer.* 2001;92:2247–2258.
2. Mouridsen H, Sun Y, Gershanovich M, et al. Superiority of letrozole to tamoxifen in the first-line treatment of advanced breast cancer: evidence from metastatic subgroups and a test of functional ability. *Oncologist.* 2004;9:489–496.
3. Stopeck AT, Lipton A, Body JJ, et al. Denosumab compared with zoledronic acid for the treatment of bone metastases in patients with advanced breast cancer: a randomized, double-blind study. *J Clin Oncol.* 2010;28:5132–5139.
4. Finn RS, Crown JP, Lang I, et al. The cyclin-dependent kinase 4/6 inhibitor palbociclib in combination with letrozole versus letrozole alone as first-line treatment of oestrogen receptor-positive, HER2-negative, advanced breast cancer (PALOMA-1/TRIO-18): a randomised phase 2 study. *Lancet Oncol.* 2015;16:25–35.

Question 16
1. Gilard V, Alexandru C, Proust F, Derrey S, Hannequin P, Langlois O. Pituitary metastasis: is there still a place for neurosurgical treatment? *J Neurooncol.* 2016;126(2):219–224.
2. Komninos J, Vlassopoulou V, Protopapa D, et al. Tumors metastatic to the pituitary gland: case report and literature review. *J Clin Endocrinol Metab.* 2004;89:574–580.

Question 18
1. Swain SM, Baselga J, Kim SB, et al. Pertuzumab, trastuzumab, and docetaxel in HER2-positive metastatic breast cancer. *N Engl J Med.* 2015;372:724–734.
2. Dang C, Iyengar N, Datko F, et al. Phase II study of paclitaxel given once per week along with trastuzumab and pertuzumab in patients with human epidermal growth factor receptor 2-positive metastatic breast cancer. *J Clin Oncol.* 2015;33. 442–427.

Question 20
1. Finn RS, Crown JP, Lang I, et al. The cyclin-dependent kinase 4/6 inhibitor palbociclib in combination with letrozole versus letrozole alone as first-line treatment of oestrogen receptor-positive, HER2-negative, advanced breast cancer (PALOMA-1/TRIO-18): a randomised phase 2 study. *Lancet Oncol.* 2015;16:25–35.

Question 22
1. Perez E, Lerzo G, Pivot X, et al. Efficacy and safety of ixabepilone (BMS-247550) in a phase II study of patients with advanced breast cancer resistant to an anthracycline, a taxane, and capecitabine. *J Clin Oncol.* 2007;25:3407–3414.
2. Carrick S, Parker S, Wilcken N, Ghersi D, Marzo M, Simes J, et al. Single agent versus combination chemotherapy for metastatic breast cancer. *Cochrane Database Syst Rev.* 2005;(2):CD003372.

Question 24
1. Verma S, Miles D, Gianni L, et al. Trastuzumab emtansine for HER2-positive advanced breast cancer. *N Engl J Med.* 2012;367:1783–1791.
2. Giordano SH, Temin S, Kirshner JJ, et al. Systemic therapy for patients with advanced human epidermal growth factor receptor 2-positive breast cancer: American Society of Clinical Oncology clinical practice guideline. *J Clin Oncol.* 2014;32:2078–2099.

Question 26
1. Amir E, Miller N, Geddie W, et al. Prospective study evaluating the impact of tissue confirmation of metastatic disease in patients with breast cancer. *J Clin Oncol*. 2012;30:587–592.
2. Pustzai L, Viale G, Kelly CM, Hudis CA. Estrogen and HER-2 receptor discordance between primary breast cancer and metastasis. *Oncologist*. 2010;15:1164–1168.

Question 27
1. Carlson RW, Theriault R, Schurman CM, et al. Phase II trial of anastrozole plus goserelin in the treatment of hormone receptor-

positive, metastatic carcinoma of the breast in premenopausal women. *J Clin Oncol*. 2010;28:3917–3921.
2. Park IH, Ro J, Lee KS, et al. Phase II parallel group study showing comparable efficacy between premenopausal metastatic breast cancer patients treated with letrozole plus goserelin and postmenopausal patients treated with letrozole alone as first-line hormone therapy. *J Clin Oncol*. 2010;28:2705–2711.
3. Cristofanelli M, Turner NC, Bondarenko I, et al. Fulvestrant plus palbociclib versus fulvestrant plus placebo for treatment of hormone-receptor-positive, HER2-negative metastatic breast cancer that progressed on previous endocrine therapy (PALOMA-3): final analysis of the multicenter, double-blind, phase 3 randomised controlled trial. *Lancet Oncol*. 2016;17:425–439.

Premalignant Breast Cancer Conditions and In Situ Disease

QUESTIONS

1. Which of the following is correct regarding atypical hyperplasia?
   A. Women who have had a benign breast biopsy demonstrating atypical hyperplasia (AH) are at about a twofold increased risk for developing breast cancer when compared with the reference population.
   B. Atypical hyperplasia is associated with a generalized increased risk of ipsilateral but not contralateral breast cancer.
   C. A higher risk of breast cancer is seen in women who have a greater number of foci of atypical hyperplasia and in those with a lesser degree of involution of the background lobular units.
   D. The surgical management of atypical hyperplasia requires negative margins.
   E. Atypical ductal hyperplasia (ADH) shares some of the cytologic and architectural features of high-grade ductal carcinoma in situ.

2. Which of the following is correct regarding atypical hyperplasia?
   A. Atypical hyperplasia (AH) is managed as an indicator lesion for subsequent risk of developing invasive ductal or lobular carcinoma.
   B. ALH, although histologically similar to lobular carcinoma in situ, is less extensive and associated with a higher risk of breast cancer.
   C. Chemoprevention with selective estrogen receptor modulators or aromatase inhibitors should be discussed with women diagnosed with AH, only if they have family history of breast cancer.
   D. Annual screening MRI is recommended for women with a previous diagnosis of AH.
   E. If AH is found at the surgical margin, regardless of the type of initial breast biopsy, a wide local excision is recommended to achieve negative margins.

3. A 54-year-old healthy female underwent a routine mammogram and was found to have microcalcifications in the lower inner quadrant of her left breast. She then underwent a core needle biopsy that revealed atypical ductal hyperplasia. She has been reading about atypical hyperplasia and has questions about her risk of developing invasive cancer in the future. You tell her:
   A. Atypical hyperplasia (AH) is found in approximately 50% of biopsies with benign findings.
   B. The Breast Cancer Risk Assessment Tool (BCRAT) is commonly used to estimate the risk of breast cancer both for women with AH or those with lobular carcinoma in situ.
   C. Women who are diagnosed with AH have a substantially increased risk for developing breast cancer that is approximately 4 times that of the reference population.
   D. ADH is more common than ALH and is associated with a higher risk of subsequent breast cancer than ALH.
   E. Atypical hyperplasia is associated with an increased risk of ipsilateral but not contralateral breast cancer.

4. A 53-year-old postmenopausal female with newly diagnosed atypical ductal hyperplasia presents to your office to discuss the role of chemoprevention. Her mother was diagnosed with breast cancer at the age of 59. She does not have other family members with a history of breast cancer. She has heard about the role of selective estrogen receptor modulators (SERM) or aromatase inhibitors (AI) for women with atypical hyperplasia, but she is concerned with the associated side effects. She asks you about the evidence available on the use of these agents for breast cancer prevention.
   A. Analyses of data from the subgroup of women with atypical hyperplasia (AH) enrolled in four randomized placebo-controlled trials of SERMs or aromatase inhibitors for chemoprevention showed relative-risk reductions ranging from 41% to 79%.
   B. Available data from randomized trials in the chemoprevention setting suggest a greater benefit of aromatase inhibitors (AIs) and tamoxifen in the total population than in the subgroup of women with AH.
   C. Most guidelines, including National Comprehensive Cancer Network (NCCN) and American Society of Clinical Oncology (ASCO), recommend that the use of a chemopreventive agent, either an SERM or an AI, should be discussed with women with a 5-year projected absolute risk of breast cancer of 5% or higher.
   D. All SERMs are associated with an increased risk of endometrial cancer, with a significant excess incidence of 5.5 per 1000 women.
   E. Vasomotor symptoms are seen in many women who receive treatment with SERMs or AIs, with attributable risks of 6 per 1000 to 11 per 1000.

5. Which of the following statements is correct regarding lobular carcinoma in situ?
   A. Lobular carcinoma in situ (LCIS) is an invasive lesion that arises from the lobules and terminal ducts of the breast.
   B. In most circumstances LCIS is identified clinically, mammographically, or by gross pathologic examination.
   C. LCIS is a benign lesion of the breast further classified as proliferative without atypia.
   D. The absolute risk of developing invasive breast cancer in women with LCIS is approximately 1% per year.
   E. LCIS is more often detected in postmenopausal than premenopausal women.

6. What characteristics distinguish lobular carcinoma in situ (LCIS) from ductal carcinoma in situ (DCIS)?
   A. Classic LCIS is considered to be a risk marker, while ductal carcinoma in situ (DCIS) is considered a precursor lesion of invasive breast cancer.
   B. The loss of expression of e-cadherin, a transmembrane protein that mediates epithelial cell adhesion, is a marker of DCIS.
   C. Radiation therapy is part of the management of some variants of LCIS.
   D. There are data regarding the benefit of aromatase inhibitors for chemoprevention in DCIS but not in LCIS.
   E. It is recommended that premenopausal patients diagnosed with LCIS undergo genetic counseling and testing.

7. A 42-year-old female found to have suspicious calcifications of the left breast underwent a core needle biopsy that showed LCIS. She subsequently underwent an excisional biopsy. The final pathology revealed LCIS with no evidence of invasive cancer. She is otherwise healthy and does not have any significant comorbidity. She is very concerned and wants to do everything to reduce the risk of developing cancer.
   Which is the most appropriate next step?
   A. Whole breast radiation
   B. Ovarian suppression and anastrozole
   C. Tamoxifen
   D. Observation
   E. Bilateral MRI annually

8. A 55-year-old female was found on screening mammogram to have suspicious microcalcifications in the right breast measuring approximately 1.1 cm in size. She underwent an excisional biopsy and was diagnosed with lobular carcinoma in situ (LCIS). One of the margins was positive for LCIS. There was no evidence of invasive cancer. She is willing to undergo any treatment that could improve her outcome. What do you recommend?
   A. Bilateral mastectomy
   B. Lumpectomy
   C. Radiation
   D. Wide local excision to achieve negative margins
   E. Risk/benefit discussion of chemoprevention with either tamoxifen or an aromatase inhibitor

9. Which of the following statements regarding pleomorphic lobular carcinoma in situ is correct?
   A. Pleomorphic LCIS often demonstrates central necrosis and calcifications which can frequently also be found in classic LCIS.
   B. If pleomorphic LCIS is identified at a surgical margin, a re-excision should be considered to obtain negative margins, regardless the type of initial breast biopsy.

C. Radiation therapy is routinely recommended for pleomorphic LCIS.
D. Use of E-cadherin immunohistochemistry is not helpful in differentiating between pleomorphic LCIS and DCIS.
E. Pleomorphic lobular carcinoma in situ is, in most cases, hormone receptor negative.

10. A 46-year-old healthy premenopausal female undergoes a screening mammogram and is found to have a cluster of microcalcifications in the right upper outer quadrant, for which biopsy is recommended. She does not have a family history of breast or ovarian cancer. Core needle biopsy is performed and reveals pleomorphic LCIS. Your recommendations include:
    A. Lumpectomy followed by whole breast radiation
    B. Lumpectomy, followed by whole breast radiation and then tamoxifen
    C. Surgical excision. If negative margins are not achieved, re-excision is recommended.
    D. Testing for HER2
    E. Surveillance without need for further surgical management

11. The following statement about ductal carcinoma in situ (DCIS) is correct:
    A. It is diagnosed more commonly than invasive breast cancer.
    B. It is associated with metastatic breast cancer in 20% of the cases.
    C. Its incidence significantly increased from the 1970s to the early 2000s.
    D. Most patients present with a palpable abnormality.
    E. It is not associated with BRCA1 or BRCA2 mutations.

12. The following feature is associated with higher risk criteria for DCIS:
    A. Older age
    B. Tumor measuring 5–10 mm
    C. Positive hormone receptors
    D. Presence of comedo necrosis and absence of gland formation
    E. Surgical margins greater than 5 mm

13. A 60-year-old woman who was diagnosed 9 years ago with ductal carcinoma in situ of the left breast, status post-lumpectomy, radiation, and 5 years of tamoxifen relocated from a different state. She now presents to your office to establish care. Her physical exam is unremarkable, except for mild breast asymmetry and the presence of a surgical scar from her previous left lumpectomy. She brings her most recent mammogram done 2 days ago, which reveals a few small areas of microcalcifications at the lumpectomy site. There is also asymmetry and distortion in the parenchyma of her left breast. The mammogram report states "BI-RADS zero." Given the findings on mammogram, she is worried that she has a recurrence of her ductal carcinoma in situ or a new invasive breast cancer. What is the best course of action?
    A. Reassure the patient that her physical exam is unremarkable and that her mammogram is benign
    B. Ensure that previous mammograms are obtained in a timely fashion for proper comparison and definitive plan of care
    C. Obtain a biopsy of the area of distortion in her left breast to rule out DCIS or invasive cancer
    D. Obtain computerized tomography scans of the chest, abdomen, and pelvis, plus bone scan
    E. Recommend that she undergo a left breast mastectomy

14. A 50-year-old asymptomatic woman presents for her first screening mammogram. It reveals suspicious microcalcifications spanning a 1.0 cm area in the upper outer quadrant of her right breast. Ultrasound evaluation is normal. A biopsy performed under stereotactic guidance reveals proliferation of abnormal epithelial cells within the mammary ductal system. These cells are large, pleomorphic with frequent mitotic figures, and many of them had multiple prominent nucleoli. The lesion has an area of central necrosis. There is no evidence of invasion into the surrounding stroma on routine light microscopic examination. Estrogen and progesterone receptors are tested and highly positive in the lesion. What is the most appropriate next step in management?
- **A.** Right lumpectomy with right sentinel lymph node biopsy followed by postlumpectomy radiation
- **B.** Right lumpectomy without right sentinel lymph node biopsy followed by postlumpectomy radiation
- **C.** Neoadjuvant chemotherapy followed by surgery
- **D.** Endocrine therapy with tamoxifen
- **E.** Endocrine therapy with an aromatase inhibitor

15. A 38-year-old premenopausal woman was treated with a right mastectomy for DCIS. The surgical margins were free of disease. Estrogen and progesterone receptors were positive. She is of Ashkenazi Jewish heritage. After genetic counseling, she underwent genetic testing. No genetic abnormalities were found. She presents to your office 4 weeks after mastectomy for postsurgical treatment planning and consideration of additional treatments. You recommend:
- **A.** Complete staging with PET-CT scan
- **B.** Postmastectomy radiation
- **C.** Adjuvant chemotherapy
- **D.** Endocrine therapy with an aromatase inhibitor
- **E.** Observation with routine mammograms

16. A 42-year-old woman presents to you for consultation to discuss treatment options after a lumpectomy for a left breast ductal carcinoma in situ (DCIS). Pathology revealed ductal carcinoma in situ, cribiform pattern, intermediate to high nuclear grade, with associated necrosis, measuring approximately 2.5 cm in the greatest diameter. Margins were uninvolved by DCIS. Estrogen receptor was positive 100%, and progesterone receptor was negative. Her medical history was otherwise unremarkable. What would you recommend?
- **A.** Postlumpectomy radiation and tamoxifen for 5 years
- **B.** Tamoxifen for 5 years
- **C.** Observation
- **D.** Adjuvant chemotherapy
- **E.** Hysterectomy with bilateral salpingo-oophorectomy

17. A 60-year-old postmenopausal woman who is a current smoker presents for a second opinion after being unable to tolerate anastrozole, letrozole, or exemestane due to severe hot flashes and disabling join pains. Her medical history is significant for hypertension since the age of 50, requiring three antihypertensive agents, saddle pulmonary embolism 8 years ago, and major depression with a previous suicidal attempt at the age of 35. DCIS was diagnosed 9 months ago, and following lumpectomy and radiation endocrine therapy, was recommended by her primary oncologist. Pathology was remarkable for a 1.5-cm focus of ductal carcinoma in situ, solid pattern, and intermediate nuclear grade, with scant necrosis and negative margins. Estrogen and progesterone receptors were positive in greater than 90% of the cells. The patient had prolonged pain and discomfort after lumpectomy, requiring narcotics. She states "the surgery affected her health and energy in a terrible way." Her depression is severe and has been well controlled in the past 6 years on fluoxetine/olanzapine combination. Her oncologist suggested discontinuing endocrine therapy at this point. What would you do?
- **A.** Switch to chemotherapy with docetaxel and cyclophosphamide for four cycles
- **B.** Recommend right mastectomy
- **C.** Recommend bilateral mastectomies
- **D.** Switch to tamoxifen
- **E.** Agree with your colleague and recommend observation with routine mammograms

18. A 52-year-old woman underwent a right lumpectomy for DCIS. She presents to you for a second opinion to discuss whether she needs additional treatment as her "margins were close." You review the pathology report and slides at your multidisciplinary meeting. The DCIS measured 2.2 cm, and there was no evidence of invasive disease. The closest margin was posterior, and the DCIS was 2 mm from the margin. Estrogen receptor was strongly positive in 90% of the cells. You recommend:
- **A.** Observation and routine follow-up with mammograms
- **B.** Re-excision in order to obtain more widely negative margins, followed by postlumpectomy whole breast radiation and consideration of subsequent endocrine therapy
- **C.** Right mastectomy
- **D.** Postlumpectomy whole breast radiation and consideration of subsequent endocrine therapy
- **E.** Adjuvant chemotherapy with cyclophosphamide, methotrexate, and 5-fluorouracil (CMF)

19. A 55-year-old postmenopausal woman without significant family history of breast or ovarian cancer presents to your office after completion of whole breast irradiation following left lumpectomy for DCIS. Pathology of the DCIS was remarkable for comedonecrosis. Estrogen and progesterone receptors were tested and negative. Margins were clear. There was no invasive component. The DCIS lesion measured 0.8 cm. She has no comorbidities. Her physical exam is notable for mild postradiation skin rash. She wants to know what else she could do to treat this DCIS. What do you recommend?
- **A.** Anastrozole for 5 years
- **B.** Tamoxifen for 5 years
- **C.** Observation with routine mammograms
- **D.** Mastectomy
- **E.** Adjuvant chemotherapy with cyclophosphamide, methotrexate and 5-fluorouracil (CMF)

20. A 37-year-old premenopausal African American woman presents with a lump in her right breast. She also has right axillary discomfort. Mammogram reveals a large area of microcalcifications. Subsequent right breast ultrasound is unremarkable; however, there are several enlarged lymph nodes in the right axilla, with the largest measuring 3 cm. A stereotactic biopsy of right breast lesion reveals DCIS. Breast MRI reveals an area of enhancement corresponding to the area of calcifications on mammogram, as well as suspicious matted nodes in the right axilla. No other abnormalities are noted. An ultrasound-guided biopsy of right axillary lymph nodes reveals hormone receptor positive HER2 negative invasive ductal carcinoma. A clip was placed in the breast and node at the time of the biopsies. The most appropriate treatment plan should include:

A. Observation only, with routine mammograms
B. Right lumpectomy and whole breast radiation followed by tamoxifen for 5 years
C. Right lumpectomy and subsequent observation with routine mammograms
D. Bilateral mastectomies and bilateral salpingo-oophorectomies
E. Chemotherapy, surgery, postoperative radiation, and adjuvant endocrine therapy

ANSWERS

1. C

The number of separate foci of atypical hyperplasia (with greater numbers of foci associated with a higher risk) and the extent of normal regression (involution) of background lobular units stratifies risk amongst women with atypical hyperplasia. The greater the degree of involution, the lower the risk. Regarding answer A, women who have had a benign breast biopsy that demonstrates atypical hyperplasia are at a substantially increased risk for developing breast cancer—approximately 4 times that of the reference population. In terms of answer B, atypical hyperplasia is associated with a generalized increased risk of ipsilateral and contralateral breast cancer. The surgical management of AH does not require negative margins (answer D). Atypical ductal hyperplasia (ADH) shares some of the cytologic and architectural features of low-grade, and not high-grade, ductal carcinoma in situ (answer E).

2. A

AH is an indicator lesion for subsequent risk of both invasive ductal or lobular CA. The management of AH includes discussion of chemoprevention strategies to decrease the risk of developing breast cancer in the future. Regarding answer B, ALH is associated with a lower risk of breast cancer when compared with LCIS. In terms of answer C, chemoprevention with selective estrogen receptor modulators or aromatase inhibitors should be discussed with women diagnosed with AH, regardless of their family history. Current guidelines do not recommend annual screening MRI in women with AH. Additionally, the surgical management of AH does not require negative margins (answer E).

3. C

Women who have had a benign breast biopsy that demonstrates AH are at a substantially increased risk for developing breast cancer—approximately 4 times that of the reference population. Regarding answer A, AH is found in approximately 10% of biopsies with benign findings. Regarding answer B, BCRAT cannot accurately calculate breast cancer risk for women with a medical history of any breast cancer, DCIS, or LCIS. Regarding answer D, ADH and ALH occur with equal frequency and confer similar risks of subsequent breast cancer. Regarding answer E, AH is associated with an increased risk of ipsilateral and contralateral breast cancer. In the Nurses' Health Study, approximately 60% of cancers that developed in premenopausal women with AH occurred in the ipsilateral breast.

4. A

Available data from four large randomized clinical trials of chemoprevention with SERMs or AIs (NSABP P1, MAP.3, IBIS-I and IBIS-II) suggested an even greater benefit than in the total population treated with active agent in those trials. Regarding answer E, vasomotor symptoms are seen in many women who receive treatment with SERMs or AIs, with attributable risks of 67 per 1000 with an AI (MAP.3 trial) to 117 per 1000 with tamoxifen (NSABP P-1 trial).

Tamoxifen, but not the other SERMs, is associated with an increased risk of endometrial cancer, with a significant excess incidence of 5.5 per 1000 women (and a lower risk in premenopausal women than in postmenopausal women; answer E). Available data from NSABP P1, MAP.3, IBIS-I, and IBIS-II suggest a greater benefit of aromatase inhibitors (AI) and tamoxifen in the subgroup of women with AH than in the total population (answer B). Regarding answer C, most guidelines, including the National Comprehensive Cancer Network (NCCN) and American Society of Clinical Oncology (ASCO), recommend that the use of a chemopreventive agent, either an SERM or an AI, should be discussed with women, with a 5-year projected absolute risk of breast cancer of 1.7% or higher.

5. D

The absolute risk of developing invasive breast cancer in women with LCIS is approximately 1% per year. answer A is false because LCIS is not an invasive lesion. Regarding answer B, LCIS is typically an incidental microscopic finding and is rarely identified clinically, by mammographic screening, or by gross pathologic examination. LCIS is detected more often in premenopausal than postmenopausal women, suggesting a hormonal influence in the development or maintenance of these lesions. LCIS is classified as a proliferative lesion with atypia along with ADH and ALH. Examples of proliferative lesions without atypia include moderate or florid ductal hyperplasia of the usual type, sclerosing adenosis, radial scar, and intraductal papilloma or papillomatosis.

6. A

Subsequent breast cancers after a diagnosis of LCIS are both of ductal and lobular phenotype, which has led to the acceptance of LCIS as a marker of increased risk rather than a true precursor lesion. The loss of expression of e-cadherin is a marker of LCIS and infiltrating lobular carcinoma (LC; answer B). LCIS is a marker of increased risk and not a malignant or premalignant lesion; thus there are no data to support the use of radiation therapy for patients with LCIS, including pleomorphic LCIS (answer C). Regarding answer D, data from the IBIS-II study support that anastrozole effectively reduces the incidence of breast cancer in high-risk postmenopausal women, including those with LCIS. Regarding answer E, it is recommended that premenopausal patients diagnosed with DCIS (and not LCIS) undergo genetic counseling and testing.

7. C

Data from NSABP P1, a large randomized trial comparing tamoxifen to placebo in high-risk women, showed that tamoxifen decreased the risk of developing invasive breast cancer by 49%. Similarly, the NSABP P2 comparing raloxifene to tamoxifen for chemoprevention in postmenopausal high-risk women showed raloxifene to be as effective as tamoxifen. Women with LCIS were well represented in both of these studies, comprising 6.2% of 13,338 participants in NSABP P1 and 9.2% of 19,747 participants in P2 trial. In both subsets, chemoprevention reduced the risk of developing breast cancer by more than 50%. Overall results were confirmed in a systemic review for the USPSTF. Regarding answer A, as LCIS is a marker of increased risk and not a malignant or premalignant lesion, there is no indication for radiation therapy. Anastrozole is a consideration in postmenopausal women with LCIS, but ovarian suppression and anastrozole would not be indicated for chemoprevention purposes in premenopausal women (answer B). There are insufficient data to support annual screening with MRI for women who are of an elevated risk due to LCIS (answer E). While surveillance is an appropriate option, this patient expresses a desire to do everything she can to reduce her risk of developing breast cancer; thus answer C is the most appropriate recommendation for this patient.

8. E

Atypical lobular hyperplasia (ALH) and LCIS are both associated with an increased risk of breast cancer, and the use of tamoxifen in these patients is associated with an approximately 40% risk reduction of invasive breast cancer. If LCIS is identified by a core needle biopsy, an excision biopsy must be performed to exclude the presence of invasive cancer. However, if LCIS is diagnosed on an excisional breast biopsy, no further local therapy (surgery or radiation) is required. Although consideration of bilateral total mastectomy is an option for a woman with LCIS without additional risk factors, it is not a recommended approach for most of these women.

9. B

Re-excision of positive margins for pleomorphic LCIS is recommended, given evidence supporting a greater potential of pleomorphic LCIS than classic LCIS to develop into invasive carcinoma. However, outcome data regarding treatment of patients with pleomorphic LCIS are lacking, due in part to a paucity of histologic categorization of variants of LCIS. Current recommendations do not endorse radiation therapy for PLCIS.

10. C

Re-excision of positive margins for pleomorphic LCIS (PLCIS) is endorsed by the NCCN guidelines and other societies, given evidence supporting a greater potential for PLCIS than classic LCIS to develop into invasive lobular carcinoma. In addition, ipsilateral recurrence of PLCIS or of invasive breast cancer has been estimated at 3.8%–19.4% of patients, suggesting that PLCIS may represent a precursor lesion to invasive cancer, rather than a marker for increased breast cancer risk. However, outcome data regarding treatment of patients with pleomorphic LCIS are lacking, due in part to a paucity of histologic categorization of variants of LCIS. Current recommendations do not endorse radiation therapy for PLCIS. There are no data to support testing for HER2 in classic LCIS, pleomorphic LCIS, or DCIS outside a clinical trial. Surveillance without surgical management is not indicated for PLCIS, for the reasons previously mentioned.

11. C

Since the implementation of mammographic screening, the incidence of DCIS in the United States significantly increased from 6/100,000 women in the 1970s to 32/100,000 women in 2004, and then reached a plateau. DCIS accounts for approximately one-fourth of breast cancers diagnosed in the United States every year. The risk of development of metastases in a patient diagnosed with pure DCIS is very low, below 1%. The majority of cases of DCIS are detected only on imaging studies. DCIS has been associated with deleterious mutations in BRCA1 and BRCA2 genes.

12. D

Comedo carcinoma is a type of DCIS. It is more often associated with invasion than other types. The degree of comedo necrosis in patients with DCIS appears to be a strong predictor for the risk of ipsilateral breast recurrence after treatment. High-grade lesions are composed of solid nests of neoplastic cells without evidence of gland formation, and typically exhibit aneuploidy and lack estrogen and progesterone receptors (answer C). These lesions are at higher risk of recurrence. The larger the lesion, the worse the prognosis (answer B). Younger age has been implicated with higher risk of death from breast cancer in patients with DCIS. In a recent publication of consensus guidelines on margins for breast-conserving surgery with whole breast irradiation in DCIS by the Society of Surgical Oncology, American Society for Radiation Oncology, and American Society of Clinical Oncology, a 2-mm margin was accepted as a new standard. Margins less than 2 mm are associated with a higher risk of local recurrence (answer E).

13. B

According to guidelines from the American College of Radiology, mammographic reports must incorporate the Breast Imaging Reporting and Data System (BI-RADS) assessment in order to clarify mammography reports and to facilitate communication with other physicians. BI-RADS zero is used when a mammogram has nonspecific abnormalities and additional views or ultrasound are required to complete the evaluation. It is also used when a comparison with prior mammograms is needed for a definitive report. Since the nonspecific abnormalities could still represent invasive or noninvasive disease, the request for previous films and proper comparison should happen within a matter of days. It would be inappropriate to reassure patient and obtain the next mammogram in 6 or 12 months (answer A), or to go straight to biopsy (answer C). A biopsy would be the next step with BI-RADS 4 or 5 (Table 14C.1). Systemic staging with imaging would be appropriate if the patient had a diagnosis of locally advanced invasive breast cancer (answer D). Left mastectomy would be an option after histologic diagnosis of left breast DCIS or invasive breast cancer in this patient (answer E).

14. B

This patient has a nonpalpable, asymptomatic area of microcalcifications. Pathology confirms hormone receptor positive ductal carcinoma. Both mastectomy and lumpectomy are appropriate definitive treatments for patients with DCIS and are associated with similar survival. Mastectomy is felt to be an overly aggressive treatment for many women. Approximately 70% of women with newly diagnosed DCIS are managed with breast-conserving surgery. Similar to what is seen in invasive disease, lumpectomy as compared with mastectomy is associated with a higher risk of local recurrence, even when combined with radiation therapy. A long-term follow-up report from the NSABP B-17 and B-24 randomized clinical trials for women with DCIS revealed that after 15 years, invasive ipsilateral breast tumor recurrence occurred in 19.4% of patients who underwent lumpectomy alone, compared with 8.5% of patients who received lumpectomy, radiation, and tamoxifen. After mastectomy, the local recurrence rate is estimated at approximately 2%. The use of sentinel lymph node (SLN) mapping in DCIS is controversial. If mastectomy is performed, most agree SLN mapping should be done at the time of surgery. If the patient is treated with lumpectomy, it is most appropriate to postpone sentinel lymph node biopsy and only do it if invasive carcinoma is

TABLE 14C.1 BI-RADS Assessment Categories (American College of Radiology)

Category 0	Mammography: Ultrasound and MRI	Incomplete— Need additional Imaging evaluation and/or prior mammograms for comparison Incomplete— Need additional imaging evaluation
Category 1	Negative	
Category 2	Benign	
Category 3	Probably benign	
Category 4	Suspicious	Mammography and ultrasound: — Category 4A: Low suspicion for malignancy Category 4b: Moderate suspicion for malignancy Category 4c: High suspicion for malignancy
Category 5	Highly suggestive of malignancy	
Category 6	Known biopsy proven malignancy	

seen. Neoadjuvant chemotherapy is not indicated in DCIS (answer E). Endocrine therapy can be discussed after the definitive surgery (answers D and E).

15. E

Disease recurrence is estimated to happen in only 1%–2% of patients after mastectomy for DCIS. Therefore post-mastectomy clinical follow-up typically includes history, physical examination, and routine mammogram. The use of tamoxifen in premenopausal women with ER/PR positive DCIS and after unilateral mastectomy may be considered, with an aim of preventing new primary contralateral DCIS or invasive breast cancer. This option was not presented in the question. Aromatase inhibitor is not an appropriate treatment option for premenopausal patients (answer D). Adjuvant chemotherapy is not indicated, since the risk of systemic recurrence is extremely low (answer C). Likewise, there is no role for systemic staging with PET-CT scans (answer A). Radiation therapy significantly reduces the risk of in-breast recurrence. However, after mastectomy, radiation therapy is not indicated for patients with DCIS (answer B) and would only be considered if margins are involved.

16. A

After lumpectomy for DCIS, radiation therapy reduces the risk of in-breast DCIS and invasive disease recurrence. In a metaanalysis of four randomized trials involving 3925 women, after breast conserving surgery for DCIS, there was significant benefit from the addition of radiation therapy on ipsilateral breast event incidence (HR = 0.49; 95% CI 0.41–0.58). In a 15-year follow-up from the NSABP B-17 study, the addition of radiation to lumpectomy improved the rates of ipsilateral invasive (19.4 vs. 8.9%) and DCIS (4.9 vs. 2.5%) recurrences when compared with lumpectomy alone. However, there was no benefit in terms of breast cancer–specific mortality at 10 years (0.9 vs. 0.8%), or of overall survival (84 vs. 83%). With regard to endocrine therapy after surgery, in a metaanalysis of 3375 patients with DCIS treated with or without tamoxifen, endocrine therapy led to a significant reduction in the risk of ipsilateral and contralateral DCIS, as well as contralateral invasive disease. However, there was no benefit of tamoxifen in all-cause mortal. There has been an ongoing debate about the overtreatment of DCIS, particularly for those with good prognosis DCIS. Given this patient's young age, the presence of necrosis, and the high nuclear grade, tamoxifen alone or observation would not be appropriate recommendations (answer B and C, respectively). Adjuvant chemotherapy is not indicated, since the risk of systemic recurrence is extremely low (answer D). Hysterectomy with bilateral salpingo-oophorectomy is not indicated as treatment for DCIS (answer E).

17. E

The treatment of DCIS with aromatase inhibitors is supported by the results of the phase III IBIS-II trial, in which patients with hormone receptor positive locally excised DCIS were treated with tamoxifen or anastrozole for 5 years. Anastrozole met the noninferiority aim for that trial. In a metaanalysis of 3375 patients with operated DCIS and subsequently treated with or without tamoxifen, endocrine therapy lead to a significant reduction of the risk of ipsilateral and contralateral DCIS, and contralateral invasive cancer. However, there was no benefit of tamoxifen on all-cause mortality. The concomitant use of selective serotonin reuptake inhibitors (SSRIs) with tamoxifen is controversial. Pharmacologic interactions have been described between tamoxifen and certain SSRIs with studies, suggesting that fluoxetine significantly decreases the plasma concentrations of the active metabolite endoxifen, thereby potentially affecting tamoxifen's overall efficacy. However, a recent study evaluating outcomes of the 16,887 breast cancer survivors, in which 8099 used antidepressants, there was no statistically significant increased risk of subsequent recurrence in women who concurrently used paroxetine or fluoxetine and tamoxifen. Tamoxifen increases the risk of thromboembolic events, in particular in women older than 55 years old, smokers, overweight/obese, hypertensive, and with family history of coronary artery disease. In this patient with personal history of pulmonary embolism and multiple additional risk factors for tamoxifen-related thromboembolic complications, it would be appropriate to recommend against tamoxifen as a choice of endocrine therapy for DCIS (answer D). Chemotherapy is not indicated as adjuvant treatment for DCIS (answer A). Right mastectomy would be potentially appropriate if the patient were interested in maximal risk reduction, even if this led to additional surgery. Unilateral mastectomy would decrease the risk of in-breast recurrence to approximately 2% (answer B). Bilateral mastectomies would decrease the overall lifetime risk of breast cancer to 2% (answer C) and is typically recommended when there is bilateral disease requiring mastectomy, or prophylactically for BRCA1/2 mutation carriers. Neither unilateral nor bilateral mastectomy has been shown to impact mortality in women with DCIS. Given the overall excellent prognosis in patients with DCIS and this patient's comorbidities, close observation including routine mammogram without additional surgeries or systemic therapies would be the most acceptable choice.

18. D

In a recent publication of consensus guidelines on margins for breast conserving surgery with whole breast irradiation in DCIS by the Society of Surgical Oncology, American Society for Radiation Oncology, and American Society of Clinical Oncology, a 2-mm margin was accepted as a new standard. The 2-mm margin minimizes the risk of ipsilateral breast tumor recurrence compared with smaller negative margins. More widely clear margins do not significantly decrease ipsilateral breast tumor recurrence compared with the 2-mm margins. Thus, in this case, next steps would include radiation and consideration of endocrine therapy for secondary chemoprevention.

19. C

In women with hormone receptor negative DCIS, endocrine therapy does not affect the risk of recurrence. This was demonstrated by the NSABP B-24 study, in which patients with hormone receptor positive DCIS treated with tamoxifen had significant decreases in any subsequent breast cancer events compared with patients receiving placebo after surgery and radiation (HR 0.58, 95% CI 0.42–0.81); however, no significant benefit was observed in those with hormone negative DCIS. Subsequent breast cancer events included ipsilateral or contralateral in-situ or invasive breast cancers. Local treatment with lumpectomy and radiation therapy is considered adequate, without additional need for mastectomy (answer D). There is no role for chemotherapy due to low risk and overall good prognosis (answer E).

20. E

Diagnostic core biopsy of a breast lesion may detect DCIS, but can miss an associated invasive component. Invasive carcinoma has been reported in 10%–20% of excision specimens following a biopsy diagnosis of DCIS. If breast cancer is diagnosed, management of the invasive disease takes priority over DCIS. With proven invasive carcinoma metastatic to lymph nodes, the most likely scenario is of an occult invasive right breast cancer. With multiple abnormal matted lymph nodes, the most appropriate treatment would include neoadjuvant chemotherapy, surgery, postoperative radiation, and adjuvant endocrine therapy. Another possible option would be surgery first, followed by chemotherapy, radiation therapy, and adjuvant endocrine therapy.

REFERENCES

Question 1

1. Hartmann LC, Degnim AC, Santen RJ, Dupont WD, Ghosh K. Atypical hyperplasia of the breast—risk assessment and management options. *N Eng J Med.* 2015;372(1):78–89.
2. Hartmann LC, Sellers TA, Frost MH, et al. Benign breast disease and the risk of breast cancer. *N Engl J Med.* 2005;353(3):229–237.
3. Rageth CJ, O'Flynn EA, Comstock C, et al. First International Consensus Conference on lesions of uncertain malignant potential in the breast (B3 lesions). *Breast Cancer Res Treat.* 2016;159(2):203–213.
4. Pinder SE, Ellis IO. The diagnosis and management of pre-invasive breast disease: ductal carcinoma in situ (DCIS) and atypical ductal hyperplasia (ADH)—current definitions and classification. *Breast Cancer Res.* 2003;5(5):254–257.

Question 2

1. Lopez-Garcia MA, Geyer FC, Lacroix-Triki M, Marchió C, Reis-Filho JS. Breast cancer precursors revisited: molecular features and progression pathways. *Histopathology.* 2010;57(2):171–192.
2. Nelson HD, Smith ME, Griffin JC, Fu R. Use of medications to reduce risk for primary breast cancer: a systematic review for the U.S. Preventive Services Task Force. *Ann Intern Med.* 2013;158(8):604–614.
3. Cuzick J, Sestak I, Forbes JF, et al. Anastrozole for prevention of breast cancer in high-risk postmenopausal women (IBIS-II): an international, double-blind, randomised placebo-controlled trial. *Lancet.* 2014;383(9922):1041–1048.
4. Schwartz T, Cyr A, Margenthaler J. Screening breast magnetic resonance imaging in women with atypia or lobular carcinoma in situ. *J Surg Res.* 2015;193(2):519–522.
5. Rageth CJ, O'Flynn EA, Comstock C, et al. First International Consensus Conference on lesions of uncertain malignant potential in the breast (B3 lesions). *Breast Cancer Res Treat.* 2016;159(2):203–213.

Question 3

1. Hartmann LC, Degnim AC, Santen RJ, Dupont WD, Ghosh K. Atypical hyperplasia of the breast—risk assessment and management options. *N Engl J Med.* 2015;372(1):78–89.
2. Collins LC, Baer HJ, Tamimi RM, Connolly JL, Colditz GA, Schnitt SJ. Magnitude and laterality of breast cancer risk according to histologic type of atypical hyperplasia: results from the Nurses' Health Study. *Cancer.* 2007;109(2):180–187.

Question 4

1. Hartmann LC, Degnim AC, Santen RJ, Dupont WD, Ghosh K. Atypical hyperplasia of the breast—risk assessment and management options. *N Engl J Med.* 2015;372(1):78–89.

Question 5

1. Fisher B, Constantino JP, Wickerham DL, et al. Tamoxifen for prevention of breast cancer: report of the National Surgical Adjuvant Breast and Bowel Project P-1 Study. *J Natl Cancer Inst.* 1998;90(18):1371–1388.
2. Chen YY, Hwang ES, Roy R, et al. Genetic and phenotypic characteristics of pleomorphic lobular carcinoma in situ of the breast. *Am J Surg Pathol.* 2009;33(11):1683–1694.

Question 6

1. Oppong BA, King TA. Recommendations for women with lobular carcinoma in situ (LCIS). *Oncology.* 2011;25(11):1051–1056. 1058.
2. Cuzick J, Sestak I, Forbes JF, et al. Anastrozole for prevention of breast cancer in high-risk postmenopausal women (IBIS-II): an international, double-blind, randomised placebo-controlled trial. *Lancet.* 2014;383(9922):1041–1048.

Question 7

1. Fisher B, Costantino JP, Wickerham DL, et al. Tamoxifen for prevention of breast cancer: reports of the National Surgical Adjuvant Breast and Bowel Project P-1 Study. *J Natl Cancer Inst.* 1998;90(18):1371–1388.
2. Vogel VG, Costantino JP, Wickerham DL, et al. Effects of tamoxifen vs raloxifene on the risk of developing invasive breast cancer and other disease outcomes: the NSABP Study of Tamoxifen and raloxifene (STAR) P-2 Trial. *JAMA.* 2006;295(23):2727–2741.
3. Nelson HD, Smith ME, Griffin JC, Fu R. Use of medications to reduce risk for primary breast cancer: a systematic review for the U.S. Preventive Services Task Force. *Ann Intern Med.* 2013;158(8):604–614.

Question 8

1. Nelson HD, Smith ME, Griffin JC, Fu R. Use of medications to reduce risk for primary breast cancer: a systematic review for the U.S. Preventive Services Task Force. *Ann Intern Med.* 2013;158(8):604–614.
2. *NCCN Breast Cancer Risk Reduction, version 1.* 2016.

Question 9

1. Chen YY, Hwang ES, Roy R, et al. Genetic and phenotypic characteristics of pleomorphic lobular carcinoma in situ of the breast. *Am J Surg Pathol.* 2009;33(11):1683–1694.

Question 10

1. Chen YY, Hwang ES, Roy R, et al. Genetic and phenotypic characteristics of pleomorphic lobular carcinoma in situ of the breast. *Am J Surg Pathol*. 2009;33(11):1683–1694.

Question 11

1. Brinton LA, Sherman ME, Carreon JD, Anderson WF. Recent trends in breast cancer among younger women in the United States. *J Natl Cancer Inst*. 2008;100:1643–1648.
2. Virnig BA, Tuttle TM, Shamliyan T, Kane RL. Ductal carcinoma in situ of the breast: a systematic review of incidence, treatment, and outcomes. *J Natl Cancer Inst*. 2010;102:170–178.
3. Siegel RL, Miller KD, Jemal A. Cancer statistics, 2015. *CA Cancer J Clin*. 2015;(65):5–29.
4. Foukakis T, Åström G, Lindström L, Hatschek T, Bergh J. When to order a biopsy to characterise a metastatic relapse in breast cancer. *Ann Oncol*. 2012;23:x349–x353.
5. Roses RE, Arun BK, Lari SA, et al. Ductal carcinoma-in-situ of the breast with subsequent distant metastasis and death. *Ann Surg Oncol*. 2011;18:2873–2878.
6. Siegel R, Ward E, Brawley O, Jemal A. Cancer statistics, 2011: the impact of eliminating socioeconomic and racial disparities on premature cancer deaths. *CA Cancer J Clin*. 2011;61:212–236.
7. Claus EB, Petruzella S, Matloff E, Carter D. Prevalence of BRCA1 and BRCA2 mutations in women diagnosed with ductal carcinoma in situ. *JAMA*. 2005;293:964–969.

Question 12

1. Schwartz GF, Patchefsky AS, Finklestein SD, et al. Nonpalpable in situ ductal carcinoma of the breast. Predictors of multicentricity and microinvasion and implications for treatment. *Arch Surg*. 1989;124:29–32.
2. Silverstein MJ, Waisman JR, Gamagami P, et al. Intraductal carcinoma of the breast (208 cases). Clinical factors influencing treatment choice. *Cancer*. 1990;66:102–108.
3. Fisher ER, Dignam J, Tan-Chiu E, et al. Pathologic findings from the National Surgical Adjuvant Breast Project (NSABP) eight-year update of Protocol B-17: intraductal carcinoma. *Cancer*. 1999;86:429–438.
4. Narod SA, Iqbal J, Giannakeas V, Sopik V, Sun P. Breast cancer mortality after a diagnosis of ductal carcinoma in situ. *JAMA Oncol*. 2015;1:888–896.
5. Morrow M, Van Zee KJ, Solin LJ, et al. Society of Surgical Oncology–American Society for Radiation Oncology–American Society of Clinical Oncology Consensus Guideline on Margins for Breast-Conserving Surgery with Whole-Breast Irradiation in Ductal Carcinoma In Situ. *Ann Surg Oncol*. 2016;23:3801–3810.

Question 13

1. Erbas B, Provenzano E, Armes J, Gertig D. The natural history of ductal carcinoma in situ of the breast: a review. *Breast Cancer Res Treat*. 2006;97(2):135–144.

Question 14

1. Collins LC, Laronga C, Wong JS. Ductal carcinoma in situ: treatment and prognosis. In UpToDate. Wolters Kluwer 2016. https://www.uptodate.com.
2. Hwang ES. The impact of surgery on ductal carcinoma in situ outcomes: the use of mastectomy. *J Natl Cancer Inst Monogr*. 2010;2010:197–199.
3. Wapnir IL, Dignam JJ, Fisher B, et al. Long-term outcomes of invasive ipsilateral breast tumor recurrences after lumpectomy in NSABP B-17 and B-24 randomized clinical trials for DCIS. *J Natl Cancer Inst*. 2011;103:478–488.
4. Lee LA, Silverstein MJ, Chung CT, et al. Breast cancer-specific mortality after invasive local recurrence in patients with ductal carcinoma-in-situ of the breast. *Am J Surg*. 2006;192:416–419.
5. Schouten van der Velden AP, van Vugt R, Van Dijck JA, Leer JW, Wobbes T. Local recurrences after different treatment strategies for ductal carcinoma in situ of the breast: a population-based study in the East Netherlands. *Int J Radiat Oncol Biol Phys*. 2007;69:703–710.
6. Bannani S, Rouquette S, Bendavid-Athias C, Tas P, Levêque J. The locoregional recurrence post-mastectomy for ductal carcinoma in situ: incidence and risk factors. *Breast*. 2015;24:608–612.
7. Sakr R, Barranger E, Antoine M, Prugnolle H, Daraï E, Uzan S. Ductal carcinoma in situ: value of sentinel lymph node biopsy. *J Surg Oncol*. 2006;94:426–430.

Question 15

1. Lee LA, Silverstein MJ, Chung CT, et al. Breast cancer-specific mortality after invasive local recurrence in patients with ductal carcinoma-in-situ of the breast. *Am J Surg*. 2006;192:416–419.
2. Schouten van der Velden AP, van Vugt R, Van Dijck JA, Leer JW, Wobbes T. Local recurrences after different treatment strategies for ductal carcinoma in situ of the breast: a population-based study in the East Netherlands. *Int J Radiat Oncol Biol Phys*. 2007;69:703–710.
3. Bannani S, Rouquette S, Bendavid-Athias C, Tas P, Levêque J. The locoregional recurrence post-mastectomy for ductal carcinoma in situ: incidence and risk factors. *Breast*. 2015;24:608–612.

Question 16

1. Goodwin A, Parker S, Ghersi D, Wilcken N. Post-operative radiotherapy for ductal carcinoma in situ of the breast—a systematic review of the randomised trials. *Breast*. 2009;18:143–149.
2. Wapnir IL, Dignam JJ, Fisher B, et al. Long-term outcomes of invasive ipsilateral breast tumor recurrences after lumpectomy in NSABP B-17 and B-24 randomized clinical trials for DCIS. *J Natl Cancer Inst*. 2011;103:478–488.
3. Staley H, McCallum I, Bruce J. Postoperative tamoxifen for ductal carcinoma in situ. *Cochrane Database Syst Rev*. 2012;10:CD007847.

Question 17

1. Forbes JF, Sestak I, Howell A, et al. Anastrozole versus tamoxifen for the prevention of locoregional and contralateral breast cancer in postmenopausal women with locally excised ductal carcinoma in situ (IBIS-II DCIS): a double-blind, randomised controlled trial. *Lancet*. 2016;387:866–873.
2. Staley H, McCallum I, Bruce J. Postoperative tamoxifen for ductal carcinoma in situ. *Cochrane Database Syst Rev*. 2012;10:CD007847.
3. Jin Y, Desta Z, Stearns V, et al. CYP2D6 genotype, antidepressant use, and tamoxifen metabolism during adjuvant breast cancer treatment. *J Natl Cancer Inst*. 2005;97:30–39.
4. Haque R, Shi J, Schottinger JE, et al. Tamoxifen and antidepressant drug interaction among a cohort of 16 887 breast cancer survivors. *J Natl Cancer Inst*. 2016;108. doi: https://doi.org/10.1093/jnci/djv 337.
5. Decensi A, Maisonneuve P, Rotmensz N, et al. Effect of tamoxifen on venous thromboembolic events in a breast cancer prevention trial. *Circulation*. 2005;111:650–656.
6. Lee LA, Silverstein MJ, Chung CT, et al. Breast cancer-specific mortality after invasive local recurrence in patients with ductal carcinoma-in-situ of the breast. *Am J Surg*. 2006;192:416–419.
7. Schouten van der Velden AP, van Vugt R, Van Dijck JA, Leer JW, Wobbes T. Local recurrences after different treatment strategies for ductal carcinoma in situ of the breast: a population-based study in the East Netherlands. *Int J Radiat Oncol Biol Phys*. 2007;69:703–710.
8. Bannani S, Rouquette S, Bendavid-Athias C, Tas P, Levêque J. The locoregional recurrence post-mastectomy for ductal carcinoma in situ: incidence and risk factors. *Breast*. 2015;24:608–612.

Question 18

1. Morrow M, Van Zee KJ, Solin LJ, et al. Society of Surgical Oncology–American Society for Radiation Oncology–American Society of Clinical Oncology Consensus Guideline on Margins for Breast-Conserving Surgery with Whole-Breast Irradiation in Ductal Carcinoma In Situ. *Ann Surg Oncol*. 2016;23:3801–3810.

Question 19

1. Allred DC, Anderson SJ, Paik S, et al. Adjuvant tamoxifen reduces subsequent breast cancer in women with estrogen receptor-positive ductal carcinoma in situ: a study based on NSABP protocol B-24. *J Clin Oncol*. 2012;30:1268–1273.

Question 20

1. Brennan ME, Turner RM, Ciatto S, et al. Ductal carcinoma in situ at core-needle biopsy: meta-analysis of underestimation and predictors of invasive breast cancer. *Radiology*. 2011;260:119–128.
2. Lara JF, Young SM, Velilla RE, Santoro EJ, Templeton SF. The relevance of occult axillary micrometastasis in ductal carcinoma in situ: a clinicopathologic study with long-term follow-up. *Cancer*. 2003;98:2105–2113.

Non-Small Cell Lung Cancer

QUESTIONS

1. A 76-year-old gentleman has a 40-pack-year history of cigarette smoking and elects to undergo routine lung cancer screening with low-dose CT of the chest, which reveals a 3-cm left lower lobe mass. The patient undergoes a CT-guided lung biopsy, which establishes a diagnosis of squamous non-small cell lung cancer (NSCLC).

   What is the next step in the patient's management?
   A. Mediastinoscopy
   B. Positron emission tomography (PET) scan
   C. Proceed to surgical management
   D. Pulmonary function tests
   E. Observation

2. In the above 76-year-old gentleman, a PET scan does not reveal any other sites of metastatic disease and a mediastinoscopy does not reveal the presence of carcinoma cells in the mediastinal or hilar lymph nodes.

   What stage is the patient's cancer?
   A. Stage I
   B. Stage IIA
   C. Stage IIB
   D. Stage III
   E. Stage IV

3. The above patient has pulmonary function tests, which are normal. What would be the recommended management of this patient's NSCLC?
   A. Observation
   B. Surgery with wedge resection
   C. Surgery with lobectomy
   D. Stereotactic body radiation therapy (SBRT)
   E. Proton therapy

4. A 64-year-old woman presents to her local emergency room with a 1-week history of hemoptysis and dyspnea on exertion on a background of a 50-pack-year history of cigarette smoking. A CT scan of the chest demonstrated a 7.2-cm lung mass in the right upper lobe and possible mediastinal lymph node enlargement. Biopsy of the lung lesion shows lung adenocarcinoma. A PET-CT shows extensive uptake in the mass but a low level of uptake in the mediastinal nodes. An MRI brain is normal. Mediastinoscopy and lymph node sampling reveal no evidence of cancer.

   What stage is this patient's cancer?
   A. Stage IV
   B. Stage IIIA
   C. Stage II
   D. Stage IB
   E. Stage IA

5. What is the optimum treatment strategy for a patient with stage II NSCLC, as per the above case?
   A. Systemic chemotherapy alone
   B. Stereotactic radiosurgery (SRS)
   C. Combination radiation and chemotherapy
   D. Surgical resection alone
   E. Surgical resection followed by chemotherapy

6. A 38-year-old woman is referred to you following resection of her primary lung cancer. Left lobectomy and mediastinal lymph node dissection yielded a 1.5-cm adenocarcinoma with 0/2 R hilar lymph nodes and 0/4 right paratracheal lymph nodes involved.

   Which of the following do you recommend at this time?
   A. Epidermal growth factor receptor (EGFR) mutation testing and treatment with targeted therapy if positive
   B. Prophylactic cranial irradiation
   C. Adjuvant cisplatin + vinorelbine
   D. Adjuvant carboplatin alone
   E. None of the above

7. A 55-year-old gentleman has a resected right-sided lung adenocarcinoma measuring 4 cm with 2 lymph nodes at the right hilum and 0/4 mediastinal lymph nodes involved with tumor. His tumor is found to have a KRAS mutation.

   What is the stage of the patient's cancer, and what do you recommend in terms of further management?
   A. Stage II: Adjuvant cisplatin + vinorelbine
   B. Stage I: Observation
   C. Stage II: Adjuvant targeted therapy
   D. Stage III: Adjuvant immunotherapy
   E. Stage IV: Erlotinib

8. A 24-year-old never-smoker presents with a 6-cm right-sided lung adenocarcinoma that is metastatic to the bone, adrenals, and liver. He has focal pain from a bony metastasis despite treatment with palliative radiation. Scant material was obtained from tumor sampling of the primary lesion. His tumor should be prioritized for testing of which of the following alterations?
   A. ERCC1
   B. Anaplastic lymphoma kinase (ALK) rearrangement
   C. KRAS
   D. EGFR
   E. B and D

9. A 59-year-old gentleman is found to have a lung lesion on a routine screening CT scan; he is clinically asymptomatic. The nodule is spiculated, 1 cm in size, and centrally located.

Which factors in this case are more likely to favor a diagnosis of lung cancer?
   A. Age of patient
   B. Spiculated lesion
   C. Location of lesion
   D. Size of lesion
   E. All of the above

10. The most common histologic subtype of NSCLC is:
   A. Large cell histology
   B. Large cell neuroendocrine tumor
   C. Adenocarcinoma
   D. Squamous carcinoma
   E. Small cell carcinoma

11. A 67-year-old gentleman undergoes a right upper lobe lobectomy for a recently diagnosed lung adenocarcinoma. The pathologic report reveals a 2-cm lung adenocarcinoma, TTF-1 positive, with surgical margins that are free of cancer. Eight lymph nodes were removed at the time of surgery, and none were found to contain cancer cells, and no visceral pleural involvement was seen. What do you do next?
   A. Observation
   B. Adjuvant radiation therapy
   C. Adjuvant chemotherapy with carboplatin and pemetrexed
   D. Adjuvant chemotherapy with cisplatin and vinorelbine
   E. PD-L1 testing on the tumor sample

12. A 54-year-old gentleman presents to the oncology clinic for an opinion on adjuvant treatment options. He was diagnosed recently with Stage IIB left lung adenocarcinoma. He underwent a LUL lobectomy 4 weeks ago and has recovered well. In looking over his pathology report, you notice a 6-cm adenocarcinoma that is well differentiated. He had an R1 resection. Peribronchial, hilar, and mediastinal LN are removed, and 1 ipsilateral hilar LN is found to be involved with cancer. He is not a candidate for any more surgery. ECOG PS is 0. What do you recommend?
   A. Carboplatin+ Paclitaxel
   B. Observation
   C. Send for EGFR, ALK, and ROS1 testing
   D. Cisplatin + Pemetrexed
   E. Cisplatin + Pemetrexed, and referral to radiation oncology

13. A 60-year-old male presents to his primary care physician with chest pain and has a 4-cm left lower lobe lesion on CT. Pathology reveals atypical cells but no confirmatory evidence for a malignancy, and PET/CT shows no other lesions. What would you recommend now?
   A. Repeat CT Chest with IV contrast in 2 months
   B. Repeat biopsy
   C. Refer to thoracic surgery
   D. Stereotactic radiation therapy (SBRT)
   E. Discharge to PCP

14. A 90-year-old gentleman with multiple medical comorbidities presents with dyspnea and is found to have a 2-cm right upper lobe lung lesion on CT chest, with no metastatic disease on PET-CT and negative mediastinal staging. His FEV1= 1L. What would you recommend for management of this lesion?

   A. Thoracic surgery
   B. Single agent chemotherapy alone
   C. SBRT
   D. Observation
   E. Platinum doublet chemotherapy

15. A 60-year-old male presents to clinic for a recommendation regarding adjuvant therapy for a resected 5-cm left lung lesion with no involvement of lymph nodes in the hilum or mediastinum. What stage is his cancer, and what do you recommend?
   A. Stage IA: Observation
   B. Stage IA: Consider chemotherapy with platinum doublet chemotherapy
   C. Stage IB: Observation
   D. Stage IB: Consider chemotherapy with platinum doublet chemotherapy
   E. C or D

16. The above patient's tumor undergoes molecular testing and is found to harbor an EMLA-ALK rearrangement. What do you recommend now?
   A. Adjuvant erlotinib
   B. Adjuvant crizotinib
   C. Adjuvant chemotherapy carboplatin + pemetrexed
   D. Adjuvant carboplatin + paclitaxel
   E. Adjuvant ceritinib

17. You elect to proceed with a plan to administer adjuvant chemotherapy with carboplatin and pemetrexed. What supportive care recommendations would you institute in preparation for commencement of chemotherapy?
   A. Administer folic acid supplementation
   B. Administer folic acid and vitamin B12 supplementation
   C. Administer folic acid and vitamin B12 supplementation and counsel against use of nonsteroidal antiinflammatory drugs
   D. Administer multivitamins
   E. Arrange palliative care consultation

18. The above patient develops new bilateral leg swelling with discoloration while receiving chemotherapy. Which of the following agents is likely to be the cause of this treatment-related side effect?
   A. Carboplatin
   B. Pemetrexed
   C. Ondansetron
   D. Dexamethasone
   E. Folic Acid

19. A 45-year-old woman has newly diagnosed stage II lung adenocarcinoma; however, the tumor is centrally located and will require a pneumonectomy to achieve complete surgical resection. What is the risk of mortality from surgical resection in this case?
   A. 10%
   B. 5%
   C. 2%
   D. 1%
   E. <1%

20. Risk factors for the development of NSCLC include:
   A. Obesity
   B. Genetic susceptibility
   C. Family history
   D. Diet
   E. Occupational radon exposure

21. A primary care physician refers a 50-year-old gentleman for evaluation of a 2-cm left upper-lobe ground-glass opacity that is biopsy-positive for AIS. The patient is white, has never smoked, and is in excellent health. A chest CT scan shows that she has multiple enlarged left-sided mediastinal nodes; otherwise, the findings are normal. Biopsy of the mediastinal nodes is positive for adenocarcinoma. You stage this disease as stage IIIA (T1N2) and recommend:
    A. Concurrent chemotherapy and radiation
    B. Surgery followed by chemotherapy
    C. Upfront chemotherapy followed by surgery
    D. Erlotinib
    E. Radiation therapy followed by crizotinib

22. A 57-year-old female current smoker presents with a 6-month history of weight loss and cough. A CT of the chest reveals a 6c left-sided lung mass and enlarged/bulky mediastinal nodes that is confirmed by PET, with no disease outside the chest. Biopsy of the mass reveals squamous cell cancer with involvement of ipsilateral left-sided lymph nodes on mediastinal staging. Which of the following management strategies is most likely to lead to a survival benefit?
    A. Concurrent chemotherapy with 60 Gy of thoracic radiation delivered over 5–6 weeks
    B. Surgical resection followed by postoperative radiation therapy
    C. Surgery resection followed by postoperative chemotherapy and sequential radiation therapy
    D. Thoracic radiation alone
    E. Chemotherapy followed by thoracic radiation therapy

23. A 52-year-old female never-smoker presents with hemoptysis and a 4-cm mass on CT of the chest in the right lung. PET imaging demonstrates FDG-avid disease at the right upper and right lower paratracheal lymph nodes, and fine needle aspirations confirms the presence of metastatic adenocarcinoma. MRI brain is negative for disease. She is now referred for treatment. What is the most appropriate management?
    A. Neoadjuvant cisplatin + etoposide followed surgical resection
    B. Neoadjuvant cisplatin + pemetrexed followed by surgical resection
    C. EGFR mutation testing and neoadjuvant erlotinib if positive
    D. Definitive radiation therapy with concurrent weekly carboplatin + paclitaxel
    E. Primary surgical resection followed by adjuvant chemotherapy

24. A 40-year-old woman presents to the oncology clinic for a discussion regarding adjuvant treatment options. She underwent a right lower lobe lobectomy 4 weeks prior and was found to have two separate lung lesions within the right lower lobe resection specimen. Pathologic evaluation revealed both lesions as squamous cell carcinomas, and of 12/12 lymph nodes sampled, none revealed the presence of cancer cells. The patient has recovered well from her surgery and her KPS=90%. What is the patient's tumor stage and optimum treatment options?
    A. Stage I: Observation
    B. Stage I: Adjuvant Cisplatin + Paclitaxel
    C. Stage II: Adjuvant Cisplatin + Paclitaxel
    D. Stage III: Adjuvant Cisplatin + Pemetrexed
    E. Stage III: Adjuvant Cisplatin + Docetaxel followed by radiation

25. A 52-year-old gentleman with a 40-pack-year smoking history has a chest CT for persistent cough, which shows a 6-cm RUL mass with enlarged right and left lung hilar lymphadenopathy. The left hilar LN is biopsied and shows lung adenocarcinoma. Mutational analysis reveals an EGFR exon 21 mutation L858R. A PET-CT shows no evidence of distant metastasis. What stage cancer does the patient have, and what is your optimal choice of therapy?
    A. Stage IIIB: Erlotinib 100 mg daily
    B. Stage IIIA: Chemoradiation with Carboplatin/Etoposide
    C. Stage IIIA: Surgery followed by adjuvant Cisplatin/Pemetrexed
    D. Stage IIIA: Surgery followed by adjuvant Cisplatin/Etoposide
    E. Stage IIIB: Chemoradiation with Cisplatin/Etoposide

26. A 48-year-old male with an ECOG PS=1 presents to his local ER with chest pain radiating to the left shoulder for months, left hand muscle atrophy, and left-sided eye ptosis. CT of the chest demonstrated a 7-cm lesion in the left lung apex, and biopsy reveals a lung adenocarcinoma in the superior sulcus. Discussion at a multidisciplinary meeting reveals that the tumor is surgically resectable. What treatment do you recommend?
    A. Surgical resection followed by adjuvant Cisplatin/Pemetrexed
    B. Neoadjuvant chemotherapy (Cisplatin/Pemetrexed) followed by surgery and then adjuvant radiation depending on pathologic assessment of the surgical specimen
    C. Neoadjuvant chemoradiation followed by surgery +/− additional chemotherapy
    D. Concurrent chemotherapy (Cisplatin/Etoposide) with Thoracic Radiation

27. An 82-year-old lifelong smoker presents to the medical oncology clinic for an opinion regarding optimum management strategies for stage IV KRAS-mutant NSCLC. What do you tell him about the biology of KRAS-mutant NSCLC?
    A. This is the most common genomic alteration seen in lung adenocarcinoma.
    B. This genomic alteration confers a poor prognosis.
    C. This type of NSCLC can be treated with targeted therapy.
    D. Treatment for this condition is administered with curative intent.
    E. A and B

28. A 35-year-old female Taiwanese never-smoker is diagnosed with metastatic NSCLC. Genomic analysis using which of the following tests is most likely to guide her choice of therapy?
    A. KRAS mutation
    B. VEGFR mutation
    C. EGFR mutation
    D. BRAF mutation
    E. PIK3CA mutation

29. A 73-year-old gentleman with stage IV lung adenocarcinoma is referred to you after completion of first-line cisplatin/pemetrexed chemotherapy. His tumor molecular profiling reveals an EML4-ALK rearrangement. What is the incidence of this genomic alteration in lung adenocarcinoma?
    A. 20%
    B. 10%–15%

C. 50%

D. 3%–5%

E. <1%

30. A 60-year-old gentleman is found to have a right-sided 1-cm mass and a left lower lobe 3-cm mass on CT chest. Mediastinoscopy reveals that all sampled LN do not contain cancer cells, and PET-CT and MRI brain show that these are the only two abnormal lesions. Both lesions undergo biopsy and show adenocarcinoma with EGFR exon 19 deletion. What is the optimum treatment for this patient?

A. Cisplatin + Pemetrexed

B. Concurrent chemotherapy and thoracic radiation

C. Chemotherapy followed by thoracic radiation

D. First-line erlotinib

E. Surgical resection of left and right lung lesions

31. A 50-year-old never-smoker has a chest CT that reveals a 4-cm mass in the right upper lobe of the lung. A PET-CT reveals distant disease with multiple liver and bone lesions, with biopsy that confirms adenocarcinoma, TTF-1 positive. What is the next step in management?

A. Carboplatin/Paclitaxel/Bevacizumab

B. Cisplatin/Pemetrexed

C. ERCC-1 testing

D. EGFR and ALK testing

E. KRAS testing

32. A 60-year-old gentleman presents to his PCP for dyspnea and is found to have a left-sided lung mass on CT, and biopsy reveals low grade/typical carcinoid tumor. A PET-CT is ordered and reveals no other evidence of disease. Which of the following is a true statement?

A. This patient should be managed with surgery alone.

B. This patient should have radiation therapy alone.

C. This patient should be observed only.

D. This patient should be offered surgery followed by adjuvant chemotherapy.

E. Patients with pulmonary carcinoid often present with the carcinoid syndrome.

33. A 42-year-old man who is a lifelong never-smoker, presents with a persistent cough. Chest CT reveals a 2.8-cm mass in the right lung. A PET-CT reveals distant disease with 10 liver lesions, and biopsy of one of these lesions shows TTF-1 positive adenocarcinoma. Molecular testing reveals a ROS1 rearrangement.

How common is this genomic alteration found in NSCLC?

A. 10%

B. 20%

C. 5%

D. 1%–2%

E. <0.5%

34. A 30-year-old never-smoker presents with newly diagnosed lung adenocarcinoma and is found to have an EML4-ALK rearrangement. What is the gold standard for diagnosis of ALK rearrangements?

A. Fluorescent in situ hybridization (FISH)

B. Immunohistochemistry (IHC)

C. Next generation sequencing

D. Hotspot genetic testing

E. Circulating tumor DNA testing

35. A 42-year old patient with stage IIIB NSCLC is treated with concurrent chemoradiation with cisplatin and etoposide and 60 Gy of thoracic radiation. Three weeks into therapy, the patient complains of difficulty swallowing and chest discomfort. What is the likely diagnosis and recommended management?

A. Pulmonary embolus, anticoagulation

B. Myocardial infarction, thrombolysis

C. Radiation skin toxicity, topical emollients

D. Radiation esophagitis, lidocaine mouthwashes

E. Radiation pneumonitis, corticosteroids

36. In the same 42-year-old patient, 3 months after completion of concurrent chemoradiation the patient complains of increasing dyspnea on exertion. A CT of the chest reveals new interstitial infiltrates. The patient denies chest pain, hemoptysis, sputum production, purulent sputum, and has no fevers on clinical examination. What is the likely diagnosis and recommended management?

A. Pulmonary embolus, anticoagulation

B. Myocardial infarction, thrombolysis

C. Radiation skin toxicity, topical emollients

D. Radiation esophagitis, lidocaine mouthwashes

E. Radiation pneumonitis, corticosteroids

37. Systemic treatment for stage III NSCLC may be delivered either neoadjuvantly or adjuvantly. The potential benefits of neoadjuvant therapy do NOT include:

A. Superior survival outcomes compared with adjuvant therapy

B. Improved therapy completion rates

C. Early treatment of micrometastatic disease

D. Improved tolerability

E. A and D

38. Which of the following agents is not a tyrosine kinase inhibitor used in the treatment of EGFR-mutant NSCLC?

A. Erlotinib

B. Gefinitib

C. Everolimus

D. Afatinib

E. Osimertinib

39. The following antiangiogenic therapies have demonstrated a benefit in response and survival in NSCLC:

A. Bevacizumab

B. Ramucirumab

C. A and B

D. Temozolamide

E. Aflibercept

40. The following chemotherapy regimens used in the management of NSCLC are considered of high emetogenic potential:

A. Carboplatin + Paclitaxel

B. Carboplatin + Paclitaxel + Bevacizumab

C. Cisplatin + Pemetrexed

D. Carboplatin + Pemetrexed + Bevacizumab

E. Docetaxel + Ramucirumab

41. A 70-year-old current smoker presents to his primary care physician with a 2-month history of cough, sore throat, and dyspnea on exertion. Antibiotics are given without resolution of the patient's symptoms. A chest x-ray is performed showing a new 5-cm left lung mass. Staging whole body PET scan shows uptake in the right adrenal gland, L ileum, and fourth rib. MRI of the brain shows a 3-cm lesion in the right frontal lobe with surrounding vasogenic edema. The lesion is not hemorrhagic. The patient has no neurologic symptoms. His

KPS is 80%. What treatment would be most appropriate for this patient?
A. Carboplatin + Pemetrexed
B. Whole brain radiation therapy
C. Carboplatin + paclitaxel + bevacizumab
D. Referral to neurosurgery for craniotomy, resection of metastasis, and postoperative radiation therapy
E. Best supportive care

42. A 54-year-old never-smoker has newly diagnosed squamous cell lung cancer metastatic to the liver, lung, and bone. She attends oncology clinic for a second opinion regarding treatment. Her sister was diagnosed with metastatic colon cancer and has been treated with bevacizumab + FOLFOX with stable disease for 1.5 years. The patient is furious that her primary oncologist has refused to treat her with this drug. Which of the following best supports her oncologist's recommendation?
A. Patients with squamous cell lung cancer do not have an overall survival benefit from bevacizumab.
B. Patients with squamous cell lung cancer were never treated with bevacizumab as part of a clinical trial of the drug.
C. Patients with squamous cell lung cancer treated with bevacizumab risk the development of severe pulmonary hemorrhage.
D. B and C
E. None of the above

43. A 62-year-old gentleman with a 60-pack-year smoking history has a PET-CT that reveals multiple liver lesions and bilateral lung disease. One of the liver lesions is biopsied and demonstrates squamous cell cancer that is p40 positive without any other histologic components. Which of the following would be your preferred management choice?
A. Carboplatin + Paclitaxel + Bevacizumab
B. Test for EML4-ALK mutation
C. Test for EGFR mutation
D. Carboplatin + Paclitaxel
E. Cisplatin + Pemetrexed

44. A 33-year-old gentleman develops dyspnea and back pain and is found to have multiple lung and liver lesions on a CT of the chest/abdomen/pelvis. A biopsy of one of the liver lesions reveals lung adenocarcinoma, which tests positive for an EGFR exon 21 L858R mutation.
What treatment do you recommend for this patient?
A. Erlotinib
B. Cisplatin+Pemetrexed
C. Erlotinib + Bevacizumab
D. Afatinib
E. Nivolumab

45. The above patient begins treatment with erlotinib and has a substantial reduction in all areas of disease. Unfortunately, his 12-month CT scan shows new pulmonary nodules and an increase in the size of the primary lung lesion. He consents to rebiopsy. Which of the following genetic lesions is most likely to be present?
A. ALK rearrangement
B. MET amplification
C. PIK3CA mutation
D. EGFR T816Q mutation
E. EGFR T790M mutation

46. The above patient's tumor biopsy reveals transformation to small cell lung cancer. What do you explain to the patient about this occurrence and your choice of treatment?

A. Transformation to small cell lung cancer is common and should be treated with a new targeted agent.
B. Transformation to small cell lung cancer is uncommon and should be treated with a platinum/etoposide.
C. Transformation to small cell lung cancer is uncommon and should be treated with a platinum/pemetrexed.
D. Transformation to small cell lung cancer is common and should be treated with a platinum/etoposide.
E. Transformation to small cell lung cancer is common and should be treated with an immunotherapy.

47. A 55-year-old gentleman with stage IV ALK-arranged NSCLC commences first-line crizotinib and sustains a partial response to therapy but develops a characteristic toxicity seen with this agent. The toxicity in question is:
A. Weight loss
B. Abdominal pain
C. Seizures
D. Visual changes
E. Bleeding

48. A 78-year-old woman with 40-pack-year smoking history, mild chronic obstructive pulmonary disease, and recently diagnosed stage IV squamous cell carcinoma is referred to you for initial therapy. Her functional status is ECOG 1. Which of the following do you recommend?
A. Erlotinib
B. Crizotinib
C. Platinum/paclitaxel
D. Platinum/pemetrexed
E. Best supportive care

49. A 58-year-old gentleman presents with a 6-month history of progressive cough and dyspnea, on a background of 30 pack-years of cigarette smoking. PET-CT demonstrates increased uptake in a right middle lobe mass, bones, and liver lesions. He undergoes a biopsy of a liver lesion that demonstrates squamous cell carcinoma, TTF-1 negative, and p40 positive. MRI of the brain is negative for metastatic disease. His ECOG performance status is 1. He will begin first-line chemotherapy next week. In addition to chemotherapy, what other intervention may lead to a survival benefit?
A. Referral to radiation oncology
B. Referral to thoracic surgery
C. Referral to palliative care
D. Referral to psychiatry
E. Referral to nutrition

50. A 73-year-old woman with a 100-pack-year smoking history is diagnosed with stage IV NSCLC with squamous histology. She receives carboplatin and paclitaxel for six cycles and then develops progressive disease. She has an excellent performance status. Which of the following is the most appropriate treatment option for this patient?
A. Gemcitabine
B. Docetaxel
C. Nivolumab
D. Vinorelbine
E. Best supportive care

51. What targeted agent should be used for the treatment of ROS-1 rearranged NSCLC
A. Erlotinib
B. Crizotinib
C. Ceritinib
D. Afatinib
E. Dabrafenib

52. A 55-year-old Asian male has stage IV ALK-rearranged NSCLC and develops new metastatic disease to the brain after first-line crizotinib. The patient has an ECOG PS=1 and is symptomatic with headache. What is the optimum therapy?
    A. Whole brain radiation and continue crizotinib
    B. Switch to cisplatin/pemetrexed chemotherapy
    C. Switch to alectinib
    D. Switch to erlotinib
    E. Best supportive care

53. A 66-year-old Jamaican woman presents with newly diagnosed stage IV lung adenocarcinoma that possess a BRAF V600E mutation. What is your treatment of choice for this patient?
    A. Cisplatin/Pemetrexed
    B. Carboplatin/Paclitaxel
    C. Vemurafenib
    D. Dabrafenib/Trametinib
    E. Erlotinib

54. A 58-year-old male has stage IV NSCLC and develops progressive disease in the lung and liver after receipt of therapy with first-line platinum doublet chemotherapy. Which one of the options below is NOT a second-line treatment option for NSCLC?
    A. Docetaxel
    B. Nivolumab
    C. Pembrolizumab
    D. Docetaxel/Ramucirumab
    E. Panitumumab

55. A 54-year-old male has stage IV NSCLC and is receiving maintenance pemetrexed therapy and develops progressive disease in the brain with three isolated lesions with mild vasogenic edema. The patient is mildly symptomatic with headache. Which one of the options below would you recommend?
    A. SRS to brain metastases and continue maintenance pemetrexed
    B. Whole brain radiation therapy
    C. Switch to nivolumab
    D. Switch to erlotinib
    E. Best supportive care

56. A 76-year-old male comes to see you to discuss treatment options for advanced lung squamous cell cancer involving the liver. His ECOG PS=0, and he has no comorbid conditions. He lives independently and can perform all his ADLs and IADLs. Which therapy is best for him?
    A. Best supportive care
    B. Weekly Paclitaxel
    C. Single agent Carboplatin

    D. Cisplatin + Pemetrexed
    E. Carboplatin + Paclitaxel

57. A 36-year-old Japanese woman develops a persistent cough for 8 weeks and has innumerable bilateral lung lesions on CT chest. A PET-CT shows no disease outside of the lung, and her brain MRI was negative. A peripheral lung lesion was biopsied and demonstrated lung adenocarcinoma with an exon 19 mutation in EGFR. Of note, her breathing is getting more labored. Which of the following treatments is best to start at this time?
    A. Erlotinib
    B. Erlotinib + Bevacizumab
    C. Carboplatin + Pemetrexed
    D. Afatinib
    E. A or E

58. A 72-year-old gentleman with a 100-pack-year smoking history presents with dyspnea CT Chest with IV contrast shows a 5-cm left lung lesion and no enlarged mediastinal or hilar lymph nodes, but a right-sided pleural effusion, which when drained demonstrated squamous cell lung cancer cells. A PET-CT shows no other evidence of other disease. What treatment would you recommend?
    A. Mediastinoscopy
    B. Surgery and adjuvant chemotherapy
    C. Radiation (SBRT) given the solitary mass
    D. Palliative chemotherapy
    E. Erlotinib 150 mg daily

59. A 59-year-old male has advanced lung adenocarcinoma with metastases in the lungs, liver, adrenals, and bone. He spends 90% of the day in bed or at rest and his family assist him with self-care activities. What do you recommend in terms of optimum management?
    A. Best supportive care only
    B. SBRT to primary lung lesion
    C. Single agent carboplatin
    D. Single agent Paclitaxel
    E. Erlotinib

60. A 50-year-old never-smoker has ALK-positive stage IV lung adenocarcinoma treated with first-line crizotinib for 18 months but then develops progressive disease in the lungs and liver. Which of the following treatment options would you recommend for this patient?
    A. Ceritinib
    B. Cisplatin alone
    C. Cisplatin + Pemetrexed
    D. Carboplatin + Pemetrexed
    E. SBRT to progressive lesions.

ANSWERS

1. B

Full body imaging will rule out the presence of widely metastatic disease and should be completed prior to staging of the mediastinum or other standard diagnostic evaluation required for surgical management such as option D. Patients should undergo complete staging prior to proceeding with surgical management.

2. A

The patient has stage I NSCLC. As per AJCC lung cancer staging, the patient has a tumor that is less than 5 cm in

size with no hilar (N1), ipsilateral mediastinal (N2), or contralateral lymph nodes involves (N3), and no metastatic disease (M1). Therefore, the stage is T1N0, stage IA non-small cell lung cancer.

3. C

Surgical resection is the gold standard management approach for patients with localized NSCLC that is suitable for surgery. In medically unfit patients, SBRT may be used instead of surgery with similar survival outcomes. Lobectomy is the current preferred surgical approach in patients with localized lung cancer. Proton therapy is not used as a standard of care in patients with lung cancer.

4. C

The patient has a primary lung cancer greater than 7 cm in size with no hilar or mediastinal lymph node involvement. The stage is T3N0, stage IIB disease.

5. E

Three randomized trials comparing adjuvant chemotherapy with surgery alone have demonstrated a survival benefit for adjuvant chemotherapy for patients with stage II–IIIA NSCLC. Although earlier studies were negative, an updated metaanalysis confirmed the benefit of adjuvant cisplatin-based adjuvant chemotherapy. The role of adjuvant therapy for stage IB is debated. One study that included patients with IB was statistically negative (*P*-value = .10), but a trend towards improved overall survival was seen (hazard ratio 0.8). In addition, patients in this study received carboplatin and not cisplatin. The role of postoperative radiation therapy is not indicated for patients with node-negative disease.

6. C

Studies have shown a 5% absolute survival benefit for adjuvant platinum doublet chemotherapy after surgery in stage II–IIIA NSCLC. The original chemotherapy regimen studied was cisplatin and vinorelbine.

7. A

This patient has T1N1, stage IIA NSCLC and should receive adjuvant chemotherapy.

8. E

It is now standard clinical care to assess patients with newly diagnosed stage IV lung adenocarcinoma for the presence of EGFR and ALK at a minimum. The patient's age and history as a never-smoker support a potential diagnosis of an oncogene-addicted NSCLC. KRAS mutations confer a poor prognosis, and there are no targeted therapies for patients with this genomic alteration. ERCC1 was examined for its potential role in predicting response to chemotherapy.

9. E

All of the above. Centrally located spiculated lesions in patients with a smoking history are suspicious for bronchogenic carcinoma, regardless of patient symptoms.

10. C

Adenocarcinoma is the most common histologic subtype of NSCLC and accounts for approximately 80% of cases of NSCLC.

11. A

This patient has stage IA disease. There is no role of adjuvant therapy. The Lung Adjuvant Cisplatin Evaluation collected and pooled data from the five largest trials (4584 patients) of cisplatin-based chemotherapy in completely resected patients that were conducted after the 1995 NSCLC metaanalysis. For stage IA disease, there was no benefit of giving chemotherapy

12. E

The role of targeted therapy is currently being studied in the early stage setting (stage I, II, III NSCLC) but is not considered standard of care at this time. Radiation therapy plays a role for patients with R1/R2 disease (who are not further surgery candidates) and possibly for patients with N2 disease (PORT analysis data set). The LACE metaanalysis examined five randomized studies (4584 patients) for the benefit conferred by adjuvant cisplatin-based chemotherapy

for resected NSCLC and demonstrated a benefit in stage II and III disease, with a 5-year absolute benefit of 5% from adjuvant chemotherapy alone.

13. C

With his smoking history, size of this lesion, and atypical cells on biopsy, there is a concern for lung cancer. Of note, often adenocarcinoma in situ (formerly known as bronchoalveolar carcinomas) and lung carcinoid tumors are not FDG-avid. In addition, even if a repeat biopsy is done and is negative, we cannot confidently exclude malignancy.

14. C

Patients with stage I NSCLC who are considered medically inoperable may be treated with SBRT rather than standard surgical management and have demonstrated similar outcomes in terms of survival and local control compared with patients who have stage I NSCLC treated with surgery.

15. D

In a subset of patients with stage IB NSCLC where the primary tumor is greater than 5 cm, patients may derive benefit from adjuvant chemotherapy. However, observation and surveillance is also a reasonable option supported by phase III data.

16. D

There are no clinical studies that demonstrate a survival benefit for targeted therapy used in early stage lung cancers. The answer thus remains D.

17. C

Standard supportive therapy for patients commencing pemetrexed requires folic acid and vitamin B12 supplementation and should not be administered together with nonsteroidal antiinflammatory drugs.

18. B

A described side effect of pemetrexed includes bilateral leg swelling.

19. B

The incidence of severe complications and mortality after pneumonectomy is estimated at 5%.

20. E

Occupational exposures such as cigarette smoking, radon, asbestos, arsenic, nickel, aromatic hydrocarbons, and chloromethyl ethers are associated with the development of lung cancer.

21. A

The treatment of stage III disease includes a local therapy such as radiation therapy and chemotherapy concurrently. The Southwestern Oncology Group conducted a phase III study of maintenance gefitinib after concurrent chemoradiotherapy and docetaxel and found an inferior survival on the gefitinib arm, which was a result of tumor progression and not toxicity. Thus, in the absence of other data, maintenance erlotinib is not recommended.

22. A

This patient has bulky, multilevel mediastinal disease, making her cancer stage IIIA (N2) and inoperable. Adjuvant therapy has been explored for the treatment of patients with stage II and microscopic IIIA disease, but not for patients with bulky stage IIIA or stage IIIB cancer. Findings from two randomized studies have shown a survival advantage for concurrent chemoradiation therapy compared with a sequential approach. In a Japanese trial, two cycles of mitomycin-C/vindesine/cisplatin (MVP) were given concurrently or sequentially with radiation therapy at 56 Gy. Patients in either arm who had a disease response received another two cycles of MVP after radiation therapy was completed. In a confirmatory randomized trial conducted by the Radiation Therapy Oncology Group, the combination of cisplatin, vinblastine, and radiation therapy was compared with sequential chemoradiation therapy. Both studies demonstrated a survival advantage for concurrent chemoradiation therapy compared with a sequential approach.

23. D

The patient has bulky N2 disease and is likely to be inoperable. In this case, the concurrent combination of chemotherapy and radiation would this be preferred. Neoadjuvant therapy prior to surgery is a treatment option in patients with earlier stage resectable NSCLC. The utility of molecular testing in earlier stage NSCLC is not known, and targeted therapy in this population is only being delivered in the context of clinical studies.

24. C

T3: Separate nodule in primary lobe. The patient's stage is T3N0, stage II NSCLC. The patient should be treated with adjuvant platinum doublet chemotherapy alone.

25. E

Stage IIIB: Chemoradiation with Cisplatin/Etoposide RTOG 94-10 randomly assigned 610 patients to either concurrent chemoradiation (Cisplatin/Vinblastine or Cisplatin/Etoposide) or sequential chemotherapy and radiation (Cisplatin/Vinblastine→RT)

The 5-year OS was significantly higher in the concurrent regimen compared with the sequential treatment (16% and 13% in concurrent arms vs. 10% sequential arm).

26. D

The patient has an operable superior sulcus tumor. These are located in the lung apex and are often found to involve either the first or second rib, chest wall, or the thoracic inlet. Symptoms from lesions in this location include shoulder pain, atrophy of hand muscles, and subclavian vein obstruction can occur. Neoadjuvant chemoradiation (with hopes of surgery) is the standard of care Horner syndrome, which the patient describes with symptoms of myosis, anhydrosis, and ptosis. If completely resected, the 5-year survival rate is over 50%.

27. E

KRAS mutant NSCLCs are known to portend a poor prognosis and can be found in approximately 25% of patients with lung adenocarcinoma.

28. C

KRAS mutations are found in approximately 25% of lung adenocarcinomas. At this time, they do not appear to predict for lack of benefit with targeted agents. Although there is interest in vascular endothelial growth factor (VEGF) receptor alterations, they do not guide therapy with antiangiogenic drugs. Up to 50% of female, Asian never-smokers have mutations in the EGFR receptor, which might guide future therapy with EGFR targeted therapy.

29. D

EML4-ALK translocations occur in 3%–5% of lung cancer cases. For these tumors, crizotinib, an orally available ALK inhibitor, results in disease control rates of approximately 80%.

30. E

The patient has two separate primary cancers. Each would be stage I since mediastinal staging is negative; therefore, management would be with curative intent with surgery.

31. D

EGFR mutations are normally found in patients with nonsquamous histologies, and EGFR exon 19 deletions and the point mutation L858R in exon 21 predict for response to EGFR tyrosine kinase inhibitors. EML4-ALK is a genomic alteration found in 3%–5% of patients with nonsquamous NSCLC, and crizotinib is an approved therapy with demonstrated improved efficacy in these patients compared with chemotherapy. This patient's tumor sample should undergo molecular testing to assess for the presence of an actionable genomic alteration.

32. A

If found to be stage I carcinoid, surgical resection followed by observation would represent optimal management. Neuroendocrine tumors such as carcinoid tumors account for 1%–2% of lung tumors. Most lung neuroendocrine tumors are asymptomatic.

33. D

This is a rare genomic alteration seen in approximately 1% of patients with lung adenocarcinoma.

34. D

Flourescent in-situ hydridization (FISH) testing is the gold standard companion diagnostic test for the diagnosis of EML4-ALK rearrangements. Immunohistochemistry can be used, however FISH remains the gold standard.

35. D

Radiation esophagitis is a common side effect of this management approach and occurs in up to 50% of patients who receive this treatment. This should be treated with lidocaine mouthwashes.

36. E

Radiation pneumonitis is a common side effect of this management approach and occurs in almost 30% of patients approximately 3 months after completion of therapy. This should be treated with tapered doses of corticosteroids.

37. E

The potential benefits of delivering upfront chemotherapy include improved therapy completion rates, theoretical early treatment of micrometastatic disease, and assessment of pathologic response to therapy. Equivalent survival benefits are seen whether therapy is delivered adjuvantly or neoadjuvantly.

38. C

Everolimus is an MTOR inhibitor. Erlotinib and gefitinib are first-generation tyrosine kinase inhibitors, afatinib is an irreversible tyrosine kinase inhibitor against EGFR, while osimertinib is a mutant-specific tyrosine kinase inhibitor that blocks T790M.

39. C

Both bevacizumab and ramucirumab have demonstrated survival benefits when combined with chemotherapy in late phase studies in patients with advanced NSCLC. In the first-line setting, the combination of carboplatin/paclitaxel/bevacizumab improved overall survival by 2 months (10.3 vs. 12.3 months, P = .003), while the second-line setting in the REVEL study demonstrated a 1.5-month benefit in overall survival compared with docetaxel alone in patients who had received platinum doublet chemotherapy first-line.

40. C

Cisplatin-based chemotherapy regimens are of high emetogenic potential.

41. D

Proceeding to surgery for the patient's brain lesion will be both diagnostic and therapeutic for this patient. The tissue obtained during the procedure will allow for histologic diagnosis of likely cancer, and it will also allow for the treatment of a brain lesion with edema.

42. C

Early clinical trials examined the use of bevacizumab in patients with squamous cell lung cancers and cases of fatal pulmonary hemorrhage were reported. A randomized phase II study evaluated the addition of bevacizumab to carboplatin and paclitaxel in patients with advanced NSCLC, and showed improved response rates. However, the bleeding risk with bevacizumab was higher. Bleeding arose from centrally located tumors close to major blood vessels. It was felt that squamous histology conferred an increased risk of bleeding in part as they often occur near central vessels. Therefore, patients with squamous lung cancers should not receive this agent for safety reasons.

43. D

Bevacizumab and Pemetrexed are indicated for NSCLCs with nonsquamous histology. A randomized phase II study evaluated the addition of bevacizumab to carboplatin and paclitaxel in patients with advanced NSCLC, and showed improved response rates. EGFR and ALK alterations are rarely found in tumors with squamous histology. Thus, of the options above, Carboplatin + Paclitaxel would be a reasonable regimen.

44. A

Erlotinib. The Phase III EURTAC enrolled patients with treatment naïve, advanced NSCLC with EGFR mutations (exon 19 deletion or L858R mutation in exon 21) to either erlotinib 150 mg per day or Cisplatin + Docetaxel or Gemcitabine. PFS favored the erlotinib arm (9.7 months vs. 5.2 months; P < .0001).

45. E

Approximately 40%–50% of patients with EGFR-mutant NSCLC will develop acquired resistance to first-generation EGFR inhibition by developing the gatekeeper mutation T790M.

46. B

In a minority of patients with EGFR-mutant NSCLC, patients will develop acquired resistance through a mechanism termed epithelial-to-mesenchymal transition where NSCLC appears to morphologically change to SCLC. At that time, patients should be treated with platinum/etoposide combination therapy.

47. D

Crizotinib is relatively well tolerated, and clinical trials of this agent have included patients with performance status up to ECOG 3. The principal toxicities of crizotinib include nausea, diarrhea, transaminitis, and visual changes (e.g., floaters and flashing lights).

48. C

The selection of chemotherapy for advanced NSCLC is based on performance status and medical comorbidities. In fit elderly patients, first-line platinum-based doublet chemotherapy is well tolerated and demonstrates efficacy. Single-agent docetaxel or erlotinib monotherapy are reasonable options for second-line therapy. The use of pemetrexed is restricted to nonsquamous histologies because of lower efficacy in squamous cell NSCLC.

49. C

In a study of early palliative care versus chemotherapy, Temel and colleagues demonstrated improved quality of life, decreased depressive symptoms, and improved survival despite less aggressive end-of-life care with early palliative care.

50. C

Single agent nivolumab is an anti-PD-1 immunotherapy that has demonstrated response rates of approximately 20% and an improvement in overall survival of 3 months in the second-line setting in patients with squamous NSCLC who progress after chemotherapy.

51. B

Crizotinib demonstrated a 73% response rate in a study of 50 patients treated with this agent with ROS-1 rearranged NSCLC and an improved progression-free survival of 19.2 months.

52. C

Alectinib is an ALK inhibitor licensed for the treatment of ALK-rearranged NSCLC after progression on crizotinib. A pooled analysis of two studies demonstrated a CNS response of 61% for this agent and CNS duration of response of 9.1 months. Therefore, alectinib would be the treatment of choice in this patient.

53. D

A phase II study of the combination of dabrafenib/trametinib in patients with stage IV BRAF V600E+ NSCLC demonstrated a response rate of 63%.

54. E

Panitumumab is an EGFR monoclonal antibody used in the treatment of colorectal cancer.

55. A

In patients with advanced NSCLC whose systemic disease remain unchanged with focal growth in an isolated number of lesions, local therapy to these lesions may be considered alongside continuation of the current systemic therapy. This approach is used for the subset of patients termed to have oligometastatic progression, which usually refers to progression in between 1 and 5 isolated lesions. In this case, the patient would be treated with SRS to the three new brain lesions, and systemic therapy would be continued.

56. E

Platinum doublet chemotherapy should be considered given the patient's performance status. A phase III study of elderly patients aged 70+ years who had locally advanced or metastatic NSCLC with an adequate performance status had an improved survival outcome with doublet compared with single-agent chemotherapy (10.3 vs. 6.2 months; $P < .0001$).

57. E

Either erlotinib (EURTAC study) or Afatinib (LUNG LUX 3 study) are suitable treatment options for this patient. The Phase III EURTAC study randomized patients with newly diagnosed advanced EGFR-mutant NSCLC (exon 19 deletion or L858R mutation in exon 21) to either erlotinib or platinum doublet chemotherapy, and a benefit in PFS was seen in the erlotinib arm (9.7 months vs. 5.2 months; $P < .0001$).

58. D

The patient has stage IV NSCLC due to the presence of the confirmed malignant pleural effusion. The patient should be treated with palliative chemotherapy since the histology is squamous in a patient with a significant smoking history, and the presence of an EGFR mutation is unlikely.

59. A

In patients with advanced lung cancer who have a driver mutation (i.e., EGFR, ALK, ROS1) and have an ECOG PS=3–4, one could consider administration of targeted therapy. However, for a patient with an ECOG PS of 3–4, chemotherapy is unlikely to be of benefit.

60. A

Several next-generation ALK-TKIs such as ceritinib and alectinib are treatment options in crizotinib-refractory settings and have demonstrated superior outcomes compared with chemotherapy in the second-line setting. Ceritinib demonstrated a 58% response rate and a 7-month progression free survival in the second-line setting after crizotinib failure in patients with stage IV ALK-rearranged NSCLC.

REFERENCES

Question 6

1. Arriagada R, Bergman B, Dunant A, et al. Cisplatin-based adjuvant chemotherapy in patients with completely resected non-small cell lung cancer. *N Engl J Med*. 2004;350:351–360.

Questions 1–20

1. *American Joint Council on Cancer Staging*. Lung Cancer Staging Guidelines. 7th ed. <https://www.nccn.org/professionals/physician_gls/pdf/nscl.pdf>; 2017 Accessed 17.04.17.
2. Zhang Y, Sun Y, Wang R, et al. Meta-analysis of lobectomy, segmentectomy, and wedge resection for stage I non-small cell lung cancer. *J Surg Oncol*. 2015;111(3):334–340.
3. Douillard JY, Rosell R, De Lena M, et al. Adjuvant vinorelbine plus cisplatin versus observation in patients with completely resected stage IB-IIIA non-small cell lung cancer (Adjuvant Navelbine International Trialist Association [ANITA]): a randomized controlled trial. *Lancet Oncol*. 2006;7:719–727.
4. Strauss G, Herndon J, Maddaus MA, et al. Adjuvant chemotherapy in stage IB non-small-cell lung cancer (NSCLC): update of Cancer and Leukemia Group B (CALGB) protocol 9633. *Proc Am Soc Clin Oncol*. 2006;24(abstr 7007):S365.
5. Winton T, Livingston R, Johnson D, et al. Vinorelbine plus cisplatin vs. observation in resected non-small cell lung cancer. *N Engl J Med*. 2005;352:2589–2597.
6. Arriagada, Bergman B, Dunant A, et al. Cisplatin-based adjuvant chemotherapy in patients with completely resected non-small cell lung cancer. *N Engl J Med*. 2004;350:351–360.
7. Hotta K, Matsuo K, Ueoka H, Kiura K, Tabata M, Tanimoto M. Role of adjuvant chemotherapy in patients with resected non-small cell lung cancer: reappraisal with a meta-analysis of randomized controlled trials. *J Clin Oncol*. 2004;22:3860–3867.
8. PORT Meta-analysis Trialists Group. Postoperative radiotherapy in non-small-cell lung cancer: systematic review and meta-analysis of individual patient data from nine randomized controlled trials. *Lancet*. 1998;352:257–263.
9. Furuya K, Murayama S, Soeda H, et al. New classification of small pulmonary nodules by margin characteristics on high-resolution CT. *Acta Radiol*. 1999;40(5):496–504.
10. Pignon JP, Tribodet H, Scagliotti GV, et al. Lung adjuvant cisplatin evaluation: a pooled analysis by the LACE Collaborative Group. *J Clin Oncol*. 2008;26(21):3552–3559.
11. Raz DJ, He B, Rosell R, Jablons DM. Bronchioloalveolar carcinoma: a review. *Clin Lung Cancer*. 2006;7(5):313–322.
12. Sun B, Brooks ED, Komaki RU, et al. 7-year follow-up after stereotactic ablative radiotherapy for patients with stage I non-small cell lung cancer: results of a phase 2 clinical trial. *Cancer*. 2017. [Epub ahead of print.].
13. British Columbia Cancer Agency Treatment Guidelines. <http://www.bccancer.bc.ca/drug-database/site/Drug%20Index/Pemetrexed_monograph_1July2011.pdf>; 2017 Accessed 17.04.17.
14. Shapiro M, Swanson SJ, Wright CD, et al. Predictors of major morbidity and mortality after pneumonectomy utilizing the Society for Thoracic Surgeons General Thoracic Surgery Database. *Ann Thorac Surg*. 2010;90(3):927–934.
15. Osann KE. Epidemiology of lung cancer. *Curr Opin Pulm Med*. 1999;4(4):198–204.

Questions 21–40

1. *National Cancer Control Network*. Non-small cell lung cancer guidelines. Version 5.2017. <https://www.nccn.org/professionals/physician_gls/pdf/nscl.pdf>; 2017 Accessed 17.04.17.
2. *American Joint Council on Cancer Staging*. Lung cancer staging guidelines. 7th ed. <https://cancerstaging.org/references-tools/deskreferences/Pages/default.aspx>; 2017 Accessed on 17.04.17.
3. Kelly K, Chansky K, Gaspar LE, et al. Phase III trial of maintenance gefitinib or placebo after concurrent chemoradiotherapy and docetaxel consolidation in inoperable stage III non-small-cell lung cancer: SWOG S0023. *J Clin Oncol*. 2008;26:2450–2456.
4. British Columbia Cancer Agency Treatment Guidelines. <http://www.bccancer.bc.ca/drug-database/site/Drug%20Index/Pemetrexed_monograph_1July2011.pdf>; 2017 Accessed 17.04.17.
5. Curran Jr WJ, Paulus R, Langer CJ, et al. Sequential vs. concurrent chemoradiation for stage III non-small cell lung cancer: randomized phase III trial RTOG 9410. *J Natl Cancer Inst*. 2011;103(19):1452–1460.
6. Foroulis CN, Zarogoulidis P, Darwiche K, et al. Superior sulcus (Pancoast) tumors: current evidence on diagnosis and radical treatment. *J Thorac Dis*. 2013;5(suppl 4):S342–S358.
7. Yang CH, Yu CJ, Shih JY, et al. Specific EGFR mutations predict treatment outcome of stage IIIB/IV patients with chemotherapy-naive non-small cell lung cancer receiving first-line gefitinib monotherapy. *J Clin Oncol*. 2008;26:2745–2758.
8. Inoue A, Suzuki T, Fukuhara T, et al. Prospective phase II study of gefitinib for chemotherapy-naive patients with advanced non-small cell lung cancer with epidermal growth factor receptor gene mutations. *J Clin Oncol*. 2006;24:3340–3346.
9. Fukuoka M, Wu Y, Thongprasert S, et al. Biomarker analyses from a phase III, randomized, open-label, first-line study of gefitinib (G) versus carboplatin/paclitaxel (C/P) in clinically selected patients (pts) with advanced non-small cell lung cancer (NSCLC) in Asia (IPASS). *J Clin Oncol*. 2009;27(abstr 8006):15s.
10. Kwak EL, Bang YJ, Camidge DR, et al. Anaplastic lymphoma kinase inhibition in non-small cell lung cancer. *N Engl J Med*. 2010;363:1693–1703.
11. Shaw AT, Yeap BY, Mino-Kenudson M, et al. Clinical features and outcome of patients with non-small cell lung cancer who harbor EML4-ALK. *J Clin Oncol*. 2009;27:4247–4253.
12. Camidge DR, Kono SA, Flacco A, et al. Optimizing the detection of lung cancer patients harboring anaplastic lymphoma kinase (ALK) gene rearrangements potentially suitable for ALK inhibitor treatment. *Clin Cancer Res*. 2010;16:5581–5590.
13. Ulivi P, Zoli W, Capelli L, Calistri D, Amadori D, Chiadini E. Target therapy in NSCLC patients: relevant clinical agents and tumour molecular characterisation. *Mol Clin Oncol*. 2013;1(4):575–581.

14. Bertino EM, Confer PD, Colonna JE, Ross P, Otterson GA. Pulmonary neuroendocrine/carcinoid tumors: a review article. *Cancer*. 2009;115(19):4434–4441.
15. Bergethon K, Shaw AT, Ou SH, et al. ROS1 rearrangements de ne a unique molecular class of lung cancers. *J Clin Oncol*. 2012;30:863–870.
16. Naidoo J, Drilon A. Molecular diagnostic testing in non-small cell lung cancer. *Am J Hematol Oncol*. 2014;10:4–11.
17. Sandler A, Gray R, Perry MC, et al. Paclitaxel-carboplatin alone or with bevacizumab for non-small-cell lung cancer. *N Engl J Med*. 2006;355(24). 2542–2450.
18. Garon EB, Ciuleanu TE, Arrieta O, et al. Ramucirumab plus docetaxel versus placebo plus docetaxel for second-line treatment of stage IV non-small-cell lung cancer after disease progression on platinum-based therapy (REVEL): a multicentre, double-blind, randomised phase 3 trial. *Lancet*. 2014;384(9944):665–673.

Questions 41–60

1. Johnson DH, Fehrenbacher L, Novotny WF, et al. Randomized phase II trial comparing bevacizumab plus carboplatin and paclitaxel with carboplatin and paclitaxel alone in previouslyuntreated locally advanced or metastatic non-small-cell lung cancer. *J Clin Oncol*. 2004;22(11):2184–2191.
2. Sandomenico C, Costanzo R, Carillio G, et al. Bevacizumab in non small cell lung cancer: development, current status and issues. *Curr Med Chem*. 2012;19(7):961–971.
3. Rosell R, Carcereny E, Gervais R, et al. Erlotinib versus standard chemotherapy as first-line treatment for European patients with advanced EGFR mutation-positive non-small-cell lung cancer (EURTAC): a multicentre, open-label, randomised phase 3 trial. *Lancet Oncol*. 2012;13(3):239–246.
4. Kuiper JL, Heideman DA, Thunnissen E, et al. Incidence of T790M mutation in (sequential) rebiopsies in EGFR-mutated NSCLC-patients. *Lung Cancer*. 2014;85(1):19–24.
5. Campo M, Gerber D, Gainor JF, et al. Acquired resistance to first-line afatinib and the challenges of prearranged progression biopsies. *J Thorac Oncol*. 2016;11(11):2022–2026.
6. *National Cancer Control Network*. Non-small cell lung cancer guidelines. Version 7.2017. <https://www.nccn.org/professionals/physician_gls/pdf/nscl.pdf>; 2017 Accessed 17.04.17.
7. Oser MG, Niederst MJ, Sequist L, et al. Transformation from non-small-cell lung cancer to small-cell lung cancer: molecular drivers and cells of origin. *Lancet Oncol*. 2015;16(4): e165–e172.
8. Kwak EL, Bang YJ, Camidge DR, et al. Anaplastic lymphoma kinase inhibition in non-small cell lung cancer. *N Engl J Med*. 2010;363:1693–1703.
9. Shaw AT, Yeap BY, Mino-Kenudson M, et al. Clinical features and outcome of patients with non-small-cell lung cancer who harbor EML4-ALK. *J Clin Oncol*. 2009;27:4247–4253.
10. Quoix E, Zalcman G, Oster JP, et al. Carboplatin and weekly paclitaxel doublet chemotherapy compared with monotherapy in elderly patients with advanced non-small cell lung cancer: IFCT-0501 randomized, phase 3 trial. *Lancet*. 2011;378: 1079–1088.
11. Scagliotti GV, Parikh P, von Pawel J, et al. Phase III study comparing cisplatin plus gemcitabine with cisplatin plus pemetrexed in chemotherapy-naive patients with advanced-stage non-small cell lung cancer. *J Clin Oncol*. 2008;26:3543–3551.
12. Temel JS, Greer JA, Muzikansky A, et al. Early palliative care for patients with metastatic non–small-cell lung cancer. *New Engl J Med*. 2010;363:733–742.
13. Brahmer J, Paz-Ares L, Horn L, et al. Nivolumab versus docetaxel in advanced squamous-cell non-small-cell lung cancer. *N Engl J Med*. 2015;373(2):123–135.
14. Shaw AT, Ou SH, Bang YJ, et al. Crizotinib in ROS1-rearranged non-small-cell lung cancer. *N Engl J Med*. 2014;371:1963–1971.
15. Gadgeel SM, Shaw AT, Govindan R, et al. Pooled analysis of CNS response to alectinib in two studies of pretreated patients with ALK-positive non-small-cell lung cancer. *J Clin Oncol*. 2016;34(34):4079–4085.
16. Planchard D, Kim TM, Mazieres J, et al. Dabrafenib plus trametinib in patients with previously treated BRAF(V600E)-mutant metastatic non-small cell lung cancer: an open-label, multicentre phase 2 trial. *Lancet Oncol*. 2016;17(7):984–993.
17. Rosell R, Carcereny E, Gervais R, et al. Erlotinib versus standard chemotherapy as first-line treatment for European patients with advanced EGFR mutation-positive non-small-cell lung cancer (EURTAC): a multicentre, open-label, randomised phase 3 trial. *Lancet Oncol*. 2012;13(3):239–246.
18. Herbst RS, Ansari R, Bustin F, et al. Efficacy of bevacizumab plus erlotinib versus erlotinib alone in advanced non-small-cell lung cancer after failure of standard first-line chemotherapy (BeTa): a double-blind, placebo-controlled, phase 3 trial. *Lancet*. 2011;377(9780):1846–1854.
19. Shaw AT, Ou SH, Bang YJ, et al. Ceritinib in ALK-rearranged non-small-cell lung cancer. *N Engl J Med*. 2014;370(13): 1189–1197.

Small Cell Lung Cancer

QUESTIONS

1. A 49-year-old male has finished 6 cycles of carboplatin plus etoposide for extensive stage small cell lung cancer. A restaging PET-CT scan shows that the index liver lesion has decreased from 6 to 2 cm. The other bilateral lung lesions (at baseline all between 3 and 4 cm) are completely gone. His brain at baseline is negative.
   What treatment would you now offer?
   A. Referral to radiation oncology for prophylactic cranial irradiation
   B. Referral to surgery for resection of the solitary liver lesion
   C. Two additional cycles of carboplatin plus etoposide
   D. CyberKnife to the liver lesion
   E. Consolidation chemotherapy with topotecan

2. A 63-year-old male presented shortness of breath. A CT scan revealed with a 6-cm R hilar mass, enlarged subcarinal lymphadenopathy causing mild compression of his bilateral mainstem bronchi, liver lesions, and lytic bone lesions. EBUS of his station 7 and 4R lymph nodes reveal small cell lung carcinoma. His staging brain MRI reveals four-subcentimeter intracranial masses without edema or mass effect. He does not have neurological symptoms.
   What do you recommend?
   A. Referral to radiation oncology to initiate WB radiotherapy urgently
   B. Initiate treatment with carboplatin/etoposide
   C. Referral to radiation oncology for CyberKnife radiotherapy to the four lesions
   D. Concurrent WB radiotherapy and carboplatin plus etoposide
   E. Initiate treatment with topotecan

3. A 55-year-old female presented to the ED with shortness of breath. A CT scan revealed with a 6-cm R hilar mass, enlarged subcarinal lymphadenopathy causing mild compression of the bilateral mainstem bronchi, liver lesions, and lytic bone lesions. EBUS of station 7 and 4R lymph nodes reveal

small cell lung carcinoma. Her staging brain MRI is negative for intracranial metastases. She initiates therapy with cisplatin plus etoposide, and after 6 cycles her restaging studies show an overall partial response to therapy. Her R hilar mass is now 2 cm, and her liver lesions have resolved. Her follow-up brain MRI is negative. Her ECOG PS is 1.
What do you recommend?
A. Two additional cycles of cisplatin plus etoposide
B. Maintenance nivolumab
C. Maintenance topotecan
D. Observation
E. Referral to radiation oncology to discuss PCI and thoracic radiotherapy

4. A 62-year-old female is staged with T2N2M0 SCLC based on brochoscopic biopsy, PET-CT scan and brain MRI. You are ready to start her on chemotherapy with cisplatin plus etoposide. She has also met with radiation oncology and has completed pulmonary function tests and simulation. She will receive radiation and part of her therapy.
Of the following choices, when would be the best time to start radiation therapy?
A. Radiation therapy first, then start chemotherapy after her radiotherapy is completed
B. Begin concurrent radiotherapy early, ideally with cycle 1 or 2 of chemotherapy
C. Start radiotherapy immediately after she's completed 4 cycles of chemotherapy
D. Wait four weeks after she completed 4 cycles of chemotherapy, then start radiotherapy
E. Add radiation only if she has persistent disease after 4 cycles of chemotherapy

5. A 65-year-old female smoker, presents with chest pain. As part of her evaluation she has a CXR with shows left hilar fullness. A CT confirms a 4 cm LUL mass, and left hilar lymph nodes measuring 2.4 cm. A staging PET-CT reveals FDG-activity in a 4 cm LUL mass and FDG-activity of a left hilar lymph node. There is no evidence of disease in the abdomen or pelvis. Her brain MRI reveals no intracranial lesions. Her EBUS confirms SCLC of the LUL and 10L LN. FNA of the subcarinal and right hilar lymph nodes show benign lymphoid tissue only. Her stage is T2aN1M0 (Limited stage) SCLC. Her comprehensive metabolic panel is within normal limits. Her CBC is notable for mild anemia with a HCT of 31.5. Her CrCl is > 60, she denies neuropathy or hearing loss. Her ECOG PS is 1.
What treatment do you recommend at this time?
A. Left upper lobectomy with thoracic lymphadenectomy followed by adjuvant carboplatin plus etoposide
B. Cisplatin plus etoposide with concurrent daily radiation starting at cycle 1 or 2
C. Cisplatin plus etoposide x 4 cycles followed by radiation after chemotherapy is completed.
D. Carboplatin plus etoposide with concurrent daily radiation starting at cycle 1 or 2
E. Cisplatin plus etoposide followed by thoracic radiotherapy

6. A 56 year old male, smoker sustained a fall at work and is found to have an opacity on CXR. A CT confirms a 2 cm RLL mass. A staging PET/CT reveals FDG-activity in a 2 cm RLL, without FDG-activity elsewhere. He undergoes EBUS with sampling of 10R, 7 and 10L, all sites show benign lymphoid tissue only. He is taken to the OR and frozen path shows small cell carcinoma. He is then treated with completion lobectomy and thoracic lymphadenectomy. His final pathologic staging is T1a N0Mx small cell lung carcinoma, margin negative.

He recovers well post-operatively and you are seeing him in clinic for the first time. What do you recommend at this time?
A. Surveillance, he's had a completion lobectomy for a stage I SCLC
B. Adjuvant radiation, you will refer him to radiation oncology
C. Adjuvant chemotherapy with cisplatin plus etoposide
D. Concurrent chemoradiation with cisplatin plus etoposide
E. Maintenance topotecan

7. A 50-year-old female smoker was found to have an opacity on CXR. A CT confirms a 2 cm RLL mass. A staging PET/CT reveals FDG-activity in a 2.2 cm RLL, without FDG-activity elsewhere. She undergoes EBUS with sampling of 10R, 7 and 10L, all sites show benign lymphoid tissue only. She is taken to the OR and frozen path shows small cell carcinoma. She then undergoes a completion lobectomy and thoracic lymphadenectomy. Her final pathology shows a 2.3 cm RLL SCLC and with metastases to the right hilar lymph nodes. All other lymph nodes are negative. She recovers well post-operatively and you are seeing her in clinic for the first time. What do you recommend at this time?
A. Surveillance, she had a completion lobectomy for a stage IIA SCLC
B. Adjuvant radiation only. You will refer her to radiation oncology
C. Adjuvant chemotherapy only with cisplatin plus etoposide
D. Concurrent chemoradiotherapy for lymph node positive disease.
E. Maintenance topotecan

8. A 76-year-old male smoker with a history of diabetes and chronic renal insufficiency is found to have a 2 cm RLL mass on screening chest CT. A staging PET/CT reveals FDG-activity in a 2.2 cm RLL mass, without FDG-activity elsewhere. He undergoes EBUS with sampling of 10R, 7 and 10L, all sites show benign lymphoid tissue only. He is taken to the OR and frozen path shows small cell carcinoma. He is then treated with completion lobectomy and thoracic lymphadenectomy. His final pathologic staging is T1N0Mx small cell lung carcinoma, margin negative.
He recovers well post-operatively and you are seeing him in clinic for the first time. His symptoms are notable for G1 peripheral neuropathy, hearing loss, and his calculated creatinine clearance is 40. Otherwise his ECOG PS is 1 and he would like to be aggressive with his care. What do you recommend at this time?
A. Surveillance, he's had a completion lobectomy for a stage 1 SCLC
B. Adjuvant radiation, you will refer him to radiation oncology
C. Adjuvant chemotherapy with cisplatin plus etoposide
D. Adjuvant chemotherapy with carboplatin plus etoposide.
E. Maintenance topotecan

9. A 72-year-old female smoker presents a cough and has a CXR which shows a large RUL mass. A follow-up CT chest reveals a 5.6cm RUL mass, bilateral hilar and mediastinal lymph node enlargement. Liver masses are also identified on her her chest CT. A PET/CT reveals widespread FDG-avid lesions including her RUL mass, thoracic lymph nodes, multiple liver metastases and bone lesions. She undergoes biopsy of a liver lesion which reveals mixed small cell lung carcinoma and lung adenocarcinoma. Her brain MRI is negative.

At baseline, she has hearing aides for minor hearing loss and Grade 1 neuropathy from her Type 2 diabetes. The latter is well controlled on Glucophage. She is quite symptomatic from her cancer and wants to start therapy. Which therapy do you offer her?

A. Carboplatin plus pemetrexed
B. Carboplatin, pemetrexed plus pembrolizumab
C. Cisplatin plus docetaxel
D. Nivoumab plus ipilimumab
E. Carboplatin plus Etoposide

10. A 67-year-old female smoker presents to the ED with mild confusion and right arm weakness. A head CT shows a left parietal mass with edema. A MRI with gadolinium reveals, in addition to a 2 cm left parietal mass, multiple bilateral subcentimeter intracranial lesions. She is started on steroids with improvement in her neurologic symptoms. She has a CT CAP which reveals a 3cm RUL mass, right hilar lymph node involement, liver lesions. She undergoes biopsy of a liver lesion which reveals small cell lung carinoma. Her labs are WNL. On consultation she does not currently have symptoms related to her intrathracic or hepatic disease. What do you recommend at this time?

A. Initiate treatment with temozolomide
B. Initiate systemic therapy with nivolumab plus ipilimumab
C. Referral to neurosurgery to resect her 2 cm left parietal mass
D. Referral to radiation oncology to initiate whole brain radiation. Start systemic chemotherapy after completion of whole brain
E. Initiate systemic therapy with carboplatin plus etoposide

ANSWERS

1. A

He has had a good response to chemotherapy for his extensive stage small cell lung cancer. A randomized study evaluated PCI in patients with extensive stage small cell lung cancer who had a response to chemotherapy.

Patients who received PCI had a lower risk of symptomatic brain metastases (HR = 0.27; $P < .001$). While OS was not a primary endpoint, the 1-year OS rate was 27.1% versus 13.3% in favor of the PCI group.

2. D

He is asymptomatic from his intracranial metastases but has respiratory symptoms due to his large mediastinal mass. SCLC is very responsive to systemic chemotherapy. Concurrent whole brain radiotherapy and chemotherapy is generally not recommended due to significant combined toxicities. In this scenario, it would be reasonable to initiate chemotherapy urgently and follow closely for the development of neurologic symptoms.

3. E

A randomized study evaluated PCI in patients with extensive stage small cell lung cancer who had a response to chemotherapy. Patients who received PCI had a lower risk of symptomatic brain metastases (HR = 0.27; $P < .001$). While OS was not a primary endpoint, the 1-year OS rate was 27.1% versus 13.3% in favor of the PCI group, and PCI dosing is lower than WB RT. The radiation oncologist should also discuss thoracic radiotherapy. A randomized study evaluated the benefit of consolidation thoracic radiotherapy in ES SCLC patients who had a response to chemotherapy and showed an improvement in 2-year OS and 6-month progression free-survival.

4. B

She has limited stage SCLC. The recommended therapy is concurrent chemoradiotherapy. Concurrent chemotherapy is superior to sequential chemotherapy followed by radiation. Data has shown that the early implementation of radiation for limited stage small cell lung cancer is associated with better survival. A decreased time between the first day of chemotherapy and the last day of chest radiotherapy is associated with improved survival in limited stage disease.

5. B

She has limited stage SCLC with N1 involvement (Stage IIA). Recommended therapy is concurrent chemoradiotherapy. In select patients with T1N0 (stage 1) disease, surgical resection followed by chemotherapy is a reasonable option, however, cannot be recommended with N1 involvement. Concurrent chemotherapy is superior to sequential chemotherapy followed by radiation. Cisplatin is preferred over carboplatin in patients treated with curative intent

6. C

He has Stage I SCLC with T1a primary tumor. For all patients with small cell lung cancer, regardless of stage, platinum-based chemotherapy is recommended. In the curative setting cisplatin is preferred. The recommendation is for 4 cycles of adjuvant cisplatin plus etoposide.

7. D

She has stage IIA SCLC with a final pathology of T1bN1. For all patients with small cell lung cancer, regardless of stage, platinum-based chemotherapy is recommended. Because she has hilar lymph node involvement, she is recommended to receive concurrent radiotherapy. In the curative setting cisplatin is preferred. The recommendation is for 4 cycles of adjuvant cisplatin plus etoposide.

8. D

This patient has had surgical resection with a lobectomy and mediastinal lymph node dissection for a Stage I SCLC with T1a primary tumor. For all patients with small cell lung cancer, regardless of stage, platinum-based chemotherapy is recommended. In the curative setting cisplatin is preferred. The recommendation is for 4 cycles of adjuvant cisplatin plus etoposide. In the absence of margin positive resection or lymph node involvement, there is no known role for radiation.

9. E

This patient has extensive stage mixed small cell lung cancer with her biopsy showing components of small cell lung cancer and adenocarcinoma. Approximately 10% of all SCLC cases contain mixed history, most commonly with lung squamous cell or adenocarcinoma. The recommended therapy for patients with mixed small cell lung is identically to those with pure SCLC: a platinum agent plus etoposide.

10. D

This patient has extensive stage small cell lung cancer and presented with symptomatic brain metastases. Small cell lung cancer is exquisitely sensitive to radiotherapy and chemotherapy. She does not have clear symptoms related to her systemic disease. The recommendation is to start with whole brain radiotherapy then initiate chemotherapy with platinum plus etoposide after completion of radiotherapy. If she had symptoms attributable to her systemic disease, and had a good ECOG PS, then one could consider concurrent WBRT plus chemotherapy with platinum plus etoposide

REFERENCES

Question 1

1. Slotman B, Faivre-Finn C, Kramer G, et al. Prophylactic cranial irradiation in extensive small-cell lung cancer. *N Engl J Med.* 2007;357(7):664–672.

Question 3

1. Slotman B, van Tinteren H, Praag JO, et al. Use of thoracic radiotherapy for extensive stage small-cell lung cancer: a phase 3 randomised controlled trial. *Lancet.* 2015;385:36–42.

2. Slotman B, Faivre-Finn C, Kramer G, et al. Prophylactic cranial irradiation in extensive small-cell lung cancer. *N Engl J Med.* 2007;357(7):664–672.

Question 4

1. De Ruysscher D., et al. Time between the first day of chemotherapy and the last day of chest radiation is the most important predictor of survival in limited-disease small-cell lung cancer. J Clin Oncol. 2006;24(7):1057–1063.

Question 5

1. NCCN SCLC guidelines.

Question 7

1. SCLC NCCN 2017 guidelines.

Question 9

1. NCCN SCLC 2017 guidelines.

Question 10

1. NCCN SCLC 2017 guidelines.

Mesothelioma

QUESTIONS

1. Which chemotherapy demonstrated a survival advantage in malignant pleural mesothelioma compared with cisplatin alone?
   A. Pemetrexed plus cisplatin
   B. Gemcitabine plus cisplatin
   C. Paclitaxel plus cisplatin
   D. Vinorelbine plus cisplatin

2. Which surgery is preferred for stage 2 pleural mesothelioma?
   A. Extrapleural pneumonectomy
   B. Pleurectomy
   C. Either surgery
   D. Surgery is not indicated for stage 2 pleural mesothelioma.

3. Which chemotherapy is the standard first-line treatment for mesothelioma?
   A. Vinorelbine and cisplatin
   B. Gemcitabine and cisplatin
   C. Pemetrexed and cisplatin
   D. None of the above
   E. All of the above are standard options.

4. Which exposure is mesothelioma associated with?
   A. Second-hand smoke exposure
   B. Silica exposure
   C. Human papillomavirus
   D. Asbestos exposure.

5. Which viral infection has been possibly associated with mesothelioma?
   A. Human papillomavirus
   B. SV 40
   C. Herpes virus
   D. Flu virus

6. Which factor is associated with poor prognosis in patients diagnosed with malignant pleural mesothelioma?
   A. Normal LDH
   B. Elevated platelet count
   C. Female gender
   D. Localized disease

7. Diagnosis of malignant mesothelioma is best and most reliably made on which type of test?

A. Cytology specimen from pleural fluid
B. Circulating tumor cells in the blood
C. Fine needle aspirate of the pleural disease
D. Surgical biopsy

8. Which chemotherapy is approved for use for second-line chemotherapy for malignant mesothelioma?
   A. Nalvelbine
   B. Gemcitabine
   C. Pemetrexed
   D. No chemotherapy is approved for use by the FDA.

9. What pattern of immunohistochemical staining is most commonly seen in malignant pleural mesothelioma biopsies?
   A. Calretinin, WT-1, and cytokeratin positive and CEA negative
   B. WT-1 and cytokeratin positive and calretinin and CEA negative
   C. Cytokeratin and CEA positive and calretinin and WT-1 negative
   D. All of the stains are negative.

10. A 71-year-old man presents with a tumor that involves the ipsilateral pleural surfaces and the ipsilateral lung parenchyma on scan. No adenopathy is seen on computed tomography (CT) or positron emission tomography (PET). What stage is the mesothelioma?
    A. Stage 1
    B. Stage 2
    C. Stage 3
    D. Stage 4

11. During the surgical evaluation for a patient with pleural mesothelioma, which of the following is NOT a routinely recommended test?
    A. PFTs including DLCO
    B. Cardiac stress test
    C. Perfusion scanning
    D. Mediastinoscopy or EBUS FNA of mediastinal lymph nodes

12. A 56-year-old woman presents with shortness of breath and is found to have a left pleural effusion and pleural thickening on CT scan. On CT, she does not have any evidence of mediastinal adenopathy. Biopsy is positive for epithelioid mesothelioma. She is staged as T2N0M0 after the staging workup has been completed. What is the recommended treatment?
    A. Combination chemotherapy only
    B. Single agent chemotherapy if deemed not a surgical candidate
    C. Radiation to the chest for palliation
    D. Pleurectomy/decortication

13. A 74-year-old man presents with shortness of breath and right-sided chest wall pain. Evaluation reveals large chest wall mass that is eroding into the ribs, pleural thickening, and mediastinal adenopathy. Biopsy reveals epithelioid mesothelioma. Staging of the mesothelioma reveals T4, N2, M0 tumor. What therapy do you recommend?
A. Pleurectomy
B. Extrapleural pneumonectomy
C. Pemetrexed and cisplatin
D. Gemcitabine and carboplatin

14. A 74-year-old man presents with shortness of breath and right-sided chest wall pain. Evaluation reveals large chest wall mass that is eroding into the ribs, pleural thickening, and mediastinal adenopathy. Biopsy reveals epithelioid mesothelioma. Staging of the mesothelioma reveals T4, N2, M0 tumor. Labs reveal platelet count of 550K, elevated white blood cell count, Cr of 2.0 with an estimated CrCl of 30, and normal liver function tests. What therapy do you recommend?
A. Pleurectomy
B. Vinorelbine and cisplatin
C. Pemetrexed and cisplatin
D. Gemcitabine and carboplatin

15. A 66-year-old man presents with shortness of breath and right-sided chest wall pain. Evaluation reveals large chest wall mass that is eroding into the ribs, pleural thickening, and mediastinal adenopathy. Biopsy reveals epithelioid mesothelioma. Staging of the mesothelioma reveals T4, N2, M0 tumor. He was treated with pemetrexed and cisplatin for 6 cycles, and his disease is now progressing. What FDA-approved therapy do you recommend?
A. Gemcitabine
B. Vinorelbine
C. Sunitinib
D. There is no FDA approved therapy.

16. Which histological subtype of mesothelioma has a better outcome or prognosis?
A. Epithelioid
B. Sarcomatoid
C. Biphasic
D. They all have poor outcomes.

17. What screening tests for malignant pleural mesothelioma have been shown to decrease the mortality due to the disease?
A. Low-dose CT
B. Serum osteopontin
C. Chest x-rays
D. No screening tests have shown a decrease in mortality.

18. What is the biggest risk factor for developing mesothelioma?
A. Smoking
B. Radiation exposure
C. Asbestos exposure
D. Radon exposure

19. What is the median overall survival in a patient diagnosed with malignant pleural mesothelioma?
A. 6 weeks
B. 6 months
C. 12 weeks
D. 12 months

20. In which situation does radiation NOT play a role in treatment of malignant pleural mesothelioma?
A. Definitive treatment of stage 1 mesothelioma
B. Palliative treatment for chest wall pain
C. Adjuvant radiation after extrapleural pneumonectomy
D. Radiation to the site of a pleural procedure to prevent tract recurrence

---

ANSWERS

1. A
In this trial, patients with unresectable malignant pleural mesothelioma were randomized to either pemetrexed and cisplatin or cisplatin alone. Pemetrexed and cisplatin resulted in a significant 3-month survival advantage.

2. B
Dr. Flores et al. compared extrapleural pneumonectomy (EPP) with pleurectomy and found that patients who underwent pleurectomy had a better survival than those who underwent extrapleural pneumonectomy. They did not find any statistical difference in survival between pleurectomy versus EPP by stage. Pleurectomy is now the commonly recommended surgery for mesothelioma.

3. C
Pemetrexed and cisplatin is the FDA-approved regimen for pleural mesothelioma based on the phase 3 study published by Dr. Vogelzang et al. comparing cisplatin as a single agent versus pemetrexed and cisplatin.

4. D
Mesothelioma has been associated with asbestos exposure based on data from the 1960s. Malignant mesothelioma of the pleura, peritoneum, and tunica vaginalis are recognized as being associated with asbestos exposure.

5. B
Dr. Carbone et al. reported finding evidence of Simian virus 40 infection in mesothelioma specimens. A clear association of causality has yet to be proven.

6. B
Elevated platelet count is associated with poor prognosis in addition to elevated LDH, male gender, and metastatic disease.

7. D
A surgical biopsy more reliably gives a diagnosis and confirmation of subtype of mesothelioma compared with the other methodologies. Unfortunately, pleural fluid cytology can be negative or indeterminate. Fine needle aspirates do not consistently yield enough tissue to determine histological subtype.

8. D
No phase 3 study has been performed to show that single-agent chemotherapy improves survival over placebo or best supportive care in the second-line treatment setting.

9. A

Calretinin, WT-1, and cytokeratin stains typically are positive, while CEA is typically negative. The important goal of immunohistochemical staining is to be able to distinguish mesothelioma from adenocarcinoma. Electromicroscopy, however, is the gold standard for diagnosis, although it is not typically needed.

10. B

Based on International Mesothelioma Interest Group Staging of Mesothelioma, this tumor is T2N0M0, that is, stage 2 disease.

11. C

Per the NCCN guidelines, the following is recommended for surgical evaluation in patients with clinical stage 1–3 epithelial or mixed histology mesothelioma: PFTs including DLCO, PET-CT, mediastinoscopy, or EBUS FNA of mediastinal lymph nodes and cardiac-stress test. Perfusion scanning is only recommended if the FEV1 is less than 80% predicted on PFTs.

12. D

Stage 2 mesothelioma is typically amenable to surgical resection either by extrapleural pneumonectomy or by pleurectomy. Chemotherapy without surgical resection is only recommended if the patient is not a surgical candidate or if the patient refuses chemotherapy.

13. C

Standard chemotherapy for unresectable mesothelioma is pemetrexed and cisplatin. Surgery would not play a role in this treatment as the cancer is unresectable.

14. D

Standard chemotherapy for unresectable mesothelioma when creatinine clearance is less than 45, is not pemetrexed, and is cisplatin. Pemetrexed is renally cleared and is not recommended if creatinine clearance is less than 45. Instead, gemcitabine and carboplatin would be reasonable choices. Cisplatin is also not recommended if the creatinine is elevated, as it can lead to worsening renal dysfunction.

15. D

There is no FDA-approved second-line treatment for pleural mesothelioma. There are small clinical trials that have demonstrated minimal activity of gemcitabine and vinorelbine. However, there are no phase 3 studies demonstrating a survival advantage compared with the best supportive care.

16. A

Epithelioid histology has better outcomes than those with either sarcomatoid or mixed (biphasic) histology.

17. D

No screening tests have demonstrated a decrease in mortality.

18. C

Asbestos exposure is the most common risk factor for the development of malignant mesothelioma. Radon and smoke exposure is not associated with the development of malignant mesothelioma. Radiation exposure has been associated with the development of mesothelioma, but it is not as common as asbestos exposure.

19. D

With treatment, the median overall survival is approximately 1 year. Unfortunately, this disease is typically not curable.

20. A

Radiation is not a definitive treatment for mesothelioma. Radiation can be used for palliation for pain or other symptoms. Radiation has also been shown to decrease the risk of local recurrence after extrapleural pneumonectomy or at the site of pleural procedure.

REFERENCES

Question 1

1. Vogelzang NJ, Rusthoven JJ, Symanowski J, et al. Phase III study of pemetrexed in combination with cisplatin versus cisplatin alone in patients with malignant pleural mesothelioma. *J Clin Oncol.* 2003;21:2636–2644.

Question 2

1. Flores RM, Pass HI, Seshan VE, et al. Extrapleural pneumonectomy versus pleurectomy/decortication in the surgical management of malignant pleural mesothelioma: results in 663 patients. *J Thorac Cardiovasc Surg.* 2008;135(3):620–626. 626.e1–626.e3.

Question 3

1. Vogelzang NJ, Rusthoven JJ, Symanowski J, et al. Phase III study of pemetrexed in combination with cisplatin versus cisplatin alone in patients with malignant pleural mesothelioma. *J Clin Oncol.* 2003;21:2636–2644.

Question 4

1. Selikoff IJ, Churg J, Hammond EC. Asbestos exposure and neoplasia. *JAMA.* 1964;188:142.

Question 5

1. Carbone M, Pass, Rizzo P, et al. Simian virus 40-like DNA sequences in human pleural mesothelioma. *Oncogene.* 1994;9:1781–1790.

Question 6

1. Herndon JE, Green MR, Chahinian AP, Corson JM, Suzuki Y, Vogelzang NJ. Factors predictive of survival among 337 patients with mesothelioma treated between 1984 and 1994 by the Cancer and Leukemia Group B. *Chest.* 1998;113:723–731.

Question 7

1. Boutinj C, Rey F. Thoracoscopy in pleural malignant mesothelioma: a prospective study of 188 consecutive patients. Patr1: diagnosis. *Cancer.* 1993;72:389–393.

Question 8

1. NCCN guidelines Version 3.2016 Malignant Pleural Mesothelioma, NCCN.org website.
2. Abdel-Rahman O, Kelany M. Systemic therapy options for malignant pleural mesothelioma beyond first-line therapy: a systemic review. *Expert Rev Respir Med.* 2015;9:533–549.
3. Zauderer MG, Kass SL, Woo K, Sima CS, Ginsberg MS, Krug LM. Vinorelbine and gemcitabine as second- or third-line therapy for malignant pleural mesothelioma. *Lung Cancer.* 2014;84:271–274.

Question 9

1. Robinson BW, Lake RA. Advances in malignant mesothelioma. *N Engl J Med.* 2005;353:1591–1603.
2. Ordonez NG, Mackey B. Electron microscopy in tumor diagnosis: indications for its use in the immunohistochemical era. *Hum Pathol.* 1998;29:1403–1411.

Question 10

1. Rusch VW. A proposed new international TNM staging system for malignant pleural mesothelioma. From the international mesothelioma interest group. *Chest*. 1995;108:1122–1128.

Question 11

1. NCCN guidelines Version 3.2016 Malignant Pleural Mesothelioma, NCCN.org website.

Question 12

1. NCCN guidelines Version 3.2016 Malignant Pleural Mesothelioma, NCCN.org website.

Question 13

1. NCCN guidelines Version 3.2016 Malignant Pleural Mesothelioma, NCCN.org website.
2. Vogelzang NJ, Rusthoven JJ, Symanowski J, et al. Phase III study of pemetrexed in combination with cisplatin versus cisplatin alone in patients with malignant pleural mesothelioma. *J Clin Oncol*. 2003;21:2636–2644.

Question 14

1. Vogelzang NJ, Rusthoven JJ, Symanowski J, et al. Phase III study of pemetrexed in combination with cisplatin versus cisplatin alone in patients with malignant pleural mesothelioma. *J Clin Oncol*. 2003;21:2636–2644.
2. NCCN guidelines Version 3.2016 Malignant Pleural Mesothelioma, NCCN.org website.

Question 15

1. NCCN guidelines Version 3.2016 Malignant Pleural Mesothelioma, NCCN.org website.
2. Abdel-Rahman O, Kelany M. Systemic therapy options for malignant pleural mesothelioma beyond first-line therapy: a systemic review. *Expert Rev Respir Med*. 2015;9:533–549.
3. Zauderer MG, Kass SL, Woo K, et al. Vinorelbine and gemcitabine as second- or third-line therapy for malignant pleural mesothelioma. *Lung Cancer*. 2014;84:271–274.

Question 16

1. NCCN guidelines Version 3.2016 Malignant Pleural Mesothelioma, NCCN.org website
2. Galateau-Salle F, Churg A, Roggli V, et al. The 2015 World Health Organization Classification of Tumors of the Pleura: advances since the 2004 Classification. *J Thorac Oncol*. 2016;11:142–154.

Question 17

1. Scherpereel A, Astoul P, Baas P, et al. Guidelines of the European Respiratory Society and the European Society of Thoracic Surgeons for the management of malignant pleural mesothelioma. *Eur Respir J*. 2010;35:479–495.
2. Roberts HC, Patsois DA, Paul NS, et al. Screening for malignant pleural mesothelioma and lung cancer in individuals with a history of asbestos exposure. *J Thorac Oncol*. 2009;4:620–628.
3. Pass HI, Carbone M. Current status of screening for malignant pleural mesothelioma. *Semin Thorac Cardiovasc Surg*. 2009;21:97–104.

Question 18

1. Selikoff IJ, Churg J, Hammond EC. Asbestos exposure and neoplasia. *JAMA*. 1964;188:142.

Question 19

1. NCCN guidelines Version 3.2016 Malignant Pleural Mesothelioma, NCCN.org website.
2. Vogelzang NJ, Rusthoven JJ, Symanowski J, et al. Phase III study of pemetrexed in combination with cisplatin versus cisplatin alone in patients with malignant pleural mesothelioma. *J Clin Oncol*. 2003;21:2636–2644.

Question 20

1. NCCN guidelines Version 3.2016 Malignant Pleural Mesothelioma, NCCN.org website.
2. Rusch VW, Rosenzweig K, Venkatraman E, et al. A phase II trial of surgical resection and adjuvant high-dose hemithoracic radiation for malignant pleural mesothelioma. *J Thorac Cardiovasc Surg*. 2001;122:788–795.

Thymoma and Thymic Cancer

QUESTIONS

1. A 42-year-old G2P2 woman with past medical history of endometriosis presents with diffuse chest pressure and dyspnea for the past 2 months. She is treated with a course of bronchodilators, which leads to modest improvement in symptoms. She is then treated with a 5-day course of azithromycin. After an abnormal chest x-ray, she has a CT scan of the chest that demonstrates an anterior mediastinal mass measuring 6 cm × 3 cm. There are no pulmonary nodules or pleural lesions. Core needle biopsy of the anterior mediastinal mass reveals thymoma (WHO type AB). Routine complete blood count shows the following:

Leukocyte count	5000/μL
Hemoglobin	12.2 g/dL
Platelet count	412,000/μL

In addition to chest pressure and dyspnea with exertion, the patient also notes intermittent diplopia worse in the evening. Physical exam at this time is unremarkable. What is the diagnostic test most likely to determine the etiology of the patient's diplopia?
   A. MRI brain with and without gadolinium
   B. Serum testing for anti-Hu and voltage gated potassium channels
   C. Thorough physical exam including complete neurological evaluation and funduscopic exam
   D. Serum testing for anti-MuSK and acetylcholine receptor antibodies
   E. Urine pregnancy test

2. A 50-year-old man with a history of hypertension, well controlled with an angiotensin converting enzyme inhibitor, has a chest x-ray obtained at the time of an annual comprehensive health evaluation. The chest x-ray was abnormal. The patient also underwent colonoscopy as part of this comprehensive evaluation. There were no significant findings. Subsequent CT scan of the chest with intravenous contrast shows a 12-cm anterior mediastinal mass with invasion of the pericardium and multiple pleural-based lesions in the right chest. He undergoes parasternal mediastinotomy (Chamberlain procedure) for tissue diagnosis. The pathology report reveals thymoma, WHO type B1.

   The patient begins chemotherapy with cisplatin 50 mg/m^2, doxorubicin 50 mg/m^2, and cyclophosphamide 500 mg/m^2 administered q3 weeks. Prior to the third cycle of chemotherapy, a CT scan shows no evidence of progressive disease. Prior to the fifth cycle of chemotherapy, he has a CT scan of the chest that, compared with baseline, shows no significant change in the size of the anterior mediastinal mass or pleural nodules. Given the absence of response, the decision is made to discontinue therapy and monitor the patient. After 3 months, the patient returns to clinic with a CT scan of the chest demonstrating no significant change in the anterior mediastinal mass, or pleural tumors. There is no pericardial effusion on CT scan. The patient reports increasing dyspnea with exertion and palpitations. On exam, BP 118/64, HR 98 bpm. He has no lower extremity edema or jugular venous distention.

Complete blood count shows the following:

Leukocyte	6000/μL
Hemoglobin	5.0 g/dL
Platelets	295,000/μL

Which of the following is the most appropriate next step?
A. Echocardiogram
B. Bone marrow biopsy and reticulocyte count
C. Change chemotherapy to carboplatin and paclitaxel
D. Darbepoetin alfa now and then weekly until hgb is greater than 8 g/dL
E. Transfusion of washed, irradiated, packed red blood cells

3. A 65-year-old man whose only medical history was of basal cell carcinoma resected from his nose (on two occasions) presented with cough. He has no improvement after an initial course of levofloxacin 750 mg daily for 7 days. Chest x-ray was done and showed a mediastinal mass. This was followed up with a CT scan of the chest that shows a 7-cm anterior mediastinal mass. He had a parasternal mediastinotomy (Chamberlain procedure) for tissue diagnosis. The pathology report reveals thymoma, WHO type B1.

The patient undergoes surgical resection. What factor best predicts the patients long-term disease-free survival?
A. Completeness of resection
B. WHO classification of tumor histology
C. Whether the capsule surrounding the tumor has been invaded
D. Ability to tolerate 4 cycles of cisplatin-based adjuvant chemotherapy
E. In vitro chemotherapy sensitivity assay and administration of appropriate therapy

4. A 72-year-old woman with a history of hypertension and diabetes reports vague chest pressure that is not associated with exertion. After persistence of this symptom for 3 weeks, she has a CT scan of the chest with intravenous contrast. The CT shows a 12-cm anterior mediastinal mass

with invasion of the pericardium and bilateral pleural-based lesions. She undergoes CT-guided core needle biopsy of a pleural lesion. The pathology report reveals thymoma, WHO type B2.

The patient begins chemotherapy with cisplatin 50 mg/m^2, doxorubicin 50 mg/m^2, and cyclophosphamide 500 mg/m^2 administered q3 weeks. Prior to the fifth cycle of chemotherapy, he has a CT scan of the chest that shows progressive pleural disease bilaterally with new lesions present. The anterior mediastinal mass is stable. The patient notes mild, intermittent nausea in the week after chemotherapy. On days 3–8, she has moderate fatigue that resolves without intervention. For the last week, she has felt relatively well. On exam, BP 132/72, HR 84 bpm. The patient has trace bilateral lower extremity edema.

Complete blood count shows the following:

Leukocyte	5500/μL
Hemoglobin	13.0 g/dL
Platelets	315,000/μL

Which of the following is the most appropriate next step?
A. Continue cisplatin, doxorubicin, and cyclophosphamide
B. Obtain radiolabeled octreotide scan
C. Change chemotherapy to carboplatin, paclitaxel
D. Begin single-agent liposomal doxorubicin
E. Discontinue doxorubicin, but continue cisplatin and cyclophosphamide

5. A 47-year-old woman without significant past medical history presents with ptosis. She is referred to a neurologist who makes a diagnosis of myasthenia gravis, confirmed by electromyography. With initiation of pyridostigmine she has prompt improvement in symptoms. CT scan of the chest demonstrates a 3.5-cm anterior mediastinal mass. There are no enlarged lymph nodes or any evidence of pleural effusion or pleural lesions. After evaluation by a thoracic surgeon, she undergoes radical thymectomy by a median sternotomy. Her postoperative course is uneventful, and she is discharged from the hospital after 4 days. She discontinues pyridostigmine and has no recurrence of myasthenia symptoms. Review of the pathology report confirms a diagnosis of thymoma, WHO type A. The tumor is encapsulated. What is the most appropriate next step in the patient's management?
A. Begin prednisone 40 mg daily
B. Refer to radiation oncology for postoperative radiotherapy
C. Recommend 4 cycles of cisplatin, doxorubicin, cyclophosphamide given on a q3 week schedule
D. Plan follow-up CT scan of the chest in 6 months
E. Recommend 4 cycles of carboplatin, paclitaxel

ANSWERS

1. D

There is a close association between thymoma and myasthenia gravis, an autoimmune disorder that often manifests with weakness of the eyelids or extraocular muscles. Approximately 15% of patients with myasthenia gravis have a diagnosis of thymoma and approximately 50% of patients with thymoma will have myasthenia gravis at diagnosis or during the course of illness. Antibodies to acetylcholine receptor were the first described antibodies

defining myasthenia gravis. More recently, anti-MuSK antibodies have been identified in patients with myasthenia gravis who do not have acetylcholine receptor antibodies. Thymoma rarely metastasizes to the brain, and an MRI of the brain is likely to be a low yield diagnostic test in this context. Anti-hu antibodies, more common in patients with small cell lung cancer, are associated with sensory neuropathy or paraneoplastic encephalomyelitis. Physical exam is unlikely to confirm the etiology of the patient's diplopia. Urine pregnancy test would not contribute to the diagnosis of the patient's diplopia.

2. B

Pure red cell aplasia is a paraneoplastic phenomenon found in ~10% of patients with thymoma. It is an autoimmune disorder that is associated with severe anemia, inappropriately low reticulocyte count, and preserved leukocyte counts. Severe anemia beyond the amount usually seen after administration of chemotherapy should raise the possibility of this diagnosis. Pure red cell aplasia is often treated with corticosteroids, sometimes with the addition of cyclosporine. Echocardiogram is helpful for identifying heart failure that could result from doxorubicin-induced cardiomyopathy; however, the patient has no clinical evidence of heart failure, and the patient has received a relatively small dose of doxorubicin. The patient has had no radiographic response to chemotherapy, but further chemotherapy in the context of severe anemia of unknown etiology is not appropriate. Darbepoetin alfa is unlikely to be effective for the treatment of pure red cell aplasia. Transfusion of packed red blood cells would be appropriate but should be accompanied by a diagnostic plan to determine the etiology of the patient's profound anemia.

3. A

In multiple analyses, the completeness of resection has been found to be the only independent prognostic factor for patients with thymoma. WHO classification and tumor stage (as defined, in part, by capsular invasion) are prognostic factors, but they are not as predictive as completeness of surgical resection. There is no proven benefit for adjuvant chemotherapy with or without in vitro chemotherapy sensitivity testing.

4. B

After initial platinum-based chemotherapy, administration of octreotide in combination with prednisone is associated with a 30% response rate. In that trial, patients had to have octreotide avid tumors as determined by an octreotide scan. While the original study administered subcutaneous octreotide 3 times per day, currently available long-acting forms of octreotide (e.g., octreotide acetate) are reasonable to use in this context. Continuation of current chemotherapy with or without doxorubicin is inappropriate, since the patient has had progressive disease despite this chemotherapy. Changing to carboplatin/paclitaxel chemotherapy is inappropriate since the only supporting data for this regimen is in patients who have not had prior chemotherapy.

5. D

The patient has a stage I thymoma for which no adjuvant therapy is recommended. Typically, patients are managed with intermittent CT scans for the first 2 years, with annual CT scan afterward. The rationale for surveillance imaging is the early identification of pleural-based sites of recurrence that can sometimes be surgically resected. There have been no randomized clinical trials of adjuvant therapy. Neither cisplatin, doxorubicin, cyclophosphamide, nor carboplatin, paclitaxel are appropriate treatments in the adjuvant setting for patients with completely resected thymoma. Radiation therapy is typically recommended for patients with stage III thymic tumors.

REFERENCES

Question 3

1. Regnard JF, Magdeleinat P, Dromer C, et al. Prognostic factors and long-term results after thymoma resection: a series of 307 patients. *J Thorac Cardiovasc Surg*. 1996;112(2):376–384.

Question 4

1. Loehrer PJ, Wang W, Johnson DH, et al. Octreotide alone or with prednisone in patients with advanced thymoma and thymic carcinoma: an Eastern Cooperative Oncology Group Phase II Trial. *J Clin Oncol*. 2004;22(2):293–299.

Head and Neck Cancer

Peter Hammerman and Ann Gramza

QUESTIONS

1. A 57-year-old Chinese male vacationing in the United States presents to the emergency department with a nosebleed. Nasopharyngoscopy reveals a mass in the nasopharynx, which is biopsied, and confirms the diagnosis of nasopharyngeal carcinoma (NPC). Which virus is most associated with nasopharyngeal cancer?
   A. Human papillomavirus
   B. Epstein-Barr virus
   C. Hepatitis C virus
   D. Human T-lymphotropic virus
   E. Rhinovirus

2. A previously healthy 47-year-old male notes right hip pain while exercising at the gym, which persists for 2 months. Further evaluation detects a lytic lesion of his right pelvis, in addition to several other lesions of the spine. A biopsy of a bone lesion reveals EBER-positive, nonkeratinizing, undifferentiated squamous cell carcinoma. What is the most likely site of his primary cancer?
   A. Tonsil
   B. Esophagus
   C. Nasopharynx
   D. Lung
   E. Larynx

3. A previously healthy 47-year-old male notes right hip pain while exercising at the gym, which persists for 2 months. Further evaluation detects a lytic lesion of his right pelvis, in addition to several other lesions of the spine. A biopsy of a bone lesion reveals EBER-positive nonkeratinizing, undifferentiated squamous cell carcinoma. Nasopharyngoscopy reveals a mass in the nasopharynx, which is biopsied, and confirms the diagnosis of nasopharyngeal carcinoma. Which of the following is the most appropriate treatment option?
   A. Palliative care/hospice
   B. Carboplatin/5-FU/cetuximab
   C. Cisplatin/5-FU/cetuximab
   D. Pembrolizumab
   E. Cisplatin/gemcitabine

4. A 50-year-old man from China presents with recurrent serous otitis and headache. After repeated courses of antibiotics, he is referred to an otolaryngologist who performs a flexible nasopharyngoscopy and identifies a mass in the fossa of Rosenmuller. Biopsy confirms nasopharyngeal carcinoma. Imaging studies reveal no lymph node involvement or distant metastases. He is clinically staged as T1N0M0. Which of the following is the most appropriate treatment option?
   A. Surgical resection
   B. Definitive radiation

   C. Definitive radiation with concurrent chemotherapy
   D. Surgical resection followed by adjuvant radiation
   E. Surgical resection followed by adjuvant radiation with concurrent chemotherapy

5. Which patient with squamous cell carcinoma of the head and neck has the best prognosis?
   A. A patient with p16 positive base-of-tongue cancer who has never smoked
   B. A patient with p16 positive tonsil cancer who is a former 25-pack-year smoker
   C. A patient with p16 positive oral tongue cancer who has never smoked
   D. A patient with p16 negative tonsil cancer who has never smoked

6. A 56-year-old male presents to your clinic for follow-up 12 months after treatment for his T2N2c squamous cell carcinoma of the right tonsil. He was treated with concurrent chemoradiation consisting of cisplatin 100 mg/m^2 days 1, 22, and 43 of radiation. He received a total of 70 Gy of radiation. He had a restaging PET-CT 2 days ago, which was negative for evidence of disease. He notes worsening fatigue over the past few months. What is the most likely cause of his fatigue?
   A. Anemia from chemotherapy
   B. Myelodysplastic syndrome
   C. Hypothyroidism
   D. Nephrotoxicity from chemotherapy
   E. Adrenal insufficiency

7. A 55-year-old Caucasian male, who has never smoked nor drank, presents to his primary care provider with a 3-cm left neck mass. He denies any other symptoms. An ultrasound shows a 3.2-cm cystic cervical lymph node. An FNA is done of the lymph node that shows p16 positive squamous cell carcinoma. What is the most likely site of the primary?
   A. Left base of tongue
   B. Left buccal mucosa
   C. Left hypopharynx
   D. Left oral tongue
   E. Nasopharynx

8. A 60-year-old Caucasian male, who has never smoked nor drank, presents to his primary care provider with a 3-cm left neck mass. He denies any other symptoms. An ultrasound shows a 3.2-cm cystic cervical lymph node. An FNA is done of the lymph node that shows p16 positive squamous cell carcinoma. A left sided tonsil mass is identified on flexible laryngoscopy. PET-CT scan shows FDG-avid matted lymph nodes in cervical regions bilaterally. There

are no distant metastases. What is the best treatment option for this patient?
A. Surgery followed by adjuvant chemoradiation with cisplatin
B. Surgery followed by adjuvant radiation
C. Concurrent chemoradiation with cisplatin
D. Radiation alone
E. Chemotherapy with docetaxel, cisplatin, and 5-FU followed by surgery

9. A previously healthy 52-year-old Caucasian man is diagnosed with clinical stage IVb squamous cell carcinoma of the oral tongue that is surgically resectable. He has an ECOG performance status of 0, excellent social support, and normal organ function. He is referred to you for your opinion regarding treatment of his cancer. Which is the best treatment option for this patient?
A. Surgery followed by adjuvant radiation plus or minus chemotherapy depending on the final pathology
B. Radiation followed by surgery
C. Definitive concurrent chemoradiation
D. Induction chemotherapy followed by chemoradiation
E. Palliative care/hospice

10. A previously healthy 52-year-old Caucasian man has undergone surgery and reconstruction for squamous cell carcinoma of the left anterior tongue. Final pathology was T2N2b, with perineural invasion, extracapsular extension, and negative margins. He has an ECOG performance status of 0, excellent social support, and normal organ function. He is referred to you for your opinion regarding further management of his cancer. Which is the best course of management for this patient?
A. Observation with PET-CT in 3 months
B. Adjuvant radiation
C. Adjuvant chemoradiation with cisplatin
D. Adjuvant chemoradiation with cetuximab
E. Adjuvant chemotherapy

11. A 61-year-old Caucasian male with a 40-pack-year smoking history presented with an enlarged left neck cervical lymph node. Subsequent evaluation found a left sided 2.5-cm supraglottic mass, with tumor invading the medial wall of the pyriform sinus. There was no fixation of the larynx. PET-CT revealed three enlarged left sided lymph nodes in the neck, the largest measuring 3 cm. There was no clinically overt extranodal extension on imaging. Which of the following is the best treatment option?
A. Cisplatin and 5-FU induction chemotherapy followed by total laryngectomy
B. Cisplatin and 5-FU induction chemotherapy followed by radiation
C. Docetaxel, cisplatin, and 5-FU induction chemotherapy followed by surgery
D. Concurrent chemoradiation with cisplatin days 1, 22, and 43 of radiation
E. Total laryngectomy with adjuvant radiation

12. A 65-year-old male with a history of squamous cell carcinoma of the glottis returns for follow-up 2 years after his treatment with concurrent cisplatin and radiation. He had a recent PET-CT with a lesion in the larynx suspicious for recurrence. A subsequent biopsy confirms recurrent disease. There are no distant metastases. What is the most appropriate next step in his management?
A. Palliative care/hospice
B. Carboplatin, 5-FU, and cetuximab

C. Total laryngectomy
D. Re-irradiation
E. Pembrolizumab or nivolumab

13. Which of the following statements regarding HPV-associated oropharynx cancer is not correct?
A. HPV-positive tumors are often more advanced at presentation.
B. HPV positive tumors are associated with high-risk sexual behavior.
C. HPV-positive tumors do not occur in smokers.
D. HPV-positive tumors are increasing in incidence.
E. HPV-positive tumors are diagnosed using p16 immunohistochemistry.

14. A 70-year-old female with a history of locally advanced squamous cell carcinoma of the hypopharynx is treated with definitive concurrent chemoradiation using cisplatin. She has a PET-CT 4 months after treatment, which reveals a local recurrence and multiple bilateral lung metastases. She has an excellent performance status, social support, and normal laboratory studies. She would like to get further treatment for her cancer. Which of the following is the next best step in her management?
A. Total laryngectomy and resection of pulmonary nodules
B. Nivolumab
C. Carboplatin, 5-FU, cetuximab
D. Carboplatin
E. Hospice and palliative care

15. A 55-year-old female with a history of locally advanced squamous cell carcinoma of the larynx is treated with definitive concurrent chemoradiation using cisplatin. She has no evidence of disease on subsequent imaging studies until 3 years later when she is found to have several lung nodules consistent with metastatic disease. She has an excellent performance status, social support, normal laboratory studies, and desires the most effective treatment possible. Which of the following is the next best step in her management?
A. Carboplatin
B. Pembrolizumab
C. Carboplatin, 5-FU, cetuximab
D. Carboplatin and 5-FU
E. Hospice and palliative care

16. A 62-year-old Caucasian male, who has never smoked, is diagnosed with p16 positive tonsil squamous cell carcinoma, stage IVb. Which of the following is not an appropriate treatment option?
A. Transoral robotic surgery with neck dissection followed by radiation with or without cisplatin
B. Transoral robotic surgery with neck dissection followed by radiation with or without cetuximab
C. Concurrent cisplatin and radiation
D. Concurrent cetuximab and radiation
E. Cisplatin, docetaxel, and 5-FU followed by concurrent chemoradiation with carboplatin

17. A 55-year-old woman is diagnosed with parotid adenoid cystic carcinoma and is treated with surgery followed by adjuvant radiation. She was lost to follow-up. Four years after treatment is complete, a surveillance chest CT scan reveals a right upper lobe pulmonary nodule that is 8 mm and a left upper lobe pulmonary nodule that is 7 mm. A biopsy of a nodule confirms metastatic adenoid cystic carcinoma. She is asymptomatic from her disease.

What is the most appropriate management of this patient at this time?
A. Watchful waiting
B. Cyclophosphamide, doxorubicin, cisplatin
C. Paclitaxel
D. Trastuzumab
E. Vinorelbine

18. A 64-year-old man is diagnosed with surgically resectable locally advanced larynx cancer. He declines total laryngectomy and opts for a larynx preservation approach. His past medical history is significant for diabetes resulting in diabetic nephropathy, with a baseline creatinine of 1.55. What is the most appropriate therapy?
A. Cisplatin with concurrent radiation
B. Cetuximab with concurrent radiation
C. Carboplatin with concurrent radiation
D. Radiation alone
E. Docetaxel, cisplatin, and 5-FU followed by concurrent chemoradiation with carboplatin

19. A 63-year-old female presents to your clinic with locally advanced tonsil cancer to discuss treatment with concurrent chemoradiation. You would like to treat her with cisplatin. What is the major dose-limiting toxicity of cisplatin?
A. Ototoxicity
B. Neurotoxicity
C. Myelosuppression
D. Nephrotoxicity
E. Nausea and vomiting

20. A 72-year-old male with a past history significant for alcoholism and tobacco abuse presents to his dentist complaining of ill-fitting dentures. His dentist discovers a floor-of-mouth mass that is biopsied and found to be squamous cell carcinoma. In completion of his staging, he is found to have a synchronous primary. What is the most likely location of his second primary?
A. Esophagus
B. Lung
C. Head and neck
D. Cutaneous
E. Bladder

21. Which of the following stage I or II head and neck squamous cell carcinomas is least appropriate for surgical resection as the primary treatment?
A. Lip
B. Floor of mouth
C. Oral tongue
D. Larynx
E. Nasopharynx

22. Which of the following is NOT a risk factor for the development of a squamous cell carcinoma of the head and neck?
A. Human papillomavirus infection
B. Alcohol consumption
C. Epstein-Barr virus infection
D. Tobacco use
E. Fanconi anemia

23. A 68-year-old man presents with a mass in the left neck, which has grown progressively over the past 2 months. On exam, a 2-cm lesion is easily appreciated and is nontender. FNA is performed in the office and reveals squamous cell carcinoma.

Which of the following diagnostic tests is NOT likely to be informative in staging of his cancer?
A. PET-CT
B. CT of the neck
C. Fiberoptic endoscopic exam
D. CT of the chest
E. MRI of the brain

24. A 62-year-old woman originally from Hong Kong presents for evaluation of swelling in the posterior right neck of 3 months duration. She also complains of mild tinnitus on the right side. On exam, a 2-cm enlargement of at least one posterior lymph node is noted in the right neck. FNA of the right neck mass is performed along with a fiberoptic exam.
What is the likely pathological process in this case?
A. Human papillomavirus–associated head and neck squamous cell carcinoma
B. Nonkeratinizing nasopharynx cancer
C. Adenoid cystic carcinoma
D. Keratinizing nasopharynx cancer
E. Primary sinonasal carcinoma

25. Which of the following risk factors is associated with the development of squamous cell carcinomas of the head and neck?
A. Hepatitis B virus infection
B. Prior organ transplantation
C. Use of alcohol-containing mouthwash
D. BRCA2 germline mutation
E. Dental prostheses

26. A 67-year-old male is seen in a multidisciplinary clinic following the recent diagnosis of a squamous cell carcinoma of the larynx. He has well-controlled hypertension and hypercholesterolemia, but is otherwise healthy. Clinical staging is consistent with T3N1 staging, and the patient expresses an interest in organ preservation if possible. PET-CT is without evidence of distant metastases.
Which of the following treatment approaches would be most appropriate at this point?
A. Concurrent chemoradiation
B. Laryngectomy followed by adjuvant chemoradiation
C. Induction chemotherapy followed by laryngectomy
D. Partial laryngectomy followed by radiotherapy
E. Radiotherapy alone

27. A 77-year-old male with diabetes and associated chronic kidney disease and peripheral neuropathy presents for evaluation for hoarseness. A fiberoptic exam reveals a tumor infiltrating both the vocal cords and the adjacent cartilage. Imaging studies reveal no adenopathy. PET-CT is without evidence of distant metastases.
What treatment approach would be associated with the highest cure rate for this patient?
A. Radiotherapy alone
B. Total laryngectomy
C. Partial laryngectomy with adjuvant chemotherapy
D. Chemotherapy alone
E. None of the above

28. A 54-year-old male presents with a locoregionally advanced squamous cell carcinoma of the head and neck with a tonsil primary and two enlarged lymph nodes in the left neck. His past medical history includes hypertension for which he is taking lisinopril, and he is otherwise healthy. He is seen in a multidisciplinary clinic and expresses a preference for organ preservation.

Which of the following treatment approaches would be most appropriate for this patient?
A. Proton beam therapy
B. Induction chemotherapy followed by radiotherapy
C. Concurrent chemoradiotherapy
D. Primary tumor excision and bilateral neck dissection
E. Intensity modulated radiotherapy

29. A 55-year-old woman is undergoing evaluation for a newly diagnosed base-of-tongue squamous cell carcinoma with metastases to bilateral anterior cervical lymph nodes. She has been evaluated in a multidisciplinary clinic, and treatment with concurrent chemoradiotherapy has been recommended.
    Which of the following toxicities would NOT be associated with this approach?
    A. Otalgia
    B. Xerostomia
    C. Myelosuppression
    D. Dental carries
    E. Compromised nutrition

30. A 58-year-old male is seen for evaluation of a new diagnosis of a squamous cell carcinoma of the hypopharynx with bilateral anterior cervical adenopathy observed both clinically and by neck CT. Multidisciplinary evaluation is undertaken, and a recommendation is offered for induction chemotherapy followed by chemoradiotherapy or chemoradiotherapy alone.
    Induction chemotherapy followed by chemoradiotherapy is associated with which of the following in locally advanced head and neck cancer therapy compared with chemoradiotherapy alone?
    A. Improved overall survival
    B. Decreased treatment-associated toxicity
    C. Improved duration of locoregional disease control
    D. Decreased progression-free survival
    E. Reduction in the prevalence of distant metastases following therapy

31. A 57-year-old woman with locally advanced squamous cell carcinoma of the tonsil with concurrent metastasis to a left anterior cervical lymph node is preparing to begin concurrent chemoradiotherapy for definitive treatment of her disease. Her medical history is significant only for postmenopausal bleeding for which she underwent hysterectomy and for well-controlled hypertension.
    Which of the following chemotherapy regimens would be most appropriate in this case to accompany radiotherapy?
    A. Weekly carboplatin
    B. Weekly cetuximab
    C. Weekly carboplatin plus paclitaxel
    D. Bolus cisplatin given every 3 weeks
    E. Bolus cisplatin with weekly cetuximab

32. A 60-year-old woman presents for evaluation having been referred by her dentist who noted a suspicious lesion in the floor of her mouth. Examination in the office accompanied by a CT scan of the neck reveals a left-sided 3.5 cm lesion in the floor of the mouth, as well as an enlarged ipsilateral anterior cervical lymph node to 2.0 cm. PET-CT is negative for distant disease. She has no other major medical problems.
    What would be the most appropriate definitive treatment option?
    A. Induction chemotherapy followed by radiotherapy
    B. Surgical resection of the primary tumor, bilateral neck dissection, and adjuvant radiotherapy

C. Proton beam radiotherapy followed by chemotherapy
D. Definitive radiotherapy
E. Chemotherapy with cisplatin, 5-FU, and cetuximab.

33. A 54-year-old male has recently undergone surgery for the initial management of a 2.2-cm tumor arising in the hard palate. He has recovered well from surgery and is seeking recommendations regarding adjuvant therapy. His medical history is otherwise unremarkable.
    What pathologic feature(s) would portend a higher rate of disease recurrence and suggest a greater degree of benefit from the addition of chemotherapy in the adjuvant setting in an individual with head and neck squamous cell carcinoma?
    A. Age greater than 65 years
    B. Primary tumor size greater than 2.0 cm
    C. Extracapsular lymph node extension
    D. Positivity for p16
    E. Positive assay for high-risk HPV

34. A 52-year-old woman presents for medical attention with a complaint of nasal discharge. Fiberoptic examination reveals a mass in the nasopharynx without parapharyngeal extension. Biopsy of the lesion is performed and is notable for nonkeratinizing carcinoma. Additional imaging studies are performed and do not identify other sites of disease.
    What is the most appropriate treatment option for this patient?
    A. Surgical resection of the primary lesion without neck dissection.
    B. Endoscopic resection of the primary lesion
    C. Concurrent chemoradiotherapy with cisplatin
    D. Radiotherapy alone
    E. Concurrent chemoradiotherapy with cisplatin followed by adjuvant chemotherapy

35. A 56-year-old male is undergoing evaluation for bilateral posterior cervical adenopathy. Endoscopic examination and imaging studies are consistent with a primary carcinoma of the nasopharynx with bilateral lymph node metastases, and this is confirmed by fine needle aspiration. There is no evidence of distant disease. The patient is otherwise well and without significant symptoms.
    Which of the following represents a standard treatment for locally advanced nasopharynx cancer?
    A. Endoscopic resection of the primary lesion and bilateral neck dissection
    B. Proton beam radiotherapy followed by adjuvant chemotherapy
    C. Intensity modulated radiotherapy followed by adjuvant chemotherapy
    D. Induction chemotherapy followed by radiotherapy
    E. Concurrent chemoradiotherapy with or without adjuvant chemotherapy

36. A 58-year-old male presents for routine evaluation 1 year after chemoradiotherapy for locally advanced squamous cell carcinoma of the larynx. He reports that he has experienced some fatigue and cough recently, but is otherwise well. He is taking lisinopril for hypertension and simvastatin for elevated cholesterol. CT imaging of the chest with contrast indicates numerous pulmonary nodules not seen on a chest CT performed 3 months previously, as well as a new mass in the larynx adjacent to the radiation field.
    What is an appropriate first-line treatment for recurrent/metastatic carcinoma of the larynx?
    A. Cisplatin and 5-FU with or without cetuximab
    B. Single agent methotrexate
    C. Panitumumab

D. Afatinib

E. Carboplatin with gemcitabine

37. A 51-year-old male underwent treatment 9 months ago with concurrent chemoradiotherapy for an HPV-associated carcinoma of the tonsil. He has done well clinically and toxicities secondary to his treatment are limited. CT imaging performed in the context of routine post-treatment surveillance is notable for a solitary nodule in the right upper lobe of the lung measuring 1.5 cm. PET-CT demonstrates avidity in this nodule, but no other concerning sites are noted. Fiberoptic exam confirms disease-free status at the treated site.

What is the appropriate next step in treatment for this patient?

A. Referral to thoracic surgery for evaluation for resection of the lung nodule

B. Initiate chemotherapy with cisplatin and 5-FU

C. Refer for cryoablation of the lung lesion

D. Initiate chemotherapy with cetuximab

E. Refer for proton beam therapy

38. A 53-year-old female presents with a chief complaint of progressive swelling in her left parotid gland. Her medical history is otherwise unremarkable. On physical exam, a 1 to 2 cm mass associated with the left parotid gland is noted, and CT of the neck confirms this finding. There is no adenopathy on exam.

What is the most likely pathologic process in this case?

A. Pleomorphic adenoma

B. Metastatic cutaneous squamous cell carcinoma

C. Adenoid cystic carcinoma

D. Merkel cell carcinoma

E. Bacterial parotitis

39. A 59-year-old woman is seen in the office 1 year following surgical resection of a salivary duct carcinoma. She reports that she has noted some swelling in her neck as well as pain in her cervical spine. Imaging studies are performed and demonstrate cervical lymph node and spinal metastases.

Which of the following molecular features found in salivary duct cancers may be therapeutically relevant in this case?

A. EGFR gene mutation

B. BCR-ABL fusion

C. KRAS mutation

D. HER2 amplification

E. KIT mutation

40. A 61-year-old female is seen for evaluation 3 years following surgery and adjuvant radiotherapy for adenoid cystic carcinoma. She reports mild dyspnea but is otherwise well and has an ECOG performance status of zero. CT imaging done in the context of the visit reveals a 2.8 cm mass in the left lower lobe of the lung without evidence of hilar or mediastinal adenopathy. A PET-CT is performed and does not show evidence of other sites of disease.

What therapy would be associated with the greatest degree of potential long-term benefit in this case?

A. Imatinib chemotherapy

B. Chemotherapy with cisplatin, 5-FU, and cetuximab

C. Surgical resection of the left lower lobe mass

D. Proton beam therapy

E. Antiestrogen therapy with tamoxifen

41. A 61-year-old woman presents to your office for an opinion regarding management of her medullary thyroid cancer metastatic to lymph nodes and bone. She has pain associated with lymphadenopathy, and her disease is not felt to be amenable to local therapy. She is otherwise healthy, and her ECOG performance status is 0.

Which systemic therapy has been associated with increased progression-free survival in metastatic medullary thyroid cancer?

A. Imatinib

B. Doxorubicin

C. Dasatinib

D. Cabozantinib

E. Cyclophosphamide

42. A 58-year-old woman is undergoing treatment with vandetanib for metastatic medullary carcinoma of the thyroid. She reports feeling well on therapy at her first visit, 2 weeks after initiation, and is without diarrhea, fatigue, or cutaneous toxicity.

What test should be ordered at this visit given the safety profile of vandetanib?

A. Electrocardiogram

B. Echocardiogram

C. Chest x-ray

D. Tuberculin skin test

E. Stool osmolality

43. A 77-year-old male presents with a rapidly progressive neck mass with associated local discomfort and dysphagia. On exam, a bulky mass extended from the thyroid gland is appreciated. Biopsy of the mass reveals anaplastic thyroid cancer, and imaging studies (PET/CT) are without evidence of disease outside the thyroid.

What is the most appropriate management for organ confined anaplastic thyroid cancer?

A. Induction chemotherapy followed by chemoradiation

B. Proton beam therapy

C. Surgical resection followed by chemoradiation

D. mTOR inhibitor therapy

E. Radioiodine ablation

44. A 74-year-old woman is seen 6 weeks following chemoradiotherapy treatment for anaplastic thyroid cancer with cisplatin and doxorubicin. Despite an initial response to therapy, she can feel that her primary thyroid mass is now enlarging, and she is experiencing increasing shortness of breath. CT of the chest and neck reveals an enlarging mass measuring 6 cm, and associated cervical adenopathy. She asks about possible treatments, but is not interested in investigational trials.

Which of the following measures would be most appropriate at this time?

A. Re-irradiation

B. Surgical resection of residual disease

C. Chemotherapy with carboplatin and paclitaxel

D. Vemurafenib

E. Best supportive care with hospice

45. A 36-year-old woman is referred for evaluation of a solitary thyroid nodule seen on ultrasound by her primary care physician. She reports on her initial visit that her mother also had thyroid cancer at an early age. Laboratory studies are notable for an elevated calcitonin level.

Germline mutation in what gene is likely responsible for this disease process?

A. BRAF

B. EGFR

C. MET

D. ALK

E. RET

46. A 48-year-old man presents for an initial multidisciplinary evaluation of locally advanced p16 positive squamous cell carcinoma of the oropharynx with metastasis to two ipsilateral cervical lymph nodes measuring 4 cm in aggregate. Serum chemistries are within normal limits. It is planned that he begin concurrent chemoradiotherapy with cisplatin, and he asks about his prognosis.

What feature would portend a favorable prognosis in this case?

A. Age under 65
B. Male sex
C. Size of cervical lymph nodes
D. Biopsy showing p16 positivity
E. Normal serum chemistries

47. A 55-year-old male with a history of HPV-associated cancer of the oropharynx presents for evaluation 5 years after undergoing concurrent chemoradiotherapy. He has both clinically and radiographically been without evidence of disease recurrence since his treatment, and has an ECOG performance status of 0. He does report that he has had a lingering cough for the past 2 to 3 months, and a chest CT shows a new 2.6 cm mass in the right middle lobe of the lung. Transthoracic needle biopsy of the lung lesion reveals squamous cell carcinoma.

What test would be most helpful in determining whether this new lesion is a new lung cancer or a metastasis from his prior oropharynx cancer?

A. p16 immunohistochemistry
B. EGFR mutation testing
C. TTF1 immunohistochemistry
D. p63 immunohistochemistry
E. PET/CT to assess SUV

ANSWERS

1. B

World Health Organization (WHO) type III, nonkeratinizing, undifferentiated squamous cell carcinoma of the nasopharynx is associated with the Epstein-Barr virus (EBV). Human papillomavirus (HPV) has been detected in nonendemic NPC, but is not as strongly associated with NPC as EBV. The remaining choices are not associated with NPC.

2. C

The WHO divides nasopharyngeal carcinoma into three histopathologic subtypes. WHO type I is keratinizing squamous cell carcinoma; WHO type II is nonkeratinizing differentiated; WHO type III is nonkeratinizing undifferentiated squamous cell carcinoma. WHO type III is associated with the Epstein-Barr virus, has a more favorable prognosis, and is endemic to Southern China. EBV is detected in cells using in situ hybridization for Epstein-Barr virus encoded RNA (EBER). The other answers are incorrect because malignancies of these sites are not associated with the EBV virus.

3. E

This patient has metastatic nasopharyngeal carcinoma (NPC), which is a very chemotherapy-sensitive tumor, with response rates up to 80% with cisplatin-based chemotherapy regimens, and occasional long-term survivors. As a result, for a healthy younger patient, palliative care or hospice is not the best answer. Platinum combinations with cetuximab are appropriate for metastatic non-nasopharyngeal squamous cell carcinomas of the head and neck. Immunotherapeutic agents, such as pembrolizumab, are under investigation for NPC but have not yet proven efficacious. The combination of cisplatin and gemcitabine in a phase III trial was found to be superior to cisplatin and 5-FU, with a median survival of 29 months, and is considered by many to be the standard of care regimen for metastatic NPC.

4. B

This patient has stage I nasopharyngeal carcinoma (NPC) and should be treated with radiation alone. NPC is a very chemotherapy- and radiotherapy-sensitive tumor, and overall survival rates of 90% have been reported for stage I disease. Surgical resection of the primary is not first-line therapy because of the deep anatomical location of the nasopharynx and its proximity to critical structures. Definitive chemoradiation is the treatment of choice for most patients with stage II, III, IVa, and IVb NPC.

5. A

Tumor p16 expression by IHC is an excellent surrogate marker for HPV positivity in oropharynx (soft palate, tonsil, base of tongue) squamous cell carcinomas. HPV-associated tumors account for at least 70% of oropharyngeal cancers in the United States, and has been associated with a much better prognosis than is seen in HPV-negative oropharyngeal tumors. A retrospective analysis of the RTOG 0129 trial data was able to identify prognostic groups for oropharyngeal cancer based on p16 and smoking history. Patients with the best prognosis were those with p16 positive tumors and a ≤10 pack-year smoking history. Oral tongue cancer is not considered an oropharyngeal tumor, and the prognostic value of p16 or HPV positivity in this tumor type is not known.

6. C

Hypothyroidism is a known complication of external beam neck irradiation and can occur in up to 50% of patients. It typically occurs at least 1 year after completion of therapy, but can occur as early as a few months following completion of therapy. As a result, most guidelines recommend that thyroid function is assessed via TSH levels every 6 to 12 months following completion of radiation therapy. Cisplatin can result in anemia, but 1 year after treatment, it has likely resolved. Myelodysplastic syndrome can be caused by any alkylating agent, but is much less common than hypothyroidism. Nephrotoxicity is an acute toxicity from cisplatin therapy and would not arise 1 year following completion of treatment. Adrenal insufficiency can arise from hypothalamic dysfunction, but is much less likely to occur in patients radiated for tonsil cancer.

7. A

p16 positivity by immunohistochemistry is a sensitive marker for the presence of HPV in oropharynx tumors. Oropharynx tumors arise from the base of tongue, tonsil, or soft palate. The demographic for HPV-associated tumors is that of younger, male, Caucasian patients who have never smoked. They typically present with a smaller primary and more advanced neck disease than seen in HPV-negative oropharynx tumors. p16 positivity can be seen in other head and neck squamous cell carcinoma primary sites, but is much less frequent, and its clinical significance in these tumor types is not known.

8. C

The best treatment for this patient is concurrent chemoradiation with cisplatin. The presence of matted lymph nodes on the CT scan makes the probability of extranodal extension high. Extranodal extension and positive margins are the accepted indications for the addition of cisplatin to adjuvant radiation. While surgical resection of the tonsil primary with bilateral neck dissection followed by radiation with or without chemotherapy is a potential treatment option, this patient would likely require both adjuvant radiation and chemotherapy. Induction chemotherapy with docetaxel, cisplatin, and 5-FU followed by surgery is also a potential option, but the patient would still require adjuvant radiation. To avoid unnecessary toxicity, most physicians recommend employing the fewest treatment modalities possible. Radiation alone is a potential treatment option for this patient, but is typically reserved for elderly patients or those with poor performance statuses. The MACH-HN meta-analysis showed that definitive concurrent chemoradiation confers a 5-year survival benefit of 6.5% compared with radiation alone.

9. A

This patient has oral tongue cancer, which is a tumor of the oral cavity. The oral cavity extends from the skin-vermilion junction of the lips to the junction of the hard and soft palate above and to the line of circumvallate papilla of the tongue below.

The primary treatment modality for good performance status patients with locally advanced, surgically resectable disease of the oral cavity is typically surgery followed by adjuvant radiation with or without chemotherapy, depending on the final pathology. Those patients who have positive margins or extranodal extension on final pathology will require the addition of adjuvant chemotherapy to radiation. Definitive chemoradiation in these patients is avoided because the dose of radiation necessary for definitive treatment of these tumors results in significant risk of osteoradionecrosis.

10. C

This patient has a surgically resected oral cavity cancer, stage IVa. These patients have a high rate of recurrence and poor prognosis, so adjuvant radiation is recommended for most, if not all, patients with locally advanced oral cavity cancers. Factors that put patients at further high risk include extracapsular nodal spread, positive resection margins, N2 or N3 nodal disease, nodal disease in levels IV or V, perineural invasion, or vascular invasion. The presence of positive margins or extranodal extension on final pathology will require the addition of adjuvant chemotherapy to radiation. This recommendation is made based on the pooled data of two trials, EORTC 22931 and RTOG 9501, which identified the subset of patients who will benefit most from the addition of chemotherapy. Cetuximab has not been studied in the adjuvant setting; therefore concurrent chemoradiation with cisplatin is the correct answer.

11. D

This patient has supraglottic larynx cancer, stage T2N2b (IVa). For a patient such as this, functional organ preservation should be attempted via a combination of chemotherapy and radiation. This can be accomplished by concurrent chemoradiation, induction chemotherapy followed by RT alone, or sequential therapy with induction chemotherapy followed by concurrent chemoradiotherapy.

Of the answers that include chemotherapy and radiation, concurrent chemoradiation with cisplatin is the best choice. The RTOG 91-11 trial established the superiority of concurrent cisplatin with radiation over induction chemotherapy with cisplatin and 5-FU followed by radiation alone for locoregional control.

12. C

If possible, surgical salvage via total laryngectomy is recommended for patients without distant metastatic disease, as this will result in the best chance of long-term survival. Palliative care and hospice would be appropriate for a patient who is not medically fit, has unresectable disease, or who has metastatic disease. It would also be appropriate for a patient who refuses total laryngectomy or palliative chemotherapy. Re-irradiation is possible in some cases of recurrent larynx cancer. Carboplatin, 5-FU, and cetuximab is appropriate first-line chemotherapy for a patient with recurrent disease who does not want to undergo laryngectomy. Pembrolizumab or nivolumab would be appropriate for platinum refractory disease if the patient did not wish to have surgery.

13. C

All of the statements regarding HPV-positive tumors are correct with the exception of the statement that HPV-positive tumors do not occur in smokers. While HPV-negative oropharynx cancer is more common in smokers, smokers can still be diagnosed with HPV-positive tumors. Smokers have a poorer prognosis than nonsmokers with HPV-positive oropharynx cancer.

14. B

This patient has what is considered platinum refractory disease, as she has developed recurrent disease within 6 months of treatment with definitive radiation and cisplatin. Of the choices available, nivolumab is the best treatment option. It has FDA approval for the treatment of head and neck cancer that is platinum refractory. Retreatment with a platinum agent is more appropriate for those with recurrent disease who have had a longer disease-free interval following definitive treatment that included platinum therapy. Hospice and palliative care is an option, but not for a patient with a good performance status who wishes to receive further therapy. Total laryngectomy with metastasectomy is rarely an option for patients with multiple lung metastases, but can be considered for those with oligometastatic disease.

15. C

Carboplatin or cisplatin, 5-FU, and cetuximab is an appropriate first-line palliative chemotherapy regimen for patients who had an initial response and disease-free interval after initial treatment with concurrent chemoradiation that included a platinum drug. A phase III trial demonstrated an improvement in overall survival using this regimen compared with cisplatin or carboplatin and 5-FU alone. Single agent carboplatin might be an active single agent, but combination therapy is preferred for patients with good performance status. Pembrolizumab is approved for platinum refractory disease, and in this patient's case, it would be appropriate after failing a first-line platinum combination. Hospice and palliative care are reasonable choices, but not for a patient with a good performance status who wants aggressive therapy.

16. B

All of these possible treatment options are appropriate with the exception of transoral robotic surgery with neck dissection followed by radiation with or without cetuximab. Cetuximab is not approved for the treatment of locally advanced head and neck cancer in the adjuvant setting. It is an option for chemoradiation in the definitive treatment setting.

17. A

This patient was lost to follow-up, and 4 years after completion of her treatment, imaging identified two small pulmonary nodules. It is likely that her disease is very indolent, and that she may survive many years without the need for systemic therapy. Systemic therapy should be given with palliative intent, as improvement in survival has not been demonstrated. Therefore of the answer choices, watchful waiting is most appropriate. Another potential treatment option is metastasectomy in select patients with limited metastases, although there is no proven survival benefit for this approach. In a patient who has rapidly growing metastases, or significant symptoms, the most effective combination is cyclophosphamide, doxorubicin, and cisplatin (CAP). Trastuzumab can be used in salivary tumors such as mucoepidermoid carcinoma that overexpress HER-2, but HER-2 is rarely overexpressed in adenoid cystic carcinoma and therefore is not an option. Vinorelbine can be used as a single agent for patients who require palliative therapy but will not tolerate CAP. Paclitaxel is not active in adenoid cystic carcinoma.

18. B

This patient has preexisting renal insufficiency; therefore cisplatin therapy is contraindicated. Cetuximab was evaluated in a trial in which patients with locoregionally advanced cancers of the oropharynx, hypopharynx, or larynx were randomly assigned to RT with or without concurrent weekly cetuximab. The group who were treated with cetuximab had significantly better overall survival and local control compared with those receiving RT alone. Carboplatin can be used with radiation, but the level of evidence is weaker than for cetuximab. Therefore cetuximab with concurrent radiation is the most appropriate therapy.

19. D

According to cisplatin prescribing information, dose-related and cumulative renal insufficiency, including acute renal failure, is the major dose-limiting toxicity of cisplatin. Renal toxicity has been noted in 28% to 36% of patients treated with a single dose of 50 mg/m^2. It is first noted during the second week after a dose and is manifested by elevations in BUN and creatinine, serum uric acid, and/or a decrease in creatinine clearance. The other toxicities listed are also associated with cisplatin therapy and can also be severe.

20. C

The risk of second primary malignancy in patients who have had a squamous cell carcinoma of the head and neck is significantly increased compared with the age-matched general population. There is an up to a 10% risk of second primary in these patients. The risk is primarily for the development of second primaries of the aerodigestive tract, likely related to the "field cancerization" effect of tobacco and alcohol use. Second primaries are most commonly identified in the head and neck, lung, and esophageal regions. One series found that patients with larynx cancer were more likely to develop second primaries of the lung, whereas patients with squamous cell carcinoma of the oral cavity were more likely to develop second primaries in the head and neck.

21. E

Early stage (I and II) head and neck squamous cell carcinomas are typically managed by either surgery or radiation. Surgery is preferred for early stage oral cavity tumors (including lip, floor of mouth, and oral tongue) in most cases, given the risk of osteoradionecrosis from definitive radiation. Adjuvant radiation can be given if needed for high-risk disease. Tumors of the larynx or hypopharynx can be managed by either definitive RT or surgery, depending on the location of the tumor and the ability to maintain functionality. Early stage nasopharynx tumors are managed by either radiation or chemoradiation. Surgical resection of the nasopharyngeal tumor is not the primary treatment modality because of the deep anatomical location of the nasopharynx and its proximity to critical structures.

22. C

Epstein-Barr virus infection is associated with the development of nasopharynx cancer and not squamous cell carcinoma of the head and neck.

23. E

Brain metastases are unlikely to be identified at diagnosis in an individual with head and neck squamous cell carcinoma.

24. B

Nonkeratinizing nasopharynx cancer is an endemic disease process in Southeast Asia and is causally related to Epstein-Barr virus infection.

25. B

Prior solid organ or bone marrow transplantation, especially when coupled with long-term immunosuppression, increases the risk of developing head and neck squamous cell carcinoma.

26. A

Concurrent chemoradiotherapy is a standard treatment approach for individuals with locally advanced larynx cancer who desire an organ-sparing approach.

27. B

For elderly patients with significant comorbidities, which limit the ability to provide an organ-sparing approach, total laryngectomy can provide the best opportunity for long-term disease-free survival. The extent of disease in this case makes radiotherapy alone unlikely to provide a durable benefit.

28. C

Concurrent chemoradiotherapy provides at least equivalent outcomes in locally advanced head and neck cancer when compared with surgery, and provides the benefit of organ preservation in appropriately selected patients.

29. A

Otalgia is not commonly reported as a side effect in individuals undergoing concurrent chemoradiotherapy for head and neck squamous cell carcinoma. It should be noted that such treatment is associated with significant toxicities, and that aggressive management to provide support is essential to avoid interruptions in therapy and to improve the patient's quality of life.

30. E

Approaches using induction chemotherapy have been compared with concurrent chemoradiotherapy alone for the treatment of locally advanced HNSCC. These studies have, in aggregate, not suggested an improvement in treatment outcome with this approach despite a reduction in the rate of distant metastases following definitive therapy.

31. D

While it can be associated with significant toxicity, bolus cisplatin administered at $100 \, \text{mg}/\text{m}^2$ every 3 weeks during radiotherapy is the best supported chemotherapy regimen for concurrent chemoradiation in a patient with a good performance status. While other cisplatin regimens have been studied, direct comparisons to a higher dose are lacking. Carboplatin is typically reserved in cases in which an individual cannot tolerate cisplatin.

32. B

Locally advanced cancers of the oral cavity are often highly aggressive in their biology and require multidisciplinary management. For individuals with good performance status, this would combine surgical resection with appropriate adjuvant therapy.

33. C

Extracapsular lymph node extension as well as lymphovascular and perineural invasion are associated with poorer prognosis following surgery in resected HNSCC.

34. D

In an individual with early stage nasopharynx cancer (T1 in this case) radiotherapy alone is associated with a high rate of cure greater than 90% and less morbidity than many other approaches.

35. E

Concurrent chemoradiotherapy remains the standard of care for locally advanced nasopharynx cancer. Adjuvant chemotherapy following chemoradiotherapy may be beneficial in some cases and has been extensively evaluated with mixed results.

36. A

Cisplatin plus 5-FU is an active and well-established treatment regimen for initial treatment of metastatic HNSCC. Recent data from the EXTREME study have indicated further benefit with the addition of cetuximab.

37. A

For individuals with oligometastatic HNSCC, long-term survival can be achieved with aggressive management of metastases. Surgical resection of the solitary lung nodule is appropriate in this case.

38. A

Pleomorphic adenomas are the most common parotid tumor and can typically be cured with excision. Some pleomorphic adenomas can recur following surgery, and the potential does exist for malignant transformation.

39. D

HER2 amplifications are often found in salivary duct carcinomas with reports of response to anti-HER2 therapies in patients with metastatic disease.

40. C

Adenoid cystic carcinoma often can be associated with recurrent disease occurring years after the initial diagnosis, and conventional chemotherapy has limited activity in the metastatic setting. While some responses have been reported to targeted agents in this disease, local therapies are preferred in the oligometastatic setting.

41. D

Cabozantinib has been shown in a phase III trial to extend progression-free survival in MTC compared with placebo.

42. A

Vandetanib therapy has been associated with QTc prolongation, and baseline and on-treatment ECGs should be obtained as safety measures.

43. C

Anaplastic thyroid cancer, when organ confined, is amenable to combined modality treatment, and such treatment can provide a survival benefit to patients. Unfortunately, only a minority of patients have a complete resection of anaplastic thyroid cancer.

44. E

Given the rapidly progressive disease shortly after chemoradiotherapy, it is unlikely that this patient will benefit from further systemic therapy. While investigational protocols should be considered in a willing patient, it is unlikely that chemotherapy will be beneficial in this case.

45. E

RET mutations, both somatic and germline, are found in individuals with medullary thyroid cancer. Such individuals should be screened for evidence of multiple endocrine neoplasia 2.

46. D

p16 positivity has been used as a surrogate marker for HPV positivity in HNSCC, and has been shown to be an independent marker of favorable prognosis in multiple studies.

47. A

Given the history of a prior HPV-associated malignancy and the near universal loss of p16 in squamous cell carcinoma of the lung, a positive p16 immunohistochemistry would be most suggestive of a late metastatic lesion.

BIBLIOGRAPHY

Bernier J, Cooper JS, Pajak TF, et al. Defining risk levels in locally advanced head and neck cancers: a comparative analysis of concurrent postoperative radiation plus chemotherapy trials of the EORTC (#22931) and RTOG (# 9501). *Head Neck.* 2005;27(10):843.

Bonner JA, Harari PM, Giralt J, et al. Radiotherapy plus cetuximab for locoregionally advanced head and neck cancer: 5-year survival data from a phase 3 randomised trial, and relation between cetuximab-induced rash and survival. *Lancet Oncol.* 2010;11(1):21.

Gillison ML, Zhang Q, Jordan R, et al. Tobacco smoking and increased risk of death and progression for patients with p16-positive and p16-negative oropharyngeal cancer. *J Clin Oncol.* 2012;30(17):2102.

<https://www.accessdata.fda.gov/drugsatfda_docs/label/2011/018057s080lbl.pdf>.

Lin K, Patel SG, Chu PY, et al. Second primary malignancy of the aerodigestive tract in patients treated for cancer of the oral cavity and larynx. *Head Neck.* 2005;27(12):1042–1048.

Pignon JP, le Maître A, Maillard E, Bourhis J, MACH-NC Collaborative Group. Meta-analysis of chemotherapy in head and neck cancer (MACH-NC): an update on 93 randomised trials and 17,346 patients. *Radiother Oncol.* 2009;92(1):4.

Vermorken JB, Mesia R, Rivera F, et al. Platinum-based chemotherapy plus cetuximab in head and neck cancer. *N Engl J Med.* 2008;359(11):1116.

Zhang L, Huang Y, Hong S, et al. Gemcitabine plus cisplatin versus fluorouracil plus cisplatin in recurrent or metastatic nasopharyngeal carcinoma: a multicentre, randomised, open-label, phase 3 trial. *Lancet*. 2016;388(10054):1883.

Question 1

1. Chua ML, Wee JT, Hui EP, Chan AT. Nasopharyngeal carcinoma. *Lancet*. 2016;387(10022):1012–1024.

Question 3

1. Raghupathy R, Hui EP, Chan AT. Epstein-Barr virus as a paradigm in nasopharyngeal cancer: from lab to clinic. *Am Soc Clin Oncol Educ Book*. 2014:149–153.

Question 4

1. Rabinovics N, Mizrachi A, Hadar T, et al. Cancer of the head and neck region in solid organ transplant recipients. *Head Neck*. 2014;36(2):181–186.

Question 5

1. Forastiere AA, Zhang Q, Weber RS, et al. Long-term results of RTOG 91-11: a comparison of three nonsurgical treatment strategies to preserve the larynx in patients with locally advanced larynx cancer. *J Clin Oncol*. 2013;31(7):845.

Question 6

1. Grover S, Swisher-McClure S, Mitra N, et al. Total laryngectomy versus larynx preservation for T4a larynx cancer: patterns of care and survival outcomes. *Int J Radiat Oncol Biol Phys*. 2015;92(3):594–601.

Question 7

1. Pignon JP, le Maître A, Maillard E, Bourhis J, MACH-NC Collaborative Group. Meta-analysis of chemotherapy in head and neck cancer (MACH-NC): an update on 93 randomised trials and 17,346 patients. *Radiother Oncol*. 2009;92(1):4.

Question 8

1. Avila JL, Grundmann O, Burd R, Limesand KH. Radiation-induced salivary gland dysfunction results from p53-dependent apoptosis. *Int J Radiat Oncol Biol Phys*. 2009;73(2):523.
2. Duke RL, Campbell BH, Indresano AT, et al. Dental status and quality of life in long-term head and neck cancer survivors. *Laryngoscope*. 2005;115(4):678.
3. Elting LS, Cooksley CD, Chambers MS, Garden AS. Risk, outcomes, and costs of radiation-induced oral mucositis among patients with head-and-neck malignancies. *Int J Radiat Oncol Biol Phys*. 2007;68(4):1110.

Question 10

1. Adelstein DJ, Li Y, Adams GL, et al. An intergroup phase III comparison of standard radiation therapy and two schedules of concurrent chemoradiotherapy in patients with unresectable squamous cell head and neck cancer. *J Clin Oncol*. 2003;21(1):92.

Question 11

1. National Comprehensive Cancer Network (NCCN). NCCN Clinical practice guidelines in oncology.

Question 12

1. Bernier J, Domenge C, Ozsahin M, et al. Postoperative irradiation with or without concomitant chemotherapy for locally advanced head and neck cancer. *N Engl J Med*. 2004;350(19):1945.

Question 13

1. Lee AW, Sze WM, Au JS, et al. Treatment results for nasopharyngeal carcinoma in the modern era: the Hong Kong experience. *Int J Radiat Oncol Biol Phys*. 2005;61(4):1107.

Question 14

1. Blanchard P, Lee A, Marguet S, et al. Chemotherapy and radiotherapy in nasopharyngeal carcinoma: an update of the MAC-NPC meta-analysis. *Lancet Oncol*. 2015;16(6):645.

Question 15

1. Vermorken JB, Mesia R, Rivera F, et al. Platinum-based chemotherapy plus cetuximab in head and neck cancer. *N Engl J Med*. 2008;359(11):1116.

Question 16

1. Shiono S, Kawamura M, Sato T, et al. Pulmonary metastasectomy for pulmonary metastases of head and neck squamous cell carcinomas. *Ann Thorac Surg*. 2009;88(3):856.

Question 17

1. Olsen KD, Lewis JE. Carcinoma ex pleomorphic adenoma: a clinicopathologic review. *Head Neck*. 2001;23(9):705.

Question 18

1. Glisson B, Colevas AD, Haddad R, et al. HER2 expression in salivary gland carcinomas: dependence on histological subtype. *Clin Cancer Res*. 2004;10(3):944.

Question 19

1. Locati LD, Guzzo M, Bossi P, et al. Lung metastasectomy in adenoid cystic carcinoma (ACC) of salivary gland. *Oral Oncol*. 2005;41(9):890.

Question 20

1. Schoffski P, Elisei R, Muller S, et al. An international, double-blind, randomized, placebo-controlled phase III trial (EXAM) of cabozantinib (XL184) in medullary thyroid carcinoma (MTC) patients (pts) with documented RECIST progression at baseline. *J Clin Oncol*. 2012;30(suppl):5508.

Question 21

1. <http://www.accessdata.fda.gov/drugsatfda_docs/label/2011/022405s000lbl.pdf>.

Question 22

1. De Crevoisier R, Baudin E, Bachelot A, et al. Combined treatment of anaplastic thyroid carcinoma with surgery, chemotherapy, and hyperfractionated accelerated external radiotherapy. *Int J Radiat Oncol Biol Phys*. 2004;60(4):1137.

Question 23

1. Smallridge RC, Ain KB, Asa SL, et al. American Thyroid Association guidelines for management of patients with anaplastic thyroid cancer. *Thyroid*. 2012;22(11):1104–1139.

Question 24

1. Wells Jr SA, Asa SL, Dralle H, et al. Revised American Thyroid Association guidelines for the management of medullary thyroid carcinoma. *Thyroid*. 2015;25(6):567.

Question 25

1. Vokes EE, Agrawal N, Seiwert TY. HPV-associated head and neck cancer. *J Natl Cancer Inst*. 2015;107(12):djv344.

Question 26

1. Vokes EE, Agrawal N, Seiwert TY. HPV-associated head and neck cancer. *J Natl Cancer Inst*. 2015;107(12):djv344.

Esophageal Cancer

David Ilson

QUESTIONS

1. A 59-year-old woman presents with progressive solid food dysphagia and weight loss. She is found to have microcytic anemia. Endoscopy reveals a friable, partially obstructing mass in the GE junction, and a biopsy indicates well-differentiated adenocarcinoma. A CT scan of the chest and abdomen shows left supraclavicular and mediastinal adenopathy and multiple hepatic metastases. Additional testing prior to initiating therapy should include:
   A. PET scan imaging
   B. Testing of the tumor for RAS mutation
   C. Testing of the tumor for HER2 expression by immunohistochemistry
   D. MRI of the brain
   E. Testing of the tumor for EGFr mutation

2. A 75-year-old man presents with adenocarcinoma of the GE junction metastatic to liver and lymph nodes. He has hypertension and hyperlipidemia and had a myocardial infarction 5 years ago complicated by mild congestive heart failure, and he recently had an echocardiogram documenting an ejection fraction of 30%. He is ECOG 1. His biopsy tested IHC 1+ for HER2, and FISH testing showed no gene amplification. FOLFOX chemotherapy is planned. You advise the patient of which of the following?
   A. Trastuzumab can be included safely as part of chemotherapy, as cardiac toxicity is rarely if ever seen with fluoropyrimidine/platinum chemotherapy.
   B. Trastuzumab should be avoided, given the risk of increasing congestive heart failure.
   C. The patient has tested negative for HER2, and trastuzumab should not be given.
   D. Trastuzumab can be given, but anthracycline-based chemotherapy should be avoided.
   E. Lapatinib may be the preferred agent here because it targets HER1 and HER2.

3. A 39-year-old stockbroker develops episodic dysphagia and abdominal pain. He otherwise has no other past history and ran in the marathon the previous year. He undergoes an endoscopy, which reveals a friable mass in the GE junction. Endoscopic ultrasound reveals a T3N1 lesion, and there is evidence of 2–3 cm celiac lymph nodes. A CT and PET scan show no evidence of metastatic disease. He undergoes a staging laparoscopy, which grossly appears normal, but three peritoneal washings indicate a positive cytology for adenocarcinoma. What is the next step in the patient's management?
   A. Preoperative chemotherapy followed by esophagogastrectomy
   B. Preoperative combined chemoradiotherapy followed by esophagogastrectomy

C. Treatment with chemotherapy alone
   D. Upfront surgery followed by postoperative 5-FU and radiation therapy
   E. Genomic profiling of the cancer to test for targetable mutations

4. An 80-year-old patient with congestive heart failure and non-insulin-dependent diabetes and a 50 pack per year history of smoking with COPD presents with dysphagia and weight loss. Endoscopy reveals a 5-cm distal esophageal mass, with a biopsy showing poorly differentiated squamous cancer. EUS suggests a T3N0 lesion, and a CT scan and PET scan only indicate a primary esophageal mass with no metastases. He has modest chronic renal failure, with a creatinine clearance of 40. You proceed with therapy to include:
   A. Weekly carboplatin, paclitaxel, and radiotherapy
   B. Cisplatin, infusional 5-FU, and radiation therapy
   C. Chemoradiotherapy followed by esophagectomy
   D. Esophageal stent placement and supportive care
   E. Radiation therapy

5. A 39-year-old woman presenting with HER2 negative metastatic GE junction adenocarcinoma with metastases to the liver has been treated with serial chemotherapy regimens, including FOLFOX, paclitaxel plus ramucirumab, and recently FOLFIRI. She has had further disease progression in the liver. She maintains ECOG PS 1 with normal organ function and has no comorbidities. She undergoes commercial genomic profiling of her cancer, which reveals a high rate of mutations present, and methylation of the promoter of ML-H1 is documented. The patient is interested in further therapy and would like to be referred for a clinical trial. You advise her to pursue which of the following?
   A. Refer for a study evaluating an FGFr tyrosine kinase inhibitor
   B. Given the benefit from prior ramucirumab, refer for a trial evaluating regorafenib versus placebo
   C. Refer for a clinical trial comparing TAS102 to placebo
   D. Refer for a clinical trial evaluating a PD-1 checkpoint inhibitor
   E. Referral for hospice and best supportive care

6. A 65-year-old African American male with a longstanding history of smoking and daily alcohol use presents with a 25-pound weight loss and progressive solid food dysphagia. Endoscopy reveals a mass extending from 25 to 28 cm from the incisors, partially obstructing and circumferential. Biopsy reveals poorly differentiated squamous cell carcinoma. A CT scan of the chest and abdomen reveals a midthoracic esophageal mass with no evidence of metastasis, and a PET scan indicates a PET avid primary lesion. Endoscopic ultrasound suggests a T3N1 lesion with two

periesophageal lymph nodes. Bronchoscopy shows no evidence of tumor in the airway. ECOG functional status is 1, and organ function is normal. The next step in treatment of this patient should be which of the following?
A. Esophagectomy
B. Preoperative chemotherapy followed by esophagectomy
C. Radiation therapy
D. Concurrent radiation and chemotherapy with a fluoropyrimidine and a platinum agent
E. Esophageal stent placement followed by chemotherapy

7. A 75-year-old woman is found to be anemic, and on physical examination has palpable left supraclavicular adenopathy. She reports a 20-pound weight loss and intermittent solid food dysphagia. Endoscopy reveals a 5-cm mass in the distal esophageal, with a biopsy showing poorly differentiated adenocarcinoma and HER2 testing is negative. A CT scan of the chest and abdomen indicates extensive mediastinal lymphadenopathy and bulky retroperitoneal and celiac nodes. She has a history of hypertension and mild congestive heart failure, with an ejection fraction on echocardiogram of 30%. ECOG PS is 1. Your choice of chemotherapy to treat this patient is:
A. FOLFOX
B. ELF
C. EOX
D. DCF
E. 5-FU monotherapy

8. A 59-year-old woman has undergone surveillance endoscopy every 2 years over the past decade for a short segment of Barrett's esophagus. She has no medical comorbidities and now presents with a follow-up endoscopy, which shows a persistent short segment of Barrett esophagus. On four-quadrant biopsy analysis, she is found to have evidence of high-grade dysplasia on multiple biopsies, but no evidence of cancer. The optimal therapy in this patient is which of the following?
A. Esophagectomy
B. Photodynamic therapy
C. Repeat endoscopy and biopsy at 6 months
D. Radiofrequency ablation
E. Carboplatin, paclitaxel, and radiation therapy

9. A 68-year-old male with a longstanding history of smoking presents with dysphagia and weight loss. Endoscopy reveals a mass in the distal esophagus extending from 35 to 40 cm and partially obstructing. CT and PET scans indicate a bulky esophageal mass and 6 cm celiac lymph nodes, but no evidence of metastatic disease. He has hypertension and gout, but has normal organ function and maintains ECOG PS 0. A biopsy of the mass reveals a poorly differentiated, high-grade neuroendocrine tumor. You meet with the patient to discuss therapy options, and you advise him to do which of the following?
A. See a surgeon to consider esophagectomy
B. Start palliative chemotherapy with FOLFOX
C. Test the tumor for HER2 overexpression to assess for trastuzumab-based therapy
D. Consider combined chemoradiotherapy with etoposide, a platinum agent, and radiotherapy
E. Proceed with paclitaxel and carboplatin and radiation therapy followed by surgery

10. A 40-year-old advertising executive with longstanding esophageal reflux and a history of short segment Barrett esophagus is found on follow-up endoscopy to have

persistent Barrett esophagus with no dysplasia, but on biopsy there is a focus of invasive adenocarcinoma. Endoscopy otherwise shows esophagitis with no frank esophageal mass. A CT scan of the chest and abdomen is normal. Endoscopy with ultrasound suggests a possible small T1 lesion, with no evidence of regional adenopathy. The patient has no medical comorbidities. He asks about the optimal next step in therapy. Which therapy do you recommend?
A. Esophagectomy
B. Photodynamic therapy
C. Short interval follow-up endoscopy and biopsy
D. Endoscopic mucosal resection
E. Preoperative carboplatin, paclitaxel, and radiotherapy followed by esophagectomy

11. A 65-year-old man with non-insulin-dependent diabetes and hypertension has been treated for a GEJ adenocarcinoma with hepatic metastases and lung metastases. His tumor tested HER2 negative, and he had a protracted response over 8 months to capecitabine and cisplatin and now has disease progression in the lung and liver. ECOG functional status is 1, and he has normal organ function. He asks about the next choice of chemotherapy. What do you recommend to the patient?
A. Supportive care and referral to hospice
B. Paclitaxel plus ramucirumab
C. FOLFIRI
D. Gefitinib
E. Oral etoposide

12. A 38-year-old presents with solid food dysphagia and fatigue. Endoscopy reveals a mass in the GEJ extending into the gastric cardia, and a biopsy shows well-differentiated adenocarcinoma. On further questioning, he reports a maternal aunt who died of uterine cancer at 45, and his mother was treated for colon cancer at age 50. A maternal grandmother died of pancreatic cancer at age 55, and a maternal aunt was treated for breast cancer at age 70. You refer the patient and family for genetic counseling. The most likely finding on genetic testing will be:
A. BRCA mutation
B. p53 mutation
C. APC gene mutation
D. Mutation in DNA mismatch repair proteins
E. RET mutation

13. A 70-year-old patient with a HER2 positive GE junction adenocarcinoma metastatic to peritoneum and abdominal lymph nodes achieves a response to capecitabine/cisplatin/trastuzumab lasting 8 months. Disease is now progressing on therapy with new liver metastases. He has no comorbidities and maintains normal organ function with ECOG PS 1. You advise the patient that his next chemotherapy regimen should consist of which of the following?
A. TDM-1 (trastuzumab emtansine)
B. Change to paclitaxel and continue trastuzumab
C. Change to paclitaxel plus ramucirumab
D. Add epirubicin to the current regimen
E. Transition to hospice and supportive care

14. A 55-year-old lawyer was recently diagnosed with esophageal adenocarcinoma with metastatic disease to lung, mediastinum, and abdominal lymph nodes. His tumor tested HER2 negative. He has had commercial testing for genomic mutations and was told that his tumor had a p53 mutation as well as amplification of the MET receptor and the EGFr receptor. He is interested in pursuing novel

therapies. You advise him that his chemotherapy regimen should include:
- **A.** Cetuximab combined with a fluorinated pyrimidine and either cisplatin or oxaliplatin
- **B.** A MET inhibitor combined with chemotherapy
- **C.** FOLFOX
- **D.** FOLFOX plus bevacizumab
- **E.** Panitumumab combined with cabozantinib

15. An obese 55-year-old with longstanding esophageal reflux presents with progressive dysphagia and odynophagia. Endoscopy reveals a long segment of Barrett esophagus and a mass in the distal esophagus extending to the GE junction at 39–42 cm from the incisors. A biopsy shows well-differentiated adenocarcinoma. A CT scan of the chest and abdomen reveals distal esophageal thickening with no metastatic disease, endoscopy with ultrasound shows a T3N1 lesion, and a PET scan lights up the primary tumor, but there is no evidence of metastasis. The patient has hypertension and hyperlipidemia on medication, but otherwise is ECOG PS 0. The most appropriate management in this patient is which of the following?
- **A.** Esophagectomy followed by adjuvant fluoropyrimidine- and cisplatin-based chemotherapy, sequenced with postoperative fluoropyrimidine and radiation therapy
- **B.** Preoperative radiotherapy followed by esophagectomy and adjuvant chemotherapy
- **C.** Esophagectomy alone
- **D.** Preoperative weekly carboplatin, paclitaxel, and radiotherapy followed by esophagectomy
- **E.** Test the tumor for HER2 status to determine the optimal chemotherapy regimen

ANSWERS

1. C

The patient has clear metastatic disease, so PET scan imaging will not contribute to staging. CNS imaging is not routinely done in these patients unless there are neurologic symptoms. RAS and EGFr mutations are rare and have no impact on currently available therapies. HER2 is targetable by trastuzumab, and in the landmark TOGA trial, adding trastuzumab to chemotherapy in HER2 positive patients improved all outcomes including survival. All patients with metastatic disease should be tested for HER2 to determine eligibility for treatment with trastuzumab.

2. C

IHC 1+ is deemed negative expression for HER2, and some question the utility of FISH testing in this situation and reserve FISH testing only for equivocal HER2 staining that is 2+; 3+ staining is considered positive. Trastuzumab does not increase cardiotoxicity when given with fluorinated pyrimidine/platinum–based chemotherapy. Lapatinib failed to improve survival when combined with chemotherapy in a recent phase III trial in HER2 positive patients.

3. C

A positive cytology escalates the stage to stage IV, and such patients have poor short-term outcomes with upfront surgery and should be approached and treated as metastatic disease.

4. A

The patient is elderly with significant medical comorbidities and is not likely a surgical candidate for esophagectomy. That being said, he may be a candidate for primary chemoradiotherapy without surgery. The recent CROSS trial validated weekly carboplatin and paclitaxel, combined with radiotherapy as an active combined modality therapy regimen, with a tolerance and pathologic complete response rate in esophageal squamous cancer that was superior to results reported with older chemoradiotherapy regimens. This would be preferred over a cisplatin-based combination, given the patient's age and renal function. Randomized trials have suggested improvement in local tumor control, without a clear-cut improvement in survival for adding surgery to upfront chemoradiotherapy in esophageal squamous cancer.

5. D

Recent studies indicate PD-1 targeted immune checkpoint inhibitors have dramatic and often durable responses in a high percentage of patients, with various primary solid tumors in the setting of high mutation rates, resulting from either silencing of or mutation of genes that encode DNA mismatch repair proteins.

6. D

Primary surgery for a stage III esophageal squamous cancer is not recommended, given the high rate of positive margins and poor outcome. Preoperative chemotherapy failed to improve outcome in the US Intergroup Trial 113, comparing surgery alone to pre- and postoperative 5-FU and cisplatin. Radiation therapy alone led to no long-term survivors in RTOG Trial 8501, but combined concurrent 5-FU, cisplatin, and radiotherapy on this trial achieved a 25% long-term survival without surgery and is the standard of care, even without surgery. Recent studies suggest better tolerance for infusional 5-FU plus oxaliplatin and radiotherapy, and weekly carboplatin and paclitaxel is also considered acceptable chemotherapy to combine with radiotherapy.

7. A

The optimal therapy in this patient is FOLFOX. ELF is a regimen combining etoposide, leucovorin, and bolus 5-FU and has severe toxicity, limited efficacy, and is no longer in use. Although EOX and DCF are options, the patient is 75 with medical comorbidities and congestive heart failure and unlikely to tolerate a triplet regimen, and avoidance of an anthracycline is advisable. Recent studies have questioned whether adding epirubicin to two-drug chemotherapy offers any benefit, and studies in patients over the age of 65 have not shown a survival benefit for adding a taxane to a fluoropyrimidine/platinum doublet. In a patient with adequate functional status, combination chemotherapy is preferred over monotherapy.

8. D

Recent studies suggest that RFA is an acceptable, nonsurgical alternative for the initial treatment of dysplastic Barrett esophagus. Morbidity and mortality are clearly lower than as well as less invasive than surgery. Photodynamic therapy has been replaced by RFA. Chemoradiotherapy is not an appropriate treatment for dysplastic Barrett.

9. D

Extrapulmonary small cell high-grade neuroendocrine tumors are treated similar to small cell lung cancer. For limited stage disease that can be encompassed in a radiotherapy field, concurrent etoposide/platinum radiation therapy is a reasonable treatment option, even without surgery, given the high rate of systemic recurrence in this histology. Several case series indicate long-term survival in such patients treated with primary chemoradiotherapy.

10. D

For a superficial T1 esophageal cancer, an attempt at endoscopic mucosal resection should be made. For T1a lesions that rate of positivity for lymph nodes is less than 3%–5%. There is controversy about more deeply penetrating T1b lesions, which may have higher rates of nodal involvement.

11. B

After disease progression on fluorinated pyrimidine/platinum–based chemotherapy, the combination of the VEGFR2 inhibitor ramucirumab added to second-line paclitaxel was superior to paclitaxel alone, with improved PFS, OS, and response rate. FOLFIRI has limited second line activity from phase II data, and gefitinib failed to improve survival compared to placebo in a phase 3 trial.

12. D

The patient's family history is concerning for Lynch syndrome. The hallmark cancers, colon and uterine cancer, were present in two blood relatives at a young age, and Lynch syndrome can also be associated with pancreatic cancer and esophagogastric adenocarcinoma. Although gastric cancer can be seen in families with BRCA mutation, gastric cancer occurs much less frequently in these families. The family history is not suggestive of familial adenomatous polyposis, which is caused by APC gene mutation.

13. C

TDM-1, the conjugate agent combining trastuzumab with and antimicrotubule agent, failed to improve outcome compared with conventional second-line paclitaxel in a recent phase III trial. Paclitaxel plus ramucirumab is the standard of care in second-line therapy, irrespective of HER2 status. There is no evidence that continuing trastuzumab into second-line chemotherapy improves outcome. There are no data supporting the addition of epirubicin to fluorinated pyrimidine/platinum–based chemotherapy at disease progression.

14. C

Recent phase III trials failed to indicate a benefit for MET targeted agents combined with chemotherapy, and negative results were also reported for EGFr targeted agents combined with chemotherapy. Bevacizumab failed to improve survival added to first-line chemotherapy on the AVAGAST trial. Chemotherapy alone is the appropriate choice.

15. D

Although up-front esophagectomy followed by postoperative chemoradiotherapy is an option, validated by US INT 116 using 5-FU and radiotherapy postoperatively, high rates of positive margins occur with upfront surgery, and the radiation field after esophagectomy is quite large. A follow-up trial to INT116 was CALGB 80101, which indicated no benefit beyond 5-FU alone for the adjuvant chemotherapy component, so that the inclusion of cisplatin with postoperative chemoradiotherapy post op would not

be recommended. Preoperative radiation therapy has no proven role, and HER2 status does not impact on chemotherapy choice, as trastuzumab is only used in HER2 positive metastatic esophagogastric cancer. Use of carboplatin, paclitaxel, and radiotherapy as a preoperative standard was established by the Dutch CROSS trial, which indicated R0 resection and survival benefits for this approach compared with surgery alone.

REFERENCES

Question 1

1. Bang YJ, Van Cutsem E, Feyereislova A, et al. Trastuzumab in combination with chemotherapy versus chemotherapy alone for treatment of HER2-positive advanced gastric or gastro-oesophageal junction cancer (ToGA): a phase 3, open-label, randomized controlled trial. *Lancet*. 2010;376:687–697.

Question 3

1. Strong VE, D'Amico TA, Kleinberg L, Ajani J. Impact of the 7th edition AJCC staging classification on the NCCN clinical practice guidelines in oncology for gastric and esophageal cancers. *J Natl Compr Canc Netw*. 2013;11:60–66.
2. Mezhir JJ, Shah MA, Jacks LM, Brennan MF, Coit DG, Strong VE. Positive peritoneal cytology in patients with gastric cancer: natural history and outcome of 291 patients. *Ann Surg Oncol*. 2010;17:3173–3180.

Question 4

1. Stahl M, Stuschke M, Lehmann N, et al. Chemoradiation with or without surgery in patients with locally advanced squamous cell carcinoma of the esophagus. *J Clin Oncol*. 2005;23:2310–2317.
2. Bedenne L, Michel P, Bouché O, et al. Chemoradiation followed by surgery compared with chemoradiation alone in squamous cancer of the esophagus: FFCD 9102. *J Clin Oncol*. 2007;25:1160–1168.

Question 5

1. Le DT. PD-1 blockade in tumors with mismatch-repair deficiency. *N Engl J Med*. 2015;372:2509–2520.

Question 6

1. Kelsen D, Ginsberg R, Pajak TF, et al. Chemotherapy followed by surgery compared with surgery alone for localized esophageal cancer. *N Engl J Med*. 1998;339:1979–1984.
2. Herskovic A, Martz K, al-Sarraf M, et al. Combined chemotherapy and radiotherapy compared with radiotherapy alone in patients with cancer of the esophagus. *New Engl J Med*. 1992;326:1593–1598.
3. Conroy T, Galais MP, Raoul JL, et al. Definitive chemoradiotherapy with FOLFOX versus fluorouracil and cisplatin in patients with oesophageal cancer (PRODIGE5/ACCORD17): final results of a randomized, phase 2/3 trial. *Lancet Oncol*. 2014;15:305–314.

Question 7

1. Al-Batran SE, Pauligk C, Homann N, et al. The feasibility of triple-drug chemotherapy combination in older adult patients with oesophagogastric cancer: a randomized trial of the Arbeitsgemeinschaft Internistische Onkologie (FLOT65+). *Eur J Cancer*. 2013;49:835–842.
2. Guimbaud R, Louvet C, Ries P, et al. Prospective, randomized, multicenter, phase III study of fluorouracil, leucovorin, and irinotecan versus epirubicin, cisplatin, and capecitabine in advanced gastric adenocarcinoma: A French intergroup study. *J Clin Oncol*. 2014;32:3520–3526.

Question 8

1. Shaheen N, Sharma P, Overholt BF, et al. Radiofrequency ablation in Barrett's esophagus with dysplasia. *N Engl J Med*. 2009;360:2277–2788.

Question 9

1. Ku GY, Minsky BD, Rusch VW, Bains M, Kelsen DP, Ilson DH. Small-cell carcinoma of the esophagus and gastroesophageal junction: review of the Memorial Sloan-Kettering experience. *Ann Oncol*. 2008;19:533–537.

Question 10

1. Soetikno T, Kaltenbach T, Yeh R, Gotoda T, et al. Endoscopic mucosal resection for early cancers of the upper gastrointestinal tract. *J Clin Oncol*. 2005;23:4490–4498.

Question 11

1. Wilke H, Muro K, Van Cutsem E, et al. Ramucirumab plus paclitaxel versus placebo plus paclitaxel in patients with previously treated advanced gastric or gastro-oesophageal junction adenocarcinoma (RAINBOW): a double-blind, randomized phase 3 trial. *Lancet Oncol*. 2014;15:1224–1235.

Question 14

1. Waddell T, Chau I, Cunningham D, et al. Epirubicin, oxaliplatin, and capecitabine with or without panitumumab for patients with previously untreated advanced oesophagogastric cancer (REAL3): a randomized, open-label phase 3 trial. *Lancet Oncol*. 2013;14:481–489.

2. Lordick F, Kang YK, Chung HC, et al. Capecitabine and cisplatin with or without cetuximab for patients with previously untreated advanced gastric cancer (EXPAND): a randomized, open-label phase 3 trial. *Lancet Oncol*. 2013;14:1224–1235.

3. Ohtsu A, Shah MA, Van Cutsem E, et al. Bevacizumab in combination with chemotherapy as first-line therapy in advanced gastric cancer: a randomized, double-blind, placebo-controlled phase III study. *J Clin Oncol*. 2011;29:3968–3976.

Question 15

1. Macdonald J, Smalley SR, Benedetti J, et al. Chemoradiotherapy after surgery compared with surgery alone for adenocarcinoma of the stomach or gastroesophageal junction. *New Engl J Med*. 2001;345:725–730.

2. van Hagen P, Hulshof MC, van Lanschot JJ, et al. Preoperative chemoradiotherapy for esophageal or junctional cancer. *N Engl J Med*. 2012;366:2074–2084.

CHAPTER
18

Gastric Cancer

Caio Max Rocha Lima

QUESTIONS

1. Hereditary diffuse gastric cancer is linked to the following:
   A. Germline mutation in one of several DNA mismatch repair (MMR) genes
   B. Germline mutation in the STK11 gene
   C. PTEN mutation
   D. E-cadherin (CDH1) gene mutation
   E. BRCA2 mutation

2. A 49-year-old male, 1-month history of dysphagia and 12-pound weight loss. The patient's PS is 1, and he has good organ function. EGD is positive for 5 cm mass in the body of the stomach. Biopsy is positive for intestinal type adenocarcinoma. Staging CT shows multiple liver hypodense lesions and multiple lung nodules involving both lungs. Which of the following would impact the first-line treatment management of this patient?
   A. Obtain staging PET-CT scan
   B. Biopsy of the liver or lungs to confirm the diagnosis of metastatic gastric cancer
   C. Submit path for HER2 studies
   D. Submit path for KRAS mutation analysis
   E. Submit path for PDL1 expression

3. All target agents listed below led to improvement in survival in metastatic gastric adenocarcinoma, except:
   A. Cetuximab or panitumumab added to platinum and fluoropyrimidine in EGFR immunohistochemistry positive gastric cancer
   B. Ramucirumab as a single-agent second-line therapy for metastatic gastric cancer
   C. Apatinib as a single-agent third-line therapy in gastric cancer
   D. Trastuzumab added to platinum and fluoropyrimidine in HER2 positive gastric adenocarcinoma

   E. Ramucirumab in combination with paclitaxel as a second-line therapy metastatic gastric cancer

4. A 65-year-old male with progressive dysphagia and 15-pound weight loss in the past month. EGD shows a GE junction mass extending 3 cm into the cardia. Biopsy is positive for moderately differentiated adenocarcinoma. EUS is positive for a T3N1 tumor. Staging scans showed no evidence of distant metastatic disease. You chose perioperative chemotherapy (neoadjuvant therapy followed by surgery followed by adjuvant therapy) as your treatment of choice. Which of the following statement is not true?
   A. Perioperative ECF (epirubicin, cisplatin, and 5FU) improves survival compared with surgery alone
   B. Perioperative CF (cisplatin and 5FU) improves survival compared with surgery alone
   C. Perioperative ECF (epirubicin, cisplatin, and 5FU) improves survival compared with perioperative CF
   D. Perioperative FLOT improves pathologic complete response compared with ECF (epirubicin, cisplatin, and 5FU)
   E. The addition of panitumumab to perioperative ECX (epirubicin, cisplatin, and capecitabine) did not improve survival in locally advanced gastroesophageal adenocarcinomas

5. Sixty-five-year-old male transferred to your care with a history of gastric adenocarcinoma posttotal gastrectomy 8 years ago. Which of the following deficiencies would you be concerned about?
   A. Vitamin B6 (pyridoxine) deficiency
   B. Iron deficiency
   C. Vitamin B12 (Cobalamin) deficiency
   D. Vitamin B1 (thiamine) deficiency
   E. B and C are correct

ANSWERS

1. D
Lynch syndrome is an autosomal dominant disorder that is caused by a germline mutation in one of several DNA MMR genes or loss of expression of MSH2 due to deletion in the EPCAM gene. Germline mutation in the STK11 gene is associated with Peutz Jeghers syndrome. Germline mutations in PTEN are found in many patients with Cowden syndrome. Mutations in the E-cadherin (CDH1) gene mutation leads to hereditary diffuse gastric cancer. It is a germline mutation inherited in an autosomal dominant pattern. The cumulative risk for advanced diffuse-type gastric cancer is

higher in males than females with E-cadherin (CDH1) mutation, 70% and 56%, respectively. An increased risk of gastric cancer has been reported in BRCA2 mutation, but it is not associated with hereditary diffuse gastric cancer.

2. C
Based on the findings of the staging CT scans, the patient has stage IV disease, and obtaining a PET-CT scan will not change the patient's management. The EGD biopsy was positive for adenocarcinoma of the stomach, and the radiologic findings were consistent with stage IV disease, and liver or lung biopsies are not warranted. Knowing the HER2 status of this patient would impact the first-line

therapy choice. The ToGA trial showed that the addition of trastuzumab to cisplatinum and fluoropyrimidine chemotherapy improved survival in HER2-positive advanced gastric cancer patients. In this trial HER2 positive was defined as "+++" via IHC or "+" via FISH. KRAS mutation analysis is a predictor of EGFR monoclonal antibody treatment in colon cancer, but not in gastric cancer. Checkpoint inhibitors are promising agents in gastric cancer, and PDL-1 expression may become a relevant biomarker in the first-line treatment selection in the future, but at this time it does not impact on the choice for first-line therapy in gastric cancer.

3. A

Anti-EGFR therapies in combination with chemotherapy in patients with metastatic gastroesophageal cancer resulted in no improvement in survival in both the REAL-3 and the EXPAND studies. Both studies failed to demonstrate a survival advantage with either cetuximab or panitumumab in unselected patient populations. The REGARD trial showed that ramucirumab was superior to BSC as second-line therapy in metastatic gastric cancer, OS of 5.2 months versus 3.8 months (HR = 0.776, 95% CI, 0.603–0.998, $P = .047$). Apatinib was superior to BSC (6.5 months; 95% CI, 4.8–7.6 vs. 4.7 months; 95% CI, 3.6–5.4; $P = .0149$) in a randomized study that enrolled 267 patients who were previously treated with at least two lines of therapy. The RAINBOW trial showed that ramucirumab plus paclitaxel improved survival compared with paclitaxel alone as second-line therapy gastric cancer (OS 9.6 months vs. 7.4 months, HR = 0.807, $P = .017$).

4. C

This patient has T3N1 GEJ adenocarcinoma. Perioperative chemotherapy was superior to surgery alone in the MAGIC and FFCD/ACCORD trials. On the MAGIC trial, three cycles of ECF, followed by surgery, followed by 3 cycles of ECF were superior to surgery alone. On the FFCD/ACCORD trial, up to 3 cycles of CF before and after surgery were superior to surgery alone. Both trials led to improvement in resection rates and improvement in 5-year survival rates. On the FFCD/ACCORD trial, most patients had GEJ adenocarcinoma, and the HR was 0.57 in this population. In the MAGIC trial, a minority of patients had GE junction adenocarcinoma, and in this population the HR was 0.49. The MRC OE05 trial randomized patients with resectable (T1N0 and T2N0 tumors excluded) distal esophageal and GEJ adenocarcinomas to either two cycles of preoperative CF or four cycles of preoperative ECX. Overall survival was not statistically different between the two arms, and perioperative ECX was more toxic. The FLOT4 randomized phase III study comparing eight cycles of perioperative FLOT (docetaxel, 5FU, leucovorin, and oxaliplatin) to six cycles of perioperative ECF/ECX (5FU or capecitabine in combination with cisplatin and epirubicin) in adenocarcinoma of the stomach or GEJ showed pathologic complete response rates of 12.8% versus 5.1%, respectively ($P = .015$). Similarly to metastatic disease, adding panitumumab to ECX did not improve outcomes in locally advanced gastroesophageal adenocarcinomas.

5. E

Total gastrectomy will result in intrinsic factor deficiency and malabsorption of vitamin B12 (cobalamin) that will lead to pernicious anemia. The median time to cobalamin deficiency is about 15 months after total gastrectomy. Iron malabsorption and deficiency postgastrectomy may result from achlorhydria, gastric dumping, or afferent (blind) loop syndromes with or without bacterial overgrowth. Vitamin B6 and vitamin B1 deficiency are not a complication from total gastrectomy.

REFERENCES

Question 1

1. Stoffel EM, Mangu PB, Gruber SB, et al. Hereditary colorectal cancer syndromes: American Society of Clinical Oncology Clinical Practice Guideline endorsement of the familial risk-colorectal cancer: European Society for Medical Oncology Clinical Practice Guidelines. *J Clin Oncol.* 2015;33:209.
2. Lim W, Hearle N, Shah B, Murday V, et al. Further observations on LKB1/STK11 status and cancer risk in Peutz-Jeghers syndrome. *Br J Cancer.* 2003;89:308.
3. Liaw D, Marsh DJ, Li J, et al. Germline mutations of the PTEN gene in Cowden disease, an inherited breast and thyroid cancer syndrome. *Nat Genet.* 1997;16:64–67.
4. van der Post RS, Vogelaar IP, Carneiro F, et al. Hereditary diffuse gastric cancer: updated clinical guidelines with an emphasis on germline CDH1 mutation carriers. *J Med Genet.* 2015;52:361–374.
5. Hansford S, Kaurah P, Li-Chang H, et al. Hereditary diffuse gastric cancer syndrome. *JAMA Oncol.* 2015;1:23–32.
6. Easton D, Thompson D, McGuffog L, et al. The Breast Cancer Linkage Consortium. Cancer risks in BRCA2 mutation carriers. *J Natl Cancer Inst.* 1999;91:1310–1316.

Question 2

1. Bang YJ, Van Cutsem E, Feyereislova A, et al. Trastuzumab in combination with chemotherapy versus chemotherapy alone for treatment of HER2-positive advanced gastric or gastro-oesophageal junction cancer (ToGA): a phase 3, open-label, randomised controlled trial. *Lancet.* 2010;376:687–697.

Question 3

1. Waddell T, Chau I, Cunningham D, et al. Epirubicin, oxaliplatin, and capecitabine with or without panitumumab for patients with previously untreated advanced oesophagogastric cancer (REAL3): a randomised, open-label phase 3 trial. *Lancet Oncol.* 2013;14:481–489.
2. Lordick F, Kang YK, Chung HC, et al. Capecitabine and cisplatin with or without cetuximab for patients with previously untreated advanced gastric cancer (EXPAND): a randomised, open-label phase 3 trial. *Lancet Oncol.* 2013;14:490–499.
3. Fuchs CS, Tomasek J, Yong CJ, et al. Ramucirumab monotherapy for previously treated advanced gastric or gastro-oesophageal junction adenocarcinoma (REGARD): an international, randomised, multicentre, placebo-controlled, phase 3 trial. *Lancet.* 2014;383:31–39.
4. Li J, Qin S, Xu J, et al. Randomized, double-blind, placebo-controlled phase III trial of apatinib in patients with chemotherapy-refractory advanced or metastatic adenocarcinoma of the stomach or gastroesophageal junction. *J Clin Oncol.* 2016;34:1448–1454.
5. Wilke H, Muro K, Van Cutsem E, et al. Ramucirumab plus paclitaxel versus placebo plus paclitaxel in patients with previously treated advanced gastric or gastro-oesophageal junction adenocarcinoma (RAINBOW): a double-blind, randomised phase 3 trial. *Lancet Oncol.* 2014;15:1224–1235.

Question 4

1. Cunningham D, Allum W, Stenning S, et al. Perioperative chemotherapy versus surgery alone for resectable gastroesophageal cancer. *N Eng J Med.* 2006;355:11–20.
2. Ychou M, Boige V, Pignon JP, et al. Perioperative chemotherapy compared with surgery alone for resectable gastroesophageal adenocarcinoma: an FNCLCC and FFCD multicenter phase III trial. *J Clin Oncol.* 2011;29:1715–1721.
3. Alderson D, Langley R, Nankivell M, et al. Neoadjuvant chemotherapy for resectable oesophageal and junctional adenocarcinoma: results from the UK Medical Research Council randomised OEO5 trial (ISRCTN 01852072). *J Clin Oncol.* 2015;33(suppl). abstr 4002.

4. Pauligk C, Tannapfel A, Meiler J, et al. Pathological response to neoadjuvant 5-FU, oxaliplatin, and docetaxel (FLOT) versus epirubicin, cisplatin, and 5-FU (ECF) in patients with locally advanced, resectable gastric/esophagogastric junction (EGJ) cancer: data from the phase II part of the FLOT4 phase III study of the AIO. *J Clin Oncol*. 2015;33(suppl). abstr 4016.
5. Moehler M, Lordick F, Mihaljevic A, et al. The role of panitumumab in combination with ECX in perioperative chemotherapy of unselected patients with locally advanced gastroesophageal adenocarcinomas: randomized phase II study of the German Cancer Society. *J Clin Oncol*. 2015;33(suppl). abstr 4040.

Question 5

1. Hu Y, Kim H, Hyung W, et al. Vitamin B(12) deficiency after gastrectomy for gastric cancer: an analysis of clinical patterns and risk factors. *Ann Surg*. 2013;258:970–975.
2. Sutton D, Baird I, Stewart J, Croft DN, Coghill NF. Gastrointestinal iron losses in atrophic gastritis, postgastrectomy states and adult coeliac disease. *Gut*. 1971;12:869–870.

QUESTIONS

1. What is the median overall survival with second-line therapy for patients with metastatic pancreatic cancer?
   A. 4 months
   B. 6 months
   C. 8 months
   D. 10 months

2. In 2016, pancreatic cancer was the twelfth leading new cancer diagnosis, but where does it rank as a cause of cancer-related death?
   A. First
   B. Third
   C. Seventh
   D. Twelfth

3. A 64-year-old male presents with painless jaundice and, by EUS-FNA, is confirmed to have a pancreatic adenocarcinoma. CT imaging reveals a 3.5-cm mass that is causing biliary obstruction; it encases a 1-cm portion of the SMV and abuts the SMA with less than 180-degree encasement. There is no evidence of metastatic disease.
   What is the resectability staging for this patient?
   A. Resectable
   B. Borderline resectable
   C. Localized, unresectable
   D. Metastatic

4. Has adjuvant radiation been shown to potentially increase her 5-year survival rate?
   A. Yes
   B. No

5. A 57-year-old male with metastatic pancreatic cancer received first-line therapy with gemcitabine and nab-paclitaxel. He benefited from this and remained progression-free for 11 months. However, he now has clear disease progression despite an excellent performance status.
   What is an FDA-approved second-line therapy regimen for patients with metastatic pancreatic cancer?
   A. 5-Fluorouracil and irinotecan (FOLFIRI)
   B. 5-Fluorouracil and oxaliplatin (FOLFOX)
   C. Capecitabine
   D. Nanoliposomal irinotecan and 5-fluorourcacil

6. What percent of pancreatic cancers are believed to be related to a predisposing germline gene mutation?
   A. 1%–3%
   B. 7%–10%
   C. 20%–25%
   D. 40%–45%

7. What is the 5-year survival rate of patients who have undergone resection of pancreatic cancer?
   A. 3%
   B. 7%
   C. 29%
   D. 45%

8. Which of the following has not demonstrated a survival benefit as compared with the standard of care for patients with metastatic pancreatic cancer?
   A. 5-Fluorouracil, irinotecan, and oxaliplatin (FOLFIRINOX)
   B. Gemcitabine plus nab-paclitaxel
   C. GTX
   D. Gemcitabine

9. FOLFIRINOX can be a difficult regimen for patients to tolerate. Although FOLFIRINOX has demonstrated a survival benefit over single-agent gemcitabine, is there a quality-of-life benefit to FOLFIRINOX over gemcitabine?
   A. Yes
   B. No

10. A 51-year-old male of Ashkenazi Jewish descent is referred following a recent diagnosis of metastatic pancreatic adenocarcinoma with liver metastases. In assessing the family history, you learn that his mother and sister both had breast cancer before age 50 and that a maternal grandmother died of pancreatic cancer. He is referred for consideration of chemotherapy, the possible benefits of platinum-based therapy, or even a clinical trial with a PARP inhibitor.
    What do you estimate is his risk of harboring a germline mutation in one of the *BRCA* genes?
    A. 1%
    B. 3%–5%
    C. 15%–20%
    D. 35%–40%

11. A 61-year-old female is incidentally found to have a 1.5-cm mass in the head of the pancreas, with no venous or arterial involvement. She successfully undergoes a Whipple resection with 2 of 19 lymph nodes involved, and negative margins. The current standard of care adjuvant therapy would be 6 months of chemotherapy.
    What is the current standard of care as adjuvant chemotherapy for patients with resected pancreatic cancer?
    A. Modified FOLFIRINOX (5-fluorouracil, irinotecan, and oxaliplatin)
    B. Gemcitabine plus nab-paclitaxel
    C. Gemcitabine
    D. Gemcitabine plus capecitabine

12. The median overall survival for patients with metastatic pancreatic cancer receiving current standard front-line therapy (FOLFIRINOX or gemcitabine plus nab-paclitaxel) is:

A. 6–8 months
B. 8.5–11 months
C. 12.5–14 months
D. 17–18 months

ANSWERS

1. B

The median overall survival for patients treated with nano-liposomal irinotecan plus 5-fluorouracil was 6.1 months.

2. B

Pancreatic cancer is the twelfth leading cancer diagnosis in the United States, with 53,070 cases diagnosed in 2016. However, with 41,780 estimated deaths, it stands as the third leading cause of cancer-related death, behind only lung cancer (158,080 deaths) and colorectal cancer (49,190 deaths).

3. B

As detailed in the NCCN guidelines, localized pancreatic cancers are separated into resectable (with no evidence of venous or arterial contact); localized, unresectable (unreconstructable occlusion or encasement of the SMV or PV; >180 degree encasement of the SMA, celiac trunk, or hepatic artery); or, in the middle, cases involving borderline resectable tumors (short, reconstructable encasement of the SMV, and <180 degree encasement of the SMA, celiac trunk, or hepatic artery). Therapy is guided (preoperative vs. postoperative) by what is determined regarding the resectability of the tumor.

4. B

There is no proven benefit to adjuvant radiation for 5-year or overall survival. Adjuvant radiation has been shown to decrease local recurrence rates, but this has not yet translated to an improvement in survival.

5. D

FOLFIRI and FOLFOX have shown activity as second-line therapy for pancreatic cancer (although the data for FOLFOX are controversial). However, the only phase III trial to ever demonstrate benefit over a standard-of-care control arm showed that the combination of nano-liposomal irinotecan and 5-fluorouracil improved survival over 5-fluorouracil alone.

6. B

Pancreatic cancer patients harbor germline mutations in up to 7%–10% of cases. These mutations can include BRCA1/2 (3%–5%), PALB2 (1%), p16INK4 (FAMMM syndrome, <1%), PTEN (Peutz–Jehgers, <1%), ATM 9 ataxia-telangiectasia, <1%), familial adenomatous polyposis (APC <1%), and the mismatch repair genes (Lynch syndrome III, <1%).

7. C

The recent ESPAC-4 presentation revealed that the 5-year overall survival for patients who have undergone a resection for pancreatic cancer is 29%.

8. C

FOLFIRINOX and gemcitabine plus nab-paclitaxel have both been shown to improve overall (and progression-free) survival as compared with gemcitabine alone. Gemcitabine was demonstrated to improve survival over the prior standard of care (5-fluorouracil) at that time. Gemcitabine,

docetaxel (T), and capecitabine (X) (GTX) has never been tested against the standard of care in a phase III trial. Thus the correct answer is C.

9. A

Despite its greater toxicity, FOLFIRINOX clearly demonstrated an improvement in quality-of-life scores over single-agent gemcitabine.

10. C

Germline mutations in the BRCA genes can predispose patients to developing pancreatic cancer. In the unselected population of patients with pancreatic cancer, the risk of identifying a *BRCA* mutation is 3%–5%. However, that risk increases in patients of Ashkenazi Jewish descent and in cases of familial pancreatic cancer, with risks as high as 17% in the highest-risk subgroups. Thus the answer in this high-risk patient is C.

11. D

The recently presented ESPAC-4 trial demonstrated unequivocally that, over gemcitabine alone, the combination of gemcitabine and capecitabine as adjuvant therapy improves both median overall survival and the 5-year overall survival rate. Thus the correct answer is D. Modified FOLFIRINOX and gemcitabine plus nab-paclitaxel are appropriate regimens for metastatic disease but do not (yet) have any proven superiority over gemcitabine as adjuvant therapy.

12. B

The median overall survival demonstrated in multiple phase III trials where gemcitabine was either the experimental or control arm exhibited a median overall survival of 6–7 months. However, gemcitabine is not the standard of care today for the vast majority of pancreatic cancer patients. The median overall survival with current standard front-line therapy is 8.6 months with gemcitabine plus nab-paclitaxel and 11.1 months with FOLFIRINOX.

REFERENCES

Question 1
1. Wang-Gillam A, et al. *Lancet.* 2016;387:545–557.

Question 2
1. American Cancer Society. *Facts and Figures.* 2016. www.cancer.org.

Question 3
1. NCCN guidelines. *Pancreatic adenocarcinoma. v.2.* 2015. www.nccn.org. 2015 Accessed 20.03.17.

Question 4
1. Smaglo BG, Pishvaian MJ. Postresection chemotherapy for pancreatic cancer. *Cancer J.* 2012;18(6):614–623.

Question 5
1. Wang-Gillam A, et al. *Lancet.* 2016;387:545–557.

Question 6

1. Edderkaoui M, Eibl G. Risk factors for pancreatic cancer: underlying mechanisms and potential targets. *Front Physiol.* 2014;5:490.
2. Korsse SE, Harinck F, van Lier MG, et al. Pancreatic cancer risk in Peutz-Jeghers syndrome patients: a large cohort study and implications for surveillance. *J Med Genet.* 2013;50:59–64.
3. Hezel AF, Kimmelman AC, Stanger BZ, Bardeesy N, Depinho RA. Genetics and biology of pancreatic ductal adenocarcinoma. *Genes Dev.* 2006;20:1218–1249.
4. Goldstein AM, et al. Increased risk of pancreatic cancer in melanoma-prone kindreds with p16INK4 mutations. *N Engl J Med.* 1995;333:970–975.

Question 7

1. Neoptolemos JP, et al. ESPAC-4: A multicenter, international, open-label randomized controlled phase III trial of adjuvant combination chemotherapy of gemcitabine (GEM) and capecitaine (CAP) versus monotherapy gemcitabine in patients with resected pancreatic ductal adencarcinoma. *J Clin Oncol.* 2016;34 (suppl; abstr LBA4006).

Question 8

1. Conroy T, Desseigne F, Ychou M, et al. FOLFIRINOX versus gemcitabine for metastatic pancreatic cancer. *N Engl J Med.* 2011;364:1817–1825.
2. Von Hoff DD, Ervin T, Arena FP, et al. Increased survival in pancreatic cancer with nab-paclitaxel plus gemcitabine. *N Engl J Med.* 2013;369:1691–1703.
3. Burris 3rd HA, Moore MJ, Andersen J, et al. Improvements in survival and clinical benefit with gemcitabine as first-line therapy for patients with advanced pancreas cancer: a randomized trial. *J Clin Oncol.* 1997;15:2403–2413.
4. De Jesus-Acosta A, Oliver GR, Blackford A, et al. A multicenter analysis of GTX chemotherapy in patients with locally advanced and metastatic pancreatic adenocarcinoma. *Cancer Chemother Pharmacol.* 2012;69:415–424.
5. Fine RL, Fogelman DR, Schreibman SM, et al. The gemcitabine, docetaxel, and capecitabine (GTX) regimen for metastatic pancreatic cancer: a retrospective analysis. *Cancer Chemother Pharmacol.* 2008;61:167–175.

Question 9

1. Conroy T, Desseigne F, Ychou M, et al. FOLFIRINOX versus gemcitabine for metastatic pancreatic cancer. *N Engl J Med.* 2011;364:1817–1825.

Question 10

1. Hahn SA, Greenhalf B, Ellis I, et al. BRCA2 germline mutations in familial pancreatic carcinoma. *J Natl Cancer Inst.* 2003;95(3):214–221.
2. Murphy KM, Brune KA, Griffin C, et al. Evaluation of candidate genes MAP2K4, MADH4, ACVR1B, and BRCA2 in familial pancreatic cancer: deleterious BRCA2 mutations in 17%. *Cancer Res.* 2002;62(13):3789–3793.
3. Stadler ZK, Salo-Mullen E, Patil SM, et al. Prevalence of BRCA1 and BRCA2 mutations in Ashkenazi Jewish families with breast and pancreatic cancer. *Cancer.* 2012;118(2):493–499. http://dx.doi.org/10.1002/cncr.26191.
4. Lowery MA, Kelsen DP, Stadler ZK, et al. An emerging entity: pancreatic adenocarcinoma associated with a known BRCA mutation: clinical descriptors, treatment implications, and future directions. *Oncologist.* 2011;16(10):1397–1402. http://dx.doi.org/10.1634/theoncologist.2011-0185.

Question 11

1. Neoptolemos JP, et al. ESPAC-4: A multicenter, international, open-label randomized controlled phase III trial of adjuvant combination chemotherapy of gemcitabine (GEM) and capecitaine (CAP) versus monotherapy gemcitabine in patients with resected pancreatic ductal adencarcinoma. *J Clin Oncol.* 2016;34 (suppl; abstr LBA4006).

Question 12

1. Burris 3rd HA, Moore MJ, Andersen J, et al. Improvements in survival and clinical benefit with gemcitabine as first-line therapy for patients with advanced pancreas cancer: a randomized trial. *J Clin Oncol.* 1997;15:2403–2413.
2. Von Hoff DD, Ervin T, Arena FP, et al. Increased survival in pancreatic cancer with nab-paclitaxel plus gemcitabine. *N Engl J Med.* 2013;369:1691–1703.
3. Conroy T, Desseigne F, Ychou M, et al. FOLFIRINOX versus gemcitabine for metastatic pancreatic cancer. *N Engl J Med.* 2011;364:1817–1825.

Colorectal and Anal Cancer

Nilofer Azad and Christopher H. Lieu

QUESTIONS

1. A 51-year-old male presents to clinic with metastatic colorectal cancer with unresectable metastases to both lobes of the liver. He is noted to have a KRAS mutation in codon 12 and has a history of well-controlled hypertension. He is initially treated with FOLFOX in combination with bevacizumab and at 2 months has stable disease noted on CT of the abdomen and pelvis. His restaging study at 4 months reveals progression of disease in the liver. Which of the following would be the best next step in management?
   A. Irinotecan in combination with cetuximab
   B. FOLFIRI in combination with bevacizumab and panitumumab
   C. FOLFIRI in combination with bevacizumab
   D. Vemurafenib
   E. Cetuximab single-agent

2. A 65-year-old female is diagnosed with stage IIIC colon cancer and is treated with modified FOLFOX6 in the adjuvant setting following surgical resection. She is diagnosed 18 months later with metastatic colon cancer with metastases to the lungs and liver. Repeat biopsy demonstrates a NRAS mutation in codon 12 (G12D). She progresses on CAPOX in combination with bevacizumab and FOLFIRI in combination with bevacizumab. Her ECOG performance status is 1, and she desires further treatment. Which of the following is the best treatment recommendation at this time?
   A. Treatment with TAS-102
   B. Referral to hospice
   C. Treatment with panitumumab
   D. Single-agent bevacizumab
   E. Surgical resection of metastases

3. A 62-year-old male notes rectal bleeding without obstructive symptoms; colonoscopy reveals a 3-cm mass in the sigmoid colon. Biopsy confirms a moderately differentiated adenocarcinoma, and staging CT of the chest/abdomen/pelvis reveals no evidence of distant metastasis. Sigmoid colectomy is performed, revealing a 3.7-cm moderately differentiated adenocarcinoma with invasion through the muscularis propria, with all margins negative for adenocarcinoma. None of 19 lymph nodes are involved with disease. No lymphovascular or PNI is noted. The patient is staged pT3N0M0. Tumor is found to have a KRAS mutation G12V, BRAF wild-type, PIK3CA wild-type, and is also microsatellite-stable (MSS). What is the next appropriate step in management?
   A. Concurrent chemotherapy and radiation to the resection site with concurrent 5-FU
   B. Active surveillance with CEA every 3 to 6 months and CT of the chest/abdomen/pelvis every 6 to 12 months

   C. Initiation of adjuvant FOLFOX for 6 months
   D. Initiation of adjuvant FOLFIRI for 6 months
   E. Initiation of adjuvant capecitabine for 6 months

4. A 72-year-old female presents with abdominal pain and fullness. Colonoscopy reveals an ascending colonic mass without evidence of obstruction. Biopsy reveals a poorly differentiated adenocarcinoma. CT of the chest/abdomen/pelvis reveals evidence of metastatic disease to the liver and peritoneum. Mutational testing reveals wild-type RAS, BRAF V600E mutation present, MSS. Which of the following is true with regard to BRAF V600E mutated colorectal cancer?
   A. BRAF mutations are found in a majority of all colorectal cancers.
   B. BRAF mutations are associated with better prognosis and DFR.
   C. BRAF mutations are often mutually exclusive from RAS mutations.
   D. BRAF mutations are seen more frequently in left-sided colorectal cancer.
   E. Single-agent vemurafenib has been shown to be effective in treating BRAF mutant colorectal cancer.

5. A 42-year-old male presents with new rectal bleeding and the sensation of a rectal mass. He undergoes a digital rectal examination, anoscopic examination, and biopsy of an anal canal lesion, revealing squamous cell carcinoma. CT of the chest and abdomen reveals no evidence of metastatic disease. MRI of the pelvis reveals an anal canal tumor measuring 3 cm in greatest dimension. One perirectal lymph node appears enlarged. The patient is staged cT2N1M0. He is found to be HIV-negative. What is the next appropriate management step for this patient?
   A. Concurrent chemotherapy and radiation with 5-FU and mitomycin
   B. FOLFOX chemotherapy
   C. Observation
   D. Surgical resection followed by adjuvant 5-FU/cisplatin
   E. Stereotactic body radiation therapy

6. A 47-year-old female notes rectal bleeding without obstructive symptoms; colonoscopy reveals a 5-cm mass in the transverse colon. Biopsy confirms poorly differentiated adenocarcinoma, and staging CT of the chest/abdomen/pelvis reveals no evidence of distant metastasis. Sigmoid colectomy is performed revealing a 5.2-cm moderately differentiated adenocarcinoma with invasion through the muscularis propria and all margins negative for adenocarcinoma. None of 23 lymph nodes are involved with disease. No lymphovascular or PNI is noted. The patient is staged pT3N0M0. Tumor is found to be RAS wild-type, PIK3CA wild-type, and a BRAF V600E mutation is

present. Microsatellite testing reveals MSI-high. What is the next appropriate step in management?
A. Concurrent chemotherapy and radiation to the resection site with concurrent 5-FU
B. Initiation of adjuvant FOLFOX for 6 months
C. Initiation of adjuvant FOLFIRI for 6 months
D. Initiation of adjuvant pembrolizumab for 6 months
E. Active surveillance and referral to genetic counseling

7. A 65-year-old female with RAS and RAF wild-type colon adenocarcinoma is found to have bilobar metastases to the liver. She is initiated on first-line chemotherapy with FOLFOX and cetuximab. After 1 month of therapy, she presents to clinic with an acneiform rash with papules covering her face and part of her chest. She is deemed to have a grade 2 rash. Vital signs are stable, and the patient is normotensive. White blood cell count is 4.2, hemoglobin is 10.8, platelets are 175, and carcinoembryonic antigen (CEA) is 12.7. She is currently receiving no treatment for her rash. What is the next appropriate step in management?
A. Discontinuation of cetuximab and continuation of FOLFOX
B. Initiation of topical fluocinonide 0.05% cream and oral doxycycline
C. Discontinuation of FOLFOX/cetuximab and initiation of FOLFIRI/bevacizumab
D. Initiation of hydrocortisone acetate with pramoxine 1% combination
E. Referral to dermatology

8. A 71-year-old male presents with occasional rectal bleeding, pelvic pain, and mild unexplained weight loss. Digital rectal exam is unremarkable, but flexible sigmoidoscopy reveals a nonobstructing mass in the midrectum. Biopsy reveals a well-differentiated adenocarcinoma. CT imaging of the chest and abdomen reveals no evidence of distant metastatic disease. Pelvic MRI reveals a 3.4-cm midrectal tumor invading through the muscularis propria. Several perirectal lymph nodes appear enlarged. The patient is staged cT3N1bM0. Complete blood count appears within normal limits, and the creatinine is 0.7. CEA is found to be 35. Molecular testing reveals a KRAS G13D mutation. What should be the next step in management?
A. Low anterior surgical resection followed by adjuvant FOLFOX
B. Neoadjuvant therapy with FOLFOX/cetuximab followed by surgical resection
C. Neoadjuvant chemoradiation with concurrent capecitabine
D. Endoscopic mucosal resection of the primary tumor
E. Surgical resection with intraoperative radiation of the surgical bed

9. A 63-year-old female with metastatic colorectal cancer with metastases to the liver and lungs is receiving FOLFOX and bevacizumab for frontline therapy. She is here prior to cycle 2, day 1 of treatment. Her main symptoms from treatment include grade 1 fatigue, grade 1 nausea, and grade 1 cold dysesthesia 5 days following infusion. Today her physical examination is unchanged, but her blood pressure is noted to be 152/95. She wants to be treated today. Her labs are all within normal limits with the exception of her absolute neutrophil count, which is noted to be 1800. The most appropriate management of her hypertension is:
A. Discontinue bevacizumab and proceed with FOLFOX today
B. Reduce the dose of bevacizumab to 2.5 mg/kg and proceed with treatment

C. Add an antihypertensive agent today
D. Hold all treatment today and recheck her blood pressure in 1 week
E. Switch his treatment regimen to FOLFIRI/bevacizumab

10. In metastatic colorectal cancer, mutations in which of these genes confers the greatest effect on prognosis?
A. KRAS
B. NRAS
C. PIK3CA
D. BRAF
E. PTEN

11. A 40-year-old male presents with left-upper-quadrant abdominal pain and occasional diarrhea. His workup includes an abdominal CT, which reveals a mass of the splenic flexure. No other sites of metastatic disease are noted. Colonoscopy reveals a partially obstructing mass and biopsy shows poorly differentiated adenocarcinoma. Patient underwent hemicolectomy 6 weeks earlier, when pathology revealed tumor penetrating through the muscularis propria, 5 of 27 lymph nodes positive for disease; lymphovascular and perineural invasion were present (pT3N2aM0). The tumor was found to be microsatellite-high (MSI-high) with loss of MSH2 noted by immunohistochemistry (IHC). Molecular testing reveals no mutations in RAS, but a BRAF V600E mutation is present. The patient has recovered well from surgery and is interested in the next steps for treatment. In addition to referral for genetic counseling, what is the best recommendation for this patient at this time?
A. Initiation of active surveillance and repeat colonoscopy in 1 year
B. FOLFOX chemotherapy for 6 months
C. FOLFOXIRI chemotherapy for 6 months
D. Pembrolizumab for 6 months
E. FOLFOX and cetuximab for 6 months

12. A 58-year-old female is diagnosed with stage IV colon cancer with metastases to the lungs. Biopsy demonstrates a NRAS mutation in codon 12 (G12D). She progresses on CAPOX in combination with bevacizumab after 8 months on treatment. She is then treated with FOLFIRI in combination with bevacizumab but develops progression after 4 months. She is treated with regorafenib, but progression of disease is seen on her first restaging study. She is subsequently treated with TAS-102 but again has progression of disease on her first restaging study. Her ECOG performance status is 1, and she wants further treatment. Which of the following is the best treatment recommendation at this time?
A. Referral for a clinical trial
B. Referral to hospice
C. Treatment with panitumumab
D. Capecitabine with bevacizumab
E. Surgical resection of pulmonary metastases

13. Which of the following alterations is most suggestive of sporadic microsatellite instability high (MSI-high) colorectal cancer?
A. MSH2 and PMS2
B. KRAS and PIK3CA
C. MSH6 and EPCAM
D. MLH1 and BRAF
E. TP53

14. A 39-year-old HIV-positive male presents with rectal bleeding. Flexible sigmoidoscopy reveals a mass in the anal canal. Biopsy reveals squamous cell carcinoma. Pelvic MRI and CT of the chest and abdomen reveal cT3N1M0 disease.

He receives chemoradiation with concurrent 5-FU and mitomycin. Following completion of chemoradiation, surveillance CT at 6 months reveals mediastinal lymphadenopathy and lung metastases. Biopsies confirm squamous cell carcinoma, consistent with recurrent metastatic disease. Patient receives 5-FU and cisplatin chemotherapy, but restaging studies after 2 months of therapy reveal progression of disease. His current ECOG performance status is 1. What is the next best step for management of this patient?
- **A.** Obtain RAS testing and consider treatment with cetuximab
- **B.** Referral for clinical trial
- **C.** 5-FU and mitomycin chemotherapy
- **D.** Palliative radiation to several lung metastases
- **E.** Capecitabine and temozolomide

15. A 68-year-old male presents with metastatic colorectal cancer with metastases to the liver and lungs. He is found to have no mutations in KRAS exon 2 (codons 12 and 13) or BRAF. He is initiated on FOLFOX and bevacizumab with a partial response noted at 4 months. At 12 months, he is found to have progression of disease in the lungs. He is switched to FOLFIRI and bevacizumab and has stable disease for 6 months, when he is found to have progression of disease, again in the lungs. His ECOG performance status is currently 1. What is the next appropriate step for this patient?
- **A.** Initiation of cetuximab and irinotecan
- **B.** Initiation of single-agent panitumumab
- **C.** Radiation therapy to the liver and lungs
- **D.** Send the tumor for expanded RAS testing
- **E.** Restart FOLFOX bevacizumab given his prior good response

16. A 70-year-old female is diagnosed with stage IV colon cancer with metastases to the liver and pelvic bones. Biopsy demonstrates no mutations in RAS or RAF. She is initially treated with FOLFOX and bevacizumab and then FOLFIRI cetuximab in the second-line setting. She is then placed on regorafenib 160 mg daily. A painful red palmar rash develops after 2 weeks of therapy. This was scored as a grade 1 reaction. Which of the following is the best treatment recommendation at this time?
- **A.** Immediate regorafenib discontinuation plus supportive care to address skin reaction
- **B.** Regorafenib dose interruption for 1 week plus supportive care
- **C.** Regorafenib dose reduction by 50% plus supportive care
- **D.** Regorafenib dose reduction by 75% plus supportive care
- **E.** Use supportive care to address skin reaction; alter dose after 1 week if no improvement

17. A 75-year-old male presents with occasional abdominal pain and fullness. CT of the abdomen and pelvis reveals what appears to be a well-circumscribed mass in the rectum and several small scattered liver lesions. Colonoscopy reveals a 4-cm mass in the rectum, and biopsy reveals well-differentiated neuroendocrine carcinoma with a Ki-67 less than 1%. Somatostatin scintigraphy reveals the primary tumor as well as several scattered liver metastases. The patient denies any history of flushing or diarrhea. What is the next best step for management?
- **A.** Initiation of lanreotide
- **B.** FOLFOX and bevacizumab
- **C.** Initiation of sunitinib
- **D.** Capecitabine and temozolomide
- **E.** Initiation of chemoradiation with concurrent capecitabine

18. Which of the following genes is associated with familial adenomatous polyposis (FAP)?
- **A.** BRAF
- **B.** MYH
- **C.** MLH1
- **D.** MSH6
- **E.** APC

19. A 27-year-old male presents with severe right-lower-quadrant pain, fever, and rebound tenderness on abdominal examination. CT abdomen/pelvis reveals an inflamed appendix, and the patient undergoes laparoscopic appendectomy. The pathology from the surgical specimen reveals a 0.9 cm focus of well-differentiated carcinoid tumor without evidence of lymphovascular or mesoappendiceal invasion. The patient has recovered well from surgery. What is the next best appropriate step for management?
- **A.** History and physical with tumor markers and consideration of CT or MRI imaging
- **B.** Recommend no further surveillance
- **C.** Referral to surgery for right hemicolectomy and lymphadenectomy
- **D.** FOLFOX chemotherapy for 6 months
- **E.** Surgical exploration and heated intraperitoneal chemotherapy (HIPEC)

20. A 71-year-old male presents for his second infusion of irinotecan and cetuximab for second-line treatment of RAS wild-type metastatic colorectal cancer following progression on FOLFOX and bevacizumab. During his first infusion 2 weeks earlier, 2 hours after the administration of irinotecan, he experienced diarrhea, emesis, diaphoresis, and abdominal cramping, which resolved approximately 4 hours later. The patient is nervous about being treated given his prior experience with the infusion. What is the next best step for managing the patient's symptoms?
- **A.** Discontinue irinotecan and continue with cetuximab alone
- **B.** Send for UGT1A1 testing
- **C.** Administration of atropine as a premedication prior to irinotecan infusion
- **D.** Discontinue cetuximab and continue irinotecan alone
- **E.** Check for DPD deficiency

21. A 42-year-old HIV-positive male presents to clinic with reports of occasional anal bleeding. Anoscopy reveals an anal margin lesion, and biopsy shows a well-differentiated squamous cell carcinoma. CT of the chest and abdomen reveals no evidence of distant metastatic disease. Pelvic MRI points to a small mass in the anal canal with no evidence of lymphadenopathy. He is staged cT1N0M0 and undergoes surgical resection of the lesion, revealing pT1 disease. Surgical margins are clear, and all margins are noted to be greater than 1 cm. What is the next best step for management?
- **A.** Routine surveillance
- **B.** Referral back to surgery for reexcision
- **C.** Chemoradiation with concurrent 5-FU/mitomycin
- **D.** Adjuvant 5-FU/cisplatin
- **E.** Short-course radiation to the surgical site

22. A 53-year-old female with KRAS-mutated metastatic colorectal cancer (G13D) received 6 cycles of mFOLFOX6 with bevacizumab. She was then treated with maintenance capecitabine and bevacizumab. Four months after initiating maintenance therapy, she is found on CT to have progression of disease with enlarging liver metastases. She has no peripheral neuropathy. What treatment option would *not* be recommended at this time?
- **A.** FOLFOX/bevacizumab

B. FOLFIRI/bevacizumab
C. FOLFIRI/ziv-aflibercept
D. FOLFIRI/cetuximab
E. FOLFIRI/ramucirumab

23. A 78-year-old female presents to her PCP for a regularly scheduled visit to manage her diabetes mellitus (DM). She has a history of poorly controlled DM with diabetic neuropathy and coronary artery disease (CAD) superimposed on a myocardial infarction 10 years earlier. Blood work shows her Hba1c to be 9.8 g/dL, creatinine at 1.5, and hemoglobin 7.9 g/dL with a MCV of 72. Iron studies reveal a ferritin of 2. She is referred for a colonoscopy to evaluate her iron-deficiency anemia. A right-sided colonic mass is found, which shows to be a moderately differentiated adenocarcinoma. She has a laparoscopic right hemicolectomy and is found to have a T3N1 colon cancer with 1/16 LN+. She is referred to oncology for adjuvant recommendations. You recommend:
    A. Adjuvant 5-FU and oxaliplatin (FOLFOX) × 4 to 6 cycles
    B. Adjuvant capecitabine × 6 cycles
    C. Adjuvant oxaliplatin × 6 cycles
    D. Watchful waiting with surveillance physical exam, blood work, and imaging every 3 to 6 months
    E. Discharge to PCP

24. A 60-year-old male in excellent health presents for his screening colonoscopy. His earlier screening colonoscopy at age 50 was unremarkable. He is found to have a friable mass of the transverse colon that is biopsy-positive for moderately well-differentiated colon cancer. At surgery, his cancer is resected and staged at T3N0 with 0/25 LN+, with no lymphovascular invasion (LVI) or perineural invasion (PNI). Baseline CEA prior to surgery is 2.4. He is referred to oncology for adjuvant therapy recommendations. You recommend:
    A. Adjuvant 5-FU and oxaliplatin (FOLFOX) × 4 to 6 cycles
    B. Adjuvant capecitabine × 6 cycles
    C. Adjuvant oxaliplatin
    D. Watchful waiting with surveillance physical exam, blood work, and imaging every 3 to 6 months
    E. Discharge to PCP

25. A 60-year-old male in excellent health presents for his screening colonoscopy. His earlier screening colonoscopy at age 50 was unremarkable. He is found to have a friable transverse colon mass that is biopsy-positive for moderately well-differentiated colon cancer. At surgery, his cancer is resected and staged at T3N0 with none of 25 lymph nodes involved, + LVI and + PNI, mismatch repair–deficient/MIS-high (MMR-d/MSI-H). Baseline CEA prior to surgery is 2.4. He is referred to oncology for adjuvant therapy recommendations. You recommend:
    A. Adjuvant 5-FU and oxaliplatin (FOLFOX) × 4 to 6 cycles owing to +LVI/PNI
    B. Adjuvant capecitabine × 6 cycles owing to +LVI/PNI
    C. Adjuvant 5-FU and oxaliplatin (FOLFOX) × 4 to 6 cycles owing to stage II disease
    D. Adjuvant capecitabine × 6 cycles owing to stage II disease
    E. Watchful waiting with surveillance physical exam, blood work, and imaging every 3 to 6 months as MMR-d/MSI-H portends an excellent prognosis

26. A 65-year-old male presents to his PCP with a 3-month history of crampy abdominal pain. He reports widespread abdominal pain 2 to 3 times a day that comes on without exacerbating factors but seems to be relieved with defecation. CT imaging is ordered, and he is found to have a sigmoid colon mass. On colonoscopy he has a near-obstructive lesion and is taken to surgery for definitive resection. Pathology reveals a T3N2a poorly differentiated cancer with 4/18 LN+, + lymphovascular invasion, − perineural invasion. His preoperative CEA is 5.3 and is normalizes postoperatively. What do you recommend as the next step for his cancer care?
    A. Adjuvant 5-FU and oxaliplatin (FOLFOX) × 4 to 6 cycles
    B. Adjuvant capecitabine × 6 cycles
    C. Adjuvant oxaliplatin
    D. Watchful waiting with surveillance physical exam, blood work, and imaging every 3 to 6 months
    E. Discharge to PCP

27. A 30-year old female presents with an 18-month history of bleeding with bowel movements that began during her first pregnancy. At that time she was diagnosed with hemorrhoids, but the rectal bleeding has persisted. She is found to have a rectal mass 8 cm from the verge that is biopsied and found to be adenocarcinoma. Full staging workup reveals a clinically staged T3N1 rectal cancer. The patient reports that she is still interested in having more children. Which of the following is *not* a true statement when you are counseling her?
    A. Standard chemoradiation therapy will likely render her infertile.
    B. Radiation dose can be modified in the regions of her ovaries and uterus to likely preserve her fertility.
    C. Prophylactic surgery to relocate her ovaries out of the radiation field can preserve her ovarian function.
    D. If the patient has a partner, prophylactic harvest of oocytes and in vitro fertilization and cryopreservation can be a successful strategy to have a biological child, though a surrogate may be necessary.
    E. Neoadjuvant chemoradiation is as effective as adjuvant chemoradiation but has fewer chronic side effects.

28. A 53-year old man presents with perirectal pain and stool caliber changes, with now 10 days of significant tenesmus with abdominal cramping at each attempt of defecation. On colonoscopy he is found to have an almost completely obstructing rectal mass at 10 cm from the anal verge. Clinical and radiological staging reveals no distant metastases with T3N1 disease. Which of the following is *not* an acceptable management strategy at this time?
    A. Immediate diverting colostomy followed by chemoradiation and then definitive resection
    B. Expedited radiation simulation, with treatment starting within the week
    C. Chemotherapy with 5-FU and oxaliplatin (FOLFOX) starting within the next week
    D. Chemoradiation with 5-fluorouracil-based chemotherapy and radiation to 5040 cGy, starting within the accepted 2- to 3-week average starting time
    E. Counseling regarding symptoms to expect with bowel obstruction

29. A 64-year-old female presents for her screening colonoscopy and is found to have a rectal mass 3 cm from the anal verge. Biopsy returns as moderately differentiated adenocarcinoma. CT scan of the chest, abdomen, and pelvis reveals no distant metastases. Which of the following should be used to stage her T and N status?
    A. The CT scan she has had is sufficient
    B. FDG-PET scan
    C. MRI of the pelvis
    D. Endoscopic ultrasound
    E. Either C or D

30. A 34-year old male presents to urgent care with rectal bleeding and pain. Blood work reveals a hemoglobin of 10.3 g/dL; on physical exam, he has a firm, palpable mass 3 cm from the anal verge. After referral to a gastroenterologist, the patient has a colonoscopy, which confirms the location of the mass; on biopsy it is found to be a rectal adenocarcinoma. MRI of the pelvis shows a T4N0 tumor with involvement of the internal anal sphincter. Which of the following is *not* accurate in terms of initial counseling about his disease?
    A. The patient will be able to avoid a permanent colostomy if he undergoes chemoradiation.
    B. There is an opportunity to avoid a permanent colostomy if he has an excellent response to preoperative chemoradiation.
    C. There is no opportunity to avoid a permanent colostomy owing to involvement of the internal anal sphincter, so he does not need preoperative chemoradiation and can go to definitive abdominoperineal resection now.
    D. He requires chemoradiation in all circumstances.
    E. A and C.

31. A 69-year-old male has recently completed neoadjuvant chemoradiation followed by a low anterior resection with diverting ileostomy. At the time of diagnosis, clinical staging with MRI revealed a T3 tumor with 4- to 5-subcentimeter lymph nodes in the perirectal area. Surgical pathology revealed a complete pathological response with none of 12 lymph nodes involved. He presents now for recommendations for care. Which of the following are reasonable options?
    A. Adjuvant chemotherapy with capecitabine
    B. Adjuvant chemotherapy with 5-FU and oxaliplatin (FOLFOX or CAPOX) × 6 cycles
    C. Watchful waiting with physical exam, blood work including tumor markers, and imaging every 4 to 6 months
    D. All are reasonable options

32. A 47-year-old female presents to an oncologist for recommendations for her care. She was recently was hospitalized for acute onset right-lower-quadrant pain and diagnosed with appendicitis. At surgery, her appendix was inflamed without perforation and an appendectomy was performed. Pathology revealed a T2, 7-mm focus of invasive adenocarcinoma with negative margins. You recommend:
    A. Diagnostic laparoscopy to assess for any signs of tumor involvement of the right colon or regional lymph nodes
    B. Completion right hemicolectomy with lymph node dissection
    C. Total colectomy
    D. Surveillance with physical exam, blood work including CEA, and scans every 4 to 6 months for the next 2 years
    E. Discharge to PCP with no further follow-up needed

33. A 23-year-old male presents to the emergency room with a large lower gastrointestinal bleed. On colonoscopy, he is found to have hundreds of polyps carpeting his colon, with a dominant, friable mass in his sigmoid colon; it is biopsied and found to be a well-differentiated adenocarcinoma. Which of the following is *not* true regarding the genetic cancer predisposition syndrome that he likely has?
    A. It arises from a mutation in the APC gene.
    B. It is autosomal dominant.
    C. It causes a predisposition to colon cancer, endometrial cancer, and ovarian cancer.
    D. It has a 100% chance of resulting in colon cancer.
    E. Patients should be referred for total colectomy.

34. A 54-year-old female presents to Medical Oncology with a new diagnosis of stage IV right-sided colon cancer with metastasis to the lungs, liver, and peritoneum. Molecular testing on the tumor shows a KRAS mutation in codon 12. Which of the following is *not* an appropriate first-line chemotherapy option for her?
    A. 5-FU and oxaliplatin (FOLFOX) with bevacizumab
    B. 5-FU and oxaliplatin (FOLFOX or CAPOX) with cetuximab
    C. 5-FU and irinotecan (FOLFIRI) with bevacizumab
    D. 5-FU, irinotecan, and oxaliplatin (FOLFOXIRI) with bevacizumab
    E. Capecitabine and oxaliplatin (CAPOX) with bevacizumab

35. A 61-year-old female presents for a follow-up visit with her medical oncologist. She was diagnosed 18 months earlier with KRAS wild-type metastatic colon cancer to the lungs and was treated with 5-FU, oxaliplatin, and bevacizumab for 12 months. Her disease progressed and has been on 5-FU, irinotecan, and cetuximab for 6 months. A CT scan taken a week earlier shows progressive disease in the lungs and new lesions in the liver. Which of the following is a reasonable next treatment option?
    A. Regorafenib
    B. Radiation to the liver lesions
    C. 5-FU, oxaliplatin, and bevacizumab
    D. Panitumumab
    E. Referral to surgery for debulking

36. A 59-year-old female with widely metastatic KRAS-mutated colorectal cancer has been treated with 5-FU, irinotecan, oxaliplatin, capecitabine, bevacizumab, and regorafenib. After discussion with her medical oncologist, she decides to move forward with therapy with TAS-102. What grade 3 side effect is she most likely to experience?
    A. Nausea and vomiting
    B. Diarrhea
    C. Neutropenia
    D. Liver function abnormalities
    E. Thrombocytopenia

37. A 44-year-old female presents for initial medical oncology consultation after a new diagnosis of colon cancer metastatic to the liver. She has seen a liver surgeon, and her disease has been deemed unresectable. You recommend systemic chemotherapy. Which of the following in *not* correct when you counsel her?
    A. Chemotherapy backbones with 5-FU and oxaliplatin (FOLFOX) versus 5-FU and irinotecan (FOLFIRI) are equivalent in the first-line setting.
    B. 5-FU, irinotecan, and oxaliplatin (FOLFOXIRI) may be superior to FOLFOX or FOLFIRI in combination with bevacizumab but the combination has added toxicity.
    C. After first-line combination chemotherapy, maintenance chemotherapy +/− bevacizumab prolongs progression-free survival (PFS) and overall survival.
    D. The average life span for a patient with metastatic colon cancer is 2½ years.
    E. Maintenance chemotherapy if the patient is stable on first-line chemotherapy prolongs PFS.

38. Which of the following are contraindications to continuing bevacizumab therapy in colon cancer patients?
    A. Deep venous thrombosis
    B. Wound dehiscence
    C. Uncontrolled hypertension

D. Moderate chronic kidney disease (glomerular filtration rate [GFR] 30 to 59 mL/min per 1.73 m²)

E. Central nervous system (CNS) metastases

39. Which of the following statements is NOT true about anti-EGFR inhibitors cetuximab and panitumumab?

A. They do not provide benefit to patients who have a mutation in KRAS, BRAF, or NRAS.

B. The acneiform rash associated with the agents almost always decreases with time on therapy.

C. Prophylaxis with sunscreen, emollients, and oral doxycycline can decrease the prevalence and severity of rash.

D. The agents can be used in combination with 5-FU and oxaliplatin (FOLFOX) and 5-FU and irinotecan (FOLFIRI) as well as single agents.

E. There is no known benefit to switching between agents once a patient has progressed on one.

40. A 71-year-old female has an appointment with her medical oncologist to discuss the next steps in her therapy. She was diagnosed with metastatic cecal cancer 2½ years earlier. Her cancer is RAS wild-type, and she has received treatment with 5-FU, oxaliplatin, irinotecan, capecitabine, bevacizumab, cetuximab, TAS-102, and, most recently, regorafenib, all with disease progression. Her performance status is ECOG 1, but she reports that she does feel her quality of life has suffered over the past 2 years owing to side effects of her chemotherapy. Options for the next step in her therapy include:

A. Supportive care with a focus on symptom management

B. Referral for a clinical trial

C. Molecular profiling for assessment of actionable mutations with available drugs

D. Counseling that insurance may or may not cover the molecular profiling and/or the drugs and that the chance of actionable mutation is slim for patients with colon cancer

E. All of the above

41. A 43-year-old male with HIV presents to his colorectal surgeon for follow-up evaluation. The patient has a long history of perianal fistulas complicated by multiple bouts of recurrent abscesses requiring surgical drainage and antibiotics over the preceding 3 years, including ICU admission for sepsis. He is currently on chronically suppressive antibiotics and has an enhancing fluid collection that has not resolved with surgical drainage over the past 6 months. On rigid proctoscopic examination, a firm mass is found along the fistula tract that is biopsied and reported as squamous cell cancer. MRI imaging confirms the mass, along with enlarged perirectal lymph nodes but no distant metastases. Radiation oncology recommends concurrent chemoradiation and consults oncology for chemotherapy recommendations. You recommend:

A. Mitomycin C days 1 and 29 and 5-fluorouracil (5-FU) infusion days 1 to 4 and 29 to 32 with growth factor support and concurrent XRT

B. Cisplatin days 1 and 29 and 5-FU infusion on days 1 to 4 and 29 to 32 and growth factor support with concurrent x-ray therapy (XRT)

C. Mitomycin C on days 1 and 29 and 5-FU infusion on days 1 to 4 and 29 to 32 with growth factor support

D. XRT alone

E. Surgery alone

42. A 54-year-old male presents to his PCP with rectal bleeding. On digital rectal exam the patient is found to have a firm, fixed 1.5-cm tumor at the dentate line, which biopsy reveals to be squamous cell cancer. On referral to a colorectal surgeon, the patient is found to have an enlarged right inguinal lymph node 1.0 cm in diameter. FDG-PET reveals a highly FDG-avid anal mass and moderately avid right inguinal lymph node. What is the next step in this patient's care?

A. Biopsy of the right inguinal lymph node

B. Mitomycin C on days 1 and 29 and 5-FU infusion on days 1 to 4 and 29 to 32 with concurrent XRT using standard radiation ports

C. Mitomycin C on days 1 and 29 and 5-FU infusion on days 1 to 4 and 29 to 32 with concurrent XRT using standard radiation ports and a boost to the inguinal lymph nodes

D. Cisplatin on days 1 and 29 and 5-FU infusion on days 1 to 4 and 29 to 32 with concurrent XRT using standard radiation ports and a boost to the inguinal lymph nodes

E. Referral back to the surgeon for an abdominoperineal resection with end colostomy and inguinal lymph node dissection

43. A 60-year-old female is diagnosed with a T3N0 squamous anal cancer 1 cm from the anal verge, confirmed by biopsy, endoscopic ultrasound (EUS), and fluorodeoxyglucose positron emission tomography (FDG-PET) evaluation during initial staging. She is treated with concurrent chemoradiation with mitomycin C on days 1 and 29 and 5-FU infusion on days 1 to 4 and 29 to 32. FDG-PET scan performed 2 months after surgery shows complete resolution of the mass and rigid anoscopy shows a scar at the tumor site that is biopsy negative for malignancy. What should be the plan going forward?

A. Refer to surgery for resection of the tumor site

B. Adjuvant chemotherapy with cisplatin and 5-fluorouracil

C. Radiation boost to scar area

D. Observation with digital rectal exam and anoscopy every 3 to 6 months for the next 5 years and annual imaging for the first 3 years

E. Discharge to PCP

44. A 56-year-old female with pain with defecation presents to a gastroenterologist for evaluation. Rigid anoscopy reveals a 1-cm mass 3 cm from the anal verge. EUS, MRI, and PET scan confirm a T1N0 lesion clinically with no distant metastases. How should this patient be treated?

A. Definitive surgical resection

B. Mitomycin C days 1 and 29 and 5-fluorouracil infusion days 1 to 4 and 29 to 32 with concurrent XRT

C. Mitomycin C days 1 and 29 and 5-fluorouracil infusion days 1 to 4 and 29 to 32

D. Radiation alone

E. Topical 5-fluorauracil per rectum

45. A 53-year-old male presents with perirectal pain, changes in stool caliber, and a 10-day history of significant tenesmus with abdominal cramping on each attempt at defecation. On colonoscopy he is found to have an almost completely obstructing rectal mass 10 cm from the anal verge. Clinical and radiological staging reveals no distant metastases with T3N1 disease. Which of the following is *not* an acceptable management strategy at this time?

A. Immediate diverting colostomy followed by chemoradiation and then definitive resection

B. Expedited radiation simulation, with treatment starting within the week

C. Chemotherapy with 5-FU and oxaliplatin (FOLFOX) starting within the next week

D. Chemoradiation with 5-FU-based chemotherapy and radiation to 5040 cGy, starting within the accepted 2- to 3-week average starting time

E. Counseling regarding symptoms to expect with bowel obstruction

46. A 69-year-old male has recently completed neoadjuvant chemoradiation followed by a low anterior resection with diverting ileostomy. At the time of diagnosis, clinical staging with MRI revealed a T3 tumor with 4- to 5-subcentimeter lymph nodes in the perirectal area. Surgical pathology revealed a complete pathological response with none of 12 lymph nodes involved. He presents now for recommendations for care. Which of the following are reasonable options?

A. Adjuvant chemotherapy with capecitabine

B. Adjuvant chemotherapy with 5-FU and oxaliplatin (FOLFOX or CAPOX) × 6 cycles

C. Watchful waiting with physical exam, blood work including tumor markers, and imaging every 4 to 6 months

D. All are reasonable options

47. A 47-year-old female presents to an oncologist for recommendations for her care. She was recently hospitalized for acute onset right-lower-quadrant pain and diagnosed with appendicitis. At surgery, her appendix was inflamed without perforation and an appendectomy was performed. Pathology revealed a T2, 7-mm focus of invasive adenocarcinoma with negative margins. You recommend:

A. Diagnostic laparoscopy to assess for any signs of tumor involvement of the right colon or regional lymph nodes

B. Completion right hemicolectomy with lymph node dissection

C. Total colectomy

D. Surveillance with physical exam, blood work including CEA, and scans every 4 to 6 months for the next 2 years

E. Discharge to PCP with no further follow-up needed

48. A 64-year old female presents for her screening colonoscopy and is found to have a rectal mass 3 cm from the anal verge. Biopsy shows a moderately differentiated adenocarcinoma. CT of the chest/abdomen/and pelvis reveals no distant metastases. Which of the following should be used to stage her T and N status?

A. The CT scan she has had is sufficient

B. FDG-PET scan

C. MRI of the pelvis

D. Endoscopic ultrasound

E. Either C or D

49. A 59-year-old female with widely metastatic KRAS-mutated colorectal cancer has been treated with 5-FU, irinotecan, oxaliplatin, capecitabine, bevacizumab, and regorafenib. After discussion with her medical oncologist, she decides to move forward with therapy with TAS-102. What grade 3 side effect is she most likely to experience?

A. Nausea and vomiting

B. Diarrhea

C. Neutropenia

D. Liver function abnormalities

E. Thrombocytopenia

ANSWERS

1. C

Second-line therapy in combination with bevacizumab is preferred presuming that there are no other absolute contraindications to anti-VEGF therapy. Treatment with an EGFR-inhibitor is contraindicated given the patient's KRAS mutation, and the combination of VEGF and EGFR inhibitors has been shown to be harmful. Vemurafenib is not approved for the treatment of metastatic colorectal cancer.

2. A

Treatment with TAS-102 is approved for refractory colorectal cancer based on results from the RECOURSE trial. On the basis of numerous retrospective studies showing a lack of benefit in patients with metastatic colorectal cancer harboring NRAS mutations. Single-agent bevacizumab is unlikely to show benefit in this patient, and surgical resection is not recommended in patients with widely distributed metastatic disease unless for palliative benefit.

3. B

This patient presents with stage II colon adenocarcinoma without high-risk features. High-risk factors for recurrence include poorly differentiated histology (exclusive of MSI-H), lymphatic/vascular invasion, bowel obstruction, less than 12 lymph nodes examined, PNI, localized

perforation, or positive margins. FOLFIRI is not an approved regimen for adjuvant therapy for colorectal cancer.

4. C

BRAF mutations are rarely seen in combination with RAS mutations; the two are thought to be mutually exclusive. BRAF mutant colorectal cancer is associated with a poorer prognosis and disease-free survival. These mutations are more frequently seen in older patients, women, and with right-sided colorectal cancer, but BRAF mutations are still found in only 5% to 10% of the patient population. Single-agent vemurafenib has not been shown to be effective in BRAF V600E mutant metastatic colorectal cancer.

5. A

Initiation of chemoradiation with concurrent 5-FU and mitomycin is the appropriate treatment for this patient. Surgery is recommended as the primary treatment for T1N0 well-differentiated lesions, but chemoradiation is the preferred initial treatment for more advanced disease. Observation, radiation alone, or systemic therapy without radiation are not recommended.

6. E

For this patient, although she has poor differentiation seen on histology (a high risk factor), the recurrence risk for MSI-high stage II colorectal cancer is low. Therefore adjuvant therapy is not warranted in this case. However, given the finding of high MSI and the patient's relatively young age at diagnosis, genetic counseling is recommended. FOLFIRI is not an approved regimen for adjuvant therapy in colorectal cancer, and pembrolizumab is not an approved therapy for use in adjuvant therapy at this time.

7. B

Development of an acneiform (papulopustular) rash is a common cutaneous adverse reaction to EGFR inhibitors. Appropriate management of a grade 2 rash would include topical corticosteroids and oral antibiotics with or without topical corticosteroids. These interventions should be attempted prior to a change in either dose, frequency, or a change in the regimen. Treatment of a grade 2 rash with low-potency topical steroids alone will be unlikely to resolve the symptoms.

8. C

As demonstrated in the German Rectal Cancer Study, the benefits of neoadjuvant as compared with adjuvant chemoradiotherapy include a superior sphincter preservation rate, a lower rate of anastomotic stenosis as a long-term complication of pelvic RT, and better local control while providing similar long-term survival. Therefore this is the recommended approach for a patient with T3 or higher disease or node-positive rectal cancer. Neoadjuvant FOL-FOX in combination with cetuximab is not a recommended regimen for preoperative therapy in cases of locally advanced rectal adenocarcinoma.

9. C

Hypertension is a common side effect of bevacizumab. The hypertension is typically managed with antihypertensive medication with good success. Given the survival benefit of bevacizumab in colorectal cancer, it is preferable to treat the side effect and proceed with therapy. Decreasing the dose may reduce efficacy and may not improve the blood pressure. A switch to FOLFIRI/bevacizumab is not indicated at this time.

10. D

BRAF V600E mutant metastatic colorectal cancer is associated with significantly decreased progression-free and overall survival, with one retrospective study showing a difference in median overall survival of 10.4 months versus 34.7 months. Mutations in KRAS and NRAS appear to be largely predictive of benefit from anti-EGFR therapy. The predictive and prognostic roles of PIK3CA and PTEN are currently unclear, with several retrospective studies showing differing results.

11. B

This patient has stage IIIB colorectal cancer; thus the recommendation in a healthy adult would be to treat with adjuvant FOLFOX for 6 months. Although the patient is MSI-high because he has positive lymph nodes and stage III disease, the recommendation would be to proceed with chemotherapy as opposed to active surveillance. Irinotecan should not be given in the adjuvant setting owing to the lack of benefit. Pembrolizumab has no indication in the adjuvant setting, though clinical trials are investigating the potential benefit in patients with MSI-high colon cancer. Cetuximab is not approved for adjuvant therapy because of the lack of an overall survival benefit.

12. A

Given that the patient has a good performance status and is motivated to continue treatment, referral for a clinical trial is the best option at this time. Given that the patient's tumor harbors a NRAS mutation, she is unlikely to benefit from EGFR-directed therapy. She has already had progression on capecitabine and bevacizumab and is unlikely to have a response. Surgical resection can sometimes be utilized in oligometastatic disease, but that is not indicated at this time.

13. D

Colorectal cancer that demonstrates microsatellite instability (MSI) is caused by either germline mismatch repair (MMR) gene mutations, or "sporadic" somatic tumor MLH1 promoter methylation, which is correlated with tumor BRAF V600E mutation status. Alterations in MSH2, MSH6, PMS2, and EPCAM are suggestive of a germline MMR. KRAS, PIK3CA, and TP53 alterations are not suggestive of MSI.

14. B

This patient presents with refractory metastatic squamous cell carcinoma of the anal canal. 5-FU and cisplatin is the only current recommended therapy for metastatic anal cancer. Given this patient's refractory disease, referral for clinical trial is the appropriate step at this point. Cetuximab is not approved for metastatic anal cancer. 5-FU with mitomycin is unlikely to be effective in this setting. Palliative radiation is not recommended at this time given that not all target lesions can be treated. Capecitabine and temozolomide are not approved for the treatment of metastatic anal cancer.

15. D

The patient's tumor was initially sent for KRAS exon 2 testing only. However, current guidelines recommend testing for additional exons in KRAS (3 and 4) as well as NRAS exons 2, 3, and 4, since mutations in these genes confer resistance to EGFR inhibitors. Radiation therapy to the liver and lungs may add limited benefit with unacceptable toxicity. FOLFOX and bevacizumab would be expected to have a low response rate given the patient's prior treatment history.

16. E

Hand-foot skin reaction is a common side effect of regorafenib therapy. If grade 1 hand-foot skin reaction is noted, regorafenib can be continued with good supportive care, including avoiding hot water, using moisturizing lotion, and wearing cotton gloves and socks at night. Grade 2 reactions can be managed by reducing the dose by 50% and giving supportive care, including the use of a moisturizing cream, clobetasol ointment twice daily, and topical analgesics. If a grade 3 reaction is noted, dosing should be interrupted and supportive care given.

17. A

This patient has been diagnosed with a well-differentiated, low-grade neuroendocrine carcinoma of the rectum with liver metastases. This appears to be a nonfunctioning tumor with no history of flushing or diarrhea. In this scenario, lanreotide has been shown to improve PFS, as shown in the CLARINET trial. FOLFOX and bevacizumab would be a reasonable regimen for colorectal adenocarcinoma. Sunitinib is approved for pancreatic neuroendocrine carcinoma. Capecitabine with temozolomide has unclear benefit in this patient population, and initiation of chemoradiation with concurrent capecitabine would be reasonable if the patient had colorectal adenocarcinoma with only locoregional disease.

18. E

FAP accounts for less than 1% of all colorectal cancers and can lead to multiple polyps in the colon and rectum. Mutations in the *APC* gene causes FAP, and most patients have a family history of the condition. Mutations in the *MYH* gene causes MYH-associated polyposis, marked by multiple precancerous polyps in the colon and rectum, similar in number to those seen in a milder form of FAP. *MLH1 and MSH6* are associated with Lynch syndrome.

19. B

Per NCCN guidelines, patients with appendiceal carcinoid tumors less than 2 cm do not require routine surveillance, and tests should be ordered only as clinically indicated. For tumors greater than 2 cm, a history and physical is recommended between 3 and 12 months after resection as well as consideration of tumor markers (5-HIAA, chromogranin) and abdominal imaging. After the first year, a history and physical and consideration of tumor markers is recommended every 6 to 12 months. FOLFOX chemotherapy is typically used for adjuvant therapy for colorectal adenocarcinomas. Surgical debulking and HIPEC is a strategy that is sometimes used for metastatic carcinoid tumors.

20. C

This patient is experiencing irinotecan-induced cholinergic hyperstimulation syndrome. The action is mediated by inhibition of acetylcholinesterase and by direct binding to and stimulation of muscarinic receptors. Symptoms can be inhibited by administration of atropine. Patients homozygous for *UGT1A1*28* are at elevated risk of neutropenia. The symptoms described by the patient do not fit the scenario typically seen with cetuximab infusion reactions. DPD deficiency can cause severe neutropenia, mucositis, and diarrhea in patients treated with 5-FU or capecitabine, but DPD deficiency has not been associated with increased toxicity to irinotecan.

21. A

Anal margin lesions (defined as the area at the anal verge including the perianal skin over a 5- to 6-cm radius from the squamous mucocutaneous junction) can be treated with either local excision or chemoradiation depending on the clinical stage. Primary treatment for patients with T1, N0 well-differentiated anal margin cancers is by local excision with adequate margins, defined as margins of 1 cm or greater. If margins are not adequate, reexcision is the preferred treatment option. Local radiation therapy with or without chemotherapy can be considered as an alternative treatment option when surgical margins are inadequate.

22. D

For this patient receiving maintenance chemotherapy with progression, a return to FOLFOX/bevacizumab would be reasonable presuming that she has grade 1 or less peripheral neuropathy. FOLFIRI in combination with bevacizumab, ziv-aflibercept, and ramucirumab would all be reasonable second-line options, given data from the TML, VELOUR, and RAISE studies respectively. Although retrospective data have shown the possibility of benefit of cetuximab in patients with G13D KRAS mutations, prospective studies have failed to show an improvement in this patient population. Therefore FOLFIRI/cetuximab would not be recommended for this patient.

23. B

The standard-of-care therapy for patients with stage III colon cancer, defined as lymph node–positive disease without metastatic disease, is oxaliplatin plus 5-FU.

However, in patients with a contraindication to oxaliplatin—for example, in this patient with existing neuropathy—studies have reported that 5-FU–based therapy alone may be used as an alternative. In particular, the X-ACT study randomized 1987 patients with resected stage III disease to capecitabine versus bolus 5-FU. The patient population that received capecitabine had equivalent 3-year disease-free survival in overall survival. Disease-free survival was 64% versus 61% with a $P = .5$, and overall survival was 81% versus 78% with a $P = .07$ favoring capecitabine.

24. D

This patient has low-risk stage II colon cancer. His cancer is well differentiated, he has an adequate lymph node dissection with 25 lymph nodes examined, and he has no lymphovascular or perineural invasion. Accordingly this patient would not be offered adjuvant chemotherapy. He should still receive surveillance for his colon cancer with physical exam, blood work including tumor marker CEA, and imaging.

25. E

This patient had a stage II colon cancer with lymphovascular and perineural invasion. Although these are considered as higher-risk features, the fact that the patient has mismatch repair-deficiency/microsatellite instability puts the patient in an excellent prognostic category. Because of their excellent prognosis, patients with stage II disease that have deficient mismatch repair should not be offered adjuvant chemotherapy.

26. A

The patient has stage III disease as defined by lymph node involvement. He also has lymphovascular and perineural invasion, but his adjuvant chemotherapy is determined by his node positivity, which makes him a stage III cancer patient. Standard-of-care adjuvant therapy is 5-FU and oxaliplatin. The standard of care is based on two major clinical trials, the MOSAIC study and the NSABP C-07 trial. Both showed an improvement in disease-free survival, and the MOSAIC study also showed an improvement in overall survival in long-term follow-up for stage III cancer patients. Capecitabine with oxaliplatin is also a reasonable adjuvant therapy regimen.

27. B

Preservation of fertility is an important issue to discuss for the patients who are still in their childbearing years and who have stage II or III rectal cancer requiring chemoradiation to help prevent local or regional recurrence. For women, the radiation port will likely cover the uterus as well as the ovaries, which can create a permanently inhospitable environment for carrying a pregnancy to term. Radiation to the ovaries can also cause ovarian failure in a high proportion of patients. Strategies to preserve fertility include surgically moving the ovaries as well as harvesting oocytes, which may be more viable if they are fertilized.

28. D

The patient has an obstructing rectal mass that is very likely to cause a bowel obstruction in the near future. A diverting colostomy followed by definitive treatment is a reasonable and safe plan for the care of this patient. If the patient is being cared for in a center where chemotherapy or radiation can be started very quickly, he could be started on chemoradiation or chemotherapy within the next few days, since to most patients have a rapid improvement in symptoms as soon as treatment with either of these modalities begins. It would not be safe to wait 2 to 3 weeks before beginning chemotherapy or chemoradiation; emergent surgery for bowel obstruction has much greater morbidity than elective correction of the obstruction.

29. E

Appropriate staging of the T and N status of rectal cancer patients is particularly important, because if such a patient has a response to neoadjuvant chemoradiation, the surgical staging is likely to understage him or her. CT scans do not provide enough pelvic visibility to properly stage rectal cancer patients. FDG-PET scans can be used to evaluate for distant disease, but also do not have enough resolution to evaluate for nodal disease; in addition, not all rectal cancer patients will have PET avid tumors. Either an MRI of the pelvis or an endoscopic ultrasound can be utilized to properly stage the T and N status of rectal cancer patients, with the caveat that endoscopic ultrasound is best used in clinical centers or with physicians with significant experience in using it for cancer staging.

30. E

The creation of a colostomy, either temporary or permanent, is a major psychological issue for patients undergoing treatment for rectal cancer. Involvement of the internal anal sphincter often requires the patient to have an abdominoperineal resection with permanent colostomy formation. However, even the patient with internal anal sphincter involvement may be able to have a permanent colostomy-sparing surgery if he or she has an excellent response to chemoradiation. Best practice is to acknowledge the real risk of a possible colostomy, but the patient should be advised that these questions will be better answered after neoadjuvant chemoradiation and perhaps even only at surgery.

31. D

The benefit of adjuvant chemotherapy in patients who undergo preoperative chemoradiation is controversial. In the EORTC 22921 study, patients who received preoperative radiation underwent randomization to four cycles of postoperative 5-FU and leucovorin versus no further therapy. In a subgroup analysis of patients who underwent a complete R0 resection, the addition of postoperative chemotherapy significantly improved overall survival in those whose tumors were downstaged to T0 from T2 but not those staged at T3/T4. However, other studies have failed to show a better outcome with postoperative chemotherapy in patients with greater downstaging. The PROCTOR/SCRIPT study, where patients underwent radiation followed by total mesorectal excision, also showed no difference in overall survival if patients received postoperative capecitabine versus observation. A phase 3 study from the United Kingdom, a clinical trial, looked at people who received postoperative capecitabine and oxaliplatin versus no adjuvant chemotherapy. There was a trend toward improved disease-free survival in those patients, but the study was closed when it had significant issues with approval. In patients with an excellent response to therapy, it is reasonable to consider treatment with 5-FU and oxaliplatin, 5-FU compound alone, or even observation.

32. B

Incidental adenocarcinoma found at the time of an appendectomy should be treated with a return to the OR for a completion hemicolectomy and lymph node dissection to accurately stage the patient's disease. Adjuvant chemotherapy can then be determined based on this staging.

33. C

FAP accounts for less than 1% of colon cancer. This is an autosomal dominant genetic predisposition syndrome resulting from a mutation in the APC gene. Such patients are at risk for developing colon cancer, with 100% penetrance usually at an average age of 45. These patients are also at increased risk for gastric cancers, adenomas, and duodenal polyps as well as thyroid cancer and CNS tumors, mostly medulloblastoma. The patient should be referred for a total colectomy owing to the complete penetrance of this genetic syndrome.

34. B

Multiple randomized phase 3 clinical trials have confirmed the equivalence of 5 fluorouracil (5-FU) and oxaliplatin chemotherapy and 5-FU and irinotecan chemotherapy in the first-line metastatic colorectal cancer setting. For all patients, the addition of the targeted agent bevacizumab has been shown to improve PFS and, in conflicting studies, overall survival. Recent studies have also shown that chemotherapy with 5-FU, irinotecan, and oxaliplatin combined with bevacizumab as compared with 5-FU, oxaliplatin, and bevacizumab may be superior in terms of overall survival. The TRIBE study as well as STEAM both suggested that quadruple chemotherapy may be more active than triplet therapy. For this patient, all of the options are reasonable except for the cetuximab, as her KRAS mutation would indicate that she would not benefit from the addition of that agent.

35. A

This patient has been treated with 5-FU, oxaliplatin, and bevacizumab as well as the second-line regimen of 5-FU, irinotecan, and cetuximab. There are no data to suggest that treatment with another anti-EGFR antibody such as panitumumab would be useful in a patient who has already progressed on cetuximab. Because this patient has disease in the lungs and the liver, treatment with radiation or surgery would also not be reasonable. There are no data suggesting that colon cancer patients are resensitized to treatments on which they have already progressed. Accordingly treatment with regorafenib, which has been FDA-approved for heavily pretreated metastatic colon cancer, would be the appropriate option.

36. C

Although all of the side effects associated with TAS-102 are known, grade 3 neutropenia, seen in 38% of patients, is most commonly a high-grade toxicity of this agent, as shown in the seminal study leading to the agent's approval.

37. C

Maintenance chemotherapy has been controversial, with conflicting results in metastatic colorectal cancer. The OPTIMOX1 and two other studies had conflicting results, with OPTIMOX1 showing maintenance 5-FU versus observation having no survival benefit, while OPTIMOX2—a trial that was halted after only 202 of 600 patients were cured—showed an improvement in PFS but not overall survival. The MRC COIN study was a trial showing that median survival was not better in the continuous arm versus the intermittent for patients treated with first-line oxaliplatin and 5-FU. The addition of bevacizumab to capecitabine as maintenance therapy in the CAIRO3 study showed improvement in PFS but not overall survival. The AIO 0207 study—which randomized patients to bevacizumab plus capecitabine versus bevacizumab versus observation—showed a possible benefit to the arms that received bevacizumab, although the benefit was very small and there was no overall survival benefit. Accordingly patients can be treated with maintenance chemotherapy. However, they should be counseled that, based on the studies that have been reported thus far, although this is likely to show a PFS benefit, it is unlikely to show an overall survival benefit.

38. B

Bevacizumab is known to increase the risk of deep venous thrombosis as well as hypertension. However, the presence of these entities in itself does not require discontinuation of therapy. Wound dehiscence is an absolute contraindication to bevacizumab therapy. Chronic kidney disease and CNS metastases are both circumstances where, based on the particular patient, an individual could be treated with bevacizumab; those with CNS metastases plus bleeding may be at higher risk versus patients with CNS metastases alone.

39. B

The EGFR inhibitors cetuximab and panitumumab do not provide benefit for the patients who have mutations in KRAS, BRAF, or NRAS. The acneiform rash associated with these agents can decrease or increase with time on therapy. Prophylaxis with sunscreen emollients and oral doxycycline have been shown to decrease the problems posed by the rash, and these agents have been shown to be useful in combination with chemotherapy backbones as well as single agents.

40. E

The patient has an excellent performance status, but as her past treatments are surveyed, she has received all of the standard treatments for her disease. The agent that she has not received, panitumumab, has no proven benefit in patients who have already progressed on cetuximab. At this point, the patient could reasonably be offered comfort care as well as referral to a clinical trial. Molecular profiling for actionable mutations leads to the finding of actionable mutation in approximately 10% of patients.

41. B

This patient has a chronic infection that is active; accordingly, therapy with mitomycin C, which is known to significantly cause prolonged neutropenia, could be particularly dangerous for this patient. Clinical trials have evaluated whether therapies with cisplatin instead of mitomycin C, 5-FU, would be reasonable as a substitution. The ACT II trials randomized 940 non-HIV infected patients to cisplatin versus mitomycin-C with 5-FU. The 3-year colostomy-free survival, progression-free survival, and overall survival are similar between the two arms. Of note, there has been another study, the RTOG 98-11 trial, showing that cisplatin may be inferior to mitomycin-C, although that trial enrolled fewer patients. Based on these data, in the scenario where the patient would be significantly at risk with prolonged neutropenia, cisplatin can be considered instead of mitomycin-C as a part of the concurrent chemoradiation regimen.

42. A

This patient has a T1 anal cancer with a right inguinal node. The inguinal node is on the borderline in terms of size. However, involvement of the right inguinal lymph node region would significantly change this patient's staging, moving it from stage I to stage III disease. Accordingly it is important to biopsy the lymph node to ascertain whether it is involved in terms of the cancer. FDG-PET can show increased SUV with both inflammation and malignancy, so it cannot distinguish whether this lymph node is benign or malignant.

43. D

Surveillance guidelines for anal cancer after treatment with concurrent chemoradiation include physical exam with inguinal node palpation, digital rectal exam, and endoscopy every 3 to 6 months for 5 years. For patients with any signs of residual cancer or T3 or T4 disease, annual imaging for the first 3 years is also reasonable.

44. A

The patient has stage III disease as defined by lymph node involvement. He also has lymphovascular and perineural invasion, but his adjuvant chemotherapy is determined by his node positivity, which makes him a stage III cancer patient. Standard-of-care adjuvant therapy is 5-FU and oxaliplatin. The standard of care is based on two major clinical trials, the MOSAIC study as well as the NSABP C-07 trial. Both of these trials showed an improvement in disease-free survival, and the MOSAIC study also showed an improvement of overall survival in long-term follow-up for stage III cancer patients. Capecitabine with oxaliplatin is also a reasonable adjuvant therapy regimen.

45. D

The patient has an obstructing rectal mass that is at high risk of causing a bowel obstruction in the near future. A diverting colostomy followed by definitive treatment is a reasonable and safe plan for taking care of this patient. If the patient is being cared for in a center where chemotherapy or radiation can be started very quickly, the patient could be started on chemoradiation or chemotherapy within the next few days, since to the majority of patients have rapid improvement in symptoms as soon as treatment with either of these modalities begins. It would not be safe to wait 2 to 3 weeks before beginning chemotherapy or chemoradiation; emergent surgery for bowel obstruction has much greater morbidity than elective correction of the obstruction.

46. D

The benefit of adjuvant chemotherapy in patients who undergo preoperative chemoradiation is controversial. In the EORTC 22921 study, patients who received preoperative radiation underwent randomization to 4 cycles of postoperative 5-FU and leucovorin versus no further therapy. In a subgroup analysis of patients who underwent a complete R0 resection, the addition of postoperative chemotherapy significantly improved overall survival in patients whose tumors were downstaged to T0 from T2 but not those that were T3/T4. However, other studies have failed to show a better outcome with postoperative chemotherapy in patients with greater down staging. The PROCTOR/SCRIPT study, where patients underwent radiation followed by total mesorectal excision, also showed no difference in overall survival if patients received postoperative capecitabine versus observation. A phase 3 study from the United Kingdom, a clinical trial, looked at people who received postoperative capecitabine and oxaliplatin versus no adjuvant chemotherapy. There was a trend toward improved disease-free survival in those patients, but the study was closed when it had significant issues with approval. In patients with an excellent response to therapy, it is reasonable to consider treatment with 5-FU and oxaliplatin, 5-FU compound alone, or even observation.

47. B

Incidental adenocarcinoma found at the time of an appendectomy should be treated with a return to the OR for a completion hemicolectomy and lymph node dissection to accurately stage the patient's disease. Adjuvant chemotherapy can then be determined based on this staging.

48. E

Appropriate staging of the T and N status of rectal cancer patients is particularly important, because if such a patient has a response to neoadjuvant chemoradiation, the surgical staging is likely to understage him or her. CT scans do not provide enough pelvic visibility to properly stage rectal cancer. FDG-PET scans can be used to evaluate for distant disease but also do not have enough resolution to evaluate for nodal disease; in addition, not all rectal cancer patients will have PET-avid tumors. Either an MRI of the pelvis or an EUS can be utilized to properly stage the T and N status of rectal cancer patients, with the caveat that EUS is best used in clinical centers or in the hands of physicians with significant experience in using it for cancer staging.

49. C

Although all of the side effects associated with TAS-102 are known, grade 3 neutropenia, seen in 38% of patients, is most commonly a high-grade toxicity of this agent, as shown in the seminal study leading to the agent's approval.

REFERENCES

Question 1
1. Bennouna J, Sastre J, Arnold D, et al. Continuation of bevacizumab after first progression in metastatic colorectal cancer (ML18147): a randomised phase 3 trial. *Lancet Oncol.* 2013;14:29–37.

Question 2
1. Mayer RJ, Van Cutsem E, Falcone A, et al. Randomized trial of TAS-102 for refractory metastatic colorectal cancer. *N Engl J Med.* 2015;372:1909–1919.

Question 4
1. Kopetz S, Desai J, Chan E, et al. Phase II pilot study of vemurafenib in patients with metastatic BRAF-mutated colorectal cancer. *J Clin Oncol.* 2015;33(34):4032–4038.

Question 8
1. Sauer R, Becker H, Hohenberger W, et al. Preoperative versus postoperative chemoradiotherapy for rectal cancer. *N Engl J Med.* 2004;351:1731–1740.

Question 10
1. Tran B, Kopetz S, Tie J, et al. Impact of BRAF mutation and microsatellite instability on the pattern of metastatic spread and prognosis in metastatic colorectal cancer. *Cancer.* 2011;117:4623–4632.

Question 13
1. Parsons MT, Buchanan DD, Thompson B, Young JP, Spurdle AB. Correlation of tumour BRAF mutations and MLH1 methylation with germline mismatch repair (MMR) gene mutation status: a literature review assessing utility of tumour features for MMR variant classification. *J Med Genet.* 2012;49:151–157.

Question 17
1. Caplin ME, Pavel M, Ćwikła JB, et al. Lanreotide in metastatic enteropancreatic neuroendocrine tumors. *N Engl J Med.* 2014;371:224–233.

Question 19
1. Kulke MH, Shah MH, Benson 3rd AB, et al. Neuroendocrine tumors, version 1.2015. *J Natl Compr Canc Netw.* 2015;13:78–108.

Question 22
1. Bennouna J, Sastre J, Arnold D, et al. Continuation of bevacizumab after first progression in metastatic colorectal cancer (ML18147): a randomised phase 3 trial. *Lancet Oncol.* 2013;14:29–37.
2. Van Cutsem E, Tabernero J, Lakomy R, et al. Addition of aflibercept to fluorouracil, leucovorin, and irinotecan improves survival in a phase III randomized trial in patients with metastatic colorectal cancer previously treated with an oxaliplatin-based regimen. *J Clin Oncol.* 2012;30:3499–3506.
3. Tabernero J, Yoshino T, Cohn AL, et al. Ramucirumab versus placebo in combination with second-line FOLFIRI in patients with metastatic colorectal carcinoma that progressed during or after first-line therapy with bevacizumab, oxaliplatin, and a fluoropyrimidine (RAISE): a randomised, double-blind, multicentre, phase 3 study. *Lancet Oncol.* 2015;16:499–508.

Hepatobiliary Cancer

Ghassan K. Abou-Alfa

QUESTIONS

1. A 64-year-old female known to have hepatitis C virus (HCV) infection due to a blood transfusion 35 years ago, presented to the hospital for abdominal discomfort. On physical examination, vital signs were BP: 110/65; pulse: 86; RR: 18; T: 98°F. Upon physical examination, the right subcostal liver could be palpated, and no other significant findings were observed. Clinical tests on admission indicated abnormal liver function, and laboratory data showed abnormally high levels of aspirate aminotransferase (AST; 186 IU/L) and alanine aminotransferase (ALT; 165 IU/L). The levels of total bilirubin were normal (0.7 mg/dL), and other tests were as follows: albumin 4 g/dL, prothrombin time 82%, and AFP 48.2 ng/mL. A triple-phase CT of the liver revealed that the tumor was in the right lobe, irregular in shape, measuring 7.6 by 8 cm, and was infiltrating the main trunk via the first branch of the portal vein. What is NOT considered an appropriate treatment option?
   A. TACE only
   B. TACE with sorafenib
   C. Sorafenib at a starting dose of 400 mg twice daily
   D. Yttrium 90 radioembolization
   E. Clinical trial

2. Which of the following is true regarding HCC?
   A. Fibrolamellar HCCs occur in cirrhotic liver only.
   B. Contrast tomography (CT) and contrast-enhanced magnetic resonance imaging (MRI) are now included in the initial screening recommendations.
   C. Ultrasound of the liver every 6 months is still the screening modality of choice in the at-risk population, with or without AFP testing.
   D. Biopsy of the liver is associated with a risk of bleeding approaching 4%.
   E. 10% of all liver malignancies are associated with cholangiocarcinoma.

3. A 72-year-old Caucasian man with a long history of alcohol consumption presented to the emergency department with 1-week duration of worsening right upper quadrant pain, itching, jaundice, and decreased oral intake. Vital signs on presentation: BP: 110/75 mm Hg; HR: 110 bpm; RR: 16; T: 96°F. On physical exam, tenderness was noted on moderate palpation in the RUQ without rebound or guarding; initial laboratory tests showed total white blood cell count of 13,000/mL, creatinine of 0.7 mg/dL, liver function tests included total bilirubin of 3.2 mg/dL, albumin level of 2.6 mg/L, AST of 184 U/L, ALT of 110 U/L, and international normalized ration (INR) of 1.35. CT scan of the abdomen showed a large heterogeneous necrotic appearing mass measuring 4.9 cm by 3 cm by 4.3 cm, occupying the right lobe. Which of the following statements is true?

   A. Right hepatectomy constitutes an appropriate approach for this patient with mortality rate less than 5%.
   B. Transarterial chemoembolization (TACE) is indicated in this case.
   C. Image-guided biopsy is indicated to confirm the diagnosis.
   D. The patient should be listed for liver transplantation, which demonstrates a 4-year survival rate of 75%.
   E. TACE plus sorafenib is indicated.

4. A 55-year-old man with established cirrhosis due to hepatitis C underwent a 6-month follow-up surveillance ultrasound. It showed a suspicious focal liver lesion. A subsequent contrast-enhanced CT scan of the abdomen confirmed a 2.5-cm focal lesion in the liver. The tumor is hypervascular, with delayed contrast washout. Until the time of evaluation, AFP was elevated to 200 ng/mL and the Child-Pugh score was B8. A previous AFP and ultrasound were normal 6 months earlier. What is the most appropriate next step?
   A. Ultrasound-guided liver biopsy
   B. MRI of the liver
   C. Liver transplant referral
   D. Repeat scan in 3 months
   E. Repeat AFP in 3 months

5. A 66-year-old male patient, known to have type II diabetes mellitus and morbid obesity, presented to the clinic with malaise, abdominal pain, and weight loss over the past few weeks. The ECOG PS is 1. Vital signs on presentation: BP: 105/75; pulse: 84; RR: 17; T: 98°F. Laboratory tests were significant for an AFP of 8440 ng/mL, normal kidney function, albumin 3.3 g/dL; INR 1.1; and total bilirubin of 1 mg/dL. A CT scan showed cirrhotic liver with a large lesion (6 × 7 cm) in the right lobe of the liver with typical radiological features of HCC. Which of the following is the best treatment modality?
   A. TACE has widespread popularity for treating unresectable HCC and is the only method of transarterial treatment that has been demonstrated to provide a survival advantage in randomized trials.
   B. Radiation therapy is associated with survival benefit and minimal toxicity.
   C. Neoadjuvant chemotherapy with doxorubicin followed by surgery.
   D. Cryoablation is well tolerated with a low local recurrence rate.
   E. Radiofrequency ablation (RFA) is similar to TACE in tumors larger than 6 cm.

6. A 65-year-old Caucasian male patient, known to be HCV positive, presented with a 3-week history of right abdominal pain and fullness in the right upper abdomen.

A dynamic CT scan of the abdomen and pelvis showed a 7-cm by 8-cm liver lesion in the right lobe, with arterial enhancement and contrast washout on delayed imaging. The tumor involves the retrohepatic IVC with lymph node involvement at the level of the porta hepatitis. The patient was started on sorafenib 400 mg twice daily. Three weeks later, he developed grade 2 skin toxicity for the first time. A suitable next step would be:

A. One-level dose adjustment to 200 mg twice daily
B. Interrupt treatment until grade 0-1 and resume at the same dose
C. Interrupt treatment until grade 0-1 and resume at 200 mg twice daily
D. Continue the same dose until grade 3 toxicity
E. Discontinue treatment

7. A 72-year-old gentleman with a long-standing history of hereditary hemochromatosis with cirrhosis, diabetes mellitus, and chronic kidney disease, presented with weight loss of approximately 30 pounds over the past 2 months and a 1-month history of productive cough and shortness of breath. The patient also complained recently of right hip pain. A CT scan of the chest, abdomen, and pelvis demonstrated a 7.2-cm by 5.3-cm right liver enhancing lesion suggestive of HCC and multiple right lower lobe lung nodules. Measured AFP was 11,200 ng/mL. The next most appropriate step includes:

A. Bone metastasis is a very common presentation in advanced HCC occurring in around 40% of patients, thus necessitating bone scintigraphy on each patient presenting with HCC
B. Sorafenib, initiated at a dose of 400 mg orally twice daily, can significantly lead to an improvement in median overall survival to 10.7 months when compared with 7.9 months for placebo
C. Sunitinib, a multitargeted TKI similar to sorafenib, carries an overall benefit and can be used as frontline therapy

D. Complete resection of the liver lesion with a right lower lobectomy carries the most beneficial outcome for the patient in terms of recurrence-free survival
E. Sorafenib benefit and risk have been shown to be the same, independent of the patient's Child-Pugh score, and has a more beneficial outcome across all stages

8. A 59-year-old male patient was admitted to the hospital with right side flank pain of 2 weeks duration. Physical examination findings upon admission were normal. Laboratory examination produced the following results: white blood cell count, 6.61×10^9/L; red blood cell count, 3.7×10^{12}/L; hemoglobin, 120 g/L; albumin, 3.9 g/dL; globulin, 26.81 g/L; total bilirubin, 0.9 μmol/L; and prothrombin time, 12.9 s. The alanine aminotransferase, aspartate aminotransferase, and lactate dehydrogenase levels were within normal ranges. Hepatitis B virus-related antigen and antibody were negative with the exception of hepatitis B e antibody (HBeAb) and hepatitis B core antibody (HBcAb), and anti-HCV antibody was negative. The α-fetoprotein was 7 ng/mL. He had a history of splenectomy and blood transfusions due to traumatic spleen rupture. However, he had no history of exposure to any hepatotoxic chemicals and no family history of liver disease. Abdominal computed tomography (CT) revealed two separate lesions in segment VI (4.5×4 cm in size) and segment VII (6×5 cm in size). What is the best next step in management?

A. Stereotactic body radiation therapy (SBRT) to both lesions
B. Surgical resection of both lesions
C. Segment VI and segment VII resection followed by adjuvant sorafenib for 6 months
D. Referral for liver transplantation because he fits the Milan criteria
E. Systemic chemotherapy

ANSWERS

1. B

This patient has a large, locally advanced HCC, with compensated liver cirrhosis and a Child-Pugh score of A5. TACE, Y90 radioembolization, and systemic therapy are all considered therapeutic options in this scenario. TACE with sorafenib did not show benefit over TACE alone in many randomized trials.

2. C

Most national and international guidelines recommend biannual liver ultrasound and AFP measurement for HCC screening. The role of newer techniques such as CT and MRI remains unclear in this setting. Liver biopsy is indicated in selected cases, and it carries a 0.4% risk of hemorrhage. Approximately 5% of all primary liver tumors are combined hepatocellular-cholangiocarcinoma.

3. D

The patient has a single lesion less than 5 cm in size, making him eligible for liver transplant evaluation. Patients who fit the Milan criteria have a 4-year survival rate of 75%. He has a Model for End-Stage Liver Disease (MELD) score of 17. The MELD consists of serum bilirubin, creatinine levels, INR levels, and recently included sodium level. It is a reliable measure of mortality risk

in patients with end-stage liver disease and is used as a disease severity index to determine organ allocation priorities. Surgical resection is reserved for patients without underlying portal hypertension, favorable anatomical criteria, and good hepatic function to leave behind an adequate liver remnant. Transarterial therapy is reserved for locally advanced disease. There is no clear data to support use of systemic therapy with TACE. Sorafenib is indicated in the advanced setting.

4. C

This patient has an established diagnosis of HCC detected on a background of liver cirrhosis based on imaging criteria and elevated AFP. Liver biopsy is not required to confirm the diagnosis, although it can be valuable in the noncurable setting. MRI and CT are both sensitive and specific diagnostic tools, and can be used interchangeably. The Milan criteria have become the standard guidelines for hepatic transplantation in patients with hepatic cirrhosis, with a single lesion less than 5 cm or no more than three tumors, all less than 3 cm, as the criteria for the best outcome after transplantation. When HCC was associated with cirrhosis of the liver, the survival rates after transplant were significantly better than those after hepatic resection. The patient has cirrhosis with a Child-Pugh score of B8, making him a candidate to be listed for transplant.

5. A

This patient has a large liver tumor with preserved hepatic function. Transarterial chemoembolization is an option for locally advanced unresectable tumors, with a survival advantage over best supportive care. Transarterial embolization with microspheres alone was shown to be comparable to chemoembolization with doxorubicin eluting beads (DEBs) in a randomized trial. Liver irradiation did not show disease control in HCC, with higher doses causing radiation hepatitis. Newer techniques to minimize tissue exposure are being investigated. Radioembolization using yttrium-90-loaded spheres also demonstrated good results in locally advanced Child-Pugh A disease. Cryoablation is not adopted in HCC due to complications and high local recurrence rate. The best results were achieved when RFA is applied in tumors less than 5 cm. A randomized trial showed that 4-year overall survival rate is similar between RFA and surgery for solitary HCC smaller than 5 cm.

6. B

One of the more common adverse events seen with sorafenib is hand-foot skin reaction, a dermatological toxicity usually localized to the pressure points of the palms and soles. Although hand-foot skin reaction is reversible and not life threatening, it can have a significant impact on a patient's quality of life and may necessitate dose modification. Hand-foot skin reaction occurred in 8% of cases in the randomized clinical trial of sorafenib versus placebo. For the first appearance of grade 2 skin toxicity, recommendation is to hold treatment until grade 0-1 and resume at the same dose. For the second appearance, it is recommended to resume at 400 mg/day. For grade 3 skin toxicity, interrupt treatment until grade 0-1 and resume at 400 mg for the first appearance, 400 mg every 2 days for the second appearance, and discontinue treatment permanently for the third appearance.

7. B

Sorafenib therapy has demonstrated overall survival benefit versus placebo in advanced HCC and is approved for first-line treatment. Safe and beneficial use is limited to Child-Pugh A and selected cases with Child-Pugh B liver function. Extrahepatic spread of HCC is mainly to the lungs followed by the bones. Bone metastasis at presentation was found to be about 10% in one retrospective series (unpublished data). Surgery has no role in the metastatic setting. Sunitinib showed an inferior outcome when compared with sorafenib in a phase III trial.

8. B

This patient has good underlying hepatic function and anatomically resectable disease. He would benefit from partial hepatectomy with overall survival benefit. Stereotactic body radiation therapy (SBRT), which delivers a high dose of radiation to the tumor and minimizes normal liver irradiation, has been studied extensively in the locally advanced or inoperable setting. However, information on optimal treatment indications, survival benefit, doses, and methods remains limited. Adjuvant sorafenib failed to add benefit when compared with surgery alone in a randomized trial. The patient does not fit the Milan criteria, with two lesions exceeding 3 cm in size.

REFERENCES

Question 1
1. Lencioni R, Llovet JM, Han G, et al. Sorafenib or placebo plus TACE with doxorubicin-eluting beads for intermediate stage HCC: the SPACE trial. *J Hepatol.* 2016;64(5):1090–1098.

Question 2
1. Chi M, Mikhitarian K, Shi C, Goff LW. Management of combined hepatocellular-cholangiocarcinoma: a case report and literature review. *Gastrointest Cancer Res.* 2012;5(6):199–202.

Question 3
1. Kamath PS, Wiesner RH, Malinchoc M, et al. A model to predict survival in patients with end-stage liver disease. *Hepatology.* 2001;33(2):464–470.

Question 4
1. Iwatsuki S, Starzl TE, Sheahan DG, et al. Hepatic resection versus transplantation for hepatocellular carcinoma. *Ann Surg.* 1991;214(3):221–229.

Question 5
1. Llovet JM, Real MI, Montaña X, et al. Arterial embolization or chemoembolization versus symptomatic treatment in patients with unresectable hepatocellular carcinoma: a randomized controlled trial. *Lancet.* 2002;359(9319):1734–1739.
2. Brown KT, Do RK, Gonen M, et al. Randomized trial of hepatic artery embolization for hepatocellular carcinoma using doxorubicin-eluting microspheres compared with embolization with microspheres alone. *J Clin Oncol.* 2016;34(17):2046–2053.
3. Salem R, Lewandowski RJ, Mulcahy MF, et al. Radioembolization for hepatocellular carcinoma using yttrium-90 microspheres: a comprehensive report of long-term outcomes. *Gastroenterology.* 2010;138(1):52–64.

4. Chen MS, Li JQ, Zheng Y, et al. A prospective randomized trial comparing percutaneous local ablative therapy and partial hepatectomy for small hepatocellular carcinoma. *Ann Surg.* 2006;243(3):321–328.

Question 6
1. Gomez P, Lacouture ME. Clinical presentation and management of hand-foot skin reaction associated with sorafenib in combination with cytotoxic chemotherapy: experience in breast cancer. *Oncologist.* 2011;16(11):1508–1519.
2. Llovet JM, Ricci S, Mazzaferro V, et al. Sorafenib in advanced hepatocellular carcinoma. *N Engl J Med.* 2008;359:378–390.

Question 7
1. Abou-Alfa GK, Amadori D, Santoro A, et al. Safety and efficacy of sorafenib in patients with hepatocellular carcinoma (HCC) and child-pugh A versus B cirrhosis. *Gastrointest Cancer Res.* 2011;4(2):40–44.
2. Cheng AL, Kang YK, Lin DY, et al. Sunitinib versus sorafenib in advanced hepatocellular cancer: results of a randomized phase III trial. *J Clin Oncol.* 2013;31(32):4067–4075.

Question 8
1. Kwon JH, Bae SH, Kim JY, et al. Long-term effect of stereotactic body radiation therapy for primary hepatocellular carcinoma ineligible for local ablation therapy or surgical resection. Stereotactic radiotherapy for liver cancer. *BMC Cancer.* 2010;10:475.
2. Bruix J, Takayama T, Mazzaferro V, et al. Adjuvant sorafenib for hepatocellular carcinoma after resection or ablation (STORM): a phase 3, randomised, double-blind, placebo-controlled trial. *Lancet Oncol.* 2015;16(13):1344–1354.

Question 9
1. Iwatsuki S, Starzl TE, Sheahan DG, et al. Hepatic resection versus transplantation for hepatocellular carcinoma. *Ann Surg.* 1991;214(3):221–229.

Neuroendocrine, Small Bowel, and Appendiceal Malignancies

Jonathan Strosberg

QUESTIONS

1. A 60-year-old African American man undergoes a routine screening colonoscopy and is found to have a 5-mm rectal polyp located 8 cm from the anal verge. He undergoes endoscopic polypectomy. Pathology reveals a submucosal neuroendocrine tumor with no mitoses identified, extending to the polyp margin. Ki-67 index is 1%. Repeat sigmoidoscopy 3 weeks later with biopsies of the scar site reveal no further evidence of disease. What would be an appropriate recommendation at this time?
   A. No further workup or treatment is necessary.
   B. Staging CT scans of the chest, abdomen, and pelvis, with referral to surgery for transanal excision if no evidence of metastases.
   C. Staging CT scans of the chest, abdomen, and pelvis, with referral to surgery for low-anterior resection if no evidence of metastases.
   D. Endoscopic ultrasound or pelvic MRI scan to evaluate for lymph node metastases.
   E. Measurement of urine 5-HIAA and serum chromogranin A. Further workup if elevated.

2. A 64-year-old man presents with acute small bowel obstruction. CT scans reveal a transition point in the mid-small intestine. He undergoes an urgent exploratory laparotomy with partial small bowel resection. Pathology reveals a 3-cm jejunal adenocarcinoma with 4/16 involved lymph nodes. No metastatic disease is noted intraoperatively. Postoperative CT scans of the chest, abdomen, and pelvis reveal no evidence of metastatic disease. Which course of treatment is most appropriate at this time?
   A. Close surveillance
   B. Adjuvant gemcitabine-cisplatin
   C. Adjuvant 5-fluorouracil and oxaliplatin (FOLFOX)
   D. Heated intraperitoneal chemotherapy (HIPEC)
   E. 5-Fluorouracil and irinoteca (FOLFIRI)

3. A 56-year-old man presented with right lower quadrant abdominal pain. A CT scan revealed a 3-cm pericecal mass. Colonoscopy was unremarkable. He underwent an exploratory laparotomy with right hemicolectomy. During surgery, he was found to have peritoneal nodules, one of which was biopsied. Pathology revealed a goblet cell carcinoid tumor of the appendix measuring 4 cm in diameter and invading the subserosa. The peritoneal nodule was positive for metastatic disease. He recovered from surgery. A postoperative PET scan 2 months later demonstrated scattered hypermetabolic peritoneal nodules. Which of the following treatments of would be most appropriate at this time?

   A. Octreotide LAR
   B. Everolimus
   C. Carboplatin-etoposide
   D. 5-Fluorouracil and oxaliplatin (FOLFOX)
   E. ^{177}Lutetium-Dotatate

4. A 58-year-old woman presents with abdominal distention and bloating. She undergoes a CT scan revealing fluid collections within the abdominal cavity with scalloping of the surface of the liver and spleen. There is a 2-cm complex lesion around the appendix. Needle aspiration of a fluid collection yields a diagnosis of adenomucinosis. Which treatment would be most appropriate at this time?
   A. Surgical debulking with or without heated intraperitoneal chemotherapy (HIPEC)
   B. 5-Fluorouracil and oxaliplatin (FOLFOX) and bevacizumab
   C. Carboplatin-etoposide
   D. Intraperitoneal cisplatin and paclitaxel
   E. No treatment. Patient can be monitored.

5. A 68-year-old man presents with severe right upper quadrant abdominal pain, dyspnea, and weight loss of 30 pounds over the past 5 months. Physical exam reveals an enlarged, tender liver. He undergoes CT scans showing diffuse liver lesions, scattered lung lesions, and thickening in the mid-transverse colon. Needle biopsy of the liver reveals poorly differentiated neuroendocrine carcinoma with a ki-67 index of 70%. Which is the most appropriate treatment regimen?
   A. 5-Fluorouracil and oxaliplatin (FOLFOX) and bevacizumab
   B. Carboplatin-etoposide
   C. Everolimus
   D. Octreotide-LAR
   E. Streptozotocin

6. A 68-year-old man presents with mild right upper quadrant abdominal pain. A CT scan of the abdomen reveals numerous liver lesions and scattered rib and vertebral lesions. Core needle biopsy of a liver lesion reveals a well-differentiated neuroendocrine tumor with a ki-67 index of 12%. Further imaging reveals a 1.8-cm left upper lobe lung lesion with hilar adenopathy. Octreoscan shows very mild (grade 1) radiotracer uptake in the liver and left hilum. Which systemic treatment would be most appropriate at this time?
   A. Octreotide LAR
   B. Lanreotide
   C. Sunitinib
   D. Everolimus
   E. Streptozotocin

7. A 39-year-old woman presents with acute appendicitis and undergoes laparoscopic appendectomy. In addition to findings of acute appendicitis, the pathology report describes a 1-cm well-differentiated carcinoid tumor in the tip of the appendix extending into the muscularis propria. The ki-67 index is 1%. The patient recovers quickly from the appendectomy and presents for consultation. Which of the following is the appropriate recommendation?
   A. No further evaluation, treatment, or follow-up necessary
   B. Right hemicolectomy for lymph node staging
   C. Perform multiphasic CT scan and Octreoscan to evaluate for metastatic disease
   D. Begin adjuvant treatment with Octreotide LAR
   E. Check serum chromogranin A and 24-hour urine 5-HIAA. Perform additional testing if abnormal.

8. A 67-year-old woman with a metastatic small bowel neuroendocrine tumor and carcinoid syndrome has been on octreotide LAR 30 mg every 4 weeks for 2 years. Prior to starting octreotide, she had significant diarrhea (averaging 6 times a day), flushing (averaging twice a day), and an elevated urine 5-HIAA of 76 mg (nl < 15). Her flushing and diarrhea improved initially, but she now reports that she is experiencing increased diarrhea and bloating. CT scans show stable liver metastases, and urine 5-HIAA is mildly elevated at 22 mg. Which treatment would be most appropriate at this time?
   A. Start pancrelipase with meals
   B. Increase the dose of octreotide LAR to 40 mg every 3 weeks
   C. Recommend hepatic transarterial embolization
   D. Begin loperamide
   E. Start simethicone and diphenoxylate-atropine

9. A 56-year-old man presents with epigastric pain and 30-lb weight loss over 3 months. Blood tests are unremarkable except for AST of 78 µg/L (nl < 35), ALT of 95 µg/L (nl < 35), and alkaline phosphatase of 306 µg/L (nl < 105). Abdominal computed tomography (CT) scan reveals innumerable liver lesions and a 3.5-cm tumor in the tail of the pancreas. Core needle biopsy of the liver reveals a well-differentiated, intermediate-grade neuroendocrine tumor with 16 mitoses per 10 high-power fields. Which of the following systemic therapies are most likely to lead to significant tumor shrinkage?
   A. Sunitinib
   B. Everolimus
   C. Lanreotide
   D. Octreotide
   E. Capecitabine + temozolomide

10. A 40-year-old woman with a history of hypothyroidism undergoes upper endoscopy after complaining of mild recurrent epigastric pain. She has tried omeprazole in the past with no relief, but does not currently take any antacids. She denies any other gastrointestinal symptoms. The procedure reveals mildly erythematous gastric mucosa and four gastric body polyps measuring about 4 to 8 mm in size. The gastroenterologist performs endoscopic polypectomy of all four lesions. Pathology reveals a low-grade carcinoid tumor. Which test should be performed next?
   A. Serum gastrin
   B. Multiphasic abdominal CT scan
   C. Somatostatin-receptor scintigraphy (Octreoscan)
   D. Capsule endoscopy
   E. Serum chromogranin A

11. A 45-year-old woman presents with severe episodic hypertension associated with headaches. She has a history of medullary thyroid carcinoma and is status post thyroidectomy at age 20. An MRI scan of the abdomen reveals a 6-cm right-sided adrenal gland tumor, hyperintense on T2 weighted sequences, and a 2-cm left-sided adrenal gland tumor with similar imaging characteristics. Germline testing is likely to reveal a mutation in which of the following genes?
   A. NF1
   B. MEN1
   C. VHL
   D. TSC1 or 2
   E. RET

12. A 56-year-old man presents with a bowel obstruction and undergoes a CT scan revealing a mesenteric tumor with numerous bilobar liver metastases. He undergoes an exploratory laparotomy with partial small bowel resection revealing a 2.3-cm well-differentiated neuroendocrine tumor of the ileum with 3 of 14 involved lymph nodes. He reports that he has been having diarrhea for the past 3 years averaging 4 times a day, and experiences facial flushing occasionally. Twenty-four-hour urine 5-HIAA is elevated at 46 mg (normal <15 mg). Which of the following treatments is most appropriate at this time?
   A. Everolimus
   B. Octreotide LAR or lanreotide
   C. Sunitinib
   D. Hepatic transarterial chemoembolization
   E. Bland hepatic transarterial embolization

13. A 78-year-old-man presents with profuse, watery diarrhea for 3 months. Blood work reveals a potassium level of 2.8 mmol/L (nl > 3.6) and a chloride level of 89 mmol/L (nl > 98). CT scans reveal a 5.5-cm tumor in the tail of the pancreas. Which blood test is likely to reveal the underlying diagnosis?
   A. Glucagon
   B. Serotonin
   C. Vasoactive intestinal peptide
   D. Gastrin
   E. Calcitonin

14. A 32-year-old woman with a history of hyperparathyroidism presents with diarrhea. An abdominal CT scan reveals three hypervascular pancreatic lesions, the largest measuring 2.5 cm in diameter, retroperitoneal adenopathy, and two liver lesions. Serum gastrin is elevated at 850 pg/mL. She begins treatment with lanreotide and high-dose proton pump inhibitor therapy. She reports a family history of neuroendocrine tumors and parathyroid surgeries. For which additional type of neoplasm is she at risk?
   A. Medullary thyroid cancer
   B. Pheochromocytoma
   C. Pituitary adenoma
   D. Paraganglioma
   E. Renal cell carcinoma

15. A 69-year-old man with a metastatic small bowel neuroendocrine tumor and carcinoid syndrome presents with mild dyspnea with exertion and lower extremity swelling. A 24-hour urine 5-HIAA is markedly elevated at 124 mg (nl < 15). On cardiac examination, he has a 2/6 systolic murmur. Which two of his cardiac valves are likely dysfunctional?
   A. Mitral and aortic
   B. Tricuspid and aortic
   C. Pulmonary and mitral

D. Tricuspid and pulmonary
E. Pulmonary and aortic

16. A 67-year-old man with metastatic ileal neuroendocrine tumor and carcinoid syndrome receives treatment with octreotide LAR 30 mg every 4 weeks. Routine 6-month CT scans demonstrate progression of liver and retroperitoneal metastases. Which of the following treatments has been shown to significantly improve progression-free survival in patients matching his clinical characteristics?
    A. ^{177}Lutetium-dotatate
    B. Everolimus
    C. Lanreotide
    D. Temozolomide
    E. High-dose octreotide

17. A 53-year-old man with metastatic rectal neuroendocrine tumor is started on everolimus 10 mg daily. After 4 weeks of treatment, he complains of occasional painful mouth sores and is prescribed a steroid mouthwash. After 3 months on treatment, he presents for follow-up scans and evaluation. He complains of dyspnea interfering with strenuous activities, and dry cough. He denies any fevers. Complete blood count is significant for mild (grade 1) leukopenia, anemia, and thrombocytopenia. CT scan reveals stable liver and bone metastases, but new infiltrates along the lung bases. Which would be the most appropriate intervention?

A. Stop everolimus and begin empiric antibiotics for atypical pneumonia. Consider resuming everolimus when pneumonia resolves.
B. Diagnostic bronchoscopy with washings is indicated.
C. Stop everolimus and initiate steroid taper. Resume everolimus at a lower dose when symptoms resolve.
D. Stop everolimus and begin sunitinib instead.
E. Continue everolimus and initiate antibiotics for atypical pneumonia.

18. The clinical picture is less consistent with infectious pneumonia, although pulmonary infection should be considered in the differential given the immunosuppressive properties of everolimus. If symptoms do not improve with treatment interruption and steroids, an infectious workup may be appropriate. Permanent discontinuation of everolimus will likely not be necessary and indeed may be detrimental given limited alternative treatment options. Sunitinib is approved for pancreatic neuroendocrine tumors (NETs), but has no proven activity in rectal NETs. The inhibitory effects of somatostatin analogs on tumor growth have been demonstrated in phase III trials in which patient population(s)?
    A. NETs of the gastrointestinal tract and lungs
    B. Midgut NETs only
    C. NETs of the colon, rectum, and small intestine
    D. Pancreatic neuroendocrine tumors only
    E. Gastrointestinal and pancreatic neuroendocrine tumors

ANSWERS

1. A
A subcentimeter, submucosal low-grade rectal NET (T1) is almost never associated with malignant behavior. Metastatic spread is associated with the size of the rectal tumor (usually >2 cm), invasiveness (typically T2 or above), and tumor grade. National Comprehensive Cancer Network (NCCN) guidelines do not recommend any further evaluation or treatment in a patient with a subcentimeter low-grade T1 rectal tumor who has undergone endoscopic resection. If there had been residual disease, endoscopic mucosal resection (EMR) or another method of endoscopic management would be appropriate. Radiographic staging and surgical resection are not recommended for small, T1 tumors. Rectal NETs are not hormonally functional, so measurement of urine 5-HIAA would not be appropriate, even in a patient with a larger or more invasive tumor. Chromogranin A measurement is also not appropriate in this scenario, where risk of malignant behavior is negligible.

2. C
Small bowel adenocarcinomas are rare, and data from prospective trials are limited. There have been no prospective studies of adjuvant chemotherapy for small bowel adenocarcinoma. However, there is evidence of activity of chemotherapy regimens used in colon cancer in the metastatic setting. Therefore adjuvant FOLFOX is recommended for stage III small bowel adenocarcinoma, similar to the recommendation for stage III adenocarcinoma of the colon.

3. D
Goblet cell carcinoid tumors, also known as adenocarcinoids, typically originate in the appendix. Pathologically, they combine features of a carcinoid tumor and adenocarcinoma, but their malignant behavior is more similar to appendiceal adenocarcinoma. Metastatic spread tends to be peritoneal. Treatment recommendations are based on case reports and small series suggesting response to regimens used in colon cancer such as FOLFOX. The role of biological agents used in colon cancer (VEGF and EGFR inhibitors) is uncertain. Octreotide LAR, everolimus, and ^{177}Lu-Dotatate are appropriate for treatment of well-differentiated NETs, not adenocarcinoids. Carboplatin plus etoposide are used in poorly differentiated neuroendocrine carcinomas.

4. A
This patient has a diagnosis of pseudomyxoma peritonei, now more commonly known as disseminated peritoneal adenomucinosis (DPAM). The condition is characterized by accumulation of mucinous material within the peritoneal cavity, typically originating in a primary appendiceal adenoma. Standard treatment consists of aggressive surgical debulking. Addition of heated intraperitoneal chemotherapy (HIPEC), typically mitomycin, allows for high concentrations of chemotherapy to accumulate within the peritoneal cavity, and appears to improve long-term outcomes, although randomized studies comparing debulking surgery with or without HIPEC have not been performed. This approach may also be useful for low-grade mucin-producing appendiceal adenocarcinomas. Patients with high-grade carcinomas, or cancers with visceral metastases, are less likely to benefit from this approach. Systemic intravenous chemotherapy is unlikely to be of benefit for a patient with DPAM. Intraperitoneal cisplatin and paclitaxel is an appropriate postoperative regimen for stage III ovarian cancer and primary peritoneal carcinoma. Observation is not an appropriate option for a symptomatic patient.

5. B

A platinum-etoposide-based regimen (either cisplatin or carboplatin) is the appropriate first-line treatment for a patient with a poorly differentiated neuroendocrine carcinoma, regardless of primary site. FOLFOX with bevacizumab is used for adenocarcinoma of the colon. Everolimus and Octreotide LAR are used in well-differentiated NETs, and streptozotocin is approved for pancreatic NET.

6. D

This patient has a metastatic lung NET. The RADIANT 4 study demonstrated improvement in PFS with everolimus compared with placebo in patients with low and intermediate-grade NETs originating in the gastrointestinal (GI) tract and lungs. Thus everolimus is an appropriate treatment choice. Octreotide LAR and lanreotide were never tested in a randomized study that included lung NETs. Although they are commonly used in patients with advanced lung NETs, they are unlikely to be active in this case: a relatively aggressive malignancy that expresses very low levels of somatostatin receptors. Sunitinib and streptozotocin are approved for advanced pancreatic NETs but have no evidence of activity in lung NETs.

7. A

Carcinoid tumors of the appendix are discovered incidentally in approximately 1 in 300 appendectomies. They are usually found in the tip of the appendix. Tumor size appears to predict malignant behavior: in one large series with long-term follow-up, none of 127 patients with tumors <2 cm in diameter developed metastatic disease. The risk of malignant behavior of a 1-cm low-grade appendiceal carcinoid tumor is negligible, and no further workup or treatment is indicated after a simple appendectomy. For tumors larger than 2 cm, completion right hemicolectomy with lymph node staging is recommended. In recent years, there have been reports of patients with tumors 1 to 2 cm in diameter who developed locoregional metastases. The risk of malignant spread appears to correlate with invasion into the mesoappendix. Consequently, hemicolectomy can be considered for select patients with tumors of intermediate size (1–2 cm) based on significant depth of invasion.

8. A

This patient likely has malabsorption and steatorrhea resulting from her octreotide treatment and its effects on pancreatic exocrine function. This is a common side effect of somatostatin analogs and should be treated with pancreatic enzymes. Given the fact that her urine 5-HIAA is only mildly elevated, it is unlikely that her diarrhea is related to progressive carcinoid syndrome. Therefore increasing the dose of octreotide or performing hepatic arterial embolization are unlikely to be of benefit. Nonspecific antidiarrheals, such as loperamide or diphenoxylate-atropine, are unlikely to be as effective as pancrelipase if the cause of the diarrhea is pancreatic malabsorption.

9. E

This patient presents with a relatively aggressive pancreatic NET. Sunitinib and everolimus are both approved for treatment of advanced, progressive pancreatic NETs based on results of phase III clinical trials, but are associated with objective radiographic response rates of less than 10% and generally result in disease stabilization. Likewise, lanreotide was compared with placebo in a randomized clinical trial of patients with gastroenteropancreatic NETs (ki67 < 10%) and demonstrated improvement in PFS. Response rates were negligible. Octreotide has never been tested in

a randomized trial of pancreatic NETs, but has a similar mechanism of action to lanreotide and almost never produces an objective radiographic response. Cytotoxic drugs, specifically temozolomide and streptozotocin-based regimens, have never been tested in randomized phase III trials, but are associated with high objective response rates in pancreatic NETs. In one series of 30 patients, the combination of capecitabine and temozolomide was associated with an objective response rate of 70%. Other retrospective series have demonstrated similar response rates. Capecitabine/temozolomide is recommended by the National Comprehensive Cancer Network (NCCN) as an option for managing pancreatic NETs and represents a particularly appropriate choice in a patient with symptoms related to high tumor burden.

10. A

Carcinoid (neuroendocrine) tumors of the stomach are categorized into three types. Type 1 gastric NETs, which represent over 80% of cases, arise in the setting of atrophic gastritis. In this condition, chronic gastric achlorhydria stimulates the G cells of the antrum to produce excess serum gastrin. Gastrin, in turn, simulates neuroendocrine cell hyperplasia and development of multifocal, polypoid carcinoid tumors. These tumors generally behave in a benign fashion. Type 2 gastric carcinoid tumors also arise in the setting of elevated serum gastrin. In these rare tumors, elevated gastrin is produced by a pancreatic or duodenal gastrinoma. As is the case with type I disease, tumors tend to be small, multifocal, and clinically indolent. Patients with type 2 gastric NETs will usually have underlying symptoms of Zollinger-Ellison syndrome such as diarrhea, heartburn, and peptic ulceration as well as radiographic evidence of an underlying gastrinoma. Sporadic gastric NETs (type 3) occur in fewer than 15% of cases and are not associated with elevated gastrin levels. These tumors have a much higher malignant potential than type 1 or type 2 tumors. Measurement of serum gastrin is the first step in the evaluation of gastric carcinoid tumors because it can distinguish type 1 and 2 (hypergastrinemic) from type 3 (normal serum gastrin). It is important to emphasize that proton pump inhibitors raise serum gastrin, leading to false positive results. The patient in this case almost certainly has type 1 gastric NETs given the presence of small multifocal tumors and absence of symptoms suggestive of Zollinger-Ellison syndrome. Serum gastrin will, almost certainly, be elevated, and the patient should be managed with endoscopic surveillance. There is no need for radiographic staging studies. Serum chromogranin A is typically elevated in the setting of atrophic gastritis and is not a useful tumor marker.

11. E

This patient has a history of medullary thyroid carcinoma and is now presenting with signs and symptoms of bilateral pheochromocytoma. The clinical picture is consistent with multiple endocrine neoplasia type 2 (MEN2), a syndrome caused by mutations in the RET gene. MEN1 is associated with tumors of the pituitary, parathyroid glands, and endocrine pancreas, as well as bronchial and thymic NETs. Von Hippel-Lindau (VHL) syndrome is associated with renal cell carcinomas; hemangioblastomas of the spinal cord, cerebellum, and retina; pheochromocytomas; and pancreatic NETs (rarely). Tuberous sclerosis and type 1 neurofibromatosis are not associated with the tumors described in this case.

12. B

The somatostatin analogs octreotide LAR or lanreotide are appropriate first-line options for patients with unresectable metastatic small bowel NETs. Both octreotide and lanreotide inhibit secretion of serotonin and other vasoactive substances, thus palliating flushing and diarrhea associated with the carcinoid syndrome. Moreover, both drugs have been shown to significantly inhibit tumor growth. The PROMID study randomized 85 patients with midgut NETs to receive octreotide LAR IM versus placebo and demonstrated a significant improvement in median time to progression from 6 months to 14.5 months. The CLARINET study randomized 204 patients with nonfunctional gastroenteropancreatic NETs to receive lanreotide 120 mg SQ versus placebo and demonstrated a 53% improvement in PFS. Everolimus was found to significantly improve PFS in patients with progressive nonfunctional NETs of the GI tract and lungs in the randomized phase III RADIANT 4 study. Although everolimus can be considered in patients with progressive tumors, it is not an appropriate first-line treatment for this patient. Various hepatic arterial embolization modalities (bland, chemo, or radioembolization) are associated with high rates of radiographic, biochemical, and symptomatic responses in patients with progressive or symptomatic liver metastases, but have not been studied in randomized controlled trials. Hepatic arterial embolization is not an appropriate first-line intervention in this case. Sunitinib is approved for treatment of advanced pancreatic NETs, but is not recommended for treatment of small bowel NET.

13. C

Pancreatic NETs producing vasoactive intestinal peptide (VIPomas) typically originate in the tail of the pancreas. VIP stimulates intestinal secretion and inhibits electrolyte and water absorption. The resulting syndrome (also known as the Verner-Morrison syndrome) is characterized by severe watery diarrhea, often exceeding 3 L a day. Other complications include hypochlorhydria, hypokalemia, and dehydration. The VIPoma syndrome often responds rapidly to somatostatin analog therapy. Although serotonin, gastrin, and calcitonin can all produce diarrhea among other symptoms, they almost never cause the severe electrolyte abnormalities that are observed with VIP secretion.

14. C

This patient has a personal and family history consistent with multiple endocrine neoplasia type 1 (MEN1). MEN1 is an autosomal dominant syndrome characterized by a predisposition to endocrine tumors of the anterior pituitary, parathyroid glands, and pancreas/duodenum. Gastrinoma is the most common type of functional pancreaticoduodenal NET in MEN1 patients. The underlying tumor suppressor gene mutation has been identified in the long arm of chromosome 11 (11q13). MEN1 encodes for menin, a nuclear protein that regulates gene transcription through chromatin remodeling. Medullary thyroid cancers pheochromocytomas (and occasionally paragangliomas) are associated with MEN2 and are caused by mutations of the RET gene. Familial paragangliomas are more often associated with mutations of the SDH enzyme complex. Hereditary renal cell carcinoma occurs in VHL, a syndrome that is also associated with pancreatic NETs.

15. D

This patient very likely has carcinoid heart disease, a condition that predominantly affects the right heart, causing fibrosis and thickening of the tricuspid and pulmonary valves. The result is typically tricuspid insufficiency and pulmonary valve stenosis, eventually leading to right heart failure. Circulating serotonin is thought to be the most important etiological factor, although other secreted substances may also contribute to the condition. The right heart valves and endocardium are most directly exposed to serotonin secreted into the systemic circulation, whereas the mitral and aortic valves are relatively spared due to inactivation of serotonin in the pulmonary circulation.

16. A

The NETTER1 study randomized patients with progressive midgut (small bowel and proximal colon) NETs to receive the radiolabeled somatostatin analog [177]Lutetium-Dotatate versus high-dose octreotide. Median PFS was not reached on the [177]Lutetium-Dotatate arm of the study versus 8 months with high-dose octreotide. The hazard ratio for PFS was 0.21, and was highly significant. Everolimus has been evaluated in two randomized studies that included ileal NETs. In the RADIANT 2 study, which randomized patients with advanced NETs and a history of carcinoid syndrome to receive everolimus plus octreotide versus placebo plus octreotide, the PFS improvement with everolimus fell narrowly short of statistical significance. In the subsequent RADIANT 4 study, which randomized patients with nonfunctional NETs to receive everolimus versus placebo, PFS was improved in a statistically significant fashion. However, the patient in this case matches the RADIANT 2 population. Temozolomide has not been studied in randomized clinical trials of midgut NET. High-dose octreotide has not been evaluated as an experimental arm in a prospective, randomized clinical study.

17. C

The clinical picture is most consistent with noninfectious pneumonitis, a condition that develops in roughly 15% of everolimus-treated patients, occurring on average approximately 3 months after onset of treatment. In asymptomatic cases, modification of treatment is not necessary. However, because the patient is symptomatic, treatment of this side effect is necessary. Standard management consists of dose interruption, often with a short course of corticosteroids. Dose reduction may be appropriate after resolution of symptoms.

18. E

The phase III PROMID study randomized patients with midgut NETs to receive octreotide LAR versus placebo, demonstrating improvement in time to progression. Subsequently, the phase III CLARINET trial randomized patients with nonfunctional gastroenteropancreatic NETs to receive lanreotide versus placebo, demonstrating improvement in PFS. Thus the antiproliferative effects of somatostatin analogs are now demonstrated based on studies that include both GI and pancreatic NETs. Randomized studies of somatostatin analogs in lung NETs are pending.

REFERENCES

Question 7

1. Moertel CG, Weiland LH, Nagorney DM, Dockerty MB. Carcinoid tumor of the appendix: treatment and prognosis. *N Engl J Med.* 1987;317:1699–1701.

Question 9

1. Yao JC, Shah MH, Ito T, et al. Everolimus for advanced pancreatic neuroendocrine tumors. *N Engl J Med.* 2011;364:514–523.

2. Raymond E, Dahan L, Raoul JL, et al. Sunitinib malate for the treatment of pancreatic neuroendocrine tumors. *N Engl J Med.* 2011;364:501–513.

Question 12

1. Rinke A, Muller HH, Schade-Brittinger C, et al. Placebo-controlled, double-blind, prospective, randomized study on the effect of octreotide LAR in the control of tumor growth in patients with metastatic neuroendocrine midgut tumors: a report from the PROMID Study Group. *J Clin Oncol.* 2009;27:4656–4663.
2. Caplin ME, Pavel M, Cwikla JB, et al. Lanreotide in metastatic enteropancreatic neuroendocrine tumors. *N Engl J Med.* 2014;371:224–233.
3. Yao JC, Fazio N, Singh S, et al. Everolimus for the treatment of advanced, non-functional neuroendocrine tumours of the lung or gastrointestinal tract (RADIANT-4): a randomised, placebo-controlled, phase 3 study. *Lancet.* 2016;387:968–977.

Question 16

1. Strosberg J, Wolin E, Chasen B, et al. NETTER-1 phase III trial: efficacy and safety results in patients with midugt neuroednocrine tumors treated with ^{177}Lu-DOTATATE. *J Clin Oncol.* 2016;34 (suppl; abstr 4005).
2. Pavel ME, Hainsworth JD, Baudin E, et al. Everolimus plus octreotide long-acting repeatable for the treatment of advanced neuroendocrine tumours associated with carcinoid syndrome (RADIANT-2): a randomised, placebo-controlled, phase 3 study. *Lancet.* 2011;378(9808):2005–2012.
3. Yao JC, Fazio N, Singh S, et al. Everolimus for the treatment of advanced, non-functional neuroendocrine tumours of the lung or gastrointestinal tract (RADIANT-4): a randomised, placebo-controlled, phase 3 study. *Lancet.* 2016;387:968–977.

Prostate Cancer

Ravi A. Madan and Jeanny B. Aragon-Ching

QUESTIONS

1. A 73-year-old male with castration-resistant prostate cancer, but negative findings on conventional imaging, has been on androgen deprivation therapy (ADT) and bicalutamide 50 mg for 3 years. Over the last 6 months his prostate-specific antigen (PSA) has risen from 10 to 20 ng/mL. The patient remains asymptomatic and otherwise in excellent health. Restaging computed tomography (CT) and a bone scan do not identify any radiographic evidence of disease. What would be the next most appropriate step in the treatment of this patient?
   A. Discontinue ADT and monitor for a withdrawal response with a PSA in 6 weeks
   B. Discontinue bicalutamide and monitor for a withdrawal response with a PSA in 6 weeks
   C. Discontinue both ADT and bicalutamide and monitor for a withdrawal response with a PSA in 6 weeks
   D. Continue bicalutamide and ADT and then add abiraterone and prednisone to his treatment regimen
   E. Order a fluorodeoxyglucose-positron emission tomography (FDG-PET) scan to further evaluate for metastatic disease

2. A 49-year-old male with metastatic castration-resistant prostate cancer (metastatic to the spine and pelvis) is currently being treated with ADT and enzalutamide 160 mg/day. The patient has been on ADT for 4 years, and the enzalutamide was begun 6 weeks ago. He is also on denosumab and antihypertensive agents. He comes to your office complaining of extreme fatigue in the past month. Upon evaluation you find that he has started no additional medications and he has no distinct cardiopulmonary complaints or findings on exam. He complains of no new pain symptoms. His PSA, which was 54.6 ng/mL upon starting treatment with enzalutamide, is now down to 9.8 ng/mL. What is the most appropriate next step in the treatment of this patient?
   A. Order a CT scan to confirm neuroendocrine dedifferentiation of the patient's tumor
   B. Order a thyroid panel and test for antithyroid antibodies
   C. Order a cosyntropin stimulation test
   D. Hold the enzalutamide for 2–4 weeks and then reevaluate the patient's symptoms
   E. Add 10 mg of prednisone to the patient's current treatment regimen.

3. A 62-year-old male comes to you for a consultation. He has Gleason 4+3 prostate cancer diagnosed in 6 of 12 cores on a recent biopsy. His PSA was 8.5 ng/mL prior to biopsy. He has seen a radiation oncologist and a urologist, but he is unclear which treatment is best for him. He feels that both doctors were just trying to extol the virtues of their respective therapies. He has hypertension and hyperlipidemia, but is otherwise healthy and taking no other medications for any other conditions. He asks your opinion on which therapy is best for him. Based on the existing data, which is the most appropriate response?
   A. There are no randomized data that identifies the most appropriate treatment for this patient
   B. Based on his relatively young age, surgery would be most appropriate
   C. Based on his comorbidities, he is not likely to live long enough to benefit from either treatment
   D. Based on his Gleason score, radiation would be most appropriate
   E. Based on his PSA, surgery would be most appropriate

4. A 56-year-old man with metastatic castration-resistant prostate cancer is under your care and is being treated with radium 223. On his most recent visit, his son, who is a medical student, came with him to discuss his father's case. He asks you, what is the proposed mechanism of action of radium 223? What is the most appropriate response?
   A. Radium 223 is a targeted alpha emitter that selectively binds to areas of increased bone turnover in bone metastases and emits high-energy alpha particles
   B. Radium 223 is a targeted beta emitter that selectively binds to areas of increased bone turnover in bone metastases and emits high-energy beta particles
   C. Radium 223 is a targeted gamma emitter that selectively binds to areas of increased bone turnover in bone metastases and emits high-energy gamma particles
   D. Radium 223 is a targeted alpha-emitting antibody that binds to prostate-specific membrane antigen (PSMA) on the prostate cancer cells
   E. Radium 223 is a targeted beta-emitting antibody that binds to PSMA on the prostate cancer cells

5. A 56-year-old male is in your office for follow-up of his biochemically recurrent prostate cancer after definitive radiation therapy. His PSA is currently up to 8.4 ng/mL, with a recent calculated PSA doubling time of about 2.5 months. He has hyperlipidemia and hypertension, and is on medication for both. In addition, he takes a daily 81-mg dose of aspirin. The patient has accepted that based on PSA doubling time, initiating ADT would be

appropriate in his case. Also, he prefers to not let his PSA rise further. What is the best schedule of ADT to initiate with this patient?
A. Continuous ADT is superior to intermittent ADT based on long-term efficacy
B. Intermittent ADT is superior to continuous ADT based on long-term efficacy
C. Continuous and intermittent ADT are equivalent based on long-term efficacy
D. Only continuous ADT will decrease the patient's PSA
E. Only intermittent ADT will decrease the patient's PSA

6. A 59-year-old male has metastatic prostate cancer that is castration-resistant. The sites of disease include spine, pelvis, and ribs. He is currently on ADT alone because he previously refused additional therapy. He now has pain requiring 10 mg of oxycodone b.i.d. with occasional extra doses of 5 mg for breakthrough pain. He wants to know which FDA approved therapies for prostate cancer have been shown to improve pain symptoms. He wants you to discuss the clinical data from each before he is willing to initiate therapy. Which of the following therapies is not likely to decrease his pain symptoms?
A. Docetaxel and prednisone
B. Enzalutamide
C. Abiraterone and prednisone
D. Sipuleucel-T
E. Radium 223

7. An 84-year-old male with metastatic castration-resistant prostate cancer recently had disease progression confirmed by PSA and imaging while on 75 mg/m² of docetaxel and 10 mg of prednisone daily. At that time his PSA was 37.6 ng/mL and he had disease on a bone scan in his pelvis (one lesion) and ribs (three lesions). He had stable pain symptoms requiring only nonsteroidal antiinflammatory drugs (NSAIDs) and otherwise had few cancer-related complaints. Based on the findings of his imaging last month, you stopped his docetaxel and prednisone with the hopes of starting him on enzalutamide when you saw him next. His previous treatments include sipuleucel-T for 1 month, abiraterone 1000 mg, and prednisone 10 mg for 2 years followed by docetaxel and prednisone for 18 months. He is now in your office for follow-up 1 month later and has had extreme fatigue over the last 2–3 weeks. His PSA remains stable at 38.1 ng/mL. What is the most appropriate next step for the management of this patient?
A. Order a TSH test to rule out thyroiditis related to previous immunotherapy
B. Restart prednisone
C. Order new scans to confirm progression of his cancer after neuroendocrine de-differentiation in the last month based on worse symptoms and discordant PSA
D. Restart docetaxel and prednisone given change of symptoms since discontinuation
E. Order hospice consultation for end-stage disease and failure to thrive

8. Which of the following patients has castration-resistant prostate cancer?
A. A 63-year-old male with newly diagnosed Gleason 8 prostate cancer whose PSA is 21 ng/mL and testosterone is 256 ng/mL, and who has yet to receive therapy (normal testosterone >180 ng/dL)
B. A 56-year-old male who was treated with radiation and just completed 2 years of ADT. His PSA is 0.03 ng/mL
C. A 66-year-old male with biochemically recurrent prostate cancer after surgery who has a rising PSA of 13.6 (testosterone = 415 ng/dL)
D. A 56-year-old patient with biochemically recurrent prostate cancer whose PSA is declining after starting ADT
E. A patient who is on bicalutamide and ADT with a rising PSA of 4.6 ng/mL (testosterone <20), and there is no radiographic evidence of disease

9. A patient with metastatic castration-resistant prostate cancer who is 73 comes to your office to initiate therapy with abirterone 1000 mg and prednisone 10 mg daily. He has previously been treated with enzalutamide and wants to defer docetaxel as long as possible. The patient's disease is metastatic to the pelvis and ribs. His wife wants to know why you recommend prednisone with the abiraterone. She says she has heard nothing good about prednisone and that her friends have had issues with ulcers, insomnia, and weight gain with prednisone in the past. How do you best reply to her concerns?
A. Tell her the prednisone is an artifact of clinical trial design and can be deferred
B. Tell her that prednisone is required for the anticancer efficacy of abiraterone
C. Tell her that prednisone is used in this regimen to minimize abiraterone treatment-related toxicity
D. Tell her that prednisone will delay disease progression in the bones
E. Tell her prednisone will increase bone density

10. A 79-year-old male with metastatic castration-resistant prostate cancer (superscan on bone scan) presents after recent progression on docetaxel 75 mg/m² every 3 weeks and prednisone 10 mg daily. He has previously developed progressive disease with confirmed radiographic findings while on enzalutamide. He has mild symptoms of pain, which is controlled with NSAIDs. You decide to initiate treatment with cabazitaxel 25 mg/m² every 3 weeks and prednisone 10 mg daily based on randomized phase III data. The patient expresses concern because of treatment-related mortality he learned about while researching the treatment online. You agree that there are some concerns and agree to modify his regimen. Which of the following modifications do you recommend?
A. Decrease dose by 50% because of his advanced age
B. Add a growth factor to decrease the risk of neutropenic infection
C. Add B12 and folate to decrease the risk of neuropathy
D. Increase his prednisone to 20 mg daily to decrease the risk of adrenal insufficiency
E. Admit the patient for each treatment to monitor for hypersensitivity reactions given previous taxane exposure

11. A 56-year-old man complains of back pain and is evaluated by his primary care doctor. Plain films of his back show osteoblastic lesions. His PSA is evaluated and found to be 124 ng/mL. A bone scan shows evidence of metastasis throughout the L-spine, in the pelvis, and in multiple ribs. Which of the follow therapies is not indicated in this patient?
A. Docetaxel
B. Androgen deprivation therapy
C. Calcium
D. Vitamin D
E. Zoledronic acid

12. A 64-year-old male with metastatic castration-resistant prostate cancer including a 2-cm metastasis in his liver, is considering options for the treatment of his disease. He has a history of coronary artery disease, an arrhythmia, seizure disorder, and hypertension. In considering treatment options for metastatic castration-resistant prostate cancer, which of the following comorbidities is a relative contraindication for enzalutamide treatment?
    A. History of coronary artery disease
    B. History of arrhythmia
    C. History of seizure disorder
    D. History of hypertension
    E. Presence of liver metastasis

13. A 65-year-old male with metastatic castration-resistant prostate cancer has recently had disease progression (three new bone lesions) while on treatment with enzalutamide 160 mg daily. His PSA was also rising from baseline (27.3 ng/mL) and is now 57.4 ng/mL. You then decide to start the patient on abiraterone 1000 mg and prednisone 10 mg daily. His PSA has continued to rise and now is 101.3 ng/mL. Restaging scans after 3 months indicates enlarging retroperitoneal lymph nodes and four new bone lesions in the ribs, spine, and pelvis. What is the most likely biologic explanation for these findings?
    A. Tumor flare that is resulting in pseudo-progression
    B. Neuroendocrine prostate cancer that is not responsive to antiandrogen therapy
    C. Castration-resistant disease does not respond to antiandrogen therapy.
    D. Changes in the androgen receptor (such as splice variants) may be driving disease progression
    E. The patient has a secondary malignancy

14. An 87-year-old male with metastatic castration-resistant prostate cancer with metastasis to the bones and liver metastasis comes to your office for a consultation. He has mild pain symptoms, but it is controlled with 10 mg of oxycodone twice daily. He still is active and helps his wife take care of their two grandchildren. He does take an occasional nap in the afternoon. He has been previously treated with standard dosing of abiraterone with prednisone, enzalutamide, and most recently docetaxel. He had documented progression on all those treatments. Which of the following treatments would be the most appropriate recommendation?
    A. Radiofrequency ablation to the liver lesion since that is a negative predictor of outcomes
    B. Retreatment with enzalutamide despite previous progression on enzalutamide
    C. Treatment with cabazitaxel despite progression on another taxane (docetaxel)
    D. Treatment with abiraterone and enzalutamide to overcome likely androgen receptor splice variant-based resistance.
    E. Referral to general surgery for evaluation of a resection of the liver metastasis

15. A 56-year-old male with castration-resistant prostate cancer is on androgen deprivation therapy alone. His scans last year demonstrated no evidence of radiographically visible disease. He presents to your office for a 3-month follow-up with a 20 lb weight loss, nausea, and increasing abdominal pain. (The patient had a screening colonoscopy last year which was negative.) His repeat PSA is 0.75 ng/mL, which is stable from his values over the previous year (range: 0.70–0.85 ng/mL). You order restaging CT and bone scan, which demonstrates liver metastases (multiple up to 3.5 cm) and several 2 cm retroperitoneal lymph nodes. The bone scan shows three new lesions in the spine. What is the most appropriate next step in treatment?
    A. Initiate therapy with bicalutamide
    B. Order a biopsy to evaluate for de-differentiated/small-cell variant prostate cancer
    C. Order a sodium-fluoride PET scan to evaluate metabolic activity in these new lesions
    D. Repeat colonoscopy to rule out colon cancer
    E. Initiate therapy with radium 223

16. An 81-year-old man with metastatic castration-resistant prostate cancer is currently under your care with stable disease and stable symptoms. He has metastasis to his spine, pelvis, and left femur. His current treatment regimen consists of a gonadotropin-releasing hormone (GnRH) agonist, daily enzalutamide 160 mg, and monthly zoledronic acid. On his most recent visit with you, he wants to review his medications and he asks, what is the benefit of the zoledronic acid? Which of the following is the most appropriate response?
    A. Zoledronic acid has been shown to extend survival in metastatic castration-resistant prostate cancer.
    B. Zoledronic acid has been shown to delay disease progression of existing bone lesions in metastatic castration-resistant prostate cancer
    C. Zoledronic acid has been shown to delay the development of additional bone lesions in metastatic castration-resistant prostate cancer
    D. Zoledronic acid has been shown to decrease skeletal complications related to metastatic castration-resistant prostate cancer
    E. Zoledronic acid has been shown to slow PSA doubling time in metastatic castration-resistant prostate cancer

17. A 64-year-old male with a PSA of 12.3 ng/dL has Gleason 4+4 adenocarcinoma of the prostate diagnosed on a biopsy. He elects to have a radical prostatectomy. Which of the following findings on the pathology report would not be an indication for adjuvant radiotherapy?
    A. Extracapsular extension
    B. Perineural invasion
    C. Seminal vesicle involvement
    D. Positive surgical margins

18. A 65-year-old male was diagnosed with prostate cancer 5 years ago and now has metastatic castration-resistant disease. Recent imaging demonstrates that his disease is limited to lymph nodes in the pelvis and retroperitoneum. The lymph nodes range in size from 1.5 to 2.5 cm. The bone scan was negative. The patient says that he searched the internet and this pattern of spread was not common. He asks you how lymph node disease impacts his prognosis. What is the most appropriate response?
    A. Retrospective data suggest that lymph-node-only disease has a more indolent course
    B. Retrospective data suggest that lymph-node-only disease is rare and has a much more aggressive course
    C. Retrospective data suggest that lymph-node-only disease is more common than expected (about 40%), and therefore imparts no prognostic information beyond general expectations
    D. Retrospective data suggest that lymph-node-only disease puts the patient at great risk for cord compression
    E. Retrospective data suggest that lymph-node-only disease puts the patient at great risk for tumor lysis syndrome if he responds to treatment

19. A 63-year-old male has metastatic castration-resistant prostate cancer and is currently considering your recommendation that he receive a radiopharmaceutical for his bone-only disease. The patient does some internet research on his own and with his daughter who works in the pharmaceutical industry. He says that he has concerns about radiopharmaceuticals in general because of the extreme marrow suppression and cytopenias he read about on the internet. How do you reply to the patient and his daughter who you are seeing in your office?
    A. Radium 223 has similar cytopenia potential to older radiopharmaceuticals, but unlike older radiopharmaceuticals (strontium and samarium) Radium 223 improves survival
    B. Radium 223 is an alpha emitter and thus has a smaller emission radius relative to older radiopharmaceuticals (strontium and samarium) and thus has less potential for cytopenias in most patients
    C. Radium 223 does not cause any cytopenia, so this question is not a concern for this patient
    D. Radium 223 will not cause cytopenia in this patient because he is younger than 65 years of age
    E. Radium 223 is no different than older agents strontium and samarium in the mechanism of action, but has better PSA responses than those therapies, so it is preferred

20. A patient with biochemically recurrent prostate cancer comes to your office with a PSA of 0.85. He was treated with surgery 6 years ago and had salvage radiation 4 years ago. His PSA has been rising slowly ever since. He is 59 years of age with hypertension, but is otherwise healthy with no other significant comorbidities. He is worried because his urologist says he needs to initiate androgen deprivation therapy when his PSA rises above 1.0 ng/mL. He is in your office today for consultation and treatment recommendations. What do you tell this patient about initiating ADT?
    A. His urologist is correct. He should begin ADT when his PSA is above 1.0 ng/mL
    B. His urologist is aggressive in his recommendations and he can wait until his PSA rises above the normal range (4.0 ng/mL)
    C. The patient should initiate ADT immediately, based on randomized data, which suggest a survival advantage for continuous ADT in patients with biochemically recurrent prostate cancer
    D. There is no clear standard of care for this population. Retrospective data suggest that PSA doubling time may be more informative than absolute PSA value in determining when to initiate ADT
    E. The patient should initiate ADT with 6 cycles of docetaxel to improve his long-term survival

21. A 56-year-old male has lower back pain. An emergency room (ER) physician does an x-ray and identifies blastic lesions in the lower spine. A subsequent PSA is found to be 153.6 ng/mL. Ultimately, a prostate biopsy yields Gleason 9 prostate cancer. CT and bone scans demonstrated metastatic disease in L3 and L4, in three ribs, sternum, and scapula. You discuss treatment recommendations for this patient. Which one of the following recommendations is not indicated?
    A. ADT
    B. Docetaxel
    C. Calcium
    D. Vitamin D
    E. Zoledronic acid

22. A 71-year-old male with metastatic castration-resistant prostate cancer has now developed progressive disease on enzalutamide. He previously progressed on abiraterone. His PSA is now 256.4 ng/mL and he has widely metastatic disease on bone scan. The patient is willing to start chemotherapy, but read online about the "new one." When you mention that you recommend docetaxel, he says that he wants to start cabazitaxel instead because it is "new" and therefore must be superior. How do you respond to this patient and his request?
    A. Tell the patient that cabazitaxel is new, but does not improve survival in prostate cancer
    B. Tell the patient that docetaxel is superior to cabazitaxel in the first-line chemotherapy setting
    C. Tell the patient that docetaxel is inferior to cabazitaxel in the first-line chemotherapy setting
    D. Tell the patient that there is no evidence that cabazitaxel is superior to docetaxel in the first-line chemotherapy setting
    E. Tell the patient that docetaxel is preferred because it is given more frequently than cabazitaxel

23. A 63-year-old male with castration-resistant prostate cancer is currently being treated with abiraterone 1000 mg and prednisone 10 mg daily. His disease has been quite stable for 6 months. His disease is metastatic to the spine, pelvis, and retroperitoneal lymph nodes. Additional medications include GnRH agonist, denosumab, calcium, vitamin D, and Norvasc for hypertension. His PSA continues to decline from an on-treatment PSA of 68.9 ng/mL. He presents to your office now. His PSA is the lowest it has been since starting abiraterone and prednisone at 12.4 ng/mL. He only has a new complaint of discomfort in his mouth. Physical examination reveals erosion of the back gums/mucosa near the molars. What is the most likely explanation for the initiating event leading to this finding?
    A. Metastatic disease to the jaw
    B. Periodontal disease unrelated to his cancer or his treatments
    C. Osteonecrosis related to denosumab
    D. Poor wound healing related to prednisone
    E. Osteonecrosis related to ADT

24. A 53-year-old male with castration-sensitive metastatic prostate cancer, with metastasis to multiple ribs, spine, scapula, and pelvis, initiates androgen deprivation therapy and 6 cycles of chemotherapy. His comorbidities include diabetes, hypertension, and hyperlipidemia. When he returns for his fourth docetaxel infusion, he reports stable dysguea and eye tearing. You also notice a coffee stain on his shirt and the patient explains that his morning coffee slipped from his hands prior to his visit. Upon further questioning, he notes that he recently has had difficulty gripping eating utensils and has had increased episodes of tripping at home. On exam you notice the patient has decreased sensation in his fingers and toes, but strength is preserved in all extremities. What is the most appropriate next step in the care of this patient?
    A. Continue ADT, but hold docetaxel due to potential taxane-related neuropathy
    B. Hold ADT, but continue docetaxel due to potential ADT-related neuropathy
    C. Continue ADT and docetaxel, but refer the patient to his internist to initiate work-up of diabetic neuropathy
    D. Check B12 and folate for dietary causes of peripheral neuropathy, but continue ADT and docetaxel
    E. Order stat MRI to evaluate the patient for cord compression

25. A 75-year-old male with metastatic castration-resistant prostate cancer is currently on treatment with abiraterone 1000 mg and prednisone 10 mg, which was initiated 2 months ago after the patient had progressive disease on docetaxel. He presents to your office with bilateral lower extremity edema, which has developed over the last month. A review of his CBC and chemistries demonstrates stable findings, including PSA. What is the most likely cause of these findings in this patient?
    A. Toxicity associated with abiraterone
    B. Toxicity associated with prednisone
    C. Deep venous thrombosis
    D. Disseminated intravascular coagulation (DIC)
    E. Lymphangitic spread of the prostate cancer

26. A 63-year-old man with metastatic castration-resistant prostate cancer discontinues docetaxel 75 mg/m² every 3 weeks and prednisone 10 mg daily for peripheral neuropathy. The patient requests a treatment holiday to recover. Three months later, the patient has stable disease based on PSA (45 ng/mL), imaging, and minimal other disease-related symptoms. Although the patient has been treated previously with abiraterone and enzalutamide, he has not yet been treated with sipuleucel-T. Which of the following statements is correct with regard to sipuleucel-T?
    A. Peripheral neuropathy precludes the use of sipuleucel-T in this patient
    B. Sipuleucel-T is a treatment option for this patient, but the patient should be prepared for the fact that PSA is unlikely to decline after this treatment
    C. There are no data that suggests sipuleucel-T can improve survival in patients already treated with docetaxel
    D. The patient's PSA of 45 is too high to derive benefit from sipuleucel-T
    E. The patient's history prednisone use has suppressed his immune system precluding potential benefit from immune-stimulating therapies like sipuleucel-T

27. A 67-year-old male with metastatic castration-resistant prostate cancer has progressive disease while on docetaxel 75 mg/m² every 3 weeks and prednisone 10 mg daily. His PSA is 77.8, he has moderate symptoms (ECOG PS 1), and metastasis to pelvic lymph nodes, liver (a single 2 cm lesion), and bone (pelvis, thoracic spine and third and fourth ribs). The patient's friend has received radium 223, so he asks you about receiving this treatment as well. Which of the following characteristics precludes this patient from receiving radium 223 based on available data?
    A. Metastatic disease in pelvic lymph nodes
    B. Previous history of chemotherapy
    C. Metastatic disease in the liver
    D. Patient requires biopsy of bone disease to initiate radium 223
    E. Patient requires severe bone pain prior to enrollment (ECOG PS 2)

28. A 62-year-old male has a radical prostatectomy and his pathology indicates T2N1 disease with 2 of 25 lymph nodes found to be positive for metastatic disease. His PSA is undetectable 2 months after surgery. The patient is concerned about these findings and wants to know what he could do now to extend his survival. The correct answer you should provide the patient is:
    A. Enzalutamide for 2 years has been shown to improve survival in TxN1 disease
    B. Androgen deprivation therapy has been shown to improve survival in TxN1 disease
    C. Docetaxel for 6 cycles has been shown to improve survival in TxN1 disease
    D. Stereotactic radiation to remaining pelvic lymph nodes has been shown to improve survival in TxN1 disease
    E. Monthly denosumab delays bone metastasis and has been shown to improve survival in TxN1 disease

29. A 63-year-old male is on androgen deprivation therapy for his biochemically recurrent prostate cancer. In the last 3 months his PSA has increased and he was found to have metastatic disease with lesions in his pelvis, scapula, and thoracic spine. The CT scan did not show evidence of visceral disease or enlarged lymph nodes. The patient has no symptoms, and is initiated on enzalutamide therapy with a PSA of 34.6 ng/mL. After 3 months of therapy, the patient's PSA drops to 4.6, but then steadily rises in the following months. After 9 months on therapy, the PSA is 41.4. The patient remains asymptomatic, with no toxicity related to the enzalutamide. In addition, the bone scan and CT scan have remained stable from baseline. What is the most appropriate next step in care of this patient?
    A. Discontinue enzalutamide, initiate docetaxel given PSA progression, which likely indicates the development androgen receptor variant-driven disease
    B. Continue enzalutamide, but add docetaxel given rising PSA
    C. Continue enzalutamide until radiographic progression or symptomatic progression
    D. Discontinue enzalutamide for rising PSA and initiate abiraterone with prednisone
    E. Discontinue enzalutamide for rising PSA and evaluate for a withdrawal response 6 weeks later

30. A 75-year-old man with metastatic castration-resistant prostate cancer presents to you with a rising PSA on androgen deprivation therapy. You are considering multiple therapies for this patient, including abiraterone 1000 mg and prednisone 10 mg daily, which has been shown to improve survival in men with metastatic castration-resistant prostate cancer. What is the proposed mechanism of action of abiraterone?
    A. Direct suppression of testicular production of androgens via 17α-hydroxylase/C17, 20-lyase (CYP17)
    B. GnRH antagonist which indirectly suppresses testicular production of androgens
    C. Androgen receptor antagonist
    D. Suppression of secondary production of androgens, including those from cells in the tumor microenvironment, via 17α-hydroxylase/C17, 20-lyase (CYP17)
    E. Emission of alpha particles that induce DNA damage

31. A 61-year-old with minimally symptomatic prostate cancer requiring rare NSAIDs was recently diagnosed with metastatic disease (to the scapula, third rib, and L2 vertebrae). He is currently on androgen deprivation therapy alone, and you speak to him about treatment with sipuleucel-T. The patient asks you about the most likely side effects. What do you tell the patient are the most common side effects from treatment with sipuleucel-T?
    A. Diarrhea and colitis
    B. Rash and fatigue
    C. Chills/fever and headache
    D. Hypothyroidism
    E. Bone pain

32. A 76-year-old male with metastatic castration-resistant prostate cancer is currently on abiraterone 1000 mg and prednisone 10 mg daily in addition to ADT. His PSA has risen in recent months and his previous scans demonstrated bone dominant disease, including lesions in the ribs, spine, pelvis, and left femur. He presents to your office with increasing lower back pain and urinary retention over the last 24 hours. You also notice that he needs help getting up from the chair to the examination table. Currently, he is only taking NSAIDs for his pain symptoms, but that has been less helpful in the last few days, and the patient is requesting narcotics for pain control. What should be your next step in working up this patient's symptoms?
    A. Straight catheterization to evaluate residual urine volume in the bladder
    B. Ultrasound of the kidneys to evaluate for hydronephrosis
    C. Refer the patient to pain and palliative consultation
    D. Initiate a trial of long-acting narcotics for pain control and follow-up in 2 weeks
    E. Schedule emergency screening spinal MRI to evaluate for cord compression

33. A 54-year-old male with metastatic castration-resistant prostate cancer is currently being treated with ADT with abiraterone 1000 mg plus prednisone 10 mg daily. His PSA has been going up over the last 6 months after declining over the previous 6 months. The patient's initial PSA was 124.6 ng/mL. After a nadir of 17.4 ng/mL, it was 24.3 ng/mL last month. The patient was seen by your partner because you were on vacation. Your partner was concerned about the rising PSA and ordered imaging with a NaF PET scan, which showed new areas of disease relative to the patient's baseline imaging (bone scan and CT scan). The patient now returns to see you to discuss the results and treatment implications. He has no new symptoms on this visit and his PSA is now 27.8 ng/mL. What is the most appropriate treatment decision for this patient?
    A. Continue the current treatment and consider repeating the CT and bone scan
    B. Continue the current treatment and consider repeating the CT but not the bone scan, since the NaF PET scan is more sensitive
    C. Discontinue the abiraterone and repeat the CT and bone scan
    D. Tell the patient that the NaF PET scan has increased sensitivity relative to the bone scan, and thus the abiraterone is no longer effective, and recommend its discontinuation
    E. Add enzalutamide to the patient's current treatment regimen since the NaF PET scan provides conclusive evidence that abiraterone alone is no longer effective

34. An 86-year-old male had a screening PSA and was found to have a PSA of 6.5. He was later biopsied and found to have Gleason 3+3 prostate cancer in 3 of 12 cores. He has a medical history of coronary artery disease (2 MIs in the last year), diabetes, and hypertension. He comes to you for consultation after speaking with a radiation oncologist about potentially curative radiation therapy. What is your most appropriate recommendation?
    A. The patient should proceed with radiation and receive 2 years of adjuvant ADT
    B. The patient should proceed with radiation and receive 3 years of adjuvant ADT
    C. The patient should proceed with radiation and receive 6 months of adjuvant ADT

    D. The patient should consider radical prostatectomy since his Gleason score is 6 given a survival advantage relative to radiation
    E. The patient should consider active surveillance or watchful waiting given his advanced age, comorbidities, and Gleason 6 disease

35. A 54-year-old male has newly diagnosed Gleason 9 prostate cancer. His screening PSA was 15.6 ng/mL and his staging scans were negative. He will not have a prostatectomy given his personal preference and after speaking with several of his friends who have had that procedure. He has seen a radiation oncologist and is now in your office to discuss potential adjuvant ADT as part of the interventions with curative intent. What do you recommend to the patient?
    A. He should reconsider surgery because randomized phase III data suggest it is more effective than radiation
    B. He should proceed with radiation therapy and 2 years of adjuvant ADT
    C. He should proceed with radiation therapy and 6 months of adjuvant ADT
    D. He should proceed with radiation therapy, but there is no role for adjuvant ADT
    E. He should consider ADT only after radiation if his PSA does not nadir to undetectable levels

36. A 73-year-old man has metastatic castration-resistant prostate cancer. He has previously been treated with abiraterone and enzalutamide, but now has progressive disease with new bone lesions. A CT scan showed 1–2 cm retroperitoneal lymph nodes. His PSA is 231.4 ng/mL. After a discussion of treatment options, the patient reveals he will adamantly refuse chemotherapy and wants to know what other options you recommend. He asks about radium 223 as a treatment option. How can you best characterize this treatment in the context of the patient's disease?
    A. Radium 223 has been shown to delay symptomatic progression and improve survival in metastatic castration-resistant prostate cancer
    B. Radium 223 has been shown to only delay symptomatic progression in metastatic castration-resistant prostate cancer
    C. Radium 223 was only associated with PSA declines in metastatic castration-resistant prostate cancer and no changes in overall survival
    D. This patient is not eligible for radium 223 due to disease in his retroperitoneal lymph nodes
    E. This patient is not eligible for radium 223 because patients only benefit if they had been previously treated with docetaxel

37. A patient you are treating is 63 years old, and was treated 4 years ago with radiation for Gleason 7 prostate cancer. You have been following him for 2 years now with biochemically recurrent prostate cancer. His PSA is now 8.9 ng/mL with a doubling time of 2 months. You recommend starting ADT and the patient agrees. He asks what other therapies he can start to help optimize his health at this time. What do you recommend to this patient?
    A. Calcium and vitamin D
    B. Selenium
    C. Daily aspirin
    D. Calcium and vitamin E
    E. Folate and B12

38. A 63-year-old male has newly diagnosed metastatic castration-resistant prostate cancer. He has a history of a stroke last year, but otherwise is now in good health with well-controlled hypertension. He has been on treatment with ADT and bicalutamide for the last 3 years, but his most recent scans demonstrate a rising PSA and two new rib lesions. The patient has no symptoms and leads an active lifestyle. He wants to live long enough to see his 15-year-old daughter graduate from high school. After a 6-week withdrawal period for the bicalutamide, what treatment is most appropriate for this patient?
A. Docetaxel and prednisone for 6 cycles
B. Docetaxel and prednisone for an indefinite period
C. Enzaluatmide
D. Abiraterone and prednisone
E. Flutamide

39. A 51-year-old male is evaluated in an ER for significant back pain. Plain films of the spine reveal several osteoblastic lesions. A subsequent PSA is found to be 596 ng/mL. The patient has a prostate biopsy confirming high-grade prostate cancer, and you are called in for a consultation with the patient. His imaging shows diffuse metastatic disease throughout the spine, ribs, and pelvis. His pain is now better controlled and he wants to know what treatment you recommend. Which the following is the most appropriate initial treatment in this patient?
A. Enzalutamide
B. Six cycles of docetaxel
C. Leuprolide
D. Degarelix
E. Abiraterone and prednisone

ANSWER

1. B
Understand the agonistic properties of bicalutamide. For patients on long-term bicalutamide, there is a documented phenomenon whereby mutations in the androgen receptor convert bicalutamide to an agonist from its primary antagonistic function. Therefore, for patients on bicalutamide, it is reasonable to confirm PSA or disease progression by having patients go through a 6-week withdrawal before starting subsequent therapy.

2. D
Understand the treatment-related toxicities of enzalutamide. The patient's increased fatigue is most likely associated with enzalutamide, which was recently initiated. Enzalutamide is associated with fatigue, which can be extreme in some patients. The treatment should be held to confirm attribution and resolve some of the fatigue. A lower dose of enzalutamide or an alternative therapy could be considered. Enzaluatmide is not commonly associated with adrenal insufficiency or hypothyroidism/thyroiditis. The addition of prednisone in this case would have unclear benefits in the absence of adrenal insufficiency. Given his rapid PSA decline and the absence of other signs of progression, neuroendocrine de-differentiation of the patient's tumor would be unlikely.

3. A
Understand the lack of randomized data comparing radiation and surgery in newly diagnosed prostate cancer. There are no clear randomized data suggesting that either treatment is superior. None of his disease characteristics favor either approach, and his comorbidities would likely not preclude surgery. Thus it best to support the patient as he makes an informed decision that best suits his personal perspective on both treatment options and associated toxicities.

4. A
Understand the proposed mechanism of action of radium 223. Radium 223 is a targeted alpha emitter that selectively binds to areas of increased bone turnover in bone metastases and emits high-energy alpha particles.

5. C
Understand the treatment options for biochemically recurrent prostate cancer. A phase 3 trial randomized patients with biochemically recurrent prostate cancer to either continuous ADT or intermittent ADT (~7 months of ADT followed by a delay in ADT until PSA recovery). There was no significant difference in median overall survival after more than 10 years of follow-up; thus, both these approaches would be acceptable in this patient. Both strategies are likely to lower the PSA in the short term.

6. D
Understand the palliative benefits of treatments for metastatic castration-resistant prostate cancer. Docetaxel, enzalutamide, abiraterone, and radium 223 have all demonstrated the ability to improve moderate pain symptoms as described in this patient. Sipuleucel-T improves overall survival, but generally does not impact short-term pain symptoms and, thus, is not indicated in patients with moderate to severe pain.

7. B
Recognize the symptoms of adrenal insufficiency in a patient who recently completed a long course of prednisone. Prolonged use of prednisone (in this case 42 months) could lead to adrenal insufficiency and should be suspected when extreme fatigue presents after discontinuation. Although blood test can be ordered, empirically restarting prednisone is likely to relive symptoms acutely. Sipuleucel-T is not associated with thyroid dysfunction. There is no clinical benefit in restarting the docetaxel in this patient, although the prednisone could be continued with subsequent therapies. While progressive disease cannot be ruled out, his stable clinical picture, except for fatigue, makes this less likely.

8. E
Understand the definition of castration-resistant prostate cancer. Only Patient E has a confirmed rising PSA despite castration levels of testosterone (patient on long term ADT). Patient D is castration sensitive and responding to ADT appropriately. Patient B has just completed ADT and likely has suppressed testosterone along with a suppressed PSA. Patient A has a rising PSA but also normal testosterone.

9. C
Understand the role of prednisone when paired with abiraterone. Abiraterone is associated with toxicities due to its activity targeting Cyp17, including edema and electrolyte disturbance. Concomitant use of prednisone is

recommended to minimize these toxicities even though it may not be required in all patients. Prednisone may actually weaken bones over time and has unclear antitumor efficacy on its own.

10. B

Understand the treatment-related morbidity and mortality associated with cabazitaxel. The randomized phase III trial with cabazitaxel in metastatic castration-resistant prostate cancer suggested the risk of neutropenia. It was seen in 94% of patients with 8% of patients having febrile neutropenia. For this reason, consideration of growth factor support may be appropriate for this patient. Although lower doses have been evaluated, there are no data supporting a 50% dose reduction due to age. The risks of neuropathy and adrenal insufficiency are not high, based on the phase III data.

11. E

Understand the therapy indicated for metastatic castration-sensitive prostate cancer. Based on phase III clinical data, this patient with high-volume metastatic castration-sensitive prostate cancer is likely to have improved survival with the combined treatment of ADT and docetaxel for 6 cycles. As with all patients on ADT, supplemental treatment with calcium and vitamin D is recommended to decrease the risk of osteoporosis or osteopenia related to castrate levels of testosterone. In a randomized study, adding zoledronic acid to ADT and docetaxel in metastatic castration-sensitive prostate cancer did not demonstrate clinical benefit.

12. C

Understand the relative contraindications for treatment with enzalutamide. Patients with a history of seizure disorder, or those with medications that substantially lower the seizure threshold, were not enrolled in the phase III trials of enzalutamide due to a concern of increased risk of seizures in those patients. For that reason, an alternative therapy should be considered in this patient if he has a history of seizure disorder. Patients with liver metastasis or cardiovascular disease were eligible for those trials.

13. D

Understand the likely mechanisms of resistance to antiandrogen therapy, including enzalutamide and abiraterone. These findings are most consistent with variants of prostate cancer that may have changes in the androgen receptor (including splice variants), which may be driving tumor growth. Pseudo-progression is not seen with antiandrogen therapy. The rising PSA makes neuroendocrine prostate cancer or a secondary malignancy less likely. Antiandrogen therapy, such as abiraterone enzalutamide, demonstrated efficacy in castration-resistant disease in large phase III trials.

14. C

Understand the therapeutic options for patients who have progressed on abiraterone enzalutamide and docetaxel in metastatic castration-resistant prostate cancer. While liver metastases are a poor prognostic finding, treating them with radiofrequency ablation or surgery is not a standard option. Retreatment with enzalutamide or retreatment with abiraterone and enzalutamide in this patient has unproven benefits. Although cabazitaxel is a taxane similar to docetaxel; it has demonstrated a benefit in time-to-progression and overall survival in patients with previous progress on docetaxel.

15. B

Understand the clinical course of de-differentiated/small-cell variant prostate cancer. This patient has a rapid acceleration of metastatic disease and clinical symptoms in the absence of a concomitant and appropriate rise in PSA. This raises concerns for de-differentiated/small-cell variant prostate cancer, and thus, a biopsy would be the appropriate next step. This pattern of spread does not fit with colon cancer despite the development of liver metastases. Neither bicalutamide therapy nor radium 223 would be indicated in this patient. Enzalutamide would be preferred over bicalutamide if the disease was thought to be responsive to an antiandrogen while liver metastases preclude the use of radium 223. A sodium fluoride PET scan will not add meaningful diagnostic information to this clinical scenario.

16. D

Understand the treatment benefits associated with zoledronic acid in metastatic castration-resistant prostate cancer. Zoledronic acid has been shown to decrease skeletal complications related to metastatic castration-resistant prostate cancer. There are no clear data suggesting that zoledronic acid lowers PSA, delays disease progression, or extends survival in metastatic castration-resistant prostate cancer.

17. B

Understand the indications for adjuvant radiation in patients who have had surgery. Extracapsular extension, seminal vesicle involvement, and positive surgical margins are all potential indications for adjuvant radiotherapy in prostate cancer. Perineural invasion carries no implications for adjuvant radiotherapy.

18. A

Understand the implications of lymph-node-only prostate cancer. Although rare, a retrospective study from TAX 327 demonstrated that patients with lymph-node-only disease have a more indolent course than patients with disease that has (also) spread to the bones and/or organs. While treatment implications of these findings are untested, the understanding of these data could inform treatment selection in some cases.

19. B

Understand the mechanism of action of radium 223 and implications for toxicity. Radium 223 is an alpha emitter, and thus has a smaller emission radius relative to older radiopharmaceuticals (strontium and samarium), and thus has less potential for cytopenias in most patients. There was no significant difference in cytopenias between radium 223 and placebo in the phase III trial. It is likely that patients with significant marrow involvement will have a greater risk of cytopenias.

20. D

Understand the approach to treating patients with biochemically recurrent prostate cancer. There is no clear standard of care for this population. Retrospective data suggest that PSA doubling time may be more informative than absolute PSA value in determining when to initiate ADT. There are no absolute values that require initiation of ADT. There are no data to support chemotherapy in this population.

21. E

Understand the treatment recommendations for castration-sensitive metastatic prostate cancer. This patient has newly diagnosed castration-sensitive metastatic prostate cancer with a high tumor volume based on the phase III study. Thus ADT with docetaxel is indicated. For all patients on ADT, calcium and vitamin D are recommended to diminish the risk/magnitude of ADT-related osteoporosis/osteopenia. Zoledronic acid is only indicated for castration-resistant disease and not in castration-sensitive metastatic prostate cancer.

22. D

Understand the data regarding cabazitaxel and docetaxel in the first line chemotherapy setting in metastatic castration-resistant prostate cancer. Docetaxel initially demonstrated improved survival in metastatic castration-resistant prostate cancer. A randomized study did not demonstrate that cabazitaxel is superior to docetaxel in first-line chemotherapy treatment for metastatic castration-resistant prostate cancer.

23. C

Understand the risk and manifestation of osteonecrosis of the jaw with the rank ligand inhibitor denosumab. Similar to zoledronic acid, densumab also carries an increased risk of osteonecrosis of the jaw. Phase III studies suggest an incidence of 5%, but the actual incidence could be higher. While poor wound healing from prednisone may contribute to the morbidity, it is likely not the initiating event. There is unclear attribution to ADT in this setting, and metastatic lesions to the jaw are less common than the incidence of osteonecrosis of the jaw.

24. A

Understand the treatment-related toxicity of docetaxel. This patient likely has taxane-related neuropathy interfering with activities of daily living. His docetaxel should be at least held until the resolution of symptoms, and discontinuing therapy should be considered in the absence of rapid improvement of his neuropathic symptoms. These symptoms are unlikely to be related to diabetes, and given their sensory nature (in the absence of motor findings) cord compression would also be unlikely. B12 and folate supplementation are unlikely to address this toxicity, nor will holding the patient's ADT.

25. A

Understand the treatment-related toxicity associated with abiraterone. This patient's bilateral lower extremity edema is most likely associated with the recent initiation of abiraterone therapy. While prednisone may cause fluid retention, it is actually included as a treatment with abiraterone to minimize side effects, such as edema. Deep venous thrombosis is unlikely to present with bilateral edema. The patient's stable PSA would make cancer-related DIC less likely. Lymphangitic spread from prostate cancer is rare and usually does not manifest itself as lower extremity edema.

26. B

Understand the potential role for sipuleucel-T in advanced prostate cancer. The phase III trial of sipuleucel-T enrolled a minority of patients after treatment with docetaxel, provided they were 3 months' removed from chemotherapy. Thus, this patient could consider sipuleucel-T, but should be educated that PSA responses are uncommon. Peripheral neuropathy is not a toxicity related to sipuleucel-T. There are no data to suggest that previous prednisone precludes possible benefit from sipuleucel-T. Clinical data suggest that patients receiving sipuleucel-T while on prednisone do not have diminished immune activation of the vaccine product. Although retrospective data suggest that patients with lower PSAs may have better clinical outcomes than patients with higher PSAs, PSA itself should not preclude the patient from the potential benefit with sipuleucel-T.

27. C

Understand the exclusion criteria for radium 223. Based on the phase III trial, patients were excluded if they had visceral disease, notably lung or liver. Pelvic lymph nodes do not qualify as visceral disease and are not exclusionary; the phase III trial enrolled patients with lymph nodes up to 3 cm. Also, chemotherapy was not an exclusion for this study, and a subsequent subgroup analysis demonstrated that previous docetaxel did not impact the efficacy of radium 223.

28. B

Understand the treatment recommendations for patients with lymph nodes that are found to be positive for metastatic disease after radical prostatectomy. A randomized study demonstrated that androgen deprivation therapy can improve survival in patients who have lymph-node-positive disease at prostatectomy compared to patients who delay androgen deprivation therapy until overt metastatic disease. There are no randomized data to support the use of enzalutamide, docetaxel, or stereotactic radiation in these patients. Although denosumab delays the development of metastatic disease in patients who are nonmetastatic, its role in this specific population remains undefined.

29. C

Understand the role of PSA in determining treatment failure in patients with metastatic castration-resistant prostate cancer. This patient has a rising PSA despite stable findings on imaging and stable symptomatology. Based on the Prostate Cancer Working Group 3 criteria and the phase III trials of enzalutamide in metastatic disease, the patient should not have his treatment decisions based solely on PSA in the absence of corroborating radiographic evidence, symptomatic progression, or treatment-related toxicity. Therefore, it would be most advisable to continue enzalutamide in this patient at this time.

30. D

Understand the mechanism of action of abiraterone. Abiraterone has a proposed method of action that suggests its anticancer therapy is mediated through the suppression of secondary production of androgens, including from cells in the tumor microenvironment, via 17α-hydroxylase/C17, 20-lyase (CYP17).

31. C

Understand the toxicity profile related to sipuleucel-T. Sipuleucel-T is associated most commonly with chills, fever, and headache. There is no commonly associated bone flare or pain-related symptoms. Diarrhea/colitis, rash, and hypothyroidism are all potential autoimmune reactions seen with immune checkpoint inhibitors, but not sipuleucel-T.

32. E

Understand the clinical manifestations of cord compression in the patient with advanced prostate cancer. This patient has early signs of cord compression and documented disease in the spine, and therefore should be evaluated with an MRI. Although incontinence is often associated with cord compression, early cord compression could manifest itself with urinary and fecal retention. The increased pain and proximal muscle weakness in the legs that are manifested by the patient's difficulty getting out of the chair are consistent with cord compression. While pain symptoms should be addressed, imaging should be done urgently.

33. A

Understand the limited role of the NaF PET scan in metastatic castration-resistant prostate cancer. Although an NaF PET scan is FDA approved for metastatic castration-resistant prostate cancer, its clinical role remains undefined. It was not evaluated at baseline for this patient, so its relevance in this case is further in question since it is likely to be more sensitive than a bone scan. Furthermore, an NaF PET scan was not used as a metric for disease progression in the phase III trials of enzalutamide, so the implications of an NaF PET scan are unclear relative to the potential continued efficacy of enzalutamide. A modest rise in PSA, as in this case and in the absence of conventional radiographic imaging showing progression, should not be used as an indicator to discontinue or change therapy.

34. E

Understand the treatment recommendations for patients with Gleason 6 prostate cancer. There is no role of ADT as part of the radiation therapy for Gleason 6 disease. There are no data to support that surgery would be superior in this case. Also given his age and comorbidities, surgery would likely not be considered. Given the indolent nature of Gleason 6 disease in any patient over 75, it is unlikely that any treatment would be indicated. Especially in this patient with advanced age and comorbidities, it is likely most appropriate to recommend active surveillance or watchful waiting.

35. B

Understand the data regarding ADT in patients receiving external beam radiation for high-risk prostate cancer. This patient has high-risk prostate cancer based on Gleason 9 disease. Multiple randomized trials have demonstrated increased survival and delayed recurrence in these patients when they were treated with 2 or 3 years of ADT. There are no randomized trials that clearly show a benefit for radiation or surgery in newly diagnosed patients. The role of ADT after biochemical recurrence following radiation would not be considered curative therapy.

36. A

Understand the phase III trial data and the indications for radium 223. Randomized phase III data showed that radium 223 delayed symptomatic progression and improved survival in metastatic castration-resistant prostate cancer. Patients with lymph nodes greater than 3 cm were excluded, but this patient's lymph nodes are less than 2 cm. The phase III trial enrolled both docetaxel refractory and docetaxel naïve patients, and both populations demonstrated clinical benefit.

37. A

Understand the treatment-related toxicity of ADT. ADT is associated with an increased risk of decreased bone mineral density. It is recommended that all patients initiating ADT should have a baseline bone density scan and start calcium and vitamin D supplementation. There are no clinical data supporting the role of selenium, aspirin, vitamin E, B12, or folate in men with prostate cancer who are on ADT.

38. D

Understand the therapeutic options for metastatic castration-resistant prostate cancer. There are no clear data that flutamide improves survival in metastatic disease. Six cycles of docetaxel would be indicated for newly metastatic castration-sensitive disease, but this patient has newly metastatic castration-resistant prostate cancer. Enzalutamide is contraindicated in patients with recent CVA or low seizure threshold. Docetaxel is not ideal given the patient's low tumor burden and minimal symptoms. Abiraterone is associated with less treatment toxicity than docetaxel, and thus is most appropriate.

39. D

Understand how to initiate ADT in patients with widely metastatic disease. Because leuprolide (a GnRH agonist) may be associated with a testosterone rise before a fall, this could cause transient pain in this patient with diffuse bone disease. If leuprolide is considered, concomitant use of an AR antagonist, such as bicalutamide, should be considered for the initial treatment phase. Degarelix is a GnRH agonist and thus should not cause a flare in this patient.

REFERENCES

Question 1

1. Sartor AO, Tangen CM, Hussain MH, et al. Antiandrogen withdrawal in castrate-refractory prostate cancer: a Southwest Oncology Group trial (SWOG 9426). *Cancer.* 2008;112:2393–2400.

Question 2

1. Beer TM, Armstrong AJ, Rathkopf DE, et al. Enzalutamide in metastatic prostate cancer before chemotherapy. *N Engl J Med.* 2014;371:424–433.
2. Scher HI, Fizazi K, Saad F, et al. Increased survival with enzalutamide in prostate cancer after chemotherapy. *N Engl J Med.* 2012;367:1187–1197.

Question 4

1. Nilsson S, Larsen RH, Fossa SD, et al. First clinical experience with alpha-emitting radium-223 in the treatment of skeletal metastases. *Clin Cancer Res.* 2005;11:4451–4459.

Question 5

1. Crook JM, O'Callaghan CJ, Duncan G, et al. Intermittent androgen suppression for rising PSA level after radiotherapy. *N Engl J Med.* 2012;367:895–903.

Question 6

1. Beer TM, Armstrong AJ, Rathkopf DE, et al. Enzalutamide in metastatic prostate cancer before chemotherapy. *N Engl J Med.* 2014;371:424–433.
2. Scher HI, Fizazi K, Saad F, et al. Increased survival with enzalutamide in prostate cancer after chemotherapy. *N Engl J Med.* 2012;367:1187–1197.
3. Basch E, Loblaw DA, Oliver TK, et al. Systemic therapy in men with metastatic castration-resistant prostate cancer: American Society of Clinical Oncology and Cancer Care Ontario clinical practice guideline. *J Clin Oncol.* 2014;32:3436–3448.
4. de Bono JS, Logothetis CJ, Molina A, et al. Abiraterone and increased survival in metastatic prostate cancer. *N Engl J Med.* 2011;364:1995–2005.

5. Kantoff PW, Higano CS, Shore ND, et al. Sipuleucel-T immuno-therapy for castration-resistant prostate cancer. *N Engl J Med.* 2010;363:411–422.
6. Parker C, Nilsson S, Heinrich D, et al. Alpha emitter radium-223 and survival in metastatic prostate cancer. *N Engl J Med.* 2013;369: 213–223.
7. Ryan CJ, Smith MR, de Bono JS, et al. Abiraterone in metastatic prostate cancer without previous chemotherapy. *N Engl J Med.* 2013;368:138–148.
8. Tannock IF, de Wit R, Berry WR, et al. Docetaxel plus prednisone or mitoxantrone plus prednisone for advanced prostate cancer. *N Engl J Med.* 2004;351:1502–1512.

Question 8

1. Scher HI, Morris MJ, Stadler WM, et al. Trial design and objectives for castration-resistant prostate cancer: updated recommendations from the prostate cancer clinical trials working group 3. *J Clin Oncol.* 2016;34:1402–1418.

Question 9

1. de Bono JS, Logothetis CJ, Molina A, et al. Abiraterone and in-creased survival in metastatic prostate cancer. *N Engl J Med.* 2011;364:1995–2005.
2. Ryan CJ, Smith MR, de Bono JS, et al. Abiraterone in metastatic prostate cancer without previous chemotherapy. *N Engl J Med.* 2013;368:138–148.

Question 10

1. de Bono JS, Oudard S, Ozguroglu M, et al. Prednisone plus cabazi-taxel or mitoxantrone for metastatic castration-resistant prostate can-cer progressing after docetaxel treatment: a randomised open-label trial. *Lancet.* 2010;376:1147–1154.

Question 11

1. Sweeney CJ, Chen YH, Carducci M, et al. Chemohormonal thera-py in metastatic hormone-sensitive prostate cancer. *N Engl J Med.* 2015;373:737–746.
2. James ND, Sydes MR, Clarke NW, et al. Addition of docetaxel, zoledronic acid, or both to first-line long-term hormone therapy in prostate cancer (STAMPEDE): survival results from an adaptive, multiarm, multistage, platform randomised controlled trial. *Lancet.* 2016;387:1163–1177.

Question 12

1. Beer TM, Armstrong AJ, Rathkopf DE, et al. Enzalutamide in metastatic prostate cancer before chemotherapy. *N Engl J Med.* 2014;371:424–433.
2. Scher HI, Fizazi K, Saad F, et al. Increased survival with enza-lutamide in prostate cancer after chemotherapy. *N Engl J Med.* 2012;367:1187–1197.

Question 13

1. Antonarakis ES, Lu C, Wang H, et al. AR-V7 and resistance to enzalutamide and abiraterone in prostate cancer. *N Engl J Med.* 2014;371:1028–1038.

Question 14

1. de Bono JS, Oudard S, Ozguroglu M, et al. Prednisone plus cabazi-taxel or mitoxantrone for metastatic castration-resistant prostate cancer progressing after docetaxel treatment: a randomised open-label trial. *Lancet.* 2010;376:1147–1154.

Question 15

1. Aparicio AM, Harzstark AL, Corn PG, et al. Platinum-based chem-otherapy for variant castrate-resistant prostate cancer. *Clin Cancer Res.* 2013;19:3621–3630.

Question 16

1. Saad F, Gleason DM, Murray R, et al. Long-term efficacy of zole-dronic acid for the prevention of skeletal complications in patients with metastatic hormone-refractory prostate cancer. *J Natl Cancer Inst.* 2004;96:879–882.

Question 17

1. Wiegel T, Bartkowiak D, Bottke D, et al. Adjuvant radiotherapy versus wait-and-see after radical prostatectomy: 10-year follow-up of the ARO 96-02/AUO AP 09/95 trial. *Eur Urol.* 2014;66:243–250.

Question 18

1. Pond GR, Sonpavde G, de Wit R, Eisenberger MA, Tannock IF, Arm-strong AJ. The prognostic importance of metastatic site in men with metastatic castration-resistant prostate cancer. *Eur Urol.* 2014;65:3–6.

Question 19

1. Parker C, Nilsson S, Heinrich D, et al. Alpha emitter radi-um-223 and survival in metastatic prostate cancer. *N Engl J Med.* 2013;369:213–223.

Question 20

1. Crook JM, O'Callaghan CJ, Duncan G, et al. Intermittent androgen suppression for rising PSA level after radiotherapy. *N Engl J Med.* 2012;367:895–903.
2. Suzman DL, Zhou XC, Zahurak ML, Lin J, Antonarakis ES. Change in PSA velocity is a predictor of overall survival in men with bi-ochemically-recurrent prostate cancer treated with nonhormonal agents: combined analysis of four phase-2 trials. *Prostate Cancer Prostatic Dis.* 2015;18:49–55.

Question 21

1. Sweeney CJ, Chen YH, Carducci M, et al. Chemohormonal thera-py in metastatic hormone-sensitive prostate cancer. *N Engl J Med.* 2015;373:737–746.
2. James ND, Sydes MR, Clarke NW, et al. Addition of docetaxel, zoledronic acid, or both to first-line long-term hormone therapy in prostate cancer (STAMPEDE): survival results from an adaptive, multiarm, multistage, platform randomised controlled trial. *Lancet.* 2016;387:1163–1177.

Question 22

1. Tannock IF, de Wit R, Berry WR, et al. Docetaxel plus prednisone or mitoxantrone plus prednisone for advanced prostate cancer. *N Engl J Med.* 2004;351:1502–1512.
2. Sartor O. Cabazitaxel vs docetaxel in chemotherapy-naive (CN) patients with metastatic castration-resistant prostate cancer. *ASCO Annual Meeting Abstract.* 2016.

Question 23

1. Smith MR, Saad F, Coleman R, et al. Denosumab and bone-metastasis-free survival in men with castration-resistant prostate cancer: results of a phase 3, randomised, placebo-controlled trial. *Lancet.* 2012;379:39–46.

Questions 24

1. Tannock IF, de Wit R, Berry WR, et al. Docetaxel plus prednisone or mitoxantrone plus prednisone for advanced prostate cancer. *N Engl J Med.* 2004;351:1502–1512.
2. Sweeney CJ, Chen YH, Carducci M, et al. Chemohormonal thera-py in metastatic hormone-sensitive prostate cancer. *N Engl J Med.* 2015;373:737–746.

Questions 25

1. de Bono JS, Logothetis CJ, Molina A, et al. Abiraterone and increased survival in metastatic prostate cancer. *N Engl J Med.* 2011;364:1995–2005.
2. Ryan CJ, Smith MR, de Bono JS, et al. Abiraterone in metastatic prostate cancer without previous chemotherapy. *N Engl J Med.* 2013;368:138–148.

Question 26

1. Kantoff PW, Higano CS, Shore ND, et al. Sipuleucel-T immuno-therapy for castration-resistant prostate cancer. *N Engl J Med.* 2010;363:411–422.
2. Schellhammer PF, Chodak G, Whitmore JB, Sims R, Frohlich MW, Kantoff PW. Lower baseline prostate-specific antigen is associated with a greater overall survival benefit from sipuleucel-T in the Im-munotherapy for Prostate Adenocarcinoma Treatment (IMPACT) trial. *Urology.* 2013;81:1297–1302.

3. Small EJ, Lance RS, Gardner TA, et al. A randomized phase II trial of sipuleucel-T with concurrent versus sequential abiraterone acetate plus prednisone in metastatic castration-resistant prostate cancer. *Clin Cancer Res.* 2015;21:3862–3869.

Question 27

1. Parker C, Nilsson S, Heinrich D, et al. Alpha emitter radium-223 and survival in metastatic prostate cancer. *N Engl J Med.* 2013;369:213–223.
2. Hoskin P, Sartor O, O'Sullivan JM, et al. Efficacy and safety of radium-223 dichloride in patients with castration-resistant prostate cancer and symptomatic bone metastases, with or without previous docetaxel use: a prespecified subgroup analysis from the randomised, double-blind, phase 3 ALSYMPCA trial. *Lancet Oncol.* 2014;15:1397–1406.

Question 28

1. Messing EM, Manola J, Yao J, et al. Immediate versus deferred androgen deprivation treatment in patients with node-positive prostate cancer after radical prostatectomy and pelvic lymphadenectomy. *Lancet Oncol.* 2006;7:472–479.

Question 29

1. Beer TM, Armstrong AJ, Rathkopf DE, et al. Enzalutamide in metastatic prostate cancer before chemotherapy. *N Engl J Med.* 2014;371:424–433.
2. Scher HI, Fizazi K, Saad F, et al. Increased survival with enzalutamide in prostate cancer after chemotherapy. *N Engl J Med.* 2012;367:1187–1197.
3. Scher HI, Morris MJ, Stadler WM, et al. Trial design and objectives for castration-resistant prostate cancer: updated recommendations from the prostate cancer clinical trials working group 3. *J Clin Oncol.* 2016;34:1402–1418.

Questions 30

1. de Bono JS, Logothetis CJ, Molina A, et al. Abiraterone and increased survival in metastatic prostate cancer. *N Engl J Med.* 2011;364:1995–2005.
2. Ryan CJ, Smith MR, de Bono JS, et al. Abiraterone in metastatic prostate cancer without previous chemotherapy. *N Engl J Med.* 2013;368:138–148.

Questions 31

1. Kantoff PW, Higano CS, Shore ND, et al. Sipuleucel-T immunotherapy for castration-resistant prostate cancer. *N Engl J Med.* 2010;363:411–422.

Question 32

1. Sciubba DM, Petteys RJ, Dekutoski MB, et al. Diagnosis and management of metastatic spine disease. A review. *J Neurosurg Spine.* 2010;13:94–108.
2. Sutcliffe P, Connock M, Shyangdan D, Court R, Kandala NB, Clarke A. A systematic review of evidence on malignant spinal metastases: natural history and technologies for identifying patients at high risk of vertebral fracture and spinal cord compression. *Health Technol Assess.* 2013;17:1–274.

Question 33

1. Beer TM, Armstrong AJ, Rathkopf DE, et al. Enzalutamide in metastatic prostate cancer before chemotherapy. *N Engl J Med.* 2014;371:424–433.
2. Scher HI, Fizazi K, Saad F, et al. Increased survival with enzalutamide in prostate cancer after chemotherapy. *N Engl J Med.* 2012;367:1187–1197.
3. Scher HI, Morris MJ, Stadler WM, et al. Trial design and objectives for castration-resistant prostate cancer: updated recommendations from the prostate cancer clinical trials working group 3. *J Clin Oncol.* 2016;34:1402–1418.

Question 34

1. Albertsen PC, Hanley JA, Fine J. 20-year outcomes following conservative management of clinically localized prostate cancer. *JAMA.* 2005;293:2095–2101.

Question 35

1. Bolla M, Van Tienhoven G, Warde P, et al. External irradiation with or without long-term androgen suppression for prostate cancer with high metastatic risk: 10-year results of an EORTC randomised study. *Lancet Oncol.* 2010;11:1066–1073.
2. Zapatero A, Guerrero A, Maldonado X, et al. High-dose radiotherapy with short-term or long-term androgen deprivation in localised prostate cancer (DART01/05 GICOR): a randomised, controlled, phase 3 trial. *Lancet Oncol.* 2015;16:320–327.

Question 36

1. Parker C, Nilsson S, Heinrich D, et al. Alpha emitter radium-223 and survival in metastatic prostate cancer. *N Engl J Med.* 2013;369:213–223.

Question 37

1. Crawford ED, Shore ND, Moul JW, et al. Long-term tolerability and efficacy of degarelix: 5-year results from a phase III extension trial with a 1-arm crossover from leuprolide to degarelix. *Urology.* 2014;83:1122–1128.

Question 38

1. Beer TM, Armstrong AJ, Rathkopf DE, et al. Enzalutamide in metastatic prostate cancer before chemotherapy. *N Engl J Med.* 2014;371:424–433.
2. Basch E, Loblaw DA, Oliver TK, et al. Systemic therapy in men with metastatic castration-resistant prostate cancer: American Society of Clinical Oncology and Cancer Care Ontario clinical practice guideline. *J Clin Oncol.* 2014;32:3436–3448.

Question 39

1. Crawford ED, Shore ND, Moul JW, et al. Long-term tolerability and efficacy of degarelix: 5-year results from a phase III extension trial with a 1-arm crossover from leuprolide to degarelix. *Urology.* 2014;83:1122–1128.
2. Noguchi K, Uemura H, Harada M, et al. Inhibition of PSA flare in prostate cancer patients by administration of flutamide for 2 weeks before initiation of treatment with slow-releasing LH-RH agonist. *Int J Clin Oncol.* 2001;6:29–33.

Bladder and Other Urothelial Cancers

Ravi A. Madan and Jeanny B. Aragon-Ching

QUESTIONS

1. A 48-year-old male presents with hematuria to his urologist. Computed tomography (CT) scan revealed a visible mass in the posterior wall of the bladder with mild hydronephrosis. His creatinine was normal at 0.8. Transurethral resection of bladder tumor (TURBT) was performed showing high-grade muscle invasive transitional cell cancer (TCC). He was referred to you for further management. You discuss with the patient the following:
   A. Initiation of neoadjuvant chemotherapy followed by radical cystectomy because it has been shown to improve survival
   B. Proceed with radical cystectomy first then consider adjuvant chemotherapy only if he has pT3 or node-positive disease
   C. Proceed with concurrent chemotherapy and radiation therapy
   D. Proceed with radical cystectomy alone; there is no role for chemotherapy in this setting
   E. Proceed with radiation alone

2. A 48-year-old female with history of spina bifida and LE paralyzes who has been wheelchair-bound presents to her urologist for hematuria. She has been doing intermittent catheterization and thought it may be secondary to trauma or another urinary tract infection, which she often gets. Cystoscopy showed a dominant bladder mass, which, on TURBT, showed pure squamous bladder cancer invading the detrusor muscle. She has no apparent metastatic disease on staging scans. You counsel her with the following:
   A. You would recommend neoadjuvant chemotherapy with gemcitabine and cisplatin followed by radical cystectomy.
   B. You would recommend chemotherapy alone because she has squamous cell histology.
   C. You would recommend proceeding straight to radical cystectomy with anterior pelvic exenteration and TAH-BSO.
   D. You would recommend intravesical bacillus Calmette-Guérin (BCG) given squamous histology.
   E. You would recommend radiation alone for bladder preservation strategy.

3. A 44-year-old male presents with a suspicious upper ureteral tract/renal pelvis mass on the right, which was incidentally found after a routine surveillance scan for a preceding history of colon cancer that was resected and treated a year ago. Further ureteroscopy and biopsy showed a high-grade urothelial cancer on washings and biopsy. He undergoes definitive right nephroureterectomy and removal of bladder cuff. Upon further review of his family history, his father had a history of colon cancer diagnosed at 48 years of age. You recommend referral to genetic counseling for testing of the following:
   A. Hereditary nonpolyposis colorectal cancer (HNPCC) or Lynch syndrome
   B. Li-Fraumeni syndrome
   C. VHL syndrome
   D. Birt-Hogg-Dubé syndrome
   E. HLRCC

4. A 56-year-old male presents to the urologist with complaints of hematuria. He underwent a CT scan (Fig. 24.1) and was found to have a midline mass (inset) in the area of the dome of the bladder. Further cystoscopy showed pathology consistent with adenocarcinoma. Which of the following is the most appropriate treatment option?
   A. Intravesical chemotherapy
   B. Partial cystectomy with en bloc resection of the urachal ligament with the bladder dome and umbilectomy
   C. Neoadjuvant chemotherapy with gemcitabine and cisplatin followed by radical cystectomy
   D. Combined chemotherapy and radiation
   E. Primary systemic chemotherapy is sufficient

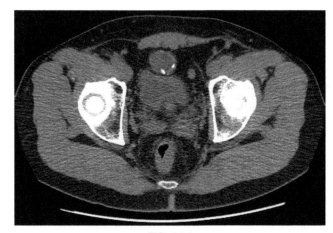

FIG. 24.1

5. A 62-year-old male presents with hematuria. Cystoscopy and TURBT showed micropapillary variant of urothelial carcinoma invading into the lamina propria. What would be the most appropriate next treatment?
   A. Consider intravesical mitomycin
   B. Consider intravesical gemcitabine
   C. Consider upfront radical cystoprostatectomy
   D. Consider TURBT and continued observation with cystoscopy every 3 months afterwards
   E. Consider palliative radiotherapy

6. A 66-year-old male presents for follow-up with a history of superficial bladder TCC. He had a prior TURBT showing T1 high-grade TCC and CIS a year prior, and received induction BCG. He presented to the urologist and was found to have + cytology on bladder wash, but there was no evidence of apparent tumor during the cystoscopy. What is the next step in management?
   A. Give intravesical mitomycin
   B. Give another induction BCG
   C. Recommend cystoprostatectomy
   D. Recommend upper tract imaging with CT urography or ureteroscopy with biopsy
   E. Continue surveillance cystoscopy in 3 months

7. A 79-year-old male presents with hematuria. His CT scan (Fig. 24.2) showed an infiltrative mass in the right kidney measuring 7 cm *(inset)* with mild hydronephrosis. Biopsy revealed TCC. No other apparent metastatic disease was seen on scans. His performance status was excellent with ECOG 0. He desires to pursue active treatment. His creatinine was 1.0. A mag-renal Lasix scan reveals only 3% function in the right kidney with 97% differential function on the left side. You recommended the following treatment:
   A. Radical nephrectomy
   B. Radical nephroureterectomy with cuff of bladder resection
   C. Chemotherapy with gemcitabine and carboplatin
   D. Cystoprostatectomy
   E. Hospice

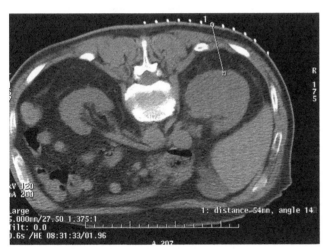

FIG. 24.2

8. A 64-year-old male presents with 3 months of pelvic pressure and pain. He undergoes cystoscopy and is found to have a bladder tumor in the posterior wall. Pathology reveals a small-cell cancer of the bladder with invasion to the detrusor muscle. His CT scan shows involvement of the bladder tumor with no lymph node involvement or extravesical involvement. His brain MRI was negative. What is your next appropriate management?
   A. Recommend neoadjuvant chemotherapy with gemcitabine and cisplatin followed by radical cystectomy
   B. Recommend chemotherapy with cisplatin and etoposide with concomitant radiation
   C. Recommend chemotherapy with MVAC
   D. Recommend upfront radical cystectomy
   E. Recommend brain prophylactic cranial irradiation

9. A 63-year-old male presented with hematuria and was found to have muscle-invasive bladder cancer. After hearing the arguments for neoadjuvant chemotherapy, he opted to proceed with upfront radical cystoprostatectomy. However, he has heard about the utility of adjuvant chemotherapy. You begin to discuss with him the following:
   A. You will offer him adjuvant chemotherapy should he have pT3 or pT4, or node-positive disease.
   B. Adjuvant chemotherapy has been shown to improve disease-free survival.
   C. Adjuvant chemotherapy trials have been largely underpowered due to insufficient accrual number of patients.
   D. Adjuvant chemotherapy has been shown in a retrospective database to improve overall survival.
   E. All of the above.

10. An 83-year-old male presented with hematuria. CT scan showed a 4-cm mass in the posterior bladder wall. He underwent TURBT showing muscle-invasive urothelial carcinoma, but had extreme difficulty with the anesthesia postoperatively. He presents to your office and expresses a desire for nonsurgical treatment. Which of the following options will potentially result in the best disease-free survival for treatment outcome?
   A. Intravesical BCG
   B. Intravesical valrubicin
   C. Intravesical gemcitabine
   D. Combined radiation and chemotherapy with mitomycin and 5FU
   E. Radiation therapy alone

11. An 85-year-old man was admitted to the hospital because of hematuria. A CT scan was ordered, which showed a 6-cm bladder wall mass along with retroperitoneal adenopathy and a focus in the liver that is indeterminate, and 2 subcentimeter lung nodules. The patient was taken to the operating room where a TURBT was performed and showed muscle-invasive urothelial carcinoma. You are then consulted. Upon your discussion of treatment, the patient and his family would like to discuss with you regarding news about promising results with immunotherapy.
   You discussed with them the following:
   A. There are promising data regarding use of PD-L1 inhibitors in advanced/metastatic bladder cancer that is refractory to therapy.
   B. There is currently no existing data regarding use of PD-L1/PD-1 inhibitors for the upfront setting.
   C. You would recommend a PD-L1 inhibitor once he gets a response to treatment.
   D. You would recommend a PD-L1 inhibitor in combination with chemotherapy.
   E. There is absolutely no role at this time for any use of PD-1 or PD-L1 inhibitors; it simply does not work.

12. A 61-year-old man was referred to you for a recently resected bladder cancer with the histology showing predominantly squamous cell cancer. Upon further history, you learn that he has been traveling to his home country in Egypt. Which of the following infections are you most concerned with?
   A. *Clonorchis sinensis*
   B. *Schistosoma haematobium*
   C. Human papillomavirus
   D. Human immunodeficiency virus
   E. None of the above

13. A 50-year-old male patient with a recent diagnosis of bladder cancer comes to you for a second opinion. He has read new and emerging therapies as well as interesting genomic alterations in bladder cancer, and wonders how it applies to him. You discuss with him about known genetic alterations on bladder cancer:
    A. The tumor suppressor gene TP53 is often implicated in invasive bladder cancer.
    B. A mutation in TSC1 has been identified in bladder cancer for which everolimus has been used as a targeted therapy.
    C. A common alteration in urothelial carcinoma is chromosome 9 deletion.
    D. Activating mutations in FGFR3 are common in noninvasive urothelial papillary bladder cancers.
    E. All of the above

14. A 62-year-old male patient with metastatic bladder urothelial cancer to the lymph nodes had undergone gemcitabine and cisplatin for 6 cycles and achieved stable disease. However, he started having impaired renal function with a creatinine of 2 as well as emerging neuropathy grade 1–2. He insists on continuing treatment. You discuss with him the following:
    A. Continue with gemcitabine and cisplatin despite the renal dysfunction and neuropathy
    B. Recommend sunitinib
    C. Recommend lapatinib
    D. Consider a clinical trial
    E. Continue cisplatin alone since he had stable disease

15. A 63-year-old patient is being referred to you for a history of penile cancer. He initially underwent penectomy, but further scans showed pelvic and retroperitoneal adenopathy with two lung nodules that was biopsy-proven metastatic penile cancer. He is being sent to you regarding consideration for chemotherapy. Which of the following would be the next best step in management with this patient?
    A. You would recommend pelvic and retroperitoneal lymph node dissection.
    B. You would recommend bleomycin alone.
    C. You would recommend surgery followed by radiation.
    D. You would recommend cisplatin-based chemotherapy, such as TIP (paclitaxel, ifosfamide and cisplatin).
    E. None of the above.

16. A 61-year-old male patient was found to have hematuria. TURBT showed detrusor muscle involvement with urothelial cancer in a papillary tumor, but with involvement of the prostate stroma. His CT scan imaging and bone scan were negative. You discussed his case with the tumor board and were asked to stage him. You assign him the following clinical stage:
    A. Stage 0
    B. Stage I
    C. Stage II
    D. Stage III
    E. Stage IV

17. A 56-year-old male patient undergoes TURBT and is found to have predominantly urothelial carcinoma with a lymphoepithelioma-like carcinoma variant. He has muscle-invasive disease. He is referred to you by the urologist for recommendations. Which of the following should you now recommend?
    A. Neoadjuvant dose-dense MVAC or gemcitabine/cisplatin followed by radical cystoprostatectomy and lymph node dissection
    B. Radical cystoprostatectomy

C. Radiation alone
D. Chemotherapy with 5FU and mitomycin with concurrent radiation
E. Any of the above approaches would be acceptable

18. A 62-year-old patient who underwent neoadjuvant chemotherapy for 4 cycles of gemcitabine and cisplatin underwent radical cystoprostatectomy and was found to have pT3 bladder cancer. He was referred to you by his primary care physician since he had also seen a radiation oncologist for consideration of adjuvant radiation. Which of the following would you discuss regarding utility of adjuvant radiation in his case?
    A. Recommend adjuvant radiotherapy now
    B. Consideration for adjuvant chemotherapy may be given
    C. Recommend chemoradiotherapy
    D. Recommend observation
    E. None of the above

19. A 40-year-old male patient presents with superficial bladder cancer. He asks you during his visit about the risk factors of developing bladder cancer. Which of the following in his medical history would you consider pertinent regarding his risk for developing bladder cancer?
    A. Smoking history
    B. Occupational history
    C. Intake of phenacetin-containing analgesics
    D. Prior exposure to drugs, such as cyclophosphamide
    E. All of the above

20. A 54-year-old male patient presents with pelvic pain and hematuria. TURBT showed pure bladder adenocarcinoma. What would be the next step in management?
    A. Neoadjuvant dose-dense MVAC or gemcitabine/cisplatin followed by radical cystoprostatectomy and lymph node dissection
    B. Referral to gastroenterology for colonoscopy and endoscopy; only proceed with radical cystoprostatectomy and lymph node dissection if negative
    C. Radiation alone
    D. Chemotherapy with 5FU and mitomycin with concurrent radiation
    E. Any of the above approaches would be acceptable

21. A 78-year-old patient with a history of small-cell bladder carcinoma was referred to you by the radiation oncologist for discussion regarding the role of PCI. He was found to have muscle-invasive bladder carcinoma 2 months ago, and on imaging had no adenopathy and no obvious metastases. His brain MRI was negative. He was started on cisplatin and etoposide. Regarding your views on PCI, you discuss with him the following:
    A. You would recommend hospice at this time.
    B. He should receive PCI before starting systemic therapy.
    C. You would recommend starting PCI at the conclusion of his chemotherapy.
    D. There is no sufficient data to recommend PCI for extrapulmonary small cell lung cancer at this time.
    E. None of the above.

22. A 58-year-old male African-American patient is referred to you for a history of urethral cancer. At the end of the visit, he asks you what risk factors he had that predisposed him to develop urethral cancer and to prevent future recurrence. You answer that the risk is associated with the following:
    A. Urethral stricture
    B. HPV status

C. Chronic inflammation
D. Repeated infection
E. All of the above

23. A 65-year-old male presents to you for another opinion from the urologist. He presented initially with microscopic hematuria and was found on TURBT to have CIS. His urologist recommends induction BCG × 6 treatments, and upon repeat cystoscopy was found to have just erythema in the bladder. You recommend the following:
A. Another induction BCG × 6
B. Observe for now and continue with maintenance BCG as planned
C. Recommend upfront radical cystectomy
D. Repeat cystoscopy; he should have undergone multiple random biopsies
E. Send a urine cytology test

24. A 62-year-old male presents with right flank pain and hematuria. He was found to have a 5 cm mass in the renal pelvis on the CT scan, with evidence of perivesical fat invasion on further MRI. Biopsy showed high-grade urothelial carcinoma on biopsy. A renal Lasix scan showed differential function of 50% on the left kidney and 50% on the right kidney. He would like to be aggressive in treating this cancer. Which of the following treatment options would you discuss with the patient?
A. Radical nephrectomy
B. Radical nephroureterectomy with cuff of bladder resection
C. Consideration for neoadjuvant gemcitabine and cisplatin followed by radical nephroureterectomy with cuff of bladder resection
D. Radical nephrectomy and cystoprostatectomy
E. Nephrostomy tube placement, and institute BCG

ANSWERS

1. A

Initiation of neoadjuvant chemotherapy followed by radical cystectomy has been shown to improve survival. Neoadjuvant chemotherapy with MVAC has historically shown improvement in overall survival in patients with muscle-invasive bladder cancer and hence would be appropriate. While several randomized studies have shown benefits in adjuvant chemotherapy where progression-free survival is beneficial, overall survival has not been uniformly seen, and studies have been largely underpowered because they suffered from insufficient accrual. Chemo-radiation as a bladder preservation strategy is an option, especially for patients who are deemed unresectable or otherwise refuse cystectomy. Radiation alone is inferior as a therapy for someone who is otherwise a surgical candidate with intent for cure.

2. C

Recommend radical cystectomy with anterior pelvic exenteration and TAH-BSO. This patient is presenting with squamous cell muscle-invasive bladder cancer. Typical risk factors for squamous cell carcinoma include chronic inflammation such as that seen in this patient. While neoadjuvant chemotherapy followed by radical cystectomy would be considered standard, especially for urothelial cancers, even in the case of variants, some other histologies, including squamous cell carcinoma, would lead to ineffective, or at times, detrimental delay of primary treatment of cystectomy.

3. A

This male patient presents with one of the cancer syndromes involved with colon cancer, with HNPCC or Lynch syndrome. HNPCC is characterized in a family with at least three cases of colon cancer, at least one of whom was diagnosed by 50 years of age, and in which individuals are affected in at least two generations. There is also a well-described increased risk of other cancers in both men and women who are HNPCC carriers, such as endometrial and ovarian cancer in women, and stomach, pancreatic, small intestine, biliary tract, ureter, and renal pelvis cancers in both men and women. Upper urinary tract tumors tend to develop at a younger age and are more likely to be in the ureter with an almost equal gender ratio in patients with Lynch syndrome.

4. B

Partial cystectomy with en bloc resection of the urachal ligament with the bladder dome and umbilicus. Urachal carcinomas are almost always adenocarcinoma in histology and frequently involve the midline or dome of the bladder due to the origin of the tumor from the urachal ligament with extension to the dome of the bladder. Clinical distinction of this tumor type with that of other urothelial cancers are important, since treatment choices with surgery or the use of chemotherapy, where there is still no great proven benefit for neoadjuvant or adjuvant approaches, may matter. Patients who present with resectable tumors can be treated with partial cystectomy with en bloc resection of the urachal ligament with the bladder dome, and removal of the umbilicus is required in order to adequately control the tumor.

5. C

Consider upfront radical cystoprostatectomy. The micropapillary variant of urothelial carcinoma is considered to be an aggressive variant. While many would recommend radical cystectomy for micropapillary bladder cancer invading the lamina propria (cT1) given the poor prognosis, contradictory small reports show some efficacy of conservative management with intravesical BCG for this disease. Mitomycin is usually used for patients during perioperative therapy with TURBT in superficial urothelial bladder cancer. While intravesical gemcitabine has been used after BCG failure, this is considered an off-label use. There is increasing interest with upfront radical cystectomy in patients presenting with micropapillary urothelial carcinoma, especially since survival is improved in those who undergo early radical cystectomy, but is compromised for those who have recurrent cystectomy, or deferred immediate cystectomy.

6. D

Recommend upper tract imaging with CT urography or ureteroscopy with biopsy. Urine cytology has variable sensitivity of about 35%–61%. However, in cases where one finds a positive urine cytology in the absence of tumors in the bladder, suspicion for an upper tract urothelial carcinoma UTUC is high. Therefore, a search for an upper tract tumor using conventional imaging, such as computed tomography (CT) urography, which involves the use of CT technology using thin slices with less than 2 mm using various protocols with improved sensitivity over intravenous urography (IVU), such as 75% versus 95.8% for CT urography. A ureteroscopy can be performed for pathological biopsy with confirmation of the diagnosis. However, the reliability for tumor staging is poor, although grading is good with correlation to the final histopathological grade of close to 90% with grade 1 or higher-grade tumors.

7. B

This patient presents with high-grade urothelial carcinoma for which the standard of care remains as surgical resection with radical nephroureterectomy and bladder cuff resection, in patients who are otherwise candidates for surgery. While there is increasing use and extrapolation from the bladder cancer data regarding neoadjuvant chemotherapy with gemcitabine and cisplatin or dd-MVAC (similar to that used in muscle-invasive bladder cancer for patients who are otherwise cisplatin-eligible) substitution of carboplatin for cisplatin would be inferior, and if perioperative chemotherapy cannot be effectively or safely delivered with the use of cisplatin, then surgery would be the most optimal approach.

8. B

Recommend chemotherapy with cisplatin and etoposide with concomitant radiation. Patients with small-cell pathology of bladder cancer are treated similarly to small-cell pathology of other sites. While regimens using gemcitabine and cisplatin or MVAC may be appropriate for urothelial cancer cell histology, cisplatin and etoposide may work better with small-cell pathology. Whereas PCI has been found beneficial in patients with limited disease of small-cell lung cancer, its use in bladder cancer is still unproven.

9. E

All of the above. Adjuvant chemotherapy in bladder cancer has been a topic of long-drawn-out controversy given several underpowered trials, and especially given lack of adequate accrual. One of the largest trials, the EORTC 30994, showed that immediate chemotherapy for patients with pT3–T4 or node-positive bladder cancer result in significant disease-free survival, but not overall survival. Conversely, a retrospective database out of the National Cancer Database (NCDB) showed an overall survival advantage, albeit with all the caveats of a retrospective analysis.

10. D

Combined radiation and chemotherapy with mitomycin and 5FU. This patient has expressed a desire for nonsurgical intervention. Given the muscle-invasive disease, intravesical treatment would be suboptimal. However, chemoradiotherapy remains an option. The BC2001 trial enrolled 360 patients who were assigned in a phase III trial to undergo either chemoradiation (regimen of 5FU 500 mg/m^2 per day during fractions 1–5 and 16–20 of radiation as well as mitomycin 12 mg/m^2 on day 1 or radiation alone). The locoregional disease-free survival was superior in the combined chemoradiotherapy group at 67% compared with 54% for the radiation group (P = .03). However, while overall survival did favor the chemoradiotherapy group, it was not statistically significant (P = 0.16).

11. A

There is promising data regarding the use of PD-L1 and PD-1 inhibitors in advanced/metastatic bladder cancer that is refractory to therapy. There is a proven role for immunotherapy in locally advanced/metastatic bladder cancer resistant to platinum therapy. A multiinstitutional phase II trial using atezolizumab an anti-PD-L1 inhibitor, showed promising objective response rates for every

specified immune cell group in the cohort of patients. The highest response rate of 27% was in the immune cell group (IC2/3) with 95% CI 19–37, P < .0001; and in all patients, regardless of their immune cell status, the response rate was 15% (95% CI 11–20, P = .0058). This has set the stage for all other PD-1/PD-L1 inhibitors in the field of bladder cancer therapy where different drugs are being used for different settings, including that of patients who are considered cisplatin-ineligible. Based on this trial, the US FDA has granted five immunotherapy drugs with accelerated approval in bladder cancer.

12. B

Schistosoma haematobium. While the majority of histological subtypes of bladder cancer are urothelial cancers, squamous cell bladder cancer is common in areas where a parasitic infection, schistosomiasis, is endemic. Clonorchis is associated with cholangiocarcinoma. While there are increasing reports of an association between HPV and bladder urothelial cancer, especially HPV16, this patient hails from and frequently visits an area endemic for schistosomiasis, which is more likely the consideration.

13. E

All of the above. Patients with urothelial carcinoma often have alterations in chromosome 9, which, when deleted, appears to be important for the initiation of bladder cancer. Other common alterations include p53 and Rb deletions, which are common in invasive bladder cancer, whereas mutations of FGFR3 are seen in noninvasive papillary cancers. A rare mutation in TSC1 had been described in a patient with bladder cancer for whom everolimus served as an effective targeted therapy using genome sequencing.

14. D

Consider a clinical trial. At this time, continued supportive care as the standard of care would be ideal. If there is a clinical trial option that looks at the question of maintenance, then it would also be appropriate. The question of maintenance after optimal treatment with chemotherapy for locally advanced or metastatic disease has been evaluated with the use of sunitinib or lapatinib, but it has been shown to be negative. Continuing further with cisplatin when he already hasdeveloped renal dysfunction and neuropathy would be inappropriate.

15. D

You would recommend cisplatin-based chemotherapy such as TIP (paclitaxel, ifosfamide, and cisplatin). Penile cancers are rare genitourinary cancers that are usually squamous cell carcinomas in histology. Treatment for stage IV penile cancers (by definition those who have pelvic or retroperitoneal or distant metastases, such as this patient) usually entails cisplatin-based chemotherapy with TIP being shown to be an active regimen. The use of bleomycin in these patients was discouraged because of toxicity. In patients with pelvic nodal disease alone, further consolidative surgery or palliative radiotherapy may be considered if sufficient responses to chemotherapy are seen. However, finding stage IV disease in penile cancer portends an ominous prognosis.

16. D

Stage III. This patient has involvement of the prostatic stroma, which elevates him to have a T4a disease, and based on the AJCC staging, this would be considered stage III disease.

17. A

Neoadjuvant dose-dense MVAC or gemcitabine/cisplatin followed by radical cystoprostatectomy and lymph node dissection. This patient presents with one of the rare urothelial carcinoma variants, urothelial carcinoma with a lymphoepithelioma-like carcinoma variant. Certain reports had suggested a favorable prognosis if lymphoepithelioma-like carcinoma was the predominant pattern, as chemotherapy seemed to yield favorable responses. Regardless, in patients with predominant urothelial carcinoma, even in the presence of a variant, treatment with neoadjuvant chemotherapy remains a reasonable approach, followed by surgery in patients who exhibit no metastatic disease.

18. D

Recommend observation. This patient was found to have persistent stage III disease but had already undergone neoadjuvant chemotherapy. While a retrospective database based on the Retrospective International Study of Cancers of the Urothelium (RISC) showed possible benefit with the use of additional adjuvant chemotherapy for residual disease despite prior receipt of neoadjuvant chemotherapy, this was a retrospective study, and there is no clear established role for further chemotherapy in the absence of overt metastatic disease. The subject of adjuvant radiation is the topic of investigation that is launched by several groups including the NRG Oncology in North America and the French GETUG-AFU, among others. While several small studies and retrospective data suggest potential benefit, it remains an investigational approach at this time.

19. E

All of the above. Risk factors for bladder cancer has historically included smoking as one of the strongest risk factors, accounting for up to 50% of cases in developed countries. However, other risk factors, such as occupation exposures to aromatic amines, environmental exposures to arsenic, drugs like chemotherapy using cyclophosphamide, urinary tract infections, and schistosomiasis (for squamous cell bladder cancer), have also been implicated.

20. B

Referral to gastroenterology for colonoscopy and endoscopy; only proceed with radical cystoprostatectomy and lymph node dissection if negative. Primary adenocarcinoma of the bladder is rare in the developed world, accounting for about 1.4% of bladder cancers undergoing radical cystectomy. It is more prevalent in the developing world, accounting for up to 11%. It is the third most common bladder cancer, after urothelial cancer and squamous cell cancer. Primary adenocarcinoma of the bladder can be histologically classified as enteric, adenocarcinoma not otherwise specified, signet ring cell, mucinous, clear cell, hepatoid, or mixed. It is crucial to rule out another primary source, such as that seen in the gastrointestinal tract. Hence, the importance of consulting with gastroenterology.

21. D

There are no sufficient data to recommend PCI for extrapulmonary small-cell lung cancer at this time. This patient presents with an aggressive histological subtype of bladder carcinoma. Treatment is often extrapolated from the small-cell cancer literature. Treatment with cranial radiation would be appropriate for overt presence of metastatic disease.

22. E

All of the above. Urethral cancers are rare cancers that occur with a rate of 5.0 per million and 2.5 per million for African Americans and whites, respectively, according to a SEER-based dataset. The most common histological subtype was transitional cell carcinoma occurring in about half the patients (55%), squamous cell carcinoma in 21.5%, and adenocarcinoma in 16.4%. There is varying incidence of the three primary histological types by race and sex.

23. B

Observe for now and continue with maintenance BCG as planned. Intravesical BCG has been the cornerstone of treatment against CIS and is recommended as first-line therapy based on the AUA and EAU guidelines, and maintenance therapy with BCG was demonstrated by the SWOG 8794 to be effective in CIS. Maintenance therapy is given as 3 weekly BCG treatments at 3 months, 6 months, and every 6 months intervals for up to 3 years. While radical cystectomy has been considered the de facto second-line option for patients who fail BCG, this patient has not exhibited failure. This patient has erythema, which is likely due to post-induction BCG. In addition, taking random biopsies are no longer considered standard. Continuation of planned maintenance BCG would be recommended with surveillance cystoscopies.

24. C

Consideration for neoadjuvant gemcitabine and cisplatin followed by radical nephroureterectomy with cuff of bladder resection. This patient presents with high-grade urothelial carcinoma for which the standard of care remains as surgical resection with radical nephroureterectomy and bladder cuff resection, in patients who are otherwise candidates for surgery. However, there is increasing use and extrapolation from the bladder cancer data regarding neoadjuvant chemotherapy with gemcitabine and cisplatin or dd-MVAC, similar to what would be used in muscle-invasive bladder cancer for patients who are otherwise cisplatin-eligible. Therefore, the National Comprehensive Cancer Network (NCCN) would also recommend consideration for neoadjuvant chemotherapy in those who are considered cisplatin-eligible.

REFERENCES

Question 1

1. Grossman HB, Natale RB, Tangen CM, et al. Neoadjuvant chemotherapy plus cystectomy compared with cystectomy alone for locally advanced bladder cancer. *N Engl J Med*. 2003;349:859–866.

Question 2

1. Willis D, Kamat AM. Nonurothelial bladder cancer and rare variant histologies. *Hematol Oncol Clin North Am*. 2015;29:237–252, viii.

Question 3

1. Crockett DG, Wagner DG, Holmang S, Johansson SL, Lynch HT. Upper urinary tract carcinoma in Lynch syndrome cases. *J Urol*. 2011;185:1627–1630.

Question 4

1. Siefker-Radtke A. Urachal adenocarcinoma: a clinician's guide for treatment. *Semin Oncol*. 2012;39:619–624.

Question 5

1. Willis DL, Fernandez MI, Dickstein RJ, et al. Clinical outcomes of cT1 micropapillary bladder cancer. *J Urol.* 2015;193:1129–1134.
2. Spaliviero M, Dalbagni G, Bochner BH, et al. Clinical outcome of patients with T1 micropapillary urothelial carcinoma of the bladder. *J Urol.* 2014;192:702–707.

Question 6

1. Colin P, Kassouf W, Konety BR, Lotan Y, Rouprêt M. Diagnosis and evaluation of upper tract urothelial carcinoma (UTUC). In: Shariat SF, Xylinas E, eds. *Upper Tract Urothelial Carcinoma.* New York, NY: Springer; 2015:31–43.
2. Wang LJ, Wong YC, Ng KF, Chuang CK, Lee SY, Wan YL. Tumor characteristics of urothelial carcinoma on multidetector computerized tomography urography. *J Urol.* 2010;183:2154–2160.
3. Soukup V, Babjuk M, Bellmunt J, et al. Follow-up after surgical treatment of bladder cancer: a critical analysis of the literature. *Eur Urol.* 2012;62:290–302.

Question 7

1. Porten S, Siefker-Radtke AO, Xiao L, et al. Neoadjuvant chemotherapy improves survival of patients with upper tract urothelial carcinoma. *Cancer.* 2014;120:1794–1799.

Question 8

1. NCCN Clinical Practice Guidelines. Bladder Cancer. Version 2. 2015.

Question 9

1. Sternberg CN, Skoneczna I, Kerst JM, et al. Immediate versus deferred chemotherapy after radical cystectomy in patients with pT3–pT4 or N+ M0 urothelial carcinoma of the bladder (EORTC 30994): an intergroup, open-label, randomised phase 3 trial. *Lancet Oncol.* 2015;16:76–86.
2. Galsky MD, Stensland KD, Moshier E, et al. Effectiveness of adjuvant chemotherapy for locally advanced bladder cancer. *J Clin Oncol.* 2016;34:825–832.

Question 10

1. James ND, Hussain SA, Hall E, et al. Radiotherapy with or without chemotherapy in muscle-invasive bladder cancer. *N Engl J Med.* 2012;366:1477–1488.

Question 11

1. Rosenberg JE, Hoffman-Censits J, Powles T, et al. Atezolizumab in patients with locally advanced and metastatic urothelial carcinoma who have progressed following treatment with platinum-based chemotherapy: a single-arm, multicentre, phase 2 trial. *Lancet.* 2016;387(10031):1909–1920.

Question 12

1. Li N, Yang L, Zhang Y, Zhao P, Zheng T, Dai M. Human papillomavirus infection and bladder cancer risk: a meta-analysis. *J Infect Dis.* 2011;204:217–223.

Question 13

1. Iyer G, Hanrahan AJ, Milowsky MI, et al. Genome sequencing identifies a basis for everolimus sensitivity. *Science.* 2012;338:221.

Question 14

1. Grivas PD, Daignault S, Tagawa ST, et al. Double-blind, randomized, phase 2 trial of maintenance sunitinib versus placebo after response to chemotherapy in patients with advanced urothelial carcinoma. *Cancer.* 2014;120:692–701.
2. Powles T, Huddart RA, Elliott T, et al. A phase II/III, double-blind, randomized trial comparing maintenance lapatinib versus placebo after first line chemotherapy in HER1/2 positive metastatic bladder cancer patients. *ASCO Meeting Abstracts.* 2015;33:4505.

Question 15

1. Pettaway CA, Pagliaro L, Theodore C, Haas G. Treatment of visceral, unresectable, or bulky/unresectable regional metastases of penile cancer. *Urology.* 2010;76:S58–S65.

Question 16

1. *AJCC Cancer Staging Manual.* 7th ed. LLC (SBM): Springer Science + Business Media; 2010.

Question 18

1. Harshman LC, Werner L, Wong Y-N, et al. Adjuvant chemotherapy for residual disease after neoadjuvant chemotherapy for muscle invasive urothelial cancer (MIUC). *ASCO Meeting Abstracts.* 2015;33:4524.
2. Christodouleas JP, Hwang WT, Baumann BC. Adjuvant radiation for locally advanced bladder cancer? A question worth asking. *Int J Radiat Oncol Biol Phys.* 2016;94:1040–1042.
3. Reddy AV, Pariser JJ, Pearce SM, et al. Patterns of failure after radical cystectomy for pT3–4 bladder cancer: implications for adjuvant radiation therapy. *Int J Radiat Oncol Biol Phys.* 2016;94:1031–1039.

Question 19

1. Jankovic S, Radosavljevic V. Risk factors for bladder cancer. *Tumori.* 2007;93:4–12.

Question 20

1. Zaghloul MS, Nouh A, Nazmy M, et al. Long-term results of primary adenocarcinoma of the urinary bladder: a report on 192 patients. *Urol Oncol.* 2006;24:13–20.

Question 21

1. Naidoo J, Teo MY, Deady S, Comber H, Calvert P. Should patients with extrapulmonary small-cell carcinoma receive prophylactic cranial irradiation? *J Thorac Oncol.* 2013;8:1215–1221.

Question 22

1. Swartz MA, Porter MP, Lin DW, Weiss NS. Incidence of primary urethral carcinoma in the United States. *Urology.* 2006;68:1164–1168.

Question 23

1. Tang DH, Chang SS. Management of carcinoma in situ of the bladder: best practice and recent developments. *Ther Adv Urol.* 2015;7:351–364.

Question 24

1. Lamm DL, Blumenstein BA, Crissman JD, et al. Maintenance bacillus Calmette-Guerin immunotherapy for recurrent TA, T1 and carcinoma in situ transitional cell carcinoma of the bladder: a randomized Southwest Oncology Group Study. *J Urol.* 2000;163:1124–1129.

CHAPTER
25

Renal Cell Carcinoma

Ravi A. Madan and Jeanny B. Aragon-Ching

QUESTIONS

1. A 53-year-old man presents with flank pain and was incidentally discovered to have an 11-cm renal mass. Upon further history and examination, you elicit the patient's personal history of cutaneous leiomyoma, and his mother and maternal grandmother had a prior history of fibroids necessitating hysterectomy. He undergoes radical nephrectomy. You expect the renal cell cancer (RCC) pathology to be the following (Fig. 25.1):
   A. Clear cell RCC
   B. Medullary RCC
   C. Papillary RCC
   D. Chromophobe RCC
   E. Oncocytoma

2. A 70-year-old male presented with metastatic kidney cancer to the lungs. He underwent treatment with sunitinib for 12 months, but has started progressing with enlargement of the target lesions. You discuss with him about switching therapies. He asks you about the benefit of immunotherapy in his situation. You tell him the following:
   A. Nivolumab showed improved overall survival compared with everolimus.
   B. Everolimus has statistically significantly better progression-free survival (PFS) compared with nivolumab.
   C. Nivolumab has similar side effects to chemotherapy.
   D. Nivolumab should be combined with pazopanib for better efficacy.
   E. Nivolumab has less overall response to everolimus.

3. A 75-year-old male was found to have metastatic clear cell kidney cancer to the lungs. His creatinine and liver function tests were all within normal limits. His LDH was normal. He underwent a prior nephrectomy 2 years ago. His performance status is 0. He presents to you for discussion regarding primary treatment of metastatic kidney cancer. You counsel him on the following:
   A. Sunitinib is superior to pazopanib in efficacy, but has more effects on fatigue and HFS.
   B. Everolimus is superior to sunitinib in efficacy, but has more effects on fatigue and HFS.
   C. Sunitinib is equally effective to pazopanib, but has more effects on hepatotoxicity.
   D. Pazopanib is equally effective to sunitinib, but has more effects on hepatotoxicity.
   E. Everolimus should be given as first-line therapy.

4. A 48-year-old African American male seeks medical attention for a history of hematuria. His medical history was significant for a history of sickle cell disease. A computed tomography (CT) scan was done which showed a 6-cm renal mass and metastatic involvement in the retroperitoneum, bone, and lungs. What histology is the most likely diagnosis?
   A. Urothelial cancer
   B. Medullary RCC
   C. Papillary kidney cancer
   D. Chromophobe kidney cancer
   E. Oncocytoma

5. A 65-year-old female presents to you for a history of resected kidney cancer. She was found to have a 10-cm clear cell RCC with Fuhrman grade IV. She had no evidence of disease on restaging scans post-nephrectomy. Which of the following is the most appropriate intervention?
   A. Start on sunitinib 50 mg 4 weeks on/2 weeks off for 1 year
   B. Start on sorafenib 800 mg daily for 1 year
   C. Observation with surveillance scans monitoring for progression
   D. Start everolimus 10 mg daily for 1 year
   E. Start pazopanib 800 mg daily

6. A 49-year-old patient was recently diagnosed with a kidney mass. He underwent radical nephrectomy with pathology revealing pT2NxMx papillary RCC. Which of the following statements is correct?
   A. Papillary RCCs make up about 75% of all kidney cancers diagnosed.
   B. Type I papillary RCCs are typically associated with *MET* alterations.
   C. Type II papillary RCCs are typically associated with VHL mutation alterations.

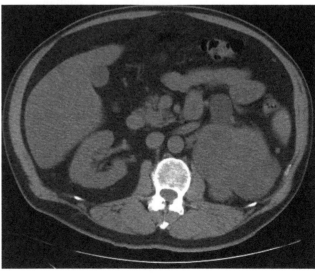

FIG. 25.1

D. Type II papillary RCCs were characterized by better survival with mutation of the gene encoding fumarate hydratase (FH).
E. None of the above are correct.

7. The VHL gene has been characterized in a hereditary kidney cancer syndrome. Which of the following is true?
A. VHL is inherited as an autosomal dominant pattern.
B. Studies of families show germline translocations involving the short arm of chromosome 3.
C. Affected family members are at risk for developing variable tumors in the kidney, retina, spinal cord, pancreas, and adrenal glands.
D. Of patients with VHL, approximately 60% would develop solid and cystic kidney lesions during their lifetime.
E. All of the above are true.

8. RCCs make up about 4% of all adult malignancies. Which of the following is true regarding the histologic subtype that makes up RCC?
A. Papillary RCC makes up the most common histologic subtype.
B. Type 2 papillary RCC is the most common hereditary subtype.
C. Sporadic clear cell RCC makes up the majority of histologic subtypes.
D. Chromophobe RCC is the most common hereditary subtype.
E. Oncocytoma is the most common histologic subtype.

9. A 78-year-old male with prior history of hypertension and stroke came for consultation regarding a history of hematuria and was found to have a 2-cm right kidney mass. His urologist recommended a partial nephrectomy. The patient is interested in this approach. You discuss that partial nephrectomy can generally be considered for the following:
A. Presence of a small less than 4 cm tumor
B. Presence of renal dysfunction
C. Presence of bilateral renal masses
D. Presence of familial kidney cancer
E. All of the above

10. A 68-year-old male presents with a large renal mass. He undergoes radical nephrectomy with pathology revealing clear cell RCC, 10 cm size, with Fuhrman grade 4. He also has laboratory tests showing anemia with hemoglobin of 8.9 g/dL, creatinine of 1.3, LDH of 211, calcium of 8.9, albumin of 4. He has recuperated well from surgery with good performance status of ECOG 0, but on a restaging scan was found to have multiple bilateral lung nodules. You calculated his MSKCCprognostic factor for choice of therapy. The factors you are considering that predict for poor overall prognosis include the following:
A. Hemoglobin of less than normal
B. Size of the renal mass
C. Clear cell histology of the kidney cancer
D. Presence of lung metastases
E. Albumin of 4

11. A 73-year-old patient presented with gross hematuria. He underwent a CT scan, which revealed a 6-cm mass, multiple retroperitoneal adenopathy, and lung nodules. He declined further surgery after a biopsy revealed clear cell RCC. He was found to have anemia, and high calcium and LDH. He also has pain and anorexia. You discuss treatment options with him and state the following:
A. He has favorable risk disease; you recommend sunitinib.
B. He has poor risk disease; you recommend high dose interleukin.

C. He has poor-risk disease; you recommend temsirolimus.
D. He has intermediate-risk disease; you recommend nivolumab.
E. He has poor-risk disease; you recommend everolimus.

12. A 59-year-old male who presented with metastatic kidney cancer went on sunitinib and had stable disease for 1 year. However, his last restaging scan showed progressive disease. He asks you about cabozantinib. You discuss with him the results of the METEOR study:
A. Cabozantinib showed overall survival advantage compared with everolimus.
B. Cabozantinib showed improvement in PFS compared with everolimus.
C. There were more dose reductions in patients undergoing cabozantinib therapy compared with everolimus.
D. Objective response rates were higher with everolimus compared with cabozantinib.
E. All of the above are correct.

13. Which of the following best describes the use of tyrosine kinase inhibitors (TKIs) in advanced RCC?
A. Cabozantinib is an oral, small-molecule TKI that targets the vascular endothelial growth factor receptor (VEGFR) as well as MET and AXL.
B. Sunitinib is a multikinase inhibitor against VEGF, PDGF and c-kit.
C. Axitinib can be given post-VEGF TKI failure.
D. Lenvatinib and everolimus can be given post-VEGF TKI failure.
E. All of the above.

14. A 72-year-old female patient was admitted to the hospital for pancytopenia, failure to thrive, stomatitis, hypercholesterolemia, shortness of breath, and cough. Her physical examination was notable for hypoxemia. Her chest x-ray is showing signs of interstitial pattern, and the pulmonologist orders a high-resolution CT scan and suspects pneumonitis after ruling out infection. The hospitalist contacted you to state that this patient has a diagnosis of metastatic kidney cancer, but the patient does not recall what drug she was on. Apart from counseling discontinuation of the drug, you also recommended starting the patient on steroids. Which drug is she likely on?
A. Sunitinib
B. Pazopanib
C. Bevacizumab
D. Interferon
E. Everolimus

15. A 56-year-old male was recently diagnosed with hereditary papillary kidney cancer. You are discussing his case with medical students. You started discussing which mutation is likely involved?
A. VHL
B. MET
C. RB1
D. SDHB
E. Folliculin (FLCN)

16. A 62-year-old male patient comes to you for a second opinion regarding his recently diagnosed metastatic papillary kidney cancer. He saw the results of a trial called Everolimus Versus Sunitinib Prospective Evaluation in Metastatic Non-Clear Cell Renal Cell Carcinoma (ESPN) for non-clear cell RCC. He wonders if the trial results are applicable to him. You discuss with him the following:
A. You will prescribe everolimus because it has shown superior efficacy against all non-clear cell RCC.

B. The unequivocal efficacy seen in this trial definitely points to the superiority of everolimus in non-clear cell RCC.

C. The median overall survival with sunitinib use was slightly better than everolimus, but is not statistically significant.

D. The majority of patients enrolled in this trial had chromophobe histology.

E. None of the above.

17. A 66-year-old male patient was being treated with metastatic kidney cancer with sunitinib for 1 year. However, upon restaging follow-up, he was found to have progression of disease in his lung lesions. He and his family are interested in immunotherapy. You describe the mechanism of action of programmed death (PD)-1 inhibitors. Which of the following is true regarding PD-1 blockade?

A. PD-1 blockade lessens secretion of T cells of more cytokines.

B. Blockade of PD-1 allows T-cell re-activation.

C. PD-1 blockade has no effect on the immune responses from regulatory T (TReg) cells.

D. PD-1 blockade does not affect T cells' metabolic program or interaction with target cells.

E. PD-1 blockade allows increased expansion of thymic T cells.

18. An 88-year-old male patient was admitted to the hospital for transient ischemic attack (TIA). Further workup was performed, which revealed a 2-cm incidental renal mass. Also, he was hospitalized 2 weeks ago for acute coronary artery disease (CAD), and has chronic kidney disease with a creatinine of 1.6–1.8. The hospitalist consults you regarding an opinion about management. Which of the following would constitute the most appropriate management for this patient?

A. Refer for radical nephrectomy

B. Refer for laparoscopic partial nephrectomy

C. Active surveillance

D. Cryoablation

E. Start sunitinib

ANSWERS

1. C

This patient is presenting with a syndrome called hereditary leiomyomatosis and renal cell carcinoma (HLRCC). This syndrome is characterized by cutaneous leiomyomata, which occurs singly or multiply in the majority of individuals; for example, uterine fibroids in women, and RCC that is usually a single tumor. The RCC is typically papillary carcinoma in character or a collecting duct tumor. These tend to be aggressive and occur in about 10%–16% of individuals. The pathogenic mechanism involves a loss of function of the FH protein with either germline pathogenic variant in FH, plus somatic variants and loss of heterozygosity in the tumor tissue. Conversely, clear cell kidney cancer is the typical RCC found in patients with VHL, whereas medullary cancers are seen in patients with sickle cell disease. While chromophobe kidney cancers can be seen in a hereditary familial syndrome called Birt-Hogg Dubé (BHD) syndrome, which is characterized also by skin lesions. The cutaneous lesions are usually fibrofolliculomas (rather than leiomyomas), pulmonary cysts, spontaneous pneumothorax, and bilateral, multifocal RCC (rather than solitary in HLRCC). Oncocytomas can grow large and may be confused with clear cell RCC because of its eosinophilic cytoplasm, but it is still largely considered a benign neoplasm in the 2004 World Health Organization classification of benign tumors.

2. A

Nivolumab is a fully human monoclonal antibody against PD-1, and on November 25, 2015, was approved by the US Food and Drug Administration for the treatment of advanced kidney cancers that have failed one line of prior antiangiogenic therapy. In the pivotal phase III trial, Checkmate 025, nivolumab was compared with everolimus in a second-line setting and was found to be superior in overall survival with a median of 25 months in those who were treated with nivolumab 3 mg/kgIV q 2 weeks versus everolimus 10 mg daily. Response rates were greater with nivolumab at 25% versus 5% with everolimus (odds ratio: 5.98; [95% confidence interval (CI), 3.68–9.72]; $P<.001$). While the median PFS was not statistically significantly different, PFS with nivolumab was better at 4.6 months compared with 4.4 months with everolimus. Nivolumab, being a checkpoint inhibitor, showed immune-related side effects, but overall grade III or IV treatment side effects occurred in 19% of patients on nivolumab versus 37% for those who received everolimus.

3. D

Treatment for metastatic/advanced kidney cancers, especially with a good Memorial Sloan Kettering Cancer Center (MSKCC) prognostic score, would be to use VEGF TKIs with either sunitinib or pazopanib. Everolimus is indicated as second-line therapy after failure post-TKI. In the COMPARZ trial, pazopanib was noninferior to sunitinib with respect to PFS (hazard ratio [HR] for progression of disease or death from any cause, 1.05; 95% CI, 0.90–1.22), meeting the predefined noninferiority margin (upper bound of the 95% CI, <1.25). Overall survival was similar (HR for death with pazopanib, 0.91; 95% CI, 0.76–1.08). However, in terms of side effects, sunitinib had a higher overall incidence of fatigue (63% vs. 55%), hand-foot syndrome (50% vs. 29%), and thrombocytopenia (78% vs. 41%); patients treated with pazopanib had a higher incidence of increased levels of alanine aminotransferase (60% vs. 43% with sunitinib). When physicians and patients were polled on their preference after an innovative crossover design, the same pattern was seen in the PISCES trial, where significantly more patients (70%) preferred pazopanib over sunitinib (22%).

4. B

Medullary RCC. While any renal cancer pathology may be seen in patients presenting with kidney mass, renal medullary cancers are an epithelial malignancy that almost exclusively occur in young black patients with the sickle cell hemoglobinopathy. These tumors are largely aggressive, and many present with advanced or metastatic disease with limited treatment options.

5. C

Observation with surveillance scans monitoring for progression. Several adjuvant studies have been conducted in patients with high-risk disease and have been found to be negative. Initial results from the ASSURE ECOG 2805 trial using adjuvant sorafenib versus sunitinib versus placebo showed no difference in terms of adjuvant therapy, making observation still the most appropriate approach for patients with optimally resected kidney cancers.

6. B

Type 1 papillary RCCs are typically associated with *MET* alterations. Type 1 and type 2 papillary renal cell carcinomas were shown to be different types of renal cancer characterized by specific genetic alterations. Type 1 tumors were associated with *MET* alterations, whereas type 2 tumors were characterized by cyclin dependence kinase inhibitor (*CDKN)2A* silencing, *SETD2* mutations, *TFE3* fusions, and increased expression of the NRF2–antioxidant response element (ARE) pathway, as had been seen in The Cancer Genome Atlas network analyses. A CpG island methylator phenotype was observed in a distinct subgroup of type 2 papillary RCC that was characterized by poor survival and mutation of the gene encoding FH.

7. E

All of the above. VHL syndrome is one of the four major autosomal dominantly inherited kidney cancer syndromes characterized by germline translocations of the distal portion of the short arm of chromosome 3, but it was initially described by Eugene von Hippel and later by Arvid Lindau. Affected individuals have a predisposition to develop tumors involving the kidney, hemangioblastomas in the cerebellum, spinal cord or retina, involvement of the inner ear, pancreas, epididymis, or pheochromocytomas of the adrenals. Of the patients with VHL studied, up to 60% may develop solid and cystic renal lesions in their lifetime, leading to the emergence of nephron-sparing surgeries as a potential strategy for these patients.

8. E

All of the above. VHL syndrome is one of the four major autosomal dominantly inherited kidney cancer syndromes characterized by germline translocations of the distal portion of the short arm of chromosome 3, but it was initially described by Eugene von Hippel and later by Arvid Lindau. Affected individuals have a predisposition to developing tumors involving the kidney, hemangioblastomas in the cerebellum, spinal cord or retina, involvement of the inner ear, pancreas, epididymis, or pheochromocytomas of the adrenals. Of the patients with VHL studied, up to 60% may develop solid and cystic renal lesions in their lifetime, leading to the emergence of nephron-sparing surgeries as a potential strategy for these patients

9. C

Sporadic clear cell RCC makes up the majority of histologic subtype. RCC affects close to 39,000 patients in the United States in 2016 alone and causes close to 13,000 deaths annually. RCC forms a unique pathological entity that spans varying histologic subtypes with clear cell RCC as the most common, making up close to 75%, and papillary RCC as the 2nd most common (type 1 pRCC making up 5% and type 2 pRCC at 10%), chromophobe and oncocytomas are rare with about a 10% incidence of all RCCs. While genetic mutations have been identified as an etiology of inherited RCC, these only account for 1-2% of all RCC cases. Majority of sporadic RCCs (up to 80%) is of clear cell histology.

10. A

Hemoglobin of less than normal. The MSKCC or the Motzer criteria for poor prognosis was based on several pretreatment factors in metastatic RCC patients, which includes a low Karnofsky performance status (<80%), a high lactate dehydrogenase level (>1.5 times the upper limit of normal), a low hemoglobin level (less than the lower limit of normal), a high corrected serum calcium

level (>10 mg/dL), and an absence of nephrectomy. The prognostic factors were used to categorize patients into favorable-, intermediate-, or poor-risk groups with corresponding median survival times of 20 months, 10 months, and 4 months, respectively.

11. C

He has poor-risk disease; you recommend temsirolimus. Using the MSKCC/Motzer prognostic model, this patient is considered to have poor-risk disease. The pivotal trial of temsirolimus versus interferon was evaluated in a phase III study involving 626 patients with previously untreated, poor-prognosis metastatic RCC with the regimen of 25 mg of intravenous temsirolimus weekly or interferon alfa (at 3 million units with provision to increase to 18 million units) 3 times weekly, or combination therapy with 15 mg of temsirolimus intravenously weekly in addition to 6 million units of interferon alfa 3 times weekly. Patients who received temsirolimus alone had a statistically significant improvement in overall survival (HR for death, 0.73; 95% CI, 0.58–0.92; *P* =.008) and PFS (*P*<.001) than did patients who received interferon alone. The median overall survival in the temsirolimus group was 10.9 months. Although high-dose intravenous interleukin-2 can occasionally result in durable remission, it can be considered only in a select group of patients as it is a toxic treatment. Everolimus is approved as a second-line treatment, as with nivolumab. While sunitinib also can be used in this setting, this patient is considered to have poor risk, rather than favorable risk, in the MSKCC prognostic criteria setting.

12. B

Cabozantinib showed improvement in PFS compared with everolimus. The METEOR trial was a phase III trial that examined cabozantinib versus everolimus in the advanced/metastatic kidney cancer population posttreatment with a VEGFR targeted therapy. The trial was positive, showing improvement in the median PFS of 7.4 months with cabozantinib versus 3.8 months with everolimus, leading to cabozantinib's approval on April 2016. The HR was 0.58 translating to a 42% reduction in the risk of progression or death with cabozantinib compared with everolimus (HR, 0.58; 95% CI, 0.45–0.75; *P*<.001). The objective response rate was also better with cabozantinib at 21% versus 5% with everolimus (*P*<.001). While a planned interim analysis showed that overall survival was longer with cabozantinib than with everolimus (HR for death, 0.67; 95% CI, 0.51–0.89; *P*=.005), it did not cross the significance boundary for the interim analysis. Adverse events were fairly manageable with dose reductions occurring in 60% of the patients who received cabozantinib, and in 25% of those who received everolimus.

13. E

All of the above. There are several currently available oral TKIs approved for first-line treatment (sunitinib or pazopanib) as well as post-failure of these drugs, which includes axitinib, cabozantinib, or lenvatinib with everolimus combination. Cabozantinib is another oral TKI against VEGFR as well as MET and AXL, which was studied in comparison to everolimus in the second-line setting.

14. E

Everolimus. Varying therapies for metastatic kidney cancer have different drug toxicity profiles, which are important to be aware of. The VEGF inhibitors have common side effects, including hypertension, hand-foot syndrome, diarrhea, cytopenias, cardiac or thyroid abnormalities, and possible bleeding or clotting problems. Everolimus, on the other hand, as a mTOR inhibitor, can result in cytopenias, hypercholesterolemia or hypertriglyceridemia, and stomatitis, but a rare, yet life-threatening, symptom could be pneumonitis. Noninfectious and nonmalignant pneumonitis occurs in up to 9.9% of patients on everolimus. The decision for treatment depends on the severity of symptoms with patients having grade 1 (asymptomatic) manifestations could have continuation of treatment without dose adjustments. Grade 2 (symptomatic, affecting ADLs) may also lead to the continuation of treatment or a reduction of the dose. However, grade 3 (which involves severe symptoms that limit self-care ADLs and oxygen requirements) as well as grade 4 (life-threatening) manifestations necessitate withdrawal of the drug and a need to administer corticosteroids after dose interruption.

15. B

MET. This patient has papillary kidney cancer, which makes up the second most common histologic subtype of papillary cancer (type 1 pRCC making up 5% and type 2 pRCC at 10%). Specifically, the papillary type 1 tumors are associated with *MET* alterations, and is one of the four major autosomal dominantly inherited kidney cancer syndromes where individuals are at risk for developing multifocal and even bilateral tumors by the fifth or sixth decade of life, whereas type 2 tumors were characterized by CDKN2A silencing, SETD2 mutations, TFE3 fusions, and increased expression of the NRF2-ARE pathway. VHL syndrome is characterized by germline translocations of the distal portion of the short arm of chromosome 3 and is associated with clear cell RCC. A recently described new RCC syndrome has been linked to germline mutation of multiple subunits (SDHB/C/D) of the Krebs cycle enzyme, succinate dehydrogenase, where individual family members developing a rare but seemingly aggressive type of clear cell kidney cancer has been described. While FLCN describes another syndrome, called BHD, the vast majority of the subtype of RCC seen in this syndrome is chromophobe or oncocytoma, and rarely of a papillary subtype, which only occurs in about 2% of patients.

16. C

The median overall survival with sunitinib use was slightly better than everolimus. The ESPN trial was a randomized phase II trial that examined the utility of sunitinib versus everolimus in improvement of PFS in first-line therapy for non-clear cell RCC. A total of 108 patients were needed to show improvement in median PFS (mPFS) from 12 weeks with sunitinib to 20 weeks with the use of everolimus. The trial was stopped early after analyses of the first 68 patients showed no statistically significant difference in the mPFS (the primary endpoint) of 6.1 months with sunitinib versus 4.1 months with everolimus (*P*=.6). While the initial analyses showed improvement in overall survival with sunitinib, final overall survival analysis showed they were also not statistically significant but with slightly better results with sunitinib at 16.2 months versus everolimus at 14.9 months (*P*=.18). The trial findings showed only very modest efficacy that precluded a recommendation for the unanimous use of everolimus, which is currently approved as a second-line treatment for non-clear cell RCCs.

17. B

Blockade of PD-1 allows T cell re-activation. The use of agents that therapeutically target the transmembrane protein PD-1 receptor or the ligand (PD-L1) has met with success in the clinic. The varying expression patterns of both PD-1 and PD-L1 are complex, with PD1 generally expressed on T cells, natural killer cells, B cells, and some myeloid cells, while PD-L1 is expressed on different nonhematopoietic cells. PD-1 functions as an inhibitory receptor; therefore, the blockade of PD-1 enhances T cell re-activation and the secretion of cytokines. It also induces the metabolic program and interaction with target cells. TReg cells may function as an inhibitor to the response of T effector cells. Therefore, the PD-1 blockade serves to relieve the suppression on effector T cells, but not necessarily further increase the expansion of thymic T cells.

18. C

Active surveillance. Active surveillance is an increasingly recognized management approach, especially for those who refuse surgery, or those who are ineligible or otherwise suboptimal candidates for surgery. The reported incidence of progression to metastatic disease can be up to 2% of patients in retrospective and prospective studies. This patient has a recent diagnosis of comorbidities, including acute TIA and recent CAD. Any surgical procedures, including radical or even partial nephrectomy or cryoablation, would not be suitable. Starting sunitinib in the absence of metastatic disease is also not recommended in this patient with multiple cardiovascular risk factors.

REFERENCES

Question 1

1. Pithukpakorn M, Toro JR. Hereditary leiomyomatosis and renal cell cancer. In: Pagon RA, Adam MP, Ardinger HH, et al., eds. Seattle, WA: GeneReviews(R); 1993.
2. Herman JG, Latif F, Weng Y, et al. Silencing of the VHL tumor-suppressor gene by DNA methylation in renal carcinoma. *Proc Natl Acad Sci U S A*. 1994;91:9700–9704.
3. Zbar B, Alvord WG, Glenn G, et al. Risk of renal and colonic neoplasms and spontaneous pneumothorax in the Birt-Hogg-Dube syndrome. *Cancer Epidemiol Biomarkers Prev*. 2002;11:393–400.
4. Comperat E, Camparo P, Vieillefond A. WHO classification 2004: tumors of the kidneys. *J Radiol*. 2006;87:1015–1024.
5. Motzer RJ, Escudier B, McDermott DF, et al. Nivolumab versus everolimus in advanced renal-cell carcinoma. *N Engl J Med*. 2015;373:1803–1813.
6. Motzer RJ, Hutson TE, Cella D, et al. Pazopanib versus sunitinib in metastatic renal-cell carcinoma. *N Engl J Med*. 2013;369:722–731.

Question 2

1. Motzer RJ, Escudier B, McDermott DF, et al. Nivolumab versus everolimus in advanced renal-cell carcinoma. *N Engl J Med*. 2015;373:1803–1813.

Question 3

1. Motzer RJ, Hutson TE, Cella D, et al. Pazopanib versus sunitinib in metastatic renal-cell carcinoma. *N Engl J Med*. 2013;369:722–731.
2. Escudier B, Porta C, Bono P, et al. Randomized, controlled, double-blind, cross-over trial assessing treatment preference for pazopanib versus sunitinib in patients with metastatic renal cell carcinoma: PISCES Study. *J Clin Oncol*. 2014;32:1412–1418.

Question 4

1. Iacovelli R, Modica D, Palazzo A, et al. Clinical outcome and prognostic factors in renal medullary carcinoma: apooled analysis from 18 years of medical literature. *Can Urol Assoc J*. 2015;9:E172–E177.
2. Baig MA, Lin YS, Rasheed J, et al. Renal medullary carcinoma. *J Natl Med Assoc*. 2006;98:1171–1174.

Question 5

1. Janowitz T, Welsh SJ, Zaki K, et al. Adjuvant therapy in renal cell carcinoma-past, present, and future. *Semin Oncol*. 2013;40:482–491.

2. Haas NB, Manola J, Uzzo RG, et al. Initial results from ASSURE (E2805): adjuvant sorafenib or sunitinib for unfavorable renal carcinoma, an ECOG-ACRIN-led, NCTN phase III trial. ASCO Meeting Abstracts 33:403

3. Haas NB. Surveillance for renal cell cancer recurrence: which patients should undergo imaging, how often, and when? *J Clin Oncol*. 2015;33:4131–4133.

Question 6

1. Linehan WM, Spellman PT, Ricketts CJ, et al. Comprehensive molecular characterization of papillary renal-cell carcinoma. *N Engl J Med*. 2016;374:135–145.

Question 7

1. Vira MA, Novakovic KR, Pinto PA, et al. Genetic basis of kidney cancer: a model for developing molecular-targeted therapies. *BJU Int*. 2007;99:1223–1229.

Question 8

1. Vira MA, Novakovic KR, Pinto PA, et al. Genetic basis of kidney cancer: a model for developing molecular-targeted therapies. *BJU Int*. 2007;99:1223–1229.

Question 9

1. Campbell SC, Novick AC, Belldegrun A, et al. Guideline for management of the clinical T1 renal mass. *J Urol*. 182:1271–1279.

Question 10

1. Motzer RJ, Bacik J, Mazumdar M. Prognostic factors for survival of patients with stage IV renal cell carcinoma: memorial sloan-kettering cancer center experience. *Clin Cancer Res*. 2004;10:6302S–6303S.

Question 11

1. Motzer RJ, Bacik J, Mazumdar M. Prognostic factors for survival of patients with stage IV renal cell carcinoma: memorial sloan-kettering cancer center experience. *Clin Cancer Res*. 2004;10:6302S–6303S.

2. Hudes G, Carducci M, Tomczak P, et al. Temsirolimus, interferon alfa, or both for advanced renal-cell carcinoma. *N Engl J Med*. 2007;356:2271–2281.

Question 12

1. Choueiri TK, Escudier B, Powles T, et al. Cabozantinib versus everolimus in advanced renal-cell carcinoma. *N Engl J Med*. 2015;373:1814–1823.

Question 14

1. Albiges L, Chamming's F, Duclos B, et al. Incidence and management of mTOR inhibitor-associated pneumonitis in patients with metastatic renal cell carcinoma. *Ann Oncol*. 2012;23:1943–1953.

Question 15

1. Linehan WM, Spellman PT, Ricketts CJ, et al. Comprehensive molecular characterization of papillary renal-cell carcinoma. *N Engl J Med*. 2016;374:135–145.

2. Ricketts CJ, Shuch B, Vocke CD, et al. Succinate dehydrogenase kidney cancer: an aggressive example of the Warburg effect in cancer. *J Urol*. 2012;188:2063–2071.

3. Pavlovich CP, Walther MM, Eyler RA, et al. Renal tumors in the Birt-Hogg-Dube syndrome. *Am J Surg Pathol*. 2002;26:1542–1552.

Question 16

1. Tannir NM, Jonasch E, Albiges L, et al. Everolimus versus sunitinib prospective evaluation in metastatic non-clear cell renal cell carcinoma (ESPN): a randomized multicenter phase 2 trial. *Eur Urol*. 2016;69:866–874.

Question 17

1. Nguyen LT, Ohashi PS. Clinical blockade of PD1 and LAG3—potential mechanisms of action. *Nat Rev Immunol*. 2015;15:45–56.

Question 18

1. Pierorazio PM, Hyams ES, Mullins JK, et al. Active surveillance for small renal masses. *Rev Urol*. 2012;14:13–19.

CHAPTER
26

Germ Cell Tumor

Ravi A. Madan and Jeanny B. Aragon-Ching

QUESTIONS

1. A 26-year-old male presents with abdominal pain. He went to the emergency room (ER) and was found to have a 4-cm retroperitoneal mass on the scan. He was also found to have a testicular mass on ultrasound. Radical orchiectomy was performed, which showed a mixed nonseminoma with 50% embryonal, 45% teratoma, and 5% seminoma. His markers, including AFP, were elevated to 300, bhCG to 150, and lactate dehydrogenase (LDH) at 500. He started with BEP, and his tumor markers declined after the third cycle to normal. His restaging computed tomography (CT) scan after chemotherapy showed persistent increase in the size of the RP mass at 2.5 cm. What is the next best step in management?
   A. Obtain a positron emission tomography (PET)-CT scan
   B. Refer for hospice; cure rates for refractory disease is low
   C. Refer for retroperitoneal lymph node dissection (RPLND) and resection of the tumor
   D. Give 2 more cycles of BEP
   E. Switch to salvage TIP

2. A 23-year-old male presents with chest pain and shortness of breath. He underwent a CT scan in the ER and was found to have a mediastinal mass (Fig. 26.1). His tumor markers, including AFP and bhCG, were elevated. His AFP was elevated to 60,300 ng/mL, bhCG was 185 mIU/mL, and his LDH was normal. His scrotal ultrasound showed no masses, and the CT of his abdomen and pelvis showed no adenopathy. You counsel him regarding his risk of disease. What is the most appropriate next step in management?
   A. Treatment with radiation because he has mediastinal disease
   B. Treatment with 3 cycles of BEP because he has good-risk disease
   C. Treatment with 4 cycles of BEP because he has poor-risk disease
   D. Referral for upfront transplant is recommended because he has high-risk disease
   E. Referral for hospice; he has an extremely poor prognosis

3. A 38-year-old man presents with painless scrotal swelling. He undergoes ultrasound and was found to have a right testicular mass. Radical orchiectomy was performed revealing a 3.5 cm pure seminoma without rete testes involvement or lymphovascular invasion. He has a negative abdominopelvic CT scan and chest x-ray, and his tumor markers were within normal limits even pre-orchiectomy. He plays the violin with the symphonic orchestra and is concerned about experiencing any neuropathic side effects. He states compliance will not be an issue. What is the next best step in management?

A. He should be offered RPLND.
B. He should be offered 3 cycles of BEP.
C. He should be offered 1 cycle of BEP.
D. He should be offered 1 cycle of carboplatin.
E. He should be offered surveillance.

4. A 28-year-old male presented to the ER with shortness of breath, headaches, and chest pain. Diagnostic work up revealed a primary mediastinal mass; AFP was elevated to 30,000 ng/mL, bhCG was 12,000 mIU/mL, and LDH was 3000. He underwent a brain MRI and was found to have a solitary parietal lesion. He proceeded with resection and primary standard chemotherapy with BEP. Which factors would predict worse overall survival in this patient with brain metastasis?
   A. Elevation of AFP >100 ng/mL
   B. Primary mediastinal extragonadal germ cell tumor
   C. hCG levels >5000 mIU/mL
   D. All of the above
   E. None of the above

5. A 45-year-old male was found to have pure seminoma on radical orchiectomy and a 5-cm retroperitoneal mass on CT scan. He underwent 3 cycles of BEP with markers all within normal limits. His repeat restaging scan at the end of restaging showed shrinkage of the mass to 1.5 cm with markers all still within normal limits. What is the next appropriate step?
   A. Obtain a PET-CT scan
   B. Continue surveillance

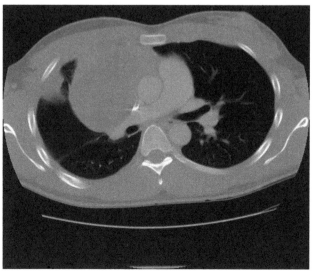

FIG. 26.1

C. Give salvage TIP
D. Refer for salvage radiation
E. Refer for high-dose therapy followed by transplant

6. A 25-year-old male was diagnosed with mixed nonseminoma (60% embryonal, 10% seminoma, 30% teratoma) and a CT scan with a 7.5-cm retroperitoneal mass and other smaller sub-centimeter RP adenopathy. His tumor markers showed the following: AFP 100 ng/mL, bhCG 12,000 mIU/mL, and LDH 200 post-orchiectomy. He received 4 cycles of BEP, and his tumor markers all normalized. He undergoes a CT scan postchemotherapy, which now shows a few pulmonary lesions at the lung bases with ground-glass appearance. His dominant RP mass is now 4 cm in size. What is your next step in management?
A. Referral for high-dose therapy and transplant
B. Switch to TIP, he now has metastatic lung disease
C. Obtain a biopsy of the lung lesion
D. RPLND with surgical resection of the retroperitoneal dominant mass
E. Surgical resection of the RP mass and the lung masses

7. A 38-year-old male patient presented with a testicular mass. Radical orchiectomy of the left revealed a pure seminoma, pathology T2 with lymphovascular invasion and size of 8 cm with rete testis involvement. He had negative disease on staging scans and negative tumor markers. He comes for consultation regarding adjuvant therapy. You discuss the following regarding adjuvant therapy for stage IB seminoma:
A. Recommendation for adjuvant chemotherapy includes use of 1 cycle of BEP.
B. Recommendation for adjuvant radiation entails use of 20 Gy of radiation.
C. Recommendation for adjuvant radiation entails use of 30 Gy of radiation.
D. Recommendation for adjuvant chemotherapy includes 2 cycles of BEP.
E. Recommendation for adjuvant chemotherapy involves 3 cycles of carboplatin.

8. A 35-year-old male presents with a 6-cm retroperitoneal mass on CT scan after presenting with mild abdominal pain. His history includes prior treatment with BEP 7 years ago for a stage II mixed nonseminoma. His tumor markers were not elevated. A biopsy of the mass reveals pathology consistent with germ cell tumor. What would be the next step in management?
A. Recommend BEP for 4 cycles
B. Referral for high-dose therapy and transplant
C. Recommend palliative care
D. Recommend surgical resection
E. Recommend gemcitabine and oxaliplatin

9. A 24-year-old male presents with painless scrotal swelling with ultrasound showing a 5-cm mass in the right testicle. He had elevated tumor markers with AFP of 654 ng/mL, bhCG of 322 mIU/mL, and LDH of 800. He undergoes radical orchiectomy with pathology showing a mixed nonseminoma (embryonal 90%, yolk sac tumor 10%), without lymphovascular invasion. His staging CT scan of the abdomen and pelvis showed some shotty retroperitoneal adenopathy that were all <1 cm. He was sent to you for consultation 6 weeks after his orchiectomy. You repeat his tumor markers, which show the following: AFP at 420 ng/mL, bhCG of 213 mIU/mL, and normal LDH at 124. You discuss the following treatment with him:
A. Recommend RPLND; he has stage IA disease
B. Recommend surveillance alone; he has stage IA disease

C. Recommend chemotherapy with BEP × 3; he has stage IS disease
D. Recommend adjuvant chemotherapy with BEP × 2; he has stage IB disease
E. Recommend chemotherapy with BEP × 4; he has stage I poor risk disease

10. A 27-year-old man recently diagnosed with testicular nonseminoma comes to you for consultation. He is concerned about the etiology of his testicular cancer and the risk factors associated with it. You discuss the following regarding known risk factors for testicular cancer:
A. His personal history of testicular cancer confers an increased risk of developing cancer in the contralateral testis.
B. Race does not contribute to any risk for testicular cancer.
C. Presence of cryptorchidism does not increase the risk for testicular cancer.
D. Infertility is not associated with testicular cancer.
E. Intratubular germ cell neoplasia is not a known risk factor for testicular cancer.

11. A 32-year-old male presents with a history of 3 months of scrotal swelling. His past medical history is only significant for intravenous drug use and alcohol drinking. Ultrasound shows a mass in the right testis, and he undergoes radical orchiectomy on the right. His pathology reveals pure embryonal carcinoma. His CT scan showed enlarged retroperitoneal adenopathy. He started with BEP, and after 3 cycles, all adenopathy had resolved. He presents 3 months later with lethargy and somnolence and is found to have elevated transaminases. His AFP is also elevated at this time. Restaging shows no adenopathy or evidence of distant disease. His LDH is elevated to 300 with a normal hCG < 2. What is your next course of management?
A. Proceed with BEP × 3
B. Refer for high-dose chemotherapy followed by transplant
C. Proceed with VIP
D. Continue supportive therapy; repeat tumor markers and LFTs in a month
E. Proceed with TIP

12. A 30-year-old white male was diagnosed with testicular cancer and a mediastinal tumor that was biopsied to show a germ cell tumor. He had elevated tumor markers with AFP of 120 ng/mL and hCG of 75 mIU/mL, and LDH of 600 post-orchiectomy. He underwent chemotherapy with BEP and after 2 cycles of chemotherapy had normalized tumor markers. He went to an urgent care center as he had a cold and cough and underwent a chest radiograph, which showed an increased size of the tumor compared with when he started, with some tracheal shift. His lung fields were otherwise clear. Which is the ideal next step in management?
A. Recommend proceeding with 2 additional cycles of BEP
B. Switch to vinblastine, ifosfamide, and cisplatin
C. Recommend surgical resection of the mass
D. Switch to high-dose chemotherapy followed by transplant rescue
E. Radiation therapy to the mediastinal mass

13. An 18-year-old patient with known Klinefelter syndrome was referred to you by the Pediatrics section after he presented with worsening symptoms of shortness of breath, dyspnea, and cough. A chest radiograph and subsequent CT scan reveals a large anterior mediastinal mass. He has

no wheezing on examination, but with pronounced gynecomastia and lack of bodily hair. You obtained basic laboratory tests, all of which were negative. He is accompanied by his parents who asked you what this mass could likely be. You respond that it is likely related to the following:

A. Hodgkin lymphoma
B. Sarcoma
C. Mediastinal germ cell tumor
D. Mediastinal thymoma
E. Mediastinal thyroid mass

14. A young male patient presents with a midline tumor. Cytogenetic studies showed an isochromosome of the short arm of chromosome 12. Which of the following is associated with this karyotypic abnormality?

    A. Germ cell tumor
    B. B-cell poorly differentiated lymphoma
    C. Neuroblastoma
    D. Rhabdomyosarcoma
    E. All of the above

15. A 28-year-old male with history of a nonseminoma with 100% embryonal carcinoma on his orchiectomy of the right and a stage IIB good-risk nonseminoma undergoes chemotherapy with 3 cycles of BEP. At the conclusion of chemotherapy, he undergoes a restaging scan, which showed a persistent, residual 2.5 cm mass in the retroperitoneum. All his tumor markers are now negative. He asks you of the likelihood that he would have a persistent, viable tumor if he were to undergo post-chemotherapy RPLND. You answer him with the following:

    A. It is most likely all viable tumor.
    B. It is most likely all necrosis.
    C. It is most likely all teratoma.
    D. It is most likely necrosis around 50%, teratoma around 35%, or viable tumor around 15%.
    E. You have no idea and no way of knowing.

16. A 25-year-old male presents for follow-up with you to set up care after moving from another state. He was treated for a stage IIA nonseminoma 4 years ago with primary chemotherapy and had been consistently followed by his oncologist with periodic scans and tumor markers. Upon review of his records, you noticed that he has had slightly elevated AFP ranging and fluctuating from 8.5 to 11 ng/mL (normal of <8 ng/mL) with normal bhCG and LDH. He also had been undergoing surveillance CT scans, which showed no adenopathy and no change. You recommend the following:

    A. Give salvage TIP
    B. Refer for high-dose therapy and auto transplant
    C. Refer for RPLND
    D. Obtain a PET-CT scan
    E. Continue observation and surveillance

17. A 25-year-old male with prior diagnosis 5 years ago with stage II nonseminoma treated with primary chemotherapy would like to go to the survivorship clinic. Which of the following is true regarding surveillance and follow-up for this patient?

    A. The risk for secondary malignant neoplasm is low because he did not receive radiation.
    B. The risk for cardiovascular disease is low because he received chemotherapy.
    C. The risk for infertility is low because he was diagnosed 5 years ago.
    D. The risk for secondary malignant neoplasm still exists since he received chemotherapy.
    E. None of the above.

18. Which of the following is true regarding infertility and testicular cancers?

    A. There is an association between infertility and testicular cancer.
    B. Men with decreased paternity or a history of infertility have an increased likelihood of testicular cancer.
    C. Infertility was initially implicated as a risk factor for TGCT only in the setting of underlying carcinoma in situ (CIS) of the testis.
    D. Men with testicular cancer and CIS often have subnormal semen quality.
    E. All of the above.

ANSWERS

1. C

Refer for RPLND for resection of the tumor. This patient presented with a mixed nonseminoma, stage IIB with good-risk disease. He was treated with 3 cycles of BEP, and while his markers all came down to normal, his restaging scan showed persistent residual mass of greater than 1 cm in size. At this time, surgical resection would be the right course of action. Obtaining further PET-CT scan would not add utility since even if this were not to be PET-avid, one would still consider disease in the retroperitoneum that would warrant resection and teratomas may not be particularly PET-avid and would need to be resected. Given negative markers and lack of confirmation that this is truly viable tumor, proceeding with salvage TIP would not be optimal. Proceeding with 2 more cycles of BEP would be erroneous, as the patient already received the appropriate number of cycles of first line BEP therapy.

2. C

Treatment with 4 cycles of BEP. Primary mediastinal germ cell tumors (GCTs), especially extragonadal ones, are rare, have an aggressive course, and always fall in the poor-risk category. Treatment with upfront BEP for 4 cycles for poor-risk germ cell tumors remains the standard of care. However, there is increasing interest in looking at upfront TIP versus BEP in this intermediate- or poor-risk population of patients, knowing that their risk for failure with a standard dose of BEP is high. Similarly, a study evaluating conventionally dosed chemotherapy with BEP compared with BEP × 2 followed by high-dose therapy and transplant for a predominantly poor-risk category of GCTs showed no improvement in overall or progression-free survival. For patients requiring salvage therapy, another trial looking at a salvage standard dose of TIP versus high-dose therapy followed by transplant is being evaluated by the Alliance trial (TIGER). Given that the patient is young, referral for treatment remains a reasonable option rather than direct referral to a hospice, although there is no clear role for radiation only with mediastinal disease, except in a palliative setting.

3. E

He should be offered surveillance. This patient is diagnosed with a stage IA pure seminoma. Several proponents of risk-adapted management of clinical stage I seminoma includes offering adjuvant carboplatin therapy for those who have known risk factors, such as size of greater than 4 cm or rete testes involvement in seminomas. However, validation of these prognostic factors was equally disputed. Regardless, surveillance would be the preferred option in this patient with no apparent risk factors.

4. D

Men with GCTs who present with brain metastases have poor overall survival. In an analysis from the global germ cell cancer group, data from 523 men who presented with primary or relapsed metastatic brain disease were found to have poor overall survival. However, the group of men who had brain metastases present at the initial diagnosis fared better than those who had it at relapse (OS at 3 years was 48% vs. 27%). Other independent adverse prognostic factors also included elevations of AFP greater than 100 ng/mL and bhCG > 5000 mIU/mL, primary mediastinal nonseminoma, and receipt of only single-modality therapy.

5. B

Continue surveillance. This patient was initially diagnosed with a stage II seminoma and was treated with standard doses of BEP × 3. All tumor markers were normalized at the conclusion of chemotherapy, but the patient has a persistent, though improved, residual mass that is now less than 3 cm. At this time, continued surveillance would be reasonable. If he had increased size to greater than 3 cm despite negative markers, then obtaining a PET-CT scan at 6 weeks or more post-chemotherapy would be appropriate in order to determine whether there is viable seminoma that would be amenable to further surgery (RPLND) or salvage chemotherapy.

6. D

RPLND with surgical resection of the retroperitoneal dominant mass. This patient has a mixed nonseminoma, intermediate-risk tumor, based on the International Germ Cell Cancer Consensus Group (IGCCCG) criteria. This patient had a good response to BEP with a decline in his tumor markers along with shrinkage of the known RP mass. Therefore, switching to TIP or performing high-dose therapy and transplant would not be appropriate. The lung nodules and ground-glass appearance likely were secondary to bleomycin toxicity. Obtaining a lung biopsy or resecting this would not be beneficial. However, findings of a residual mass in a patient with negative markers would entail resection of the RP mass.

7. B

Recommendation for adjuvant radiation entails the use of 20 Gy of radiation. While some clinicians would advocate adjuvant treatment in a risk-adapted manner, such as those patients who have increased size of greater than 4 cm or rete testes involvement, some discourage the risk-adapted approach with surveillance being the main therapeutic approach in stage I seminoma patients. For patients who opt for adjuvant therapy, the principles of adjuvant therapy for pure seminoma includes consideration for 1 cycle of carboplatin AUC of 7 or radiation using 10 fractions of 2 Gy each, with equivalent relapse-free survival rates for both groups.

8. D

Recommend surgical resection. Late relapse for nonseminomas occurs in a minority of patients (about 2%–3%), and the behavior is often clinically different and aggressive. The primary sites of involvement include the retroperitoneum or the lungs, and AFP is the primary tumor marker that is elevated. While these tumors may remain chemotherapy-sensitive, they rarely respond to or are cured with chemotherapy alone, and surgical resection would be considered the definitive therapy. Patients who were treated with surgical resection had a higher likelihood of being disease-free compared with those who are treated with chemotherapy alone.

9. C

Recommend chemotherapy with BEP × 3; he has stage IS disease. While his pathology on orchiectomy does show pT1 disease, which would put him at a stage IA, his post-orchiectomy markers have not declined according to specified half-lives, and the elevated markers at 6 weeks post-orchiectomy are worrisome for persistent disease, despite a seemingly negative scan. Therefore, he would be best treated with systemic chemotherapy that follows good-risk disease per the IGCCCG criteria.

10. A

His personal history of testicular cancer confers an increased risk of developing cancer in the contralateral testis. There are varying risk factors that contribute to the development of testicular cancer. Having had a personal history of testicular cancer results in a 12-fold increased risk, although this occurs in only approximately 2%–3% of all testicular cancer survivors. Other risk factors include cryptorchidism, family history (though this may be confounded by a shared environmental history), intratubular germ cell neoplasia, race (highest among Caucasians and lowest among African Americans or Asians), environmental exposures, and infertility.

11. D

Continue supportive therapy; repeat tumor markers and LFTs in a month. Patients who have a prior history of treated testicular cancer who present with isolated elevated AFP in the absence of any other signs or symptoms of recurrent testicular cancer has to be ruled out for conditions that could give rise to high AFP. Elevation of AFP could be secondary to hepatitis and it would be important to rule out this condition before starting them on salvage treatment for relapsed testicular cancer.

12. C

Recommend surgical resection of the mass. Growing teratoma syndrome describes a rare phenomenon with a prevalence of 1.9%–7.6%, where patients with germ cell tumors could have enlarging sites of metastases despite an appropriate response to systemic chemotherapy with decline or even normalization of tumor markers. Histology of these lesions, once resected, often reveals benign teratomas, which are important to recognize and resect given the nonresponse to chemotherapy.

13. C

Mediastinal germ cell tumor. While several tumors may occur in the mediastinum, the anterior mediastinum is usually a site for lymphomas, including Hodgkin disease and non-Hodgkin lymphoma, as well as thymoma or thymic cysts, and mediastinal germ cell tumors. Klinefelter syndrome, otherwise known as XXY, is characterized by two or more X chromosomes in males with varying physical, endocrine, and developmental manifestations. An association between a primary mediastinal germ cell tumor and Klinefelter syndrome exists. In patients with a primary mediastinal germ cell tumor, about 20% had karyotypic findings suggestive of Klinefelter syndrome, which often occurs in young males (median of 15 years of age). The findings of a young median age (18 years), nonseminomatous subtype, and a mediastinal location of the germ cell neoplasm is typically characteristic of mediastinal germ cell tumors.

14. A

Germ cell tumor. An isochromosome of the short arm of chromosome 12 [i (12p)] has been reported to be a frequent nonrandom chromosomal marker of germ cell tumors. This is present in about 80% of male germ cell tumors with evaluable cytogenetic abnormalities, and is found to have diagnostic and prognostic significance. An abnormal karyotype was more frequently seen in nonseminomatous tumors compared with seminomas. An alteration of one or more copies of i(12p), an excess 12p copy number, or a deletion on the long arm of chromosome 12 was found in as much as 25% of midline tumors of uncertain histogenesis in a study, thereby helping to establish diagnosis.

15. D

It is most likely necrosis around 50%, teratoma around 35%, or viable tumor around 15%. Post-chemotherapy RPLND remains an important treatment modality for patients who undergo primary chemotherapy and have residual disease. Several series have found that the most common histology in post-chemotherapy RPLND remains to be necrosis, in half of the cases. However, up to one-third can have a teratoma and about 10%–15% can have a viable tumor.

16. E

Continue observation and surveillance. Persistently elevated AFP post-cisplatin-based chemotherapy have usually been considered a contraindication to surgery because of presumed presence of persistent, active, germ cell elements, and post-chemotherapy RPLND is often reserved for those with negative markers and residual disease. On the other hand, second- or third-line chemotherapy is often recommended after increasing serum tumor markers. However, this patient has neither residual disease on scans, nor persistently increasing tumor markers. He has had persistently slightly elevated AFP with no indication of disease for the past 4 years now. In addition, there is the phenomenon of hereditary persistence of AFP, which may be considered, and for which no further active treatment is necessary.

17. D

The risk for a secondary malignant neoplasm still exists since he received chemotherapy. Patients with testicular cancer who undergo treatment with chemotherapy or radiation therapy can incur risks of treatment, which include second malignant neoplasms, cardiovascular disease, neurotoxicity and ototoxicity, pulmonary complications, hypogonadism, and nephrotoxicity. Therefore, continued long-term follow-up is essential in these patients.

18. E

All of the above. The association between infertility and cancer is particularly strong for testicular cancer, with an increased risk in men with oligozoospermia, in those who have demonstrated decreased paternity, or in the setting of subnormal semen quality or CIS. Therefore, it is important to evaluate and counsel men for infertility even when they are diagnosed with testicular cancer.

REFERENCES

Question 2

1. McKenney JK, Heerema-McKenney A, Rouse RV. Extragonadal germ cell tumors: a review with emphasis on pathologic features, clinical prognostic variables, and differential diagnostic considerations. *Adv Anat Pathol.* 2007;14:69–92.
2. Williams SD, Birch R, Einhorn LH, Irwin L, Greco FA, Loehrer PJ. Treatment of disseminated germ-cell tumors with cisplatin, bleomycin, and either vinblastine or etoposide. *N Engl J Med.* 1987;316:1435–1440.

3. Motzer RJ, Nichols CJ, Margolin KA, et al. Phase III randomized trial of conventional-dose chemotherapy with or without high-dose chemotherapy and autologous hematopoietic stem-cell rescue as first-line treatment for patients with poor-prognosis metastatic germ cell tumors. *J Clin Oncol.* 2007;25:247–256.

Question 3

1. Aparicio J, Germa JR, Garcia del Muro X, et al. Risk-adapted management for patients with clinical stage I seminoma: the Second Spanish Germ Cell Cancer Cooperative Group study. *J Clin Oncol.* 2005;23:8717–8723.
2. Chung PW, Daugaard G, Tyldesley S, et al. Prognostic factors for relapse in stage I seminoma managed with surveillance: a validation study. *ASCO Meeting Abstracts.* 2010;28:4535.

Question 4

1. Feldman DR, Lorch A, Kramar A, et al. Brain metastases in patients with germ cell tumors: prognostic factors and treatment options—an analysis from the Global Germ Cell Cancer Group. *J Clin Oncol.* 2016;34:345–351.

Question 7

1. Oliver RT, Mason MD, Mead GM, et al. Radiotherapy versus single-dose carboplatin in adjuvant treatment of stage I seminoma: a randomised trial. *Lancet.* 2005;366:293–300.

Question 8

1. Baniel J, Foster RS, Gonin R, Messemer JE, Donohue JP, Einhorn LH. Late relapse of testicular cancer. *J Clin Oncol.* 1995;13:1170–1176.
2. George DW, Foster RS, Hromas RA, et al. Update on late relapse of germ cell tumor: a clinical and molecular analysis. *J Clin Oncol.* 2003;21:113–122.

Question 10

1. Stevenson SM, Lowrance WT. Epidemiology and diagnosis of testis cancer. *Urol Clin North Am.* 2015;42:269–275.

Question 12

1. Logothetis CJ, Samuels ML, Trindade A, et al. The growing teratoma syndrome. *Cancer.* 1982;50:1629–1635.

Question 13

1. Nichols CR, Heerema NA, Palmer C, Loehrer Sr PJ, Williams SD, Einhorn LH. Klinefelter's syndrome associated with mediastinal germ cell neoplasms. *J Clin Oncol.* 1987;5:1290–1294.

Question 14

1. Bosl GJ, Ilson DH, Rodriguez E, Motzer RJ, Reuter VE, Chaganti RS. Clinical relevance of the i(12p) marker chromosome in germ cell tumors. *J Natl Cancer Inst.* 1994;86:349–355.

Question 15

1. Fox EP, Weathers TD, Williams SD, et al. Outcome analysis for patients with persistent nonteratomatous germ cell tumor in postchemotherapy retroperitoneal lymph node dissections. *J Clin Oncol.* 1993;11:1294–1299.
2. Sim HG, Lange PH, Lin DW. Role of post-chemotherapy surgery in germ cell tumors. *Urol Clin North Am.* 2007;34:199–217. abstract ix.

Question 16

1. Schefer H, Mattmann S, Joss RA. Hereditary persistence of alpha-fetoprotein. Case report and review of the literature. *Ann Oncol.* 1998;9:667–672.

Question 17

1. Fung C, Fossa SD, Williams A, Travis LB. Long-term morbidity of testicular cancer treatment. *Urol Clin North Am.* 2015;42:393–408.

Question 18

1. Hanson HA, Anderson RE, Aston KI, Carrell DT, Smith KR, Hotaling JM. Subfertility increases risk of testicular cancer: evidence from population-based semen samples. *Fertil Steril.* 2016;105: 322–328.e1.

Gynecological Malignancies

Susana Campos and Don S. Dizon

Ovarian Cancer and Fallopian Tube Cancer

QUESTIONS

1. A 54-year-old nulliparous woman presents to her primary care physician with increasing shortness of breath and abdominal distention. Radiographical studies reveal bilateral pleural effusions, bilateral adnexal masses, extensive omental caking, and a pelvic mass adherent to the descending colon. The patient's performance status is 1. An omental biopsy reveals a high-grade papillary serous carcinoma. A gynecological surgical oncology and medical oncology consultation is obtained. Which of the following statements describes the most appropriate recommendation from both disciplines?
   A. Upfront surgical debulking alone
   B. Given the advanced nature of the disease, palliative care is the most appropriate recommendation
   C. Neoadjuvant chemotherapy with a platinum and taxane based regimen followed by interval debulking, followed by chemotherapy
   D. Surgical debulking followed by systemic therapy with a platinum and anthracycline

2. In patients with stage IIIC or stage IV ovarian cancer who are advised to consider neoadjuvant chemotherapy with a platinum and taxane combination, all of the following statements are true *except:*
   A. The strongest independent variable predicting overall survival is the complete resection of all macroscopic disease at primary or interval debulking.
   B. Postoperative rates of adverse events are higher after primary debulking than interval debulking.
   C. Neoadjuvant chemotherapy followed by interval debulking was not inferior to primary debulking.
   D. Neoadjuvant chemotherapy followed by interval debulking was inferior to primary debulking.

3. PARP inhibitors are approved in the management of patients with:
   A. *BRCA1* mutation positive ovarian cancer, fallopian tube, or peritoneal cancer as upfront therapy
   B. *BRCA2* mutation positive ovarian cancer, fallopian tube, or peritoneal cancer as maintenance therapy
   C. *BRCA1/2* negative ovarian cancer, fallopian tube, or peritoneal cancer
   D. *BRCA1/2* mutation positive recurrent ovarian cancer, fallopian tube, or peritoneal cancer who has received three prior lines of therapy

4. Which of the following statements regarding the current guidelines regarding *BRCA* testing in patients with ovarian, fallopian tube, or peritoneal cancer is correct?
   A. All patients with epithelial ovarian cancer should undergo genetic counseling and testing for *BRCA*.
   B. Only patients less than 50 years of age who develop ovarian, fallopian tube, or peritoneal cancer should undergo *BRCA* testing.
   C. Only patients of Ashkenazi or Eastern European descent should *BRCA* testing.
   D. Only patients with a strong family history of breast or ovarian cancer should undergo *BRCA* testing.

5. Which of the following factors are associated with an increased risk for ovarian cancer (multiple answer)?
   A. Advanced age
   B. History of oral contraceptive use
   C. Nulliparity
   D. Talc powder
   E. Late age at first pregnancy

6. Which of the following statement is true?
   A. Ovarian cancer accounts for 30% of all cancers among women.
   B. The risk of ovarian cancer decreases with age.
   C. The majority of cases of ovarian cancer are diagnosed at an early stage.
   D. Ovarian cancer is associated with the highest mortality rate of any gynecological cancer.

7. Which of the following statement(s) is (are) true? Choose all correct answers.
   A. Approximately 25% of all ovarian malignancies are epithelial in origin.
   B. Approximately 90% of all ovarian malignancies are epithelial in origin.
   C. Most cases of high-grade serous carcinoma of the ovary arise in the fallopian tubes rather than the ovaries.
   D. Endometroid carcinoma of the ovary is the most common histology.

8. A 65-year-old woman presents with increasing abdominal distention. Radiographical studies reveal omental caking and bilateral adnexal masses. Her preoperative CA125 is 4323 U/mL. She is referred to a gynecological surgical oncologist and undergoes a TAH, BSO, omentectomy nodal dissection, and peritoneal biopsies. The pathology report reveals a high-grade papillary serous carcinoma involving both ovaries, the omentum, the serosa of the uterus, and 3/10 pelvic nodes measuring 3.0–3.4 cm in size. Cytology is positive for malignant cells. The stage of her disease is:
   A. Stage IIC
   B. Stage IIB

C. Stage IV
D. Stage IIIC

9. The patient in Question 8 underwent debulking surgery and was deemed NED. Adjuvant options in the management of this patient include (multiple answer):
A. Intraperitoneal/intravenous chemotherapy with a platinum and a taxane
B. Dose-dense chemotherapy with a platinum and a taxane
C. Adjuvant chemotherapy with bleomycin, etoposide, and a platinum
D. No adjuvant chemotherapy given that she is NED

10. A 34-year-old woman presents to her gynecologist for a routine annual exam. She notes transient lower abdominal pressure that is mild in character. A pelvic exam is notable for a pelvic mass in the left adnexal region. A pelvic ultrasound reveals a left-sided complex cyst with a 4.3-cm solid component. The patient is premenopausal and desires to retain fertility. A preoperative CA125 is slightly elevated at a value of 57 U/mL. She undergoes an LSO under the direction of a gynecologic surgical oncologist. Pathology reveals a *serous borderline malignancy of the left ovary*. Multiple peritoneal biopsies reveal serous borderline malignancy. Peritoneal washing are positive for malignant cells. There is no evidence of invasive implants. You counsel the patient regarding the appropriate adjuvant therapy. All the following statements are false *except:*
A. No adjuvant chemotherapy is required.
B. Strict surveillance with a CT scan of the chest, abdomen, and pelvis is mandatory every 3 months for 2 years.
C. Adjuvant chemotherapy with carboplatin and paclitaxel every 3 weeks for 6 cycles
D. Pelvic radiation therapy

11. A 21-year-old female nursing student of Northern European descent presents to her primary care physician complaining of transient abdominal distention often related to dietary indiscretions. She notes normal bowel movements. She denies any family history of breast, ovarian, or colon cancer. She is also asymptomatic. She requests that a CA125 be done as she is fearful that her symptoms may be consistent with ovarian cancer. Which of the following statements is true?
A. Inform the patient that ovarian cancer does not occur in patients less than 45 years of age
B. Order the CA125
C. Order a CA125 and a pelvic ultrasound as the combination of these two tests have a positive predictive value of 75%
D. Inform the patient that screening for ovarian cancer has not been deemed an effective strategy for the use in the general population
E. Refer this patient for genetic counseling and testing for *BRCA*

12. Which of the following statements regarding hereditary ovarian cancer are true? (multiple answer)
A. Hereditary ovarian cancer is the major cause of all ovarian neoplasms.
B. *BRCA1* and *BRCA 2* are tumor suppressor genes that play a role in the repair of DNA damage.
C. *BRCA 1* and *BRCA 2* is located in chromosomes 17 and 13, respectively.
D. Inheritance of these mutations confers a significantly increased lifetime risk for ovarian cancer.
E. Inheritance of these mutations confers a significantly increased lifetime risk for nonserous endometrial cancer.

13. A 45-year-old patient presents for a follow-up visit to her medical oncologist. She completed 6 cycles of IV/IP adjuvant chemotherapy for stage IIIC fallopian tube cancer 4 months prior. Her initial CA125 at presentation was 978 U/mL. Her CA125 at the completion of therapy was 8 U/mL. She notes mild residual neuropathy, fatigue but otherwise, a comprehensive review of systems is negative. Today's CA125 is slightly increased at a value of 15 U/mL. The patient is worried that this represents recurrent disease. Which of the following statements is current?
A. Assure the patient that her CA125 is below 35 U/mL and, as such, this cannot represent recurrent disease
B. Start treatment immediately with carboplatin as a single agent
C. Ask the patient to repeat the CA125 in 4 weeks to establish whether there is a sustained rise in the CA125
D. Inform the patient that there is an overall survival advantage to initiating therapy as soon as possible

14. Which of the following statements regarding recurrent disease is true?
A. Platinum-sensitive disease is defined as recurrence of disease after a treatment-free interval of 3 months or longer.
B. Platinum refractory disease is defined as recurrence of disease 6 months after completion of platinum chemotherapy.
C. Platinum resistant disease is defined as recurrence of disease on platinum chemotherapy less than 6 months after completion of therapy.

15. A 67-year-old musician is seen for a routine follow-up after completing chemotherapy for her stage IIIC fallopian tube 2 years ago. The patient notes that she is doing well but notes mild residual fatigue and increasing lower abdominal cramping. She notes that she can eat, drink, and eliminate without difficulty. Her CA125 at presentation was normal at a value of 12 U/mL. She has been followed closely over the past several years with a physical exam and with routine radiographical studies, as her marker has never been revealing. Her CA125 today is slightly elevated at a value of 18 U/mL. A CT of the abdomen and pelvis reveals ascites, extensive peritoneal carcinomatosis coupled with extensive disease on the serosa of the bowel. You advise the patient as such.
A. Recommend a surgical consultation given that she has a disease-free interval of 2 years
B. Recommend a bevacizumab combination given the presence of ascites
C. Recommend a platinum doublet given her disease-free interval of 2 years
D. Counsel the patient that treatment is palliative and recommend single agent therapy with liposomal doxorubicin

16. A 42-year-old woman is seen in the clinic for an initial visit after completing dose-dense chemotherapy with carboplatin and paclitaxel for stage IIC clear cell carcinoma of the ovary. Her last cycle of chemotherapy was 3 months prior. She is unsettled regarding genetic counseling, as she is an only child and has no biological children. The patient describes persistent neuropathy and increasing constipation despite routine use of laxatives. Routine chemistries reveal a normal basic metabolic profile. The calcium is slightly elevated at 10.8. The CA125 which at the end of therapy was 13 (preoperative CA125 was 43 U/mL) is now 57 U/mL. Radiographical studies reveal numerous liver metastases. All the following statements represent an appropriate treatment plan except:
A. Advise a liver biopsy to confirm recurrent clear cell carcinoma of the ovary
B. Given the clear cell carcinoma histology, check an ionized calcium level
C. Start carboplatin and paclitaxel immediately

D. Genetic counseling to assess for *BRCA1* and *BRCA2* mutation

E. Advise the patient to consider bevacizumab and liposomal doxorubicin

17. Bevacizumab has been associated with:
A. An increased survival in patients with recurrent platinum-sensitive disease
B. An increased survival in patients with recurrent platinum-resistant disease
C. An improvement in progression-free survival in patients with platinum-resistant disease and platinum-sensitive ovarian cancer
D. None of the above

18. Germ cells tumors include all of the following except:
A. Dysgerminoma
B. Choriocarcinoma
C. Endodermal sinus tumor
D. Immature teratoma
E. All of the above

19. Choriocarcinoma is associated with the following tumor marker:
A. AFP
B. LDH
C. CA19-9
D. hCG

20. A 23-year-old female presents to the emergency with severe right-lower quadrant pain. An abdominal ultrasound reveals a right 20-cm solid mass. A CT of the abdomen and pelvis reveals an isolated mass in the right adnexal region. The patient undergoes surgery and is diagnosed with a stage I, grade 1 immature teratoma of the right ovary. You advise the patient as follows:
A. You advise the patient that there is no role for adjuvant chemotherapy.
B. You recommend chemotherapy with bleomycin, etoposide, and cisplatin for 6 cycles.
C. You recommend chemotherapy with bleomycin, etoposide, and cisplatin for 4 cycles.
D. You recommend to the patient that she completes staging with a TAH, LSO, omentectomy and peritoneal, and nodal dissection.

21. Which of the following statements regarding granulosa cell tumor (GCT) of the ovary are true?
A. GCTs constitute approximately 25% of all ovarian tumors.
B. Mutation of FOXL2 is seen about 25% of adult GCT.
C. Tumor markers include estradiol and inhibin levels.
D. GCTs typically produce testosterone.

22. Which of the following statements regarding palliative care for patients with ovarian cancer is true?
A. Involves a multidisciplinary approach.
B. Bowel obstruction is common.
C. G-tube for decompression should be considered in patients with recurrent bowel obstructions.
D. Catheter placement for ascites drainage should be considered in patients with recurrent ascites.
E. All of the above.

23. Common side effects associated with liposomal doxorubicin include all of the following except:
A. Hypertension

B. Cardiac toxicity
C. Hand foot syndrome
D. Mucositis

24. *Common* mutations associated with low-grade serous carcinoma of the ovary include:
A. KRAS mutations
B. P53 mutations
C. PI3K mutations
D. ARID1A mutations

25. A 62-year-old woman is currently receiving liposomal doxorubicin (she has received three prior doses) at the FDA-approved dose of 50 mg/m^2 for platinum resistant ovarian cancer. Her CA125 has declined nicely from a value of 543 to 257 U/mL. On a follow-up visit in the clinic, she describes to her clinical provider that she has experienced mucositis that has limited her oral intake and a diffuse papular rash. You advise the patient to do the following:
A. Continue with liposomal doxorubicin at the current dose as these toxicities are self-limited
B. Discontinue the liposomal doxorubicin as she is experiencing a true allergic reaction to this agent
C. Assuming that the toxicities have resolved, decrease the dose of the liposomal doxorubicin to 40 mg/m^2
D. Refer to a dermatologist

26. An 85-year-old woman with a history of hypertension and diabetes presents with abdominal distention, fatigue, and anorexia. She notes that prior to 8 weeks ago, she was rather active in her gym class and notes that she is still working part time at a museum as a volunteer. A CT of the abdomen and pelvis reviews bilateral adnexal masses and omental caking. An omental biopsy is positive for high-grade serous carcinoma of Mullerian origin. Surgical debulking results in suboptimal cytoreduction. She recovers well from surgery despite her multiple medical conditions and notes that she has resumed her walking routine. She is now 4 weeks postoperative and presents to discuss options in her care. The appropriate treatment strategy is:
A. Inform the patient that given her advanced years and her advanced disease that chemotherapy is prohibitive due to the potential toxicity
B. Advise the patient that the standard of care is weekly paclitaxel
C. Advise the patient to consider hospice immediately
D. Advise the patient that the standard of care is a platinum and paclitaxel doublet given every 3 weeks for 6 cycles (every 21 days)

27. A 32-year-old mother of four children presents with progressive masculinization, hirsutism, temporal balding, and enlargement of the clitoris. She notes pelvic and lower back pain. The patient undergoes radiographical studies, which reveal bilateral adnexal mass and a soft tissue mass in Morrison's pouch and omental caking. She undergoes surgery and is diagnosed with stage III Sertoli-Leydig cell tumor. The appropriate treatment strategy includes:
A. No adjuvant therapy
B. Systemic adjuvant chemotherapy with carboplatin and gemcitabine
C. Systemic adjuvant chemotherapy with bleomycin, etoposide, and cisplatin for 4 cycles
D. Systemic adjuvant chemotherapy with carboplatin and paclitaxel for 6 cycles

ANSWERS

1. C

The patient has been diagnosed with an advanced stage high-grade papillary serous carcinoma most consistent with ovarian cancer. Several studies have now reported on the use of primary chemotherapy with interval debulking. Vergote et al. reported that neoadjuvant chemotherapy followed by interval debulking surgery/chemotherapy was not inferior to primary debulking surgery followed by chemotherapy as a treatment for patients with advanced ovarian cancer. Postoperative rates of adverse effects were higher after initial debulking than after interval debulking. The hazard ratio for death in the group assigned to neoadjuvant chemotherapy compared with primary surgery was 0.98 (90% CI, 0.84 to 1.13; $P = .01$). The *CHORUS study*, a phase III noninferiority, randomized trial also concluded that survival in women with stage III or IV ovarian cancer treated with primary chemotherapy was noninferior to primary surgery. Median overall survival was 22.6 months in the upfront surgery group versus 24.1 months in the neoadjuvant group. The hazard ratio for death was 0.87 in favor of the neoadjuvant group.

2. D

Neoadjuvant chemotherapy followed by interval debulking/chemotherapy is not inferior to primary debulking in patients with advanced ovarian cancer. However, the strongest independent variable predicting overall survival is the complete resection of all macroscopic disease at primary or interval debulking. Postoperative rates of adverse events are higher after primary debulking than interval debulking.

3. D

BRCA positive tumors have impaired ability to repair double-stranded DNA breaks by the homologous recombination repair pathway. These tumors are sensitive to PARP inhibition. Olaparib is the only PARP inhibitor that has been approved for patients with germline mutations in *BRCA1/2* who have received three prior lines of therapy. *Audeh et al.* conducted a phase II trial in patients with *BRCA1/2* mutations with recurrent disease. The overall response rate was 33% in patients who received olaparib at 400 mg twice daily. Side effects include nausea, fatigue, and anemia.

The SOLO-1 trial and the SOLO-2 trial are double-blinded placebo-controlled multicenter randomized clinical trials that are studying the role of olaparib as maintenance therapy in the upfront setting (SOLO-1) and in the recurrent setting (platinum sensitive; SOLO-2), respectively.

4. A

All patients diagnosed with epithelial ovarian, tubal, and peritoneal cancers should receive genetic counseling and be offered genetic testing, even in the absence of a family history.

Germline *BRCA1* and *BRCA2* mutations account for approximately 5% to 15% of invasive ovarian carcinomas. Some women with hereditary ovarian carcinoma have no immediate relatives with cancer. Over a third of women with hereditary ovarian carcinoma are older than 60. Hence, all women diagnosed with ovarian, fallopian tube, or peritoneal carcinoma, regardless of age or family history, should receive genetic counseling and be offered genetic testing. The Society of Gynecologic Oncology (SGO) advocates for genetic counseling and testing for all women with ovarian, fallopian tube, and peritoneal carcinoma.

5. A, C, and **D**

Several factors have been associated with an increased risk of ovarian cancer. These include advanced age, family history, nulliparity, estrogen replacement, talc powder, pelvic inflammatory disease, living in industrialized Western countries, and being of Jewish descent. Factors associated with a decreased risk include lactation, oral contraceptives, parity, reproductive surgery, a diet high in carotene, low alcohol consumption, and low lactose intake. Late age at first pregnancy is associated with an increased risk for breast cancer but not ovarian cancer.

6. D

Approximately 22,280 women will be diagnosed with ovarian cancer in 2016, and about 14,420 women will die from ovarian cancer. Given that about 843,000 of US women will be diagnosed with cancer in 2016, ovarian cancer accounts for about 3% of all new cancers. Epithelial ovarian cancer ranks fifth in cancer deaths among women. Of all the gynecological neoplasm(s), ovarian cancer is associated with the highest mortality rate of any gynecological cancer. The median age of diagnosis is 63 years of age. The risk of ovarian cancer increases with age. The majority of cases are diagnosed with stage III/stage IV disease.

7. B and **C**

Approximately 90 % of all ovarian malignancies are of epithelial origin. Histologic subtypes include (1) papillary serous carcinoma, (2) clear cell, (3) mucinous carcinoma, (4) endometroid carcinoma, and (5) carcinosarcoma. Evidence now supports that the fallopian tube epithelia is an etiological site for the development of most high-grade serous carcinoma. A majority of serous carcinomas appear to have in situ lesions in the distal fallopian tube. The most common histology is papillary serous carcinoma of the ovary.

8. D

Staging of ovarian cancer (Table 27.1)

9. A and **B**

Adapted from the American Cancer Society.

Several key trials have established platinum/paclitaxel as the standard of care in patients with ovarian cancer.

GOG 111, GOG 104, and GOG172 studied the role of intraperitoneal therapy in the management of patients with advanced ovarian, fallopian tube, and peritoneal cancer.

GOG 172 is the most recent published trial of intraperitoneal/intravenous chemotherapy. Patients enrolled in this trial were optimally cytoreduced. Patients were randomized to IP cisplatin/IV paclitaxel on day 1 of therapy/IP paclitaxel on day 8 of therapy versus IV cisplatin and paclitaxel (cycle = 21 days). There was an overall survival benefit with intraperitoneal therapy (overall survival was 66 vs. 50 months; $P = .03$). A Japanese GOG trial of dose-dense chemotherapy (carboplatin AUC 6 D1 and paclitaxel 80 mg/m^2 D1, 8, 15; q 21-day cycle) also demonstrated a survival benefit when compared with the traditional every 3-week administration of carboplatin and paclitaxel.

10. A

There is no proven benefit from adjuvant chemotherapy or radiation therapy even in advanced stage disease. Surgery is the cornerstone in the management of these neoplasms. Long-term follow-up of these patients is necessary because recurrences can develop years after the primary treatment. Patients should be evaluated with clinical examinations and CA125 measurements. For stage I disease, conservative surgery with unilateral salpingo-oophorectomy is viable in patients wishing to maintain their fertility. The staging for borderline malignancies of the ovary is the same as the staging for invasive ovarian cancer.

TABLE 27.1 Definition of Primary Tumor (T)

T Category	FIGO Stage	T Criteria
TX		Primary Tumor cannot be assessed
T0		No evidence of primary tumor
T1	1	Tumor limited to ovaries (one or both) or fallopian tube(s)
T1a	IA	Tumor limited to one ovary (capsule intact) or fallopian tube surface; no malignant cells in ascites or peritoneal washings
T1b	IB	Tumor limited to one or both ovaries (capsules intact) or fallopian tubes; no tumor on ovarian or fallopian tube surface; no malignant cells in ascites or peritoneal washings
T1c	IC	Tumor limited to one or both ovaries or fallopian tubes, with any of the following:
T1C1	ICI	Surgical spill
T1c2	IC2	capsule ruptured before surgery or tumor on ovarian or fallopian tube surface
T1c3	IC3	Malignant cells in ascites or peritoneal washings
T2	II	Tumor involves one or both ovaries or fallopian tubes with pelvic extension below pelvis brim or primary peritoneal cancer.
T2a	IIA	Extension and/or implants on the uterus and or fallopian tube(s) and/or ovaries
T3	III	Tumor involves one or both ovaries or fallopian tubes or primary peritoneal cancer, with microscopically confirmed peritoneal metastasis outside the pelvis and or metastasis to the retroperitoneal (pelvic and/or para-aortic) lymph nodes
T3a	IIIA2	Microscopic extrapelvic (above the pelvic brim) peritoneal involvement with or without positive retroperitoneal lymph nodes
T3b	IIIB	Macroscopic peritoneal metastasis beyond pelvis 2 cm or less in greatest dimension with or without metastasis to the retroperitoneal lymph nodes
T3c	IIIC	Macroscopic peritoneal metastasis beyond the pelvis more than 2 cm in greatest dimension with or without metastasis to the retroperitoneal lymph nodes (includes extension or tumor to capsule of liver and spleen without parenchymal involvement of either organ)

In Stage IV any distant metastasis (excludes peritoneal metastasis).
From Amin, Mahul et al. the AJCC Cancer Staging Manual. New York: Springer 2016.

11. D

The PLCO study examined the impact of screening patients with serum CA125 and transvaginal ultrasound. The trial concluded that screening was not deemed an effective strategy for use in the *general population*, and no tool is a specific screening tool. The combination of CA125 and ultrasound has a positive predictive value of 23.5%. Many other conditions also can cause an elevated CA125 level, including the following:

- Diverticulitis
- Endometriosis
- Liver cirrhosis
- Normal menstruation
- Pelvic inflammatory disease
- Urinary tract infections
- Pregnancy
- Uterine fibroids

12. B, C, D

Hereditary ovarian cancer constitutes 5% to 15 % of cases of ovarian cancers, not the majority of all ovarian neoplasms. *BRCA1* and *BRCA 2* are tumor suppressor genes that play a role in the repair of DNA damage. *BRCA1* and *BRCA2* are located in chromosomes 17 and 13, respectively. Inheritance of these mutations confers an increased lifetime risk for both ovarian and breast cancer, and these typically occur with an earlier age of onset compared with the general population. While there has been debate about whether or not *BRCA1/2* mutations increase the risk for uterine cancer, the current evidence indicates no increased risk of endometrioid endometrial carcinoma but perhaps a very small absolute increased risk of serous endometrial carcinoma.

13. C

Serologic relapse of ovarian cancer can be described based on CA125. Early treatment based solely on CA125 is not recommended based on a UK trial which enrolled 1442 women who had achieved a complete clinical remission and who underwent serial CA125 testing every 3 months but were blinded to the results. Patients whose CA125 became elevated to 2 times the upper limit of normal were randomized to early intervention versus delayed treatment (treatment was delayed until there was clinical symptoms). The study concluded that there was no difference in the overall survival of woman between the two arms (HR 1.0; 95% CI, 0.82–1.22).

14. C

Platinum-sensitive disease is defined as recurrence of disease after a treatment-free interval of 6 months or longer. Options in patient's care include a platinum doublet, for example, carboplatin and paclitaxel, or carboplatin and gemcitabine, or carboplatin and liposomal doxorubicin. Platinum refractory disease is defined as recurrence of disease during or on completion of platinum chemotherapy. Patient options include chemotherapy and bevacizumab or a clinical trial. Platinum-resistant disease is defined as recurrence of disease on platinum chemotherapy less than 6 months after the completion of chemotherapy. Patient options include chemotherapy and bevacizumab or a clinical trial.

15. C

The patient described above has platinum-sensitive disease given her disease-free interval of 2 years. Although surgery should always be considered in patients with a prolonged disease-free interval, it may not be appropriate in this patient given the fact that radiographical studies revealed ascites, extensive peritoneal carcinomatosis coupled with extensive disease on the serosa of the bowel. Bevacizumab has been associated with an increased risk of bowel perforation in patients with bowel involvement. Options in the management of this patient include carboplatin and paclitaxel, carboplatin and gemcitabine, or carboplatin and liposomal doxorubicin.

16. C

The patient has a history of clear cell carcinoma of the ovary, which can be associated with a hypercalcemic state. Her disease-free interval is at best 3 months; thus, she has platinum-resistant disease. A liver biopsy is reasonable to consider obtaining more current tissue to confirm recurrent disease and consider genomic profiling of the tumor. Given the resistant state of the disease, one option to consider is a combination of bevacizumab and liposomal doxorubicin as outlined by the AURELIA trial. It is also important to check the ionized calcium to be certain that this level remains within normal limits and does not require intervention such as aggressive hydration and the use of a bisphosphonate. Genetic counseling is now considered standard care in all patients with ovarian cancer regardless of histology. Assessing for *BRCA1* or *BRCA2* might enable the patient to be treated with a PARP inhibitor such as olaparib, which is now FDA approved for patients with a germline mutation after three prior lines of therapy.

17. C

The *OCEANs trial* was a randomized double-blind, placebo-controlled phase III trial of chemotherapy with or without bevacizumab in patients with platinum-sensitive, recurrent epithelial ovarian, primary peritoneal, or fallopian tube cancer. The combination of gemcitabine, carboplatin, and bevacizumab resulted in a statistically significant improvement in progression-free survival in patients with platinum-sensitive disease.

The *AURELIA trial* reported that the combination of bevacizumab and chemotherapy versus chemotherapy improved progression-free survival in patients with platinum-resistant disease.

18. E

Germ cell tumors of the ovary can be benign or malignant, and they typically occur in younger women between the ages of 10 and 30. They can comprise several cell types including teratomas (mature and immature), dysgerminomas, endodermal sinus tumors (also known as yolk sac tumors), and choriocarcinomas.

19. D

Tumor markers associated with Germ Cell Tumors:
1. Dysgerminoma: LDH and hCG
2. Choriocarcinoma: hCG
3. Endodermal sinus tumor: AFP
4. Embryonal carcinoma: AFP /hcG
5. Immature teratoma: usually none

20. A

Adjuvant chemotherapy is recommended for ovarian germ cell tumors except for stage I pure dysgerminoma and stage I grade 1 immature teratoma. The combination of bleomycin, etoposide, and cisplatin is the standard of care. Cycles are given every 3 weeks for a total of 3 cycles. Given the patient's age fertility, sparing surgery is of utmost importance, if the disease is localized to one ovary, as is the case here.

21. C

GCTs constitute less than 5% of all ovarian cancers. The majority are diagnosed at stage I. Mutation of FOXL2 is seen in greater than 97% of adult GCT. Tumor markers useful in the early detection of recurrence include estradiol and inhibin levels. In about half of the cases, these tumors produce estrogen and/or progesterone. Patients can present with abnormal uterine bleeding.

22. E

Palliative care for patients with advanced disease should be approached in a multidisciplinary fashion. The multiple disciplines often include medical oncology, surgical oncology (in the event of a small bowel obstruction amenable to resection or more commonly for the placement of a G-tube for decompression), pain and palliative care, social work, and in rare cases radiation oncology (brain metastases, painful liver enlargement). Ascites is often present in late stage ovarian cancer. Palliative options include repeated paracentesis or the placement of an intraabdominal catheter (Pleur X). This catheter is a tunneled indwelling peritoneal catheter used for the treatment of refractory malignant ascites. Potential complications of this catheter include erythema and or infection.

23. C

Liposomal doxorubicin is with hand foot syndrome, mucositis and a lower risk of cardiac toxicity than non-liposomal doxorubicin. There is no risk of hypertension.

24. A

KRAS, BRAF, or ERBB2 mutations are frequently associated with low-grade serous carcinoma of the ovary. P53 mutations are often found in high-grade serous carcinoma of the ovary, fallopian tube, and peritoneal cancer. PI3K mutations are often found in various tumors some of which include breast cancer, ovarian cancer, and uterine cancer. They are not commonly associated with low-grade serous carcinomas. ARID1A mutations are noted in endometriosis-associated ovarian cancers.

25. C

Liposomal doxorubicin is an FDA-approved drug for the management of patient with both platinum-sensitive and platinum-resistant ovarian cancer. Common toxicities include hand food syndrome, rash, and mucositis. Although the FDA-approved dose is 50 mg/m^2, this dose is often associated with a rash. A dose of 40 mg/m^2 is the most commonly used dose in ovarian cancer. This agent is a dose- and schedule-dependent drug. Toxicity is cumulative. Although patients can experience allergic reactions to this agent, in this case, this is most consistent with drug toxicity. The correct answer is to try to reduce the agent and to monitor the symptoms closely.

26. D

Despite the patient's advanced years, chemotherapy is not prohibitive in all cases. The patient, despite common comorbidities, appears to have had a relatively good performance status prior to her diagnosis. She has also recovered in a timely fashion from surgery. The standard of care remains that of a platinum and paclitaxel given every 3 weeks for 6 cycles. Options in elderly patients may also include single-agent carboplatin if the combination of a platinum and paclitaxel is considered prohibitive. Performance status, not age, should drive the utilization of chemotherapy in the elderly population.

27. C

Sertoli-Leydig cell tumors are rare tumors that originate from the gonadal stroma. They occur in all age groups but are most common in young women. Clinical presentation may include masculinization, hirsutism, temporal balding, and enlargement of the clitoris. Over 90% are diagnosed at stage I. Treatment included systemic adjuvant chemotherapy with bleomycin, etoposide, and cisplatin for 3–4 cycles (q 28-day cycle).

REFERENCES

Question 1
1. Vergote I, Trope C, Amant F, et al. Neoadjuvant chemotherapy or primary surgery in stage III or stage IV ovarian cancer. *N Engl J Med.* 2010;363:943–953.
2. Kehoe S, Jook J, Nankivell M, et al. Primary chemotherapy versus primary surgery for newly diagnosed advanced ovarian cancer (CHORUS): an open label, randomised, controlled, non-inferiority trial. *Lancet.* 2015;386:49–57.

Question 2
1. Vergote I, Trope C, Amant F, et al. Neoadjuvant chemotherapy or primary surgery in stage III or stage IV ovarian cancer. *N Engl J Med.* 2010;363:943–953.
2. Kehoe S, Jook J, Nankivell M, et al. Primary chemotherapy versus primary surgery for newly diagnosed advanced ovarian cancer (CHORUS): an open label, randomised, controlled, non-inferiority trial. *Lancet.* 2015;386:49–57.

Question 3
1. Audeh MW, Carmichael J, Penson RT, et al. Oral poly (ADP-ribose) polymerase inhibitor olaparib in patients with BRCA1 or BRCA2 mutations and recurrent ovarian cancer: a proof-of-concept trial. *Lancet.* 2010;376:245–251.
2. Ledermann J, Harter P, Gourley C, et al. Olaparib maintenance therapy in platinum-sensitive relapsed ovarian cancer. *N Engl J Med.* 2012;366:1382–1392.

Question 4
1. Pal T, Permuth-Wey J, Betts JA, et al. BRCA1 and BRCA2 mutations account for a large proportion of ovarian carcinoma cases. *Cancer.* 2005;104:2807–2816.
2. Schrader KA, Hurlburt J, Kalloger WE, et al. Germline BRCA1 and BRCA2 mutations in ovarian cancer. *Obstetric Gyncol.* 2012;120:235–240.
3. Walsh T, Casadei S, Lee MK, et al. Mutations in 12 genes for inherited ovarian, fallopian tube, and peritoneal carcinoma identified by massively parallel sequencing. *Proc Natl Acad Sci U S A.* 2011;108:18032–18037.

Question 5
1. Hunn J, Rodriguez GC. Ovarian cancer: etiology, risk factors, and epidemiology. *Clin Obstet Gynecol.* 2012;55(1):3–23.

Question 6
1. American Cancer Society. *Cancer Facts and Figures 2016.* Atlanta, GA: American Cancer Society; 2016.

Question 7
1. Erickson BK, Conner MG, Landen C. The role of the fallopian tube in the origin of ovarian cancer. *Am J Obstet Gynecol.* 2013;209(5):409–414.

Question 8
1. Adapted from the American Cancer Society.

Question 9
1. Armstrong D, Bundy B, Wenzel L, et al. Intraperitoneal cisplatin and paclitaxel in ovarian cancer. *N Engl J Med.* 2006;354(1):34–43.
2. Katsumata N, Yasuda M, Takahashi F, et al. Dose-dense paclitaxel once a week in combination with carboplatin every 3 weeks for advanced ovarian cancer: a phase 3, open-label, randomised controlled trial. *Lancet.* 2009;374:1331–1338.

3. Ozols R, Bundy B, Greer B, et al. Phase II trial of carboplatin and paclitaxel compared with cisplatin and paclitaxel in patients with optimally resected stage III ovarian cancer: a Gynecologic Oncology Group Study. *N Engl J Med.* 2003;21(17):3194–3200.

Question 10
1. Caldron I, Leunen K, Gorp TV, Amant F, Neven P, Vergote I. Management of borderline ovarian neoplasms. *J Clin Oncol.* 2007;25(20):2928–2937.

Question 11
1. Partridge E, Kreimer AR, Greenless RT, et al. Results from four rounds of ovarian cancer screening in a randomized trial. *Obstet Gynecol.* 2009;113(4):775–782.

Question 12
1. Prat J, Ribé A, Gallardo A. Hereditary ovarian cancer. *Hum Pathol.* 2005;36(8):861–870.
2. Shu CA, Pike MC, Jotwani AR. Uterine cancer after risk-reducing salpingo-oophorectomy without hysterectomy in women with BRCA mutations. *JAMA Oncol.* 2016;2(11):1434–1440. http://dx.doi.org/10.1001/jamaoncol.2016.1820.

Question 13
1. Rustin GJ, van der Burg ME, Griffin CL, et al. Early versus delayed treatment of relapsed ovarian cancer (MRC OV05/EORTC 55955): a randomised trial. *Lancet.* 2010;376(9747):1155–1163.

Question 14
1. Parmer MK, Ledermann JA, Colombo N, et al. Paclitaxel plus platinum—based chemotherapy versus conventional platinum—based chemotherapy in women with relapsed ovarian cancer: ICON 4/AGO-OVAR-2.2 trial. *Lancet.* 2003;361(9375):2099–2106.
2. Pfisterer J, Plante M, Vergote I, et al. Gemcitabine plus Carboplatin compared with Carboplatin in patients with platinum sensitive recurrent ovarian cancer: an intergroup trial of the AGO-OVA, the NCIC CTG, and the EORTC GCG. *J Clin Oncol.* 2006;24(29):4699–4707.
3. Wagner U, Marth C, Largillier R, et al. Final overall survival results of phase III GCIG CALYPSO trial of pegylated liposomal doxorubicin and carboplatin vs., paclitaxel and carboplatin in platinum-sensitive ovarian cancer patients. *Br J Cancer.* 2012;107(4):588–591.

Question 15
1. Parmer MK, Ledermann JA, Colombo N, et al. Paclitaxel plus platinum—based chemotherapy versus conventional platinum—based chemotherapy in women with relapsed ovarian cancer: ICON 4/AGO-OVAR-2.2 trial. *Lancet.* 2003;361(9375):2099–2106.
2. Pfisterer J, Plante M, Vergote I, et al. Gemcitabine plus Carboplatin compared with Carboplatin in patients with platinum sensitive recurrent ovarian cancer: an intergroup trial of the AGO-OVA, the NCIC CTG, and the EORTC GCG. *J Clin Oncol.* 2006;24(29):4699–4707.
3. Wagner U, Marth C, Largillier R, et al. Final overall survival results of phase III GCIG CALYPSO trial of pegylated liposomal doxorubicin and carboplatin vs., paclitaxel and carboplatin in platinum-sensitive ovarian cancer patients. *Br J Cancer.* 2012;107(4):588–591.
4. Pujade-Lauraine E, Hilpert F, Weber B, et al. Bevacizumab combined with chemotherapy for Platinum Resistant Ovarian Cancer: the AURELIA open label randomized phase III trial. *J Clin Oncol.* 2014;32(13):1302–1308.

Question 16
1. Pujade-Lauraine E, Hilpert F, Weber B, et al. Bevacizumab combined with chemotherapy for Platinum Resistant Ovarian Cancer: the AURELIA open label randomized phase III trial. *J Clin Oncol.* 2014;32(13):1302–4025.
2. Lewin S, Dezube D, Guddati A, Mittal K, Muggia F, Klein P. Paraneoplastic hypercalcemia in clear cell ovarian adenocarcinoma. *Ecancermedicalscience.* 2012;6:271.

Question 17

1. Aghajanian C, Blank S, Goff B, et al. OCEANS: a randomized double blind, placebo controlled phase III trial of chemotherapy with or without bevacizumab in patients with platinum-sensitive, recurrent epithelial ovarian, primary peritoneal or fallopian tube cancer. *J Clin Oncol*. 2012;30(17):2039–2045.
2. Pujade-Lauraine E, Hilpert F, Weber B, et al. Bevacizumab combined with chemotherapy for Platinum Resistant Ovarian Cancer: the AURELIA open label randomized phase III trial. *J Clin Oncol*. 2014;32(13):1302–1308.

Question 20

1. Matei D, Brown J, Frazier LF. Updates in the Management of Ovarian Germ Cell Tumors. 2013 ASCO educational book/asco.org/edbook.

Question 21

1. Kottarathill VD, Antony M, Nair I, Pavithran K. Recent advances in granulosa cell tumor ovary: a review. *Indian J Surg Oncol*. 2013;4(1):37–47.

Question 24

1. Vang R, Shih I-M, Kurman RJ. Ovarian low-grade and high-grade serous carcinoma: pathogenesis, clinicopathologic and molecular biologic features, and diagnostic problems. *Adv Anat Pathol*. 2009;16(5):267–282.

Question 26

1. Lambrou NC, Bristow RE. Ovarian cancer in elderly women. *Oncology (Williston Park)*. 2003;17(8):1075–1081.

Question 27

1. Homesley HD, Bundy BN, Hurteau JA, Roth LM. Bleomycin, etoposide and cisplatin combination therapy of ovarian granulosa cell tumors and other stromal malignancies: a Gynecologic Oncology Group Study. *Gynecol Oncol*. 1999;72(2):131.

Cancer of the Cervix, Uterus, Vagina, Vulva, and Gestational Choriorcinoma

QUESTIONS

1. A 45-year-old female has a history of stage II cervical cancer, for which she was treated with cisplatin-based chemoradiation. She has done well over the past 3 years, but she re-presents now with vaginal bleeding. Her pelvic examination shows a mass at the vaginal cuff, and a biopsy confirms recurrent disease. She undergoes repeat staging, and it unfortunately shows metastatic disease in her liver. A biopsy of the liver confirms the presence of metastatic squamous cell carcinoma, consistent with her primary cervical cancer. The most appropriate treatment for this patient consists of:
   A. Cisplatin 75 mg/m^2 plus paclitaxel 135 mg/m^2 for 6 cycles
   B. Carboplatin AUC 6 plus paclitaxel 175 mg/m^2 until evidence of disease progression
   C. Carboplatin AUC 2 plus paclitaxel 60 mg/m^2 administered weekly for 18 weeks
   D. Cisplatin 75 mg/m^2, paclitaxel 135 mg/m^2, and bevacizumab 15 mg/kg every 3 weeks until evidence of disease progression
   E. Hospice care

2. A 65-year-old female is diagnosed with locally advanced vulvar cancer. The primary lesion is approximately 4.5 cm in size. After presentation at a multidisciplinary tumor board, she undergoes surgical resection and node staging. The final pathology shows a 6-cm squamous cell carcinoma of the vulva with evidence for lymphovascular invasion. The margins are close, and she has no evidence of pelvic-node metastases. Which of the following statements about adjuvant therapy applies?
   A. There is no role for adjuvant therapy following surgical resection of locally advanced vulvar cancer.
   B. She is a candidate for adjuvant radiation therapy (RT) given the high-risk features present.

C. Adjuvant chemoradiation affords improved survival outcomes compared with adjuvant RT for women with locally advanced vulvar cancer.
   D. Adjuvant platinum-based chemotherapy should be administered with curative intent.
   E. A combination approach utilizing chemoradiation followed by 4 cycles of adjuvant chemotherapy is superior to adjuvant RT alone.

3. A 67-year-old female presented with vaginal bleeding. On direct questioning, she also reported a recent onset of urinary frequency, often accompanied by pain. On pelvic examination, a 5-cm mass was identified in the upper third of the vagina. Examination of the inguinal node basins showed bilateral inguinal adenopathy with nodes up to 3 cm in size appreciated. A biopsy of the vaginal mass confirmed a primary vaginal squamous cell carcinoma and a subsequent FNA of the left inguinal node was positive. Which is the most appropriate next step in her management?
   A. Primary surgical resection
   B. Primary chemoradiation using 5-FU and cisplatin
   C. Neoadjuvant chemotherapy
   D. Radiation therapy as a single modality treatment
   E. None of the above

4. A 36-year-old female presented with bleeding after intercourse and pelvic pain. She denied other symptoms. Her exam showed a cervical mass, approximately 1.5 cm in size, and biopsy of this lesion showed a grade 3 squamous cell carcinoma. She underwent surgery for cervical cancer, and final pathology showed a deeply invasive cervical lesion, 2 cm in size with evidence of lymphovascular space invasion. There was no evidence of pelvic node invasion, and surgical margins were negative. Which of the following is the most appropriate recommendation for adjuvant treatment?
   A. Whole pelvic radiation therapy
   B. Intravaginal brachytherapy
   C. Chemoradiation using weekly cisplatin
   D. Cisplatin plus gemcitabine for 6 cycles
   E. No further treatment

5. A 45-year-old woman underwent surgery with curative intent for a 3-cm cervical cancer. Final pathology showed that the parametria were microscopically involved and

3/17 pelvic nodes contained metastatic disease. She sees you for treatment recommendations. What is your recommendation?

A. Whole pelvic radiation therapy
B. Intravaginal brachytherapy
C. Chemoradiation using weekly cisplatin
D. Cisplatin plus gemcitabine for 6 cycles
E. No further treatment

6. A 39-year-old female was treated for early-stage cervical cancer 2 years previously. At that time, she was diagnosed with stage IB2 disease and received definitive chemoradiation using weekly cisplatin. She tolerated treatment without major side effects and then entered follow-up. She was doing well, until she recently presented with pelvic pain and intermittent spotting after intercourse. A pelvic examination revealed a mass at the vaginal cuff that was fixed in position. She had no evidence of lymphadenopathy. A biopsy of the mass was positive for recurrent cervical cancer and subsequent staging with FDG-PET scan was negative for metastatic disease. Treatment for this patient with curative intent would entail:

A. Pelvic exenteration
B. Neoadjuvant chemotherapy followed by resection of local disease
C. Re-irradiation of the vaginal vault
D. Chemotherapy plus bevacizumab
E. None of the above

7. A 47-year-old woman is diagnosed with vaginal cancer, stage I. She undergoes surgery and is told she needs no further treatment. She enters surveillance and wants to know about how this might have developed. Which of the following is not a risk factor for vaginal cancer?

A. Human papillomavirus infection
B. Multiple lifetime sexual partners
C. Early age at intercourse
D. Current smoking history
E. Nulliparity

8. A 60-year-old woman presents to you for a second opinion. She has a long history of vulvar carcinoma, and she has been treated multiple times in the past with resection and at other times with radiation therapy. She developed pulmonary metastases 5 months ago and has had progressive disease despite combined cisplatin and paclitaxel plus bevacizumab, vinorelbine monotherapy, and pemetrexed. She has a performance status of 3 and requires a wheelchair. Her baseline symptoms include a fairly significant neuropathy, profound nausea, and anorexia. Which is the most appropriate recommendation for this patient?

A. Proceed with a phase I clinical trial
B. Re-treatment with carboplatin and paclitaxel
C. Fourth line therapy with oral etoposide
D. Referral for radiation therapy
E. Referral for hospice and end-of-life care

9. A 60-year-old woman presented with abdominal bloating and pelvic pain. On exam, she had obvious abdominal distention and a sense of fullness in the pelvis, though no discrete mass was identified on pelvic exam. A subsequent CT scan showed a large uterine mass but no other findings. Therefore, she underwent surgical staging, including a total abdominal hysterectomy, bilateral salpingo-oophorectomy, and pelvic and para-aortic node dissection. The final pathology showed a deeply invasive serous carcinoma of the uterus. There was evidence of pelvic and para-aortic node involvement with 3/10 pelvic and 2/12 para-aortic nodes positive for metastatic disease. What do you recommend as adjuvant therapy?

A. She does not require adjuvant therapy and should proceed with surveillance.
B. She should proceed with vaginal brachytherapy.
C. She should proceed with pelvic radiation therapy.
D. She should proceed with adjuvant chemotherapy using carboplatin and paclitaxel.
E. She requires multimodality treatment, consisting of chemotherapy and radiation therapy.

10. A previously healthy 68-year-old female underwent hysterectomy for a uterine mass. The final pathology revealed a leiomyosarcoma, which was confined to the uterus. She is worried about dying from this tumor and seeks your opinion regarding adjuvant therapy. Which of the following do you recommend?

A. She does not need adjuvant chemotherapy and I recommend surveillance.
B. She should proceed with doxorubicin for 6 cycles.
C. She should proceed with fixed-dose rate gemcitabine plus docetaxel as adjuvant treatment.
D. She should undergo whole pelvic radiation therapy.
E. She requires multimodality treatment using doxorubicin followed by whole pelvic radiation therapy.

11. A 66-year-old female presents with pulmonary metastases. She has a history of stage I leiomyosarcoma for which she underwent a total hysterectomy 5 years previously. A biopsy of her lung metastasis was consistent with uterine leiomyosarcoma. What is her next best step?

A. Fixed-dose rate gemcitabine (900 mg/m^2 over 90 minutes on days 1 and 8) plus docetaxel (75 mg/m^2 on day 8)
B. Carboplatin AUC 6 + paclitaxel 175 mg/m^2
C. Doxorubicin 60 mg/m^2 + Paclitaxel 60 mg/m^2
D. Trabectidin (1.5 mg/m^2)
E. None of the above

12. A 42-year-old woman presented after having a seizure at a mall. Head CT showed a solitary lesion in her left parietal lobe. Bloodwork showed an elevated hCG >1,000,000 mIU/mL. Pelvic ultrasound was negative for pregnancy, but it did reveal an 8-cm uterine mass and bilateral ovarian theca-lutein cysts. CT of the chest, abdomen, and pelvis showed two liver lesions measuring 2 and 3 cm, respectively, and at least four lung metastases, measuring 1–2 cm in size. Per her husband, she had undergone a D&E for an early second trimester pregnancy loss about 7 months previously. He recalled the doctor telling him that the placenta was "very abnormal." Based on the picture, she was diagnosed with GTN stage IV. What is the most appropriate treatment for this patient?

A. Neurosurgery for resection of the brain metastasis
B. High-dose methotrexate
C. Hysterectomy and bilateral salpingo-oophorectomy
D. Whole brain radiation therapy
E. Systemic chemotherapy using Etoposide, high-dose methotrexate, actinomycin D (EMA) alternating with cyclophosphamide and vincristine (CO) and consultation with neurosurgery

13. A 60-year-old woman has a history of a stage IB endometrial cancer, endometrioid type, for which she underwent adjuvant radiation therapy (RT). She did well until this past month, when she developed abdominal bloating. A work-up was pursued, which included CT scan of the chest, abdomen, and pelvis. Unfortunately, this revealed omental carcinomatosis and ascites. A biopsy of the omental disease was consistent with recurrent endometrioid adenocarcinoma. She is not a surgical candidate and hence, is sent to you for

treatment recommendations. Given she has never received chemotherapy in the past, your recommendation is:
A. Carboplatin AUC = 6 and paclitaxel 175 mg/m^2 on a 21-day cycle.
B. Cisplatin 50 mg/m^2, paclitaxel 160 mg/m^2, and doxorubicin 50 45 mg/m^2 on a 21-day cycle.
C. Single agent cisplatin 75 mg/m^2.
D. A Weekly treatment using carboplatin AUC = 2 plus paclitaxel 80 mg/m^2.
E. Letrozole 2.5 mg daily.

14. A 32-year-old female presents with bleeding after intercourse. On pelvic examination, she has a 5-cm cervical lesion, which is friable and bleeds easily on palpation. A biopsy shows a high-grade squamous cell carcinoma of the cervix. Pelvic MRI confirms a bulky cervical cancer extending into the posterior wall of the uterine body (Fig. 27B.1). A staging FDG-PET scan shows no evidence of lymphadenopathy or metastatic disease. Your recommendation for treatment consists of:
A. Neoadjuvant chemotherapy using cisplatin, paclitaxel, and doxorubicin for 3 cycles followed by simple hysterectomy
B. Definitive chemoradiation using weekly cisplatin
C. Radical hysterectomy followed by adjuvant chemotherapy
D. Weekly carboplatin plus paclitaxel with radiation therapy
E. Carboplatin, paclitaxel, plus bevacizumab

15. A 56-year-old woman comes to you for a second opinion. She has been diagnosed with a stage II vulvar carcinoma and has recovered well from her surgical procedure 6 weeks previously. On review of pathology, she had excision of a 3-cm vulvar squamous cell carcinoma, the margins were clear, and there was no evidence of lymphovascular invasion. However, she only had a sentinel node biopsy, which was negative (0 of 3 nodes). Regarding further nodal evaluation, the most appropriate recommendation would be:
A. She does not require further nodal evaluation.
B. She should have a repeat sentinel node biopsy now that she is 6 weeks out from surgery.
C. She needs to proceed with a formal inguinofemoral lymphadenectomy.
D. Further imaging to evaluate the status of her lymph nodes is required.
E. She should proceed with adjuvant radiation therapy.

16. A 58-year-old woman has been diagnosed with recurrent vulvar cancer. Her prior treatment consisted of surgical resection and bilateral inguinofemoral node dissection, after which she received adjuvant RT based on high-risk pathologic features. It has been 15 months since end of treatment, and she is found with recurrent disease involving the residual vulva. A multidisciplinary tumor board has recommended she proceed with re-excision. Prior to surgery, she should undergo:
A. Head CT scan
B. Chest x-ray
C. Pelvic MRI
D. Ultrasound of the liver
E. Full-body FDG PET scan

17. A 67-year-old woman is referred for a newly diagnosed vulvar melanoma. She initially presented with nonspecific discomfort and vulvar itching. Examination showed a pigmented lesion involving the labia minora. She underwent surgery and was ultimately diagnosed with a T2aN0M0 melanoma (stage IB). She wants to know more about this disease. Which of the following are true statements about vulvar melanoma?

A. These are rare tumors of the vulva and typically occur in white women.
B. The average age at diagnosis is 60, although girls as young as 10 years have been diagnosed.
C. Staging of vulvar melanoma utilizes the same staging convention as for skin melanomas
D. In contrast to skin melanomas, vulvar melanomas have a lower rate of BRAF or NRAS mutations.
E. All of the above are true.

18. A 75-year-old female presented with vaginal bleeding, and a biopsy showed a grade 3 endometrioid adenocarcinoma. She also underwent full surgical staging, including a total abdominal hysterectomy, bilateral salpingo-oophorectomy, pelvic and para-aortic node dissection. The final pathology showed a grade 3 endometrioid carcinoma with evidence of lymphovascular invasion. The tumor was also deeply invasive to the myometrium. Her lymph nodes showed no evidence of malignancy. What do you recommend as adjuvant therapy?
A. She does not require adjuvant therapy and should proceed with surveillance.
B. She should proceed with vaginal brachytherapy.
C. She should proceed with pelvic radiation therapy.
D. She should proceed with adjuvant chemotherapy using carboplatin and paclitaxel.
E. She requires multimodality treatment, consisting of chemotherapy and radiation therapy.

19. A 70-year-old woman has metastatic uterine leiomyosarcoma, having progressed on docetaxel and gemcitabine and then on doxorubicin. She maintains an excellent performance status and desires further treatment. What do you recommend?
A. Eribulin
B. Trabectidin
C. Pazopanib
D. Best supportive care
E. All of the above

20. A 20-year-old female had undergone a dilatation and curettage for molar pregnancy 10 months ago. Her hCG had normalized as expected but most recently started to rise once more and increased exponentially from 15 to 1725 mIU/mL. Her exam showed an enlarged uterus but no other findings. This prompted a pelvic ultrasound that showed a 6-cm, complicated uterine mass. What further studies are required to formally stage this patient?
A. Chest x-ray
B. FDG- PET scan
C. Whole body CT scan
D. Brain MRI
E. Biopsy of a representative lung lesion

21. A 32-year-old woman presents with excess vaginal bleeding over the past 2 weeks, with onset 6 months after a normal spontaneous vaginal delivery. A pelvic ultrasound showed a thickened endometrium, which prompted a dilatation and curettage. Pathology from that procedure showed endometrial proliferation and evidence of intermediate trophoblast cells (Fig. 27B.2). hCG was elevated to 400 mIU/mL and subsequent staging CT of the chest and abdomen showed at least five pulmonary lesions greater than 2 cm in size. She was taken for a total abdominal hysterectomy due to bleeding, and the final pathology showed a diffuse infiltration of intermediate trophoblasts between muscle fibers and vascular channels. The cells diffusely stained positive for human placental lactogen (hPL) but less so for hCG.

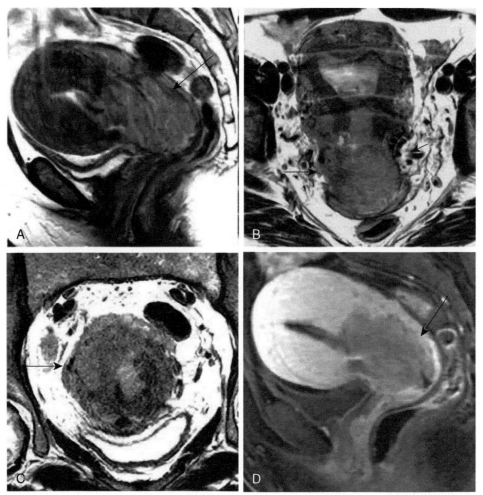

FIG. 27B.1 Cervical cancer on magnetic resonance imaging. (A) Sagittal T2-weighted image showing a heterogeneous isointense mass in the cervix extending into the posterior wall of the uterine body *(arrow)*. (B) T2-weighted image sliced coronally through the cervix showing a mass protruding into the uterine cavity *(arrow)*. (C) T2-weighted image sliced axially across the cervix showing a bulky, eccentric cervical mass on the right side with spread beyond the T2 hypointense ring of the cervical stroma into the parametrium *(arrow)*. (D) T1-weighted gadolinium-enhanced image revealing clear delineation of the mass relative to the adjacent ut erus *(arrow)*. (From Abeloff Clinical Oncology, 5th edition, figure 87.11.)

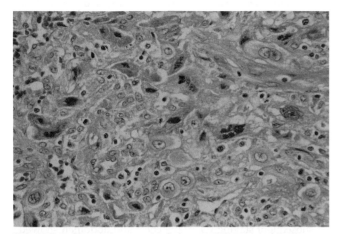

FIG. 27B.2 Photomicrograph of placental site trophoblastic tumor composed almost entirely of mononuclear cells of the intermediate trophoblast. (From Abeloff Clinical Oncology, 5th edition, figure 90.5.)

Immunohistochemistry was positive for alpha-inhibin and cytokeratin 8/18, but it was negative for smooth muscle markers. These characteristics are most consistent with:

A. Complete mole
B. Partial mole
C. Choriocarcinoma
D. Placental site trophoblastic tumor
E. Uterine sarcoma

22. A 62-year-old woman has a history of uterine fibroids. They have not really bothered her until recently, when she noticed an acute sense of fullness in her pelvic associated with pain on occasion. An ultrasound showed an 8cm uterine mass showed an irregular pattern of vessel distribution and mixed echogenicity. A subsequent CT of the pelvis confirmed a solitary mass in the uterus without associated adenopathy. Which of the following are indicative that she has a uterine leiomyosarcoma?

A. Age >60 years
B. A solitary uterine mass
C. Mixed echogenicity on the pelvic ultrasound
D. CT findings of a mass without associated adenopathy
E. None of the above

23. A 36-year-old female underwent a dilatation and curettage for suspected molar pregnancy. At the time, her hCG was 15,000 mIU/mL. Pelvic ultrasound demonstrated an enlarged uterus greater than expected for gestational age and large ovarian cysts, measuring >7 cm. Final pathology from the D&C showed a complete mole. What do you recommend for her now?

A. Observation without further treatment
B. Hysterectomy and bilateral salpingo-oophorectomy
C. Simple hysterectomy
D. Methotrexate
E. Etoposide, Methotrexate, Actinomycin-D (EMA) followed by cyclophosphamide and vincristine (CO)

ANSWERS

1. D

For patients with metastatic cervical cancer who have previously been treated with chemoradiation, chemotherapy plus bevacizumab affords a survival advantage, so the correct answer would be D. This was shown in Gynecologic Oncology Group (GOG) 240 trial, which enrolled over 450 women with primary stage 4B cervical cancer or recurrent or persistent disease (all of whom were chemotherapy naïve) and randomly assigned them to chemotherapy with or without bevacizumab. Compared with chemotherapy alone, the incorporation of bevacizumab significantly improved overall survival by almost 4 months (16.8 vs. 12.9 months, respectively; $P = 0.0132$). Therefore, the correct option is cisplatin, paclitaxel, plus bevacizumab. For those who are not candidates for bevacizumab therapy, a separate trial conducted by the Japanese Gynecologic Oncology Group (JGOG 0505) suggests that carboplatin plus paclitaxel is equivalent to cisplatin and paclitaxel and not as toxic. Hence, such patients can be spared the toxicity of cisplatin and proceed with carboplatin and paclitaxel.

2. B

She has multiple high-risk factors for recurrence, including large tumor size, presence of lymphovascular invasion, and close surgical margins. For these patients, the standard treatment consists of adjuvant RT (B). There are no randomized trials to support this recommendation, but a large retrospective study that included more than 1600 patients reported that compared with no postoperative RT, adjuvant RT was associated with a significant improvement in progression-free survival (HR 0.67, 95% CI 0.51–0.88). While it also improved overall survival at 3 years (57 vs. 51%, respectively), this was not statistically significant. There are no data to inform the use of combined modality treatment in vulvar carcinoma. However, some experts prefer chemoradiation to RT alone as an extrapolation from the treatment of cervical cancer. In the absence of data, though, RT alone should be the standard treatment approach.

3. B

Of the listed options above, the most appropriate treatment is primary chemoradiation with 5-FU and/or cisplatin (B). Although only informed by low-quality data, single institution studies consistently report improved locoregional control rates. As an example, one small study included 20 patients treated with RT alone versus 51 treated with chemoradiation. Compared with RT alone, patients treated with combined modality therapy had a higher 3-year disease-free survival rate (73% vs. 43%, $P = .011$) and overall survival (79% vs. 56%, $P = 0.037$). Given the local extent of disease, surgical resection is not recommended as she would likely not achieve a complete resection. In general, chemotherapy has a limited role in vulvar cancer management, and neoadjuvant chemotherapy would only be appropriate on a clinical trial.

4. A

This patient meets Sedlis' criteria for intermediate risk disease and should proceed with whole pelvic RT (A). The precise criteria include the presence of LVSI plus deep one-third cervical stromal invasion and tumor of any size; presence of LVSI plus middle one-third stromal invasion and tumor size ≥2 cm; presence of LVSI plus superficial one-third stromal invasion and tumor size ≥5 cm; no LVSI but deep or middle one-third stromal invasion and tumor size ≥4 cm. These criteria were used in a randomized trial of whole pelvic RT or no further treatment. Compared with follow-up only, adjuvant RT resulted in a significant reduction in the risk of recurrence (RR = 0.53, $P = .008$). Because she has undergone hysterectomy, she is not able to have vaginal brachytherapy, which requires an intact cervix for placement of the brachytherapy device. While chemoradiation has shown benefits for more advanced disease, its role for women who meet Sedlis' criteria is not yet clear, and an ongoing clinical trial being conducted by NRG Oncology hopes to address this issue. Systemic chemotherapy is not utilized in patients with intermediate risk disease.

5. C

This patient meets Peters' criteria for high-risk cervical cancer. The precise criteria include positive surgical margins; pathologically confirmed involvement of the pelvic lymph nodes; and/or microscopic involvement of the parametrium. For women with high-risk disease, adjuvant treatment consisting of chemoradiation is recommended; therefore, the correct answer is C. This is based on a trial in this population where over 100 women were randomly assigned to RT alone or RT with chemotherapy (consisting of cisplatin and 5-FU). RT resulted in a significantly lower 4-year rate of progression-free survival and overall survival. Because of toxicity, cisplatin is often used rather than cisplatin and 5-FU.

6. A

For patients with a central pelvic recurrence, as in this woman, curative treatment requires pelvic exenteration (A). The chance of cure (assuming resection to negative surgical margins and the absence of metastatic disease) approaches 50%. However, treatment is not without its risks, which include operative mortality of 3%–5% and treatment-related morbidity exceeds 50%. She is not a candidate for re-irradiation after prior chemoradiation due to the risk of severe toxicities to normal tissue, and there is no curative role for chemotherapy in this circumstance.

7. E

Vulvar carcinoma shares the same risk factors as for cervical cancer, including multiple lifetime sexual partners, early age at intercourse, and smoking. In addition, most vaginal cancers are squamous cell carcinomas and are likely mediated by human papillomavirus (HPV) infection. In one study that included almost 190 cases of invasive vaginal cancer, HPV DNA was detected in 74% of cancers with the highest detection rates in warty-basaloid subtypes of squamous cell carcinomas. Although a risk factor for breast and ovarian cancer, nulliparity is not a risk factor for vaginal carcinoma (E).

8. E

This patient has end-stage vulvar cancer and should be referred for hospice and end-of-life care (E). Her performance status disqualifies her from clinical trials and, in general, the role for chemotherapy in vulvar cancer is exceedingly limited. While treatment with chemotherapy plus bevacizumab, vinorelbine, and then pemetrexed represent reasonable extrapolations of data on their role in the management of metastatic cervical cancer, there are no data to inform the benefits of continuing with treatment after progression on multiple lines of therapy. Her symptoms are also systemic, which makes it unlikely that there is a reasonable target for treatment with radiation therapy.

9. D

This patient has stage IIIC endometrial cancer with serous histology and is at high risk for recurrence and death from disease. Therefore, she requires chemotherapy. The current standard treatment utilizes carboplatin and paclitaxel (D), which was shown to be as effective and better tolerated than the three-drug combination of cisplatin, doxorubicin, and paclitaxel in a randomized clinical trial. While some clinicians favor multimodality treatment, there are no prospective randomized trials that show it is superior to chemotherapy alone.

10. A

The most appropriate answer is A. This patient has a stage I uterine leiomyosarcoma, and there are no data to inform the benefits of any treatment versus the almost certain toxicities. Doxorubicin was compared with no further treatment in one trial; patients treated with doxorubicin had a lower recurrence risk, but this treatment showed no benefit in either progression-free or overall survival. Docetaxel and gemcitabine has been evaluated in a phase II trial ($n = 25$) and reported a 3-year progression-free survival rate of 59%. However, there was no control arm; hence, it is not possible to conclude that it should be standard of care. Finally, RT has no role in the adjuvant context. This was shown in the European Organization for the Research and Treatment of Cancer (EORTC) trial 55874. Among the 103 patients with leiomyosarcoma in this trial, there was no significant differences in disease progression rates (local or distant) between RT and observation. However, RT was associated with lower overall survival (HR 0.64, 95% CI 0.36–1.14).

11. A

For patients with metastatic leiomyosarcoma, the first-line treatment of choice is docetaxel and gemcitabine (A). This is based on a phase II trial from the Gynecologic Oncology Group (GOG 87L) that included 42 women. Docetaxel and gemcitabine resulted in an overall response rate of 36%. Doxorubicin is a reasonable alternative to docetaxel and gemcitabine, but it is usually reserved for the second-line setting. Carboplatin has minimal activity in sarcoma and plays no role in treatment of leiomyosarcoma. Trabectidin is approved for use in leiomyosarcoma following disease progression on doxorubicin; hence, is often used in third-line treatment.

12. A

This patient has a grade 2 endometrioid cancer with less than 50% myometrial invasion, consistent with stage IA endometrial cancer. These patients do not generally

require lymph node dissection given that their risk of nodal metastases is no higher than 5 percent. As a result of their excellent prognosis, no adjuvant therapy is required and the correct answer is that she should proceed with surveillance (A). While radiation therapy (RT) can reduce the risk of a local recurrence, there is no improvement in overall survival outcomes, since as stated above, the outcomes are excellent already with surgery alone. In addition, both pelvic RT and vaginal brachytherapy carry small toxicity risks, including a higher risk of secondary malignancies with pelvic RT[13] and an increase in GU complications (e.g., dysuria, frequency, and incontinence) with vaginal brachytherapy.[14]

13. A

The most appropriate treatment for this patient is carboplatin and paclitaxel (A). The data to support its use comes from Gynecologic Oncology Group trial 209 (GOG 209), which randomly assigned 1300 women to carboplatin and paclitaxel or to cisplatin, paclitaxel, and doxorubicin (TAP).[17] Compared with TAP, carboplatin and paclitaxel resulted in a similar overall response rate (51% in both arms), median progression-free survival (13 months), and overall survival (37 vs. 40 months). However, carboplatin and paclitaxel was significantly less toxic, with much lower neuropathy rates (19 vs. 26%), thrombocytopenia (12 vs. 23%), and GI side effects (6 vs. 13%).

14. B

This patient presents with a stage IB cervical cancer. For these patients, definitive treatment consists of chemoradiation using weekly cisplatin (B). Compared with RT alone, chemoradiation results in a 30% relative reduction in the risk of death, 34% reduction in the risk of disease progression, 41% reduction in the risk of a local recurrent, and an almost 20% reduction in the risk of a distant recurrence. Given her large cervical cancer, radical hysterectomy would likely show evidence of parametrial invasion or positive margins, and this would require use of adjuvant chemoradiation in the adjuvant setting that would subject her to significant risk for treatment-related toxicities. Neoadjuvant chemotherapy is not utilized in such a scenario when chemoradiation can be offered with curative intent. If used, however, the proper surgery for invasive cervical cancer consists of a radical hysterectomy. While bevacizumab is an active agent in cervical cancer, the data support its use in combination with carboplatin and paclitaxel as a first-line treatment for recurrent or metastatic cervical cancer.

15. A

For patients with vulvar cancer who undergo surgical resection and have a negative sentinel node biopsy, no further nodal evaluation is required (A). A 2005 systematic review lends support to this recommendation, with a pooled sensitivity of 97% with technectium and 95% with blue dye. In contrast, other tests for nodal evaluation (including imaging) had poorer sensitivities, ranging from 45% to less than 90%. If she had not undergone sentinel lymph node biopsy (SLNB), or if the technical capabilities to perform it were not available, the standard approach would be inguinofemoral lymphadenectomy. A repeat SLNB is never performed, and given her final pathologic findings, she does not require adjuvant treatment.

16. E

Patients with recurrent vulvar cancer should undergo full-body imaging to rule out distant metastases, which are present in up to 15% of these patients. Of the imaging modalities listed, the appropriate one is E. While the data regarding PET is limited in metastatic vulvar cancer, data in preoperative staging and radiation therapy planning for women with vulvar cancer shows that it has a high specificity of 95% and is better at identifying extranodal disease rather than disease in lymph nodes.

17. E

All of the above (E). Only 644 cases of vulvar melanoma were identified within the Surveillance Epidemiology and End Results (SEER) database between 1973 and 2003, which is a testament to the rarity of these diseases. The average age of diagnosis is 60 years, with median between 54 and 68. However, there are case reports of vulvar melanoma being diagnosed in girls as young as 10. AJCC staging for dermal melanomas is utilized for mucosal melanomas and others occurring at unusual sites, including the vulva. Vulvar melanomas have a very low rate of mutations in BRAF and neuroblastoma RAS viral oncogene homolog (NRAS) compared with dermal melanomas, though c-KIT aberrations appear to be more common, with a reported incidence of up to 40% and 6%, respectively.

18. B

This patient meets criteria for intermediate-risk endometrial cancer. One classification comes from the Gynecologic Oncology Group (GOG) and based on age and any of three pathologic factors: deep myometrial invasion, grade 2 or 3 histology, or the evidence for lymphovascular space invasion (LVSI). Intermediate risk is characterized by the presence of any one factor in women 70 years and older; two risk factors in a woman 50–69 years; and all three factors in women 18–49 years. Patients with an intermediate-risk endometrial cancer should proceed with vaginal brachytherapy (B). RT is associated with a reduction in the risk of local recurrence compared with surveillance alone (HR 0.42, 95% CI 0.21–0.83) though there is no associated improvement in overall survival. The seminal Post-Operative Radiation Therapy in Endometrial Cancer (PORTEC-2) trial provides justification for the use of vaginal brachytherapy rather than whole pelvic RT. In this trial, there were no differences in recurrence-free survival, rate of distant metastases, or 5-year survival outcomes. However, vaginal brachytherapy resulted in lower rates of treatment-related toxicity, including diarrhea.

19. E

All these options represent reasonable options for this patient. Eribulin was evaluated in a phase III trial against dacarbazine for patients with soft tissue leiomyosarcoma or adipocytic sarcoma. All patients had received at least two prior lines of therapy. Compared with dacarbazine, eribulin resulted in a statistically significant improvement in overall survival (OS, 13.5 vs. 11.5 months, respectively; $P = .0169$), although there was no statistically significant difference in progression-free survival (PFS, 5 vs. 2 months). Demetri et al. reported the phase III results comparing trabectidin to dacarbazine in patients with previously treated liposarcoma or leiomyosarcoma. Compared with dacarbazine, trabectidin resulted in a significant improvement in PFS (4.2 vs. 1.5 months, $P < .001$) though no benefit was reported in OS (median 12.4 vs. 12.9 months, $P = .37$). Finally, pazopanib was compared to placebo in a phase III trial for patients with non-adipocytic soft tissue sarcoma. Compared with placebo, there was a statistically significant benefit associated with pazopanib in terms of PFS (4.6 vs. 1.6 months, $P < 0.0001$) but not in OS (12.5 vs. 10.7

months, $P = 0.25$). Hence, the lack of an overall survival advantage with any of these therapies makes the option for supportive care an option. In addition, it is entirely reasonable to offer palliative care even if she opts to proceed with third-line therapy.

20. A

This patient has gestational trophoblastic neoplasia (GTN), which is diagnosed by her history of mole and re-elevation of her hCG level. GTN is staged using the International Federation of Gynecology and Obstetrics (FIGO) staging system:

- Stage I—Persistently elevated human chorionic gonadotropin (hCG) levels; tumor confined to the uterine corpus
- Stage II—Tumor outside of the uterus, but is not beyond the pelvis and/or vagina
- Stage III—Pulmonary metastases with or without uterine, pelvic, or vaginal involvement. Note: Detection of pulmonary metastases is determined by chest x-ray, not chest CT scan
- Stage IV—Metastatic disease beyond the lungs and pelvis and/or vagina

In addition to FIGO staging, a risk score is assigned using the World Health Organization (WHO) Prognostic Scoring System (Table 27.2), which considers eight factors: age, antecedent pregnancy, interval from last pregnancy, pretreatment serum hCG level (taken from the most recent rise), site of metastases, number of metastases, and prior systemic therapy administered.

Imaging of GTN requires a pelvic ultrasound and a chest x-ray (A). Other imaging is indicated based on the results of these two studies. If the chest x-ray is negative, she will not require additional imaging, especially since her pelvic exam was negative for vaginal extension of disease. Importantly, lesions suspected of being GTN should not be biopsied as this carries high risk of hemorrhage.

21. D

The presentation, relatively low hCG level (in consideration of the diffuse disease) and immunohistochemical stains (particularly for hPL), is consistent with a diagnosis of placental site trophoblastic tumor (PSTT). These tumors are more chemoresistant than other forms of gestational trophoblastic neoplasia (GTN); hence, both surgery and chemotherapy are the mainstays of treatment. Complete moles are typically hydropic diffusely and surrounded by hyperplastic trophoblasts. These tumors carry two sets of parental chromosomes (46XX or 46XY) and do not contain scalloping chorionic villi. In contrast, partial moles have scalloped chorionic villi and have an extra set of chromosomes attached (69XXY or 69XXX). Choriocarcinoma is made of sheets of anaplastic cytotrophoblasts and syncitiotrophoblasts and is absent of chorionic villi. The absence of smooth muscle markers essentially rules out uterine sarcoma.

22. E

There are no features on imaging that reliably distinguish a leiomyoma from a uterine sarcoma. Features suggestive of sarcoma on ultrasound, such as mixed echogenicity, central necrosis, and irregular vessel distribution, may also be found in leiomyomas.[18] In addition, the size of the mass does not reliably predict a uterine sarcoma. Finally, CT scan does not reliably differentiate a sarcoma from a leiomyoma. While the mean age at diagnosis of a uterine sarcoma is 60, these tumors can arise in women as young as 20 years. Hence, age should not be used to predict the presence of sarcomas of the uterus.

TABLE 27.2 The Modified World Health Organization Prognostic Scoring System for gestational trophoblastic neoplasms, human chorionic gonadotropin, human chorionic gonadotropin

Scores	0	1	2	4
Age	<40 years	>40 years	–	–
Antecedent pregnancy	Mole	Abortion	Term	–
Interval months from index pregnancy	<4	4–7	7–13	>13
Pretreatment serum	<1000 hCG (mIU/mL)	<10,000 hCG (mIU/mL)	<100,000 hCG (mIU/mL)	>100,000 hCG (mIU/mL)
Largest tumor size	–	3–5 cm	>5 cm	–
Site of metastases	Lung	Spleen/kidney	GI	Liver/brain
Number of metastases	–	1–4	5–8	>8
Previous failed chemotherapy	–	–	Single drug	Combination

hCG, Human chorionic gonadotropin; *GI*, gastrointestinal. From Abeloff Clinical Oncology, 5th edition.

23. D

This patient is at high risk for the development of gestational trophoblastic neoplasia (GTN) on the basis of older age, large uterine size, and the presence of large ovarian theca-lutein cysts. As a result, she should proceed with chemotherapy, and of the agents listed, the most appropriate treatment is for methotrexate. EMA-CO is indicated for the treatment of established high-risk GTN based on the World Health Organization criteria (score >7), not as prophylactic treatment after D&C. While a hysterectomy is reasonable if she is done with child-bearing, it is not required, especially given the sensitivity of GTN to chemotherapy.

REFERENCES

Question 1

1. Tewari KS, Sill MW, Long HJ, et al. Improved survival with bevacizumab in advanced cervical cancer. *N Engl J Med*. 2014;370:734–743.
2. Saito I, Kitagawa R, Fukuda H, et al. A phase III trial of paclitaxel plus carboplatin versus paclitaxel plus cisplatin in stage IVB, persistent or recurrent cervical cancer: Gynecologic Cancer Study Group/Japan Clinical Oncology Group Study (JCOG0505). *Jpn J Clin Oncol*. 2010;40:90–93.

Question 2

1. Mahner S, Jueckstock J, Hilpert F, et al. Adjuvant therapy in lymph node-positive vulvar cancer: the AGO-CaRE-1 study. *J Natl Cancer Inst*. 2015;107. http://dx.doi.org/10.1093/jnci/dju426.

Question 3

1. Miyamoto DT, Viswanathan AN. Concurrent chemoradiation for vaginal cancer. *PLoS One*. 2013;8:e65048.

Question 4

1. Sedlis A, Bundy BN, Rotman MZ, Lentz SS, Muderspach LI, Zaino RJ. A randomized trial of pelvic radiation therapy versus no further therapy in selected patients with stage IB carcinoma of the cervix after radical hysterectomy and pelvic lymphadenectomy: a Gynecologic Oncology Group Study. *Gynecol Oncol*. 1999;73:177–183.

Question 5

1. Peters 3rd WA, Liu PY, Barrett 2nd RJ, et al. Concurrent chemotherapy and pelvic radiation therapy compared with pelvic radiation therapy alone as adjuvant therapy after radical surgery in high-risk early-stage cancer of the cervix. *J Clin Oncol*. 2000;18:1606–1613.

Question 6

1. Höckel M, Dornhöfer N. Pelvic exenteration for gynaecological tumours: achievements and unanswered questions. *Lancet Oncol*. 2006;7:837–847.

Question 7

1. Alemany L, Saunier M, Tinoco L, et al. Large contribution of human papillomavirus in vaginal neoplastic lesions: a worldwide study in 597 samples. *Eur. J Cancer Oxf Engl*. 2014;50:2846–2854.

Question 9

1. Miller D. Randomized phase III noninferiority trial of first-line chemotherapy for metastatic or recurrent endometrial carcinoma: a Gynecologic Oncology Group study. In: *Society of Gynecologic Oncologists Annual Meeting*. LBA1; 2012.

Question 13

1. Rustin GJ, Newlands ES, Begent RH, Dent J, Bagshawe KD. Weekly alternating etoposide, methotrexate, and actinomycin/vincristine and cyclophosphamide chemotherapy for the treatment of CNS metastases of choriocarcinoma. *J Clin Oncol*. 1989;7:900–903.

Question 14

1. Omura GA, Blessing JA, Major F, et al. A randomized clinical trial of adjuvant adriamycin in uterine sarcomas: a Gynecologic Oncology Group Study. *J Clin Oncol*. 1985;3:1240–1245.
2. Hensley ML, Wathen JK, Maki RG, et al. Adjuvant therapy for high-grade, uterus-limited leiomyosarcoma: results of a phase 2 trial (SARC 005). *Cancer*. 2013;119:1555–1561.
3. Reed NS, Mangioni C, Malmström H, et al. Phase III randomised study to evaluate the role of adjuvant pelvic radiotherapy in the treatment of uterine sarcomas stages I and II: an European Organisation for Research and Treatment of Cancer Gynaecological Cancer Group Study (protocol 55874). *Eur J Cancer Oxf Engl*. 2008;44:808–818.

Question 15

1. Hensley ML, Maki R, Venkatraman E, et al. Gemcitabine and docetaxel in patients with unresectable leiomyosarcoma: results of a phase II trial. *J Clin Oncol*. 2002;20:2824–2831.

Question 16

1. Chemoradiotherapy for Cervical Cancer Meta-analysis Collaboration (CCCMAC). Reducing uncertainties about the effects of chemoradiotherapy for cervical cancer: individual patient data meta-analysis. *Cochrane Database Syst Rev*. 2010. http://dx.doi.org/10.1002/14651858.CD008285. Online CD008285.

Question 17

1. Selman TJ, Mann C, Zamora J, Appleyard TL, Khan K. Diagnostic accuracy of tests for lymph node status in primary cervical cancer: a systematic review and meta-analysis. *CMAJ*. 2008;178:855–862.

Question 18

1. Cohn DE, Dehdashti F, Gibb RK, et al. Prospective evaluation of positron emission tomography for the detection of groin node metastases from vulvar cancer. *Gynecol Oncol*. 2002;85:179–184.

Question 19

1. Leitao MM. Management of vulvar and vaginal melanomas: current and future strategies. Am Soc Clin Oncol Educ Book. 2014;e277–e281. doi:10.14694/EdBook_AM.2014.34.e277.

Question 20

1. Keys HM, Roberts JA, Brunetto VL, et al. A phase III trial of surgery with or without adjunctive external pelvic radiation therapy in intermediate risk endometrial adenocarcinoma: a Gynecologic Oncology Group study. *Gynecol Oncol*. 2004;92:744–751.

2. Nout RA, Smit VT, Putter H, et al. Vaginal brachytherapy versus pelvic external beam radiotherapy for patients with endometrial cancer of high-intermediate risk (PORTEC-2): an open-label, non-inferiority, randomised trial. *Lancet Lond Engl*. 2010;375:816–823.

Question 21

1. Schöffski P, Chawla S, Maki RG, et al. Eribulin versus dacarbazine in previously treated patients with advanced liposarcoma or leiomyosarcoma: a randomised, open-label, multicentre, phase 3 trial. *Lancet Lond Engl*. 2016;387:1629–1637.

2. Demetri GD, von Mehren M, Jones RL, et al. Efficacy and safety of trabectedin or dacarbazine for metastatic liposarcoma or leiomyosarcoma after failure of conventional chemotherapy: results of a phase III randomized multicenter clinical trial. *J Clin Oncol*. 2016;34:786–793.

Melanoma and Other Skin Cancers

Nikhil I. Khushalani and Sanjiv S. Agarwala

QUESTIONS

1. The most common molecular alteration seen in cutaneous melanoma involves which of the following genes?
   A. CDNK2A
   B. PI3K
   C. KIT
   D. BRAF
   E. NRAS

2. Which of the following is true regarding the cyclin-dependent kinase inhibitor 2A (*CDNK2A*) gene in melanoma?
   A. A mutation in *CDNK2A* is present in up to 40% of families with three or more cases of melanoma.
   B. The risk of developing melanoma in a *CDNK2A* mutation carrier is 30% by age 5 years.
   C. A mutation in *CDNK2A* is identified in up to 10% of patients with multiple primary melanomas.
   D. Families with germline mutations in *CDNK2A* have a higher incidence of developing pancreatic cancer.
   E. All of the above are true.

3. A 42-year-old Caucasian male presents with a mole on his abdomen that has now changed color and is intermittently bleeding over the past 4 weeks. Physical examination does not reveal any significant abnormality apart from this mole on the left midabdomen along the midclavicular line. It is 4 mm in diameter and has irregular borders. A punch biopsy reveals this to be malignant melanoma, 2.3 mm Breslow depth, ulcerated, and with brisk tumor infiltrating lymphocytes. What is the appropriate next step in management?
   A. Wide excision of the lesion with 2 cm margins and sentinel lymph node mapping
   B. Checking BRAF status on the tumor; if positive for BRAF V600E mutation, initiating therapy with vemurafenib and cobimetinib as neoadjuvant therapy
   C. Wide excision of the lesion with 2 cm margins and concurrent left superficial inguinal lymph node dissection
   D. Wide excision of the lesion with 4 cm margins plus sentinel lymph node mapping
   E. Concurrent left axillary and left superficial inguinal lymph node dissection as the location of this tumor may result in nodal spread to either of these anatomic basins

4. A 55-year-old male is referred to you after undergoing wide excision for a 1.2 mm Breslow depth melanoma from his right forearm. The tumor was not ulcerated, had a mitotic rate of less than 1 mitosis/mm², and there was no evidence of lymphovascular invasion. Lymphoscintigraphy mapped to the ipsilateral axillary nodal basin, and all three nodes retrieved were negative for metastatic spread

by routine histological and immunohistochemical staining. His physical examination reveals scars from his surgery and no evidence of lymphadenopathy. What would you now recommend for further staging of his tumor?
   A. Chest radiograph only
   B. Contrast-enhanced computed tomography (CT) imaging of the chest, abdomen, and pelvis plus contrast-enhanced magnetic resonance imaging (MRI) of the brain
   C. Whole body fluorodeoxyglucose (FDG) positron emission tomography (PET-CT) scan
   D. No radiographic staging is recommended
   E. Complete blood count, metabolic profile including liver function tests and lactate dehydrogenase (LDH) in addition to (B) above

5. Which of the following statements accurately summarizes the results of the Multicenter Selective Lymphadenectomy Trial (MSLT-1) as they relate to the primary study group (1.2–3.5 mm depth; intermediate thickness tumors)?
   A. The overall survival (OS) of the sentinel lymph node biopsy group was superior to the observation group.
   B. The 5-year disease-free survival (DFS) was similar between the biopsy group and the observation group.
   C. The most important prognostic indicator was the presence of melanoma metastases in the sentinel node.
   D. The 5-year DFS was superior in the observation group compared with the biopsy group.
   E. For patients with nodal metastases, there was no difference in 5-year survival between immediate versus delayed lymphadenectomy.

6. A 36-year-old female underwent wide excision plus sentinel lymph node mapping for melanoma on her right deltoid region after an initial biopsy revealed an ulcerated, 3.4 mm Breslow depth primary tumor, with involvement of the deep margin. There was no residual melanoma identified in the resection specimen. One of three sentinel nodes identified in the right axilla demonstrated metastatic subcapsular involvement, 1.3 mm in diameter, and without extracapsular extension (ECE). Follow-up completion lymph node dissection did not reveal any additional positive nodes among 14 retrieved in the surgical specimen. Staging CT imaging of the torso and MRI brain were negative. Hematological and biochemical parameters including serum LDH were normal. Which of the following are appropriate considerations for adjuvant therapy for this stage IIIb melanoma (T3bN1aM0)?
   A. Ipilimumab at 10 mg/kg
   B. Ipilimumab at 3 mg/kg
   C. Pembrolizumab
   D. Interferon (standard high-dose interferon alfa-2b, or pegylated interferon)
   E. A and D

7. A 45-year-old male presents to the office at the start of his third week of adjuvant intravenous induction interferon alfa-2b (20 million international units/m^2) for stage IIIc melanoma of the scalp. He complains of progressive fatigue, low-grade fever and chills that responds well to acetaminophen, anorexia, and has lost approximately 5% of his baseline weight. His absolute neutrophil count is 900/mm^3, and his platelet count is normal. His serum alanine aminotransferase (ALT) and aspartate aminotransferase (AST) are 5.4 and 7 times the upper limit of institutional normal, respectively. Serum bilirubin is normal. What would you recommend at this time?
   A. Continue with ongoing treatment as his bilirubin is normal and transaminitis is expected with this agent
   B. Discontinue intravenous interferon and immediately start him on maintenance subcutaneous interferon at 10 million international units/m^2 3 times weekly
   C. Discontinue intravenous interferon permanently due to severity of hepatic toxicity
   D. Hold interferon, repeat laboratory parameters at least weekly or more often, and restart interferon at 20% dose reduction after hepatic enzymes normalize
   E. Hold interferon, repeat laboratory parameters at least weekly or more often, and restart interferon at 50% dose reduction after hepatic enzymes normalize

8. A 67-year-old male is receiving adjuvant high-dose ipilimumab (10 mg/kg) for stage IIIb (T4aN1bM0) melanoma of the back. After his first and second doses he developed a grade 1 localized maculopapular rash over his forearms that resolved with topical steroid therapy prior to the subsequent cycle. After his third dose he noted progressive fatigue with a mild headache, but no visual disturbances or neurological symptoms or signs. On examination, he is alert and oriented, afebrile, heart rate 92 beats/min and regular, blood pressure 116/64 mm Hg, and is not orthostatic. Contrast-enhanced brain MRI is performed and shown below (Fig. 28.1). What is the most likely diagnosis?

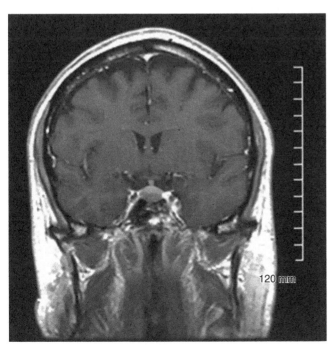

FIG. 28.1 Contrast-enhanced brain MRI. Image courtesy: Nikhil I. Khushalani, MD [Moffitt Cancer Center].

A. Brain metastases
B. Dehydration
C. Hypophysitis
D. Encephalomalacia
E. Meningitis

9. Which of the following statements regarding adjuvant ipilimumab (10 mg/kg) in stage III melanoma is correct?
   A. Ipilimumab prolongs recurrence-free survival (RFS) but not OS.
   B. Ipilimumab prolongs OS but has no impact on RFS.
   C. Ipilimumab improves RFS and OS.
   D. Ipilimumab is associated with an inferior survival compared with interferon alfa-2b.
   E. Ipilimumab is well tolerated, and 85% of patients could complete all planned therapy in the pivotal phase III trial (EORTC 18071).

10. A 51-year-old female is referred to you after undergoing right inguinal lymph node dissection for macroscopic relapse of melanoma approximately 18 months after a negative sentinel lymph node biopsy performed for a nonulcerated, 2.2 mm depth melanoma of the right anterior thigh. The dissection revealed metastatic involvement of 4 nodes out of 14 retrieved with the largest measuring 3 cm and with evidence of extracapsular extension. She wishes to understand the role of adjuvant radiotherapy in this situation. Which of the following is correct?
    A. Adjuvant radiotherapy to the nodal basin is indicated for all node-positive melanoma after completion lymph node dissection.
    B. Adjuvant radiotherapy for palpable lymph node relapse can decrease the risk of local recurrence, but has no effect on OS.
    C. Adjuvant radiotherapy improves regional control and OS after lymph node dissection for macroscopic nodal disease.
    D. Adjuvant radiotherapy does not increase the risk of lower extremity lymphedema.
    E. Both C and D.

11. A 72-year-old Asian male had undergone resection of T1b-N1a melanoma of the left ring finger 2 years ago followed by 1 year of adjuvant high-dose interferon. On a preoperative chest radiograph performed for elective right knee replacement surgery, three pulmonary nodules were identified. Whole body FDG-PET imaging confirmed the presence of four FDG-avid lung nodules, the largest in the left lower lobe measuring 2 cm. In addition, hypermetabolic left supraclavicular adenopathy was also identified. Ultrasound guided biopsy of the noted adenopathy confirmed metastatic melanoma. What is the next appropriate step in management?
    A. Send metastatic tumor tissue for molecular analysis to include at least BRAF and KIT mutational analysis
    B. Contrast imaging of the brain (MRI or CT)
    C. Complete blood count, comprehensive metabolic panel, and LDH level assessment
    D. A and C
    E. All of the above

12. A 36-year-old man has been referred for newly diagnosed stage IV melanoma from an unknown primary with metastatic involvement of the lung and liver (three focal lesions; largest 1.5 cm). He is asymptomatic. Brain imaging does not reveal metastatic disease. Molecular analysis reveals a BRAF V600K mutation. All of the following are appropriate options for first-line therapy except:
    A. Ipilimumab
    B. Pembrolizumab
    C. Ipilimumab plus nivolumab
    D. Dabrafenib plus trametinib
    E. Nivolumab

13. The above patient insists on receiving aggressive therapy no matter what the toxicity. You elect to give him combination ipilimumab (3 mg/kg) plus nivolumab (1 mg/kg) every 3 weeks. After his second dose, he calls with a 2-day history of diarrhea—seven to eight loose bowel movements per day, with associated abdominal cramping. On examination, his oral mucosa is dry. His vital signs are stable, and his abdominal examination is remarkable only for hyperactive bowel sounds. There is no tenderness or rebound. What is the appropriate next step in management?
    A. Reassure him that this is quite normal and this should settle down in a few days
    B. Give him ciprofloxacin plus metronidazole for presumed diverticulitis
    C. Start loperamide along with a BRAT diet
    D. Hospital admission for intravenous high-dose steroids
    E. Start subcutaneous octreotide 3 times per day to manage the diarrhea

14. Which of the following are common toxicities associated with the administration of high-dose interleukin-2 (IL-2)?
    A. Hypotension
    B. Tachycardia
    C. Elevated serum creatinine
    D. Peripheral edema and weight gain
    E. All of the above

15. Which of the following is true regarding the use of combination ipilimumab and nivolumab in advanced melanoma?
    A. Tumor PD-L1 status must be ascertained prior to therapy with ipilimumab plus nivolumab.
    B. Randomized trials have shown improved progression-free survival (PFS) and OS with the combination compared with ipilimumab.
    C. This combination improves PFS, but not OS compared with ipilimumab.
    D. This combination improved PFS and OS compared with nivolumab.
    E. None of the above statements are true.

16. Which of the following mutations are common in primary uveal melanoma?
    A. GNAQ and GNA11
    B. BRAF
    C. KIT
    D. NRAS
    E. PI3K

17. A 58-year-old female with melanoma of the right calf and metastatic adenopathy in the pelvic and retroperitoneal nodes was treated with nivolumab for 7 months before developing clear evidence of disease progression in the nodal basins plus new metastatic disease in the lungs. She is in good health otherwise. Next-generation sequencing of her tumor does not reveal any mutations. What would you consider for second-line therapy?
    A. Ipilimumab
    B. Dacarbazine
    C. Combination ipilimumab plus nivolumab
    D. Vemurafenib plus cobimetinib
    E. Trametinib alone

18. A 36-year-old man presents with rapidly progressive adenopathy in the right neck and supraclavicular basin over the past 6 weeks. A core needle biopsy reveals malignant melanoma. Physical examination reveals palpable adenopathy in levels 3, 4, and 5 in the right neck, the largest node measuring 3.5 cm. Staging studies demonstrate extensive pulmonary and hepatic metastatic disease in additional to the clinically obvious nodal disease. In retrospect, he notes mild dyspnea on moderate exertion over the same time frame. He has a history of melanoma resected from his upper back (right scapular area) 8 years ago but is unable to recall details of the pathology except that it was an early stage cancer. However, he notes that a lymph node sampling was not performed at that time. Laboratory data reveal grade 1 elevations in serum ALT and AST levels and an elevated serum LDH level (3.4 times upper limit of normal). Brain MRI is normal. Molecular analysis confirms the presence of BRAF V600E mutation. What would you recommend as first-line therapy for this patient?
    A. Vemurafenib
    B. Ipilimumab plus vemurafenib
    C. Cobimetinib
    D. Vemurafenib plus cobimetinib
    E. Vemurafenib plus cobimetinib plus atezolizumab

19. Which of the following signaling pathways is important in the development of sporadic and hereditary cases of basal cell carcinoma (BCC)?
    A. Epidermal growth factor receptor
    B. Mitogen-activated protein kinase (MAP kinase)
    C. Hedgehog (Hh)
    D. Vascular endothelial growth factor
    E. Mammalian target of rapamycin

20. Which of the following are phenotypic manifestations of Gorlin syndrome (nevoid basal cell carcinoma syndrome)?
    A. Odontogenic cysts
    B. Early development of multiple BCCs
    C. Palmar and plantar pits
    D. Medulloblastoma
    E. All of the above

21. A 69-year-old male with chronic sun damaged skin presented with a 9-month history of progressively enlarging ulcerative mass in the right preauricular area. On examination, there is a 7-cm ulcerated cutaneous lesion extending from the right ear to the malar area with destruction of the right tragus and exposure of the external auditory canal. Some areas of the tumor bleed easily. There is no evidence of intraoral or ocular involvement. A photomicrograph of an office biopsy performed is shown in Fig. 28.2. Your pathologist informs you that this is nodular and infiltrative BCC. Contrast CT imaging of the maxilla-facial, neck, and thoracic regions outline the locally advanced anatomy of this mass, but without any bony involvement or pulmonary metastatic disease. Multidisciplinary discussion deems this mass to be unresectable at this time. Which of

the following systemic options would you consider for this patient as first-line treatment?

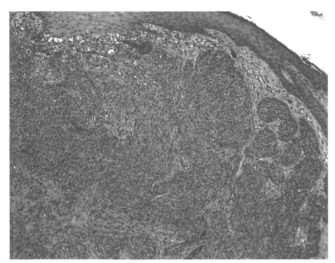

FIG. 28.2 A photomicrograph of an office biopsy performed. Image courtesy: Jane Messina, MD [Moffitt Cancer Center].

A. Vismodegib
B. Pembrolizumab
C. Cetuximab
D. Bevacizumab
E. Ipilimumab

22. All of the following increase the risk of development of cutaneous squamous cell carcinoma (SCC) except:
A. Ultraviolet light exposure
B. Chronic immunosuppression
C. PUVA (psoralen + ultraviolet A)

D. Thermal injury
E. Phenytoin

23. A 65-year-old male presents with a new violaceous nodule on the anterior aspect of the right midhigh. He thought this was a "bug-bite." Examination shows this lesion to be 1.5 cm in diameter, slightly raised, nontender, and without bleeding. There is no palpable adenopathy in the groin. Biopsy reveals uniform appearing tumor cells with hyperchromatic nuclei and minimal amounts of cytoplasm. There is no lymphovascular invasion, and the depth is 3 mm. Immunohistochemical stains demonstrate the tumor cells to be positive for cytokeratin 20 with perinuclear dot-like accentuation. What is the most likely histological diagnosis?
A. SCC
B. BCC
C. Merkel cell carcinoma (MCC)
D. Desmoplastic melanoma
E. Sebaceous gland carcinoma

24. The patient in Question 23 undergoes wide excision of the primary tumor on the thigh along with sentinel lymph node mapping and sampling. One of three lymph nodes in the right superficial inguinal basin is positive for micrometastatic disease. Staging contrast-enhanced CT imaging of the torso is negative for metastatic spread. Complete blood count and comprehensive metabolic panel, including serum LDH, are normal. What would you recommend as the next step in his management?
A. Observation
B. Intralesional injection of talimogene laherparepvec (TVEC)
C. Pembrolizumab
D. Radiotherapy to the primary site and regional nodal basin
E. Concurrent chemoradiotherapy (CRT) with cisplatin and etoposide

ANSWERS

1. D
Somatic mutations are the most common molecular alteration in cutaneous melanoma, with the majority being V600E located in exon 15. The single amino acid substitution of valine by glutamic acid in this mutation results in constitutional activation of the MAP kinase pathway causing cell growth, proliferation, and survival. Lesser common variants at BRAF V600 have also been identified. Mutations in NRAS occur in about 22% of cutaneous melanoma, while KIT mutations are seen more commonly in acral-lentiginous and mucosal melanomas.

2. E
All of the listed statements are correct. The *CDNK2A* gene is located on chromosome 9p21 and encodes for two tumor suppressor proteins, p16 and p14. It is a highly penetrant predisposition gene, and the risk for developing melanoma in a mutation carrier is as high as 67% by age 80 years.

3. A
The appropriate next step in management of an intermediate thickness melanoma without clinical evidence of nodal metastatic disease is wide excision with adequate margins plus sentinel lymph node mapping and biopsy.

Prospective surgical trials in melanoma have shown that 2 cm margins are adequate for tumors with Breslow thickness greater than 2 mm without any difference in local recurrence or OS when compared with surgery with wider margins than 2 cm. Only one study from the UK has demonstrated improvement in melanoma-specific survival but not in OS for surgical margin resection of 3 cm compared with 1 cm for tumors greater than 2 mm in depth. However, whether this is superior to a 2-cm margin is not known and thus has not been considered to be practice altering.

4. D
This is a low-risk melanoma (T2aN0 = stage Ib). The yield with cross-sectional imaging in low-risk melanoma is very low and insufficient to justify its routine use in the absence of specific symptoms or signs of concern. Imaging for staging is considered for high-risk stage II melanoma (thick tumors) or those with node involvement (stage III).

5. C
The MSLT-1 is a landmark trial that established the prognostic importance of the sentinel node in melanoma. In this trial of 1269 patients with an intermediate thickness primary tumor, the presence of melanoma metastases in

the sentinel node was associated with an inferior 5-year survival (72.3%) compared with those with a negative sentinel node where the 5-year survival was 90.2% (hazard ration for death 2.48; $P < .001$). The 5-year DFS was superior in the biopsy group compared with the observation group, but there was no difference in OS identified. In those patients with involved nodes, the 5-year survival for immediate lymphadenectomy was superior to the survival in those where lymphadenectomy was delayed. The performance of sentinel lymph node biopsy is now considered standard of care for melanomas that are thicker than 1 mm.

6. E

Interferon (high-dose and pegylated) and ipilimumab (10 mg/kg) are approved in the United States for the adjuvant treatment of stage III melanoma. High-dose interferon is also approved for melanomas thicker than 4 mm without nodal involvement. The other listed options are not approved at this time, although trials examining their efficacy in the adjuvant setting are ongoing or have completed accrual. Treatment must be individualized considering comorbidities, anticipated toxicity, and patient preference and motivation. Participation in a clinical trial of adjuvant therapy in melanoma is also very appropriate.

7. E

Toxicity is common with the use of adjuvant interferon in melanoma. Most commonly manifest as flu-like symptoms, fatigue, myelosuppression, elevated liver enzymes, thyroid dysfunction, and neuropsychiatric symptoms including depression. Approximately 50% of patients in the original Eastern Cooperative Oncology Group (ECOG) trials of adjuvant interferon required dose interruption or dose reduction. Liver toxicity is common and needs close vigilance during administration. For grade 3 elevation in transaminases (as in this case), treatment should be held until resolution with resumption at 50% dose attenuation per the approval labeling for this agent. An alternate approach based on the cumulative ECOG/Intergroup experience is 33% dose reduction upon resolution of toxicity. A second occurrence of a dose-limiting toxicity would warrant dose reduction by 66% compared with baseline, while a third occurrence would mandate discontinuation of interferon therapy.

8. C

The MRI demonstrates convex enlargement of the pituitary gland consistent with hypophysitis that is undoubtedly immune mediated from ipilimumab. Hypophysitis was seen in 16% patients treated with adjuvant ipilimumab in the EORTC 18071 trial that led to its regulatory approval. This was moderate to severe (grade 3–4) in 4.4%. This diagnosis can usually be confirmed by obtaining a hormonal panel to include thyroid profile, cortisol, ACTH, and testosterone levels for this patient.

9. C

In EORTC 18071, 951 patients with stage III melanoma (microscopic dimension of nodal involvement >1 mm) were randomized to receive adjuvant ipilimumab or placebo. Ipilimumab significantly prolonged both 5-year RFS (40.8% vs. 30.3%) and OS (65.4% vs. 54.4%) compared with placebo. It, however, has significant toxicity, and only 13.4% in the ipilimumab arm completed all planned therapy over 3 years. More than 50% of patients discontinued ipilimumab due to an adverse event, and

41.6% experienced grade 3 or 4 immune-related toxicity with this drug. While the trial comparing ipilimumab with interferon alfa-2b has been completed (ECOG 1609), results are currently pending.

10. B

The role of adjuvant radiotherapy in melanoma should be determined on an individual basis. In the phase III TROG 02.01 trial, 250 patients with palpable nodal disease (at presentation or at relapse; and without distant metastases) were randomized to receive adjuvant radiation or observation. There was significant improvement in local control with radiotherapy (adjusted hazard ratio 0.52, $P = .023$) but no difference in RFS or OS. This observation is also supported by retrospective data. There was significant increase in lower limb volumes with radiotherapy compared with placebo secondary to lymphedema ($P = .014$). In clinical practice, decisions for adjuvant nodal radiotherapy are made based on the location, number of nodes, size of involved nodes, and the presence of extracapsular extension.

11. E

After confirmation of the diagnosis of metastatic melanoma, it is important to assess the tissue for potentially actionable mutations such as *BRAF* and *KIT*. The latter is found more commonly in acral and mucosal melanomas (~20%) and may lend itself to intervention with *KIT* targeting agents such as imatinib. Brain imaging must be performed at baseline for newly diagnosed metastatic melanoma due to the high propensity of melanoma to spread to the central nervous system. Serum LDH is an important adverse prognostic marker and is incorporated into the staging of metastatic melanoma.

12. A

Ipilimumab was approved for therapy-naïve metastatic melanoma in 2011 as the first agent to improve survival in this setting. However, randomized trials conducted since then have rapidly established anti-PD1 based therapy as the standard first-line option, either singly (pembrolizumab or nivolumab) or in combination with ipilimumab (nivolumab plus ipilimumab) based on improvements in response rate, PFS, and/or OS. As this patient's tumor is BRAF V600K mutant, combination targeted therapy with BRAF and MEK inhibitors is also an appropriate first-line choice. Mutations in BRAF V600K are far less frequent than V600E but lend themselves to therapeutic inhibition by inhibitors of the MAP-kinase pathway. The approved combinations are dabrafenib plus trametinib or vemurafenib plus cobimetinib.

13. D

This patient likely has immune-mediated enterocolitis from his therapy. This is a common side effect of combination immunotherapy using these agents, and any grade diarrhea was reported in 44% of patients treated with this regimen in the phase III Checkmate 067 trial. The incidence of grade 3–4 diarrhea was 9.3%. The most appropriate step in the management of this patients' grade 3 diarrhea is prompt institution of high-dose steroids (equivalent of prednisone 1–2 mg/kg per day) along with appropriate supportive care including fluid resuscitation, bowel rest (in select cases), and excluding an infectious etiology such as clostridium difficile colitis (where clinical suspicion exists). For cases nonresponsive to steroids, other immunosuppressants such as infliximab should be given (provided there is no evidence of gastrointestinal perforation).

14. E

High-dose IL-2 causes a capillary leak syndrome that contributes to many of its toxic effects. Common adverse events include fever, chills, nausea, emesis, tachycardia, hypotension, oliguria, elevated creatinine, hyperbilirubinemia, peripheral edema, cardiac arrhythmias, and pulmonary congestion. High-dose IL-2 requires appropriate cardiopulmonary screening for eligibility and has the potential to induce durable responses in a small percentage of patients (less than 10%).

15. C

The combination of ipilimumab plus nivolumab was first approved in 2015 for unresectable or metastatic melanoma that did not harbor a BRAF V600 mutation. This indication was expanded in 2016 to advanced melanoma regardless of the BRAF status of the tumor. In Checkmate 067, the combination improved the response rate and PFS compared with ipilimumab. However, an effect on OS has yet to be reported from this phase III study. In a previous randomized phase II trial comparing the combination with ipilimumab, the OS at 2 years with the former was numerically higher than with ipilimumab alone (63.8% vs. 53.6%), but this difference did not reach statistical significance. More than half the patients on the ipilimumab arm received subsequent anti-PD1 therapy upon progression in this trial. Responses to checkpoint inhibitors have been seen in melanoma tumors with and without PD-L1 expression by immunohistochemistry. Hence, the use of this test to ascertain eligibility for combination anti-CTLA4 and anti-PD1 blockade in melanoma is not recommended.

16. A

Mutations in *GNAQ* and *GNA11* occur in approximately 83% of uveal melanomas. This results in activation of the MAP-kinase pathway. Other listed mutations are distinctly uncommon in uveal melanoma. The BRCA1-associated protein 1 (*BAP1*) is another common mutation reported in uveal melanoma and is associated with high risk of metastases.

17. A

Options for patients with BRAF-wild-type metastatic melanoma progressing on anti-PD1 therapy are limited. In the absence of a mutation in BRAF V600, vemurafenib, cobimetinib, or trametinib would not be indicated. Ipilimumab as a single agent is the most appropriate choice in this case. In a randomized phase II trial of planned sequencing of nivolumab for 12 weeks followed by ipilimumab for 12 weeks or the reverse sequence (both followed by maintenance nivolumab), the response rate and OS was higher in the former schedule. Prospective data on combination ipilimumab with an anti-PD1 agent after progression on single agent anti-PD1 therapy are lacking at this time.

18. D

This is a young patient with symptomatic metastatic melanoma and an elevated LDH, which is a poor prognostic marker. Of the listed options, combined inhibition of the MAP-kinase pathway with vemurafenib plus cobimetinib is the appropriate choice as first-line therapy. Combination BRAF and MEK inhibition has a higher response rate compared with single agent BRAF inhibitor therapy, and improves PFS and OS. In the phase III co-BRIM trial, the median PFS for combination vemurafenib plus cobimetinib was 12.3 months compared with 7.2 months with vemurafenib plus placebo (hazard ratio 0.58; $P < .001$). Similarly, median OS was also improved from 17.4 months to 22.3 months with the combination (HR 0.70; $P = .005$). Similar results have been reported for combination dabrafenib plus trametinib versus dabrafenib alone. This reinforces that a BRAF inhibitor should no longer be used as a single agent in metastatic melanoma unless there a contraindication exists for combination BRAF and MEK inhibitor therapy. Responses to the combination are often rapid leading to symptomatic improvement. While the combination of vemurafenib plus cobimetinib plus atezolizumab has demonstrated excellent preliminary efficacy in a phase 1b trial in advanced melanoma, its use remains investigational at this time and cannot be recommended outside of a clinical trial. A phase III trial of this triplet combination compared with vemurafenib plus cobimetinib has been initiated. The combination of ipilimumab and vemurafenib was shown to have a high rate of hepatotoxicity and should not be used.

19. C

Activation of the Hh signaling pathway is important for the development of BCC. Mutations in the tumor suppressor Patched (*PTCH1*) gene on chromosome 9 or activating mutations in Smoothened homolog (SMO) result in constitutive activation of this pathway, which can be inhibited by inhibitors of SMO. Vismodegib and sonidegib are examples of SMO inhibitors in clinical use for advanced BCC.

20. E

Gorlin syndrome is an autosomal dominant disorder due to germline mutations in the Patched (*PTCH1*) gene. All of the listed answers are a part of this syndrome. Early development of multiple BCCs by age 20 is a major manifestation. Patients with this condition are prone to develop medulloblastomas at an early age along with other tumors including cardiac and ovarian fibromas, fibrosarcoma, and meningioma. Odontogenic cysts (often of the mandible) and other skeletal defects (e.g., bifid ribs) are also part of this phenotypic spectrum. The Patched (*PTCH1*) gene is a tumor suppressor gene and is located on chromosome 9q22–q31.

21. A

Identification of the critical role of the Hedgehog signaling pathway in the genesis of BCC has permitted the development of targeted inhibitors of Smoothened homolog (SMO), with resultant inhibition of the Hh pathway. There are two approved oral agents for locally advanced or metastatic BCC—vismodegib and sonidegib. In an open label international trial, the response rate in BCC to vismodegib was 66.7% for locally advanced disease and 37.9% for metastatic BCC. Complete responses were observed in approximately half of the locally advanced cases. Common side effects associated with vismodegib include muscle spasms, dysgeusia, anorexia, fatigue, and alopecia. Trials of immune checkpoint inhibitors in nonmelanoma cutaneous cancers are ongoing. Cetuximab targets the epidermal growth factor receptor and has activity in cutaneous SCC. Bevacizumab is an inhibitor of VEGF and has no role in the management of advanced BCC outside of a clinical trial.

22. E

The incidence of cutaneous SCC correlates with chronic and cumulative sunlight exposure. It is the second most common skin cancer in the United States after BCC. Other risk factors include fair skin, red hair, albinism, immunodeficiency,

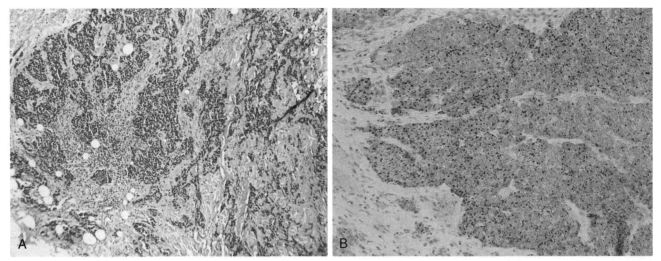

FIG. 28.3 (A) Hematoxylin-eosin stain of tumor (×10). (B) CK 20 immunostain of tumor (×10). Image courtesy: Jane Messina, MD [Moffitt Cancer Center].

chronic immunosuppression (e.g., transplant recipients), thermal injury, chronic wound (Marjolin ulcer), chemical exposure, and phototherapy with PUVA. There is no defined association between the use of phenytoin and cutaneous SCC.

23. C

This is a typical clinical and histological appearance for MCC. This most closely resembles a high-grade neuroendocrine carcinoma of the skin with small, round, basophilic cells, often with frequent mitotic figures. The perinuclear dot-like pattern for CK 20 staining is typical for MCC and seen in 80%–90% of these tumors (Fig. 28.3). These tumors are often dermal-based with involvement of the subcutaneous tissue. They have a high propensity for regional nodal and disseminated metastases.

24. D

This patient has stage IIIa (T1N1aM0) MCC of the extremity based on the size of the primary tumor and microscopic involvement of the sentinel node. These tumors are highly radiosensitive, and the use of adjuvant radiotherapy can decrease the risk of locoregional relapse. A retrospective analysis of MCC in the SEER database demonstrated improved OS with postoperative radiation compared with patients who did not receive adjuvant radiotherapy. Hence this modality is commonly considered as part of the multimodal management of localized MCC. The role of adjuvant chemotherapy is not well defined in the setting of micrometastatic nodal disease. Recent anti-PD1 or anti-PDL1 therapy with pembrolizumab or avelumab has shown promising results in advanced MCC. Regulatory approval is anticipated in this setting. However, its use in the adjuvant arena is still investigational. TVEC is oncolytic virotherapy that is approved for local treatment of unresectable cutaneous, subcutaneous, or nodal lesions in patients with melanoma recurrent after initial surgery.

Bone and Soft Tissue Sarcoma

Dennis Priebat

QUESTIONS

1. Several sarcomas are associated with specific chromosomal translocations. Which translocation is matched with the correct sarcoma?
   A. Ewing sarcoma-$t(9;22)$
   B. Myxoid/round liposarcoma-$t(12;16)$
   C. Alveolar rhabdomyosarcoma-$t(x;18)$
   D. Synovial sarcoma-$t(2;13)$
   E. Dermatofibrosarcoma protuberans-$t(11;22)$

2. Which of the following are characteristics of radiation-induced sarcomas?
   A. They respond well to imatinib.
   B. They usually have an excellent prognosis.
   C. They occur within 5 years of previous radiation.
   D. They are associated with an increased risk of glioma, breast carcinoma, and adrenocortical cancer.
   E. Osteogenic sarcoma, malignant fibrous histiocytoma of bone, and angiosarcoma are common.

3. An 18-year-old male presents to his local emergency room following a contact injury in his athletics class. Because the patient is non-weight bearing, additional studies are ordered. Plain x-rays reveal a lytic lesion (with pathological fracture) in the distal femur with a small soft tissue component. When the attending physician discusses the findings with the patient's father, he notes that the young man has had one eye removed. Following further gentle probing, the father revealed that he had been diagnosed with retinoblastoma of the eye as a young child, which was treated with chemotherapy and radiation. Given the history above, what is the most likely diagnosis for the above patient?
   A. Ewing sarcoma
   B. Giant cell tumor of bone
   C. Synovial sarcoma
   D. Osteosarcoma
   E. Chondrosarcoma

4. An ambitious medical resident was entering data into a cancer research registry and noted multiple patients with the same unusual last name. Because all patients had authorized Health Insurance Portability and Accountability Act (HIPAA) waivers for research purposes, the resident probed the records for additional information. His research yielded that the seven patients were related. Diagnoses included one patient with leukemia, one with osteosarcoma, two breast cancers, one soft tissue sarcoma of the thigh, one colon cancer, and one adrenocortical cancer. Given the familial nature and the specific diagnoses, what is most likely responsible for this high incidence of malignancies?
   A. Li-Fraumeni syndrome (LFS)
   B. Familial adenomatous polyposis
   C. Hereditary nonpolyposis cancer syndrome

   D. *BRCA1* mutation
   E. Neurofibromatosis

5. When comparing preoperative to postoperative radiation therapy (RT) for primary soft tissue sarcoma of the extremity, preoperative RT is associated with:
   A. Improved overall survival
   B. Fewer wound complications
   C. Fewer late tissue fibroses
   D. Larger radiation port size
   E. Improved local control

6. A 42-year-old female patient presents with an 8-cm mass within the left thigh. The mass is felt to be consistent with a high-grade sarcoma on MRI scan. She is referred to an orthopedic oncologist for evaluation. How should a biopsy be obtained to confirm the diagnosis?
   A. Fine-needle biopsy
   B. Tru-cut core biopsy under CT guidance
   C. Incisional biopsy oriented horizontally
   D. Excisional biopsy
   E. Incisional biopsy oriented longitudinally

7. Which sarcoma subtype commonly metastasizes to non-pulmonary sites?
   A. Synovial cell
   B. Desmoid tumor
   C. Myxoid liposarcoma
   D. Well-differentiated liposarcoma
   E. High-grade undifferentiated pleomorphic sarcoma

8. Which of the following soft tissue sarcomas carries a greater risk of lymph node involvement at the time of initial presentation?
   A. Leiomyosarcoma
   B. Dermatofibrosarcoma protuberans
   C. Well-differentiated liposarcoma
   D. Angiosarcoma
   E. High-grade undifferentiated pleomorphic sarcoma

9. A 67-year-old woman is diagnosed with a high-grade, 6-cm, synovial sarcoma of the right thigh. She has no evidence of metastases and undergoes limb-sparing surgery followed by adjuvant radiation. You would recommend the following surveillance studies:
   A. Chest, abdomen, pelvis, and right thigh CT scan
   B. Chest x-ray, MRI thigh
   C. Whole body PET-CT scan
   D. Chest CT, MRI thigh
   E. PET-CT scan, MRI thigh

10. A 55-year-old female presents with a 4-month history of intermittent abdominal pain that has worsened over the past week. A CT scan of the chest, abdomen, and pelvis

shows a 14-cm retroperitoneal mass with no evidence of lung or liver metastases, and no organ invasion. A CT-guided biopsy reveals a spindle cell sarcoma that is immunohistochemical-stain-positive for desmin and smooth muscle actin, and negative for CD117 and DOG1. Which treatment would you recommend now?

A. Neoadjuvant doxorubicin/ifosfamide
B. Neoadjuvant imatinib
C. Neoadjuvant radiation
D. Neoadjuvant doxorubicin/ifosfamide and radiation
E. Surgical resection

11. A 68-year-old man is being examined by his primary care doctor for a swollen left thigh and calf. Because the man has had a DVT in the past, the physician utilizes a hand-held Doppler and carefully palpates both calves. A large, deep-seated mass is palpated in the area of the left medial gastrocnemius. An MRI was performed, and the T2-weighted image showed a heterogeneous mass with a central region of necrosis. A needle biopsy in the outpatient clinic was performed, and benign hemorrhagic soft tissue was obtained. The next course of action for this patient would be:

A. Conclude that this is a hematoma and follow-up with the patient in 4 weeks
B. Conclude that this is a hematoma and perform an ultrasound to obtain accurate size and proximity to critical vessels
C. Remain suspicious that this is a malignant process and obtain additional tissue with Tru cut core biopsies under CT guidance
D. Remain suspicious that this is a malignant process and schedule the patient for an excisional biopsy
E. Perform a PET scan to determine if this is a mass of metastatic origin

12. A 60-year-old female patient presents to her internist complaining of shortness of breath. The physical exam is otherwise normal. She has recently retired after working as a gardener in a commercial greenhouse for 40 years. Her surgical history is significant for cholecystectomy for gallstones 8 years ago and a morcellator myomectomy 3 years ago. She is a nonsmoker. Her family history is positive for lung cancer in her father; her mother died of pancreatic cancer; and an older sister had colon cancer. A CT scan of her chest reveals small (<1 cm) bilateral pulmonary nodules. The most probable sarcoma on a differential diagnosis list would be:

A. Small cell osteosarcoma
B. Metastatic leiomyosarcoma
C. Ewing sarcoma
D. Classic chondrosarcoma
E. Angiosarcoma

13. A 42-year-old female marathon runner notes pain in the lower right thigh and a questionable mass. She sees a general surgeon who feels that this is a lipoma. She undergoes an excisional surgical resection, and a well-circumscribed 5-cm mass is removed. Pathology reveals a high-grade undifferentiated pleomorphic sarcoma with lateral and posterior margins that are positive. Which of the following would now be the appropriate treatment?

A. Above-knee amputation
B. Radiation
C. Re-resection followed by radiation
D. Doxorubicin/ifosfamide
E. Doxorubicin/ifosfamide followed by radiation

14. A 27-year-old homosexual man presents with violaceous lesions on his arms, legs, and chest, as well as two lesions on the hard palate. He was previously diagnosed with HIV disease 3 years ago and started on highly active antiretroviral therapy (HAART) therapy. He stopped taking HAART medications 7 months ago. Laboratory tests reveal positive HIV test and CD/4 count 67, viral load 132,000. He is referred for treatment. CT scans of the chest/abdomen/pelvis show a few ill-defined lung nodules, and mild lymphadenopathy of the axilla and retroperitoneum. He is afebrile and Hgb stable at 11.2. Which treatment would you recommend?

A. HAART, then imatinib
B. HAART, then doxorubicin/ifosfamide
C. HAART, then liposomal doxorubicin, if no response
D. Liposomal doxorubicin only
E. Gemcitabine/docetaxel, then restart HAART

15. Imatinib is highly efficacious for many patients with gastrointestinal stromal tumor (GIST). For which other sarcoma with a specific chromosomal translocation has it also been shown to be effective?

A. Dermatofibrosarcoma protuberans
B. Alveolar rhabdomyosarcoma
C. Myxoid liposarcoma
D. Ewing sarcoma
E. Angiosarcoma

16. A 64-year-old man is evaluated for worsening left hip pain. He has a history of multiple hereditary exostosis, and a plain radiograph shows a large, aggressive, destructive secondary chondrosarcoma arising from a previous lesion in the left proximal femur. The patient has a wide surgical resection with a limb-sparing prosthesis reconstruction. Pathology shows stage II chondrosarcoma; the margins of resection are negative. Following surgery, this patient's management should include:

A. Doxorubicin/cisplatin
B. Radiation to the deep surgical bed
C. Vincristine/doxorubicin/cyclophosphamide alternating with ifosfamide/etoposide
D. Gemcitabine/docetaxel
E. Chemotherapy or radiation therapy is not warranted for this patient

17. It is increasingly recognized that different pathological subtypes of soft tissue sarcomas have variable patterns of chemosensitivity. Match the sarcoma subtype with the appropriate known chemotherapy sensitivity.

A. Synovial sarcoma: trabectedin
B. Leiomyosarcoma: cisplatinum
C. Myxoid/round cell liposarcoma: ifosfamide
D. Scalp angiosarcoma: paclitaxel
E. Alveolar cell sarcoma: doxorubicin

18. An 18-year-old student is receiving high-dose methotrexate (MTX) during treatment for an osteosarcoma of the distal femur. He has a history of gastritis and was previously on a proton pump inhibitor. He is also a vegan and has had a poor appetite. As part of the treatment with MTX, what would you recommend?

A. Maintaining urine pH <7.0
B. Restarting proton pump inhibitor
C. Maintaining adequate hydration
D. Twenty-four hours after the start of MTX, initiate glucarpidase rescue
E. Twenty-four hours after the start of MTX, initiate folic acid rescue until the MTX level is less than 0.1 µM

19. A 30-year-old woman with recurrent osteosarcoma of the pelvis with a large soft tissue mass, previously treated with cisplatinum, doxorubicin, and high-dose MTX, is started on treatment with high-dose ifosfamide over 5 days. She is noted to have a creatinine of 1.6 and an albumin of 2.6. On the evening of the fourth day of her second cycle of treatment, she is noted to be confused, disoriented, lethargic, hallucinating, and has twitching of both hands. Her creatinine has increased to 2.1, and her serum sodium (Na) is 134. In addition to continuing hydration and urine alkalinization, you would:
A. Obtain a brain MRI and continue ifosfamide
B. Decrease the ifosfamide infusion rate and obtain a brain MRI
C. Decrease the ifosfamide infusion rate and increase the mesna dose
D. Stop ifosfamide and consider treatment with methylene blue
E. Stop ifosfamide and give phenobarbital

20. A 59-year-old female with a previous history of hepatitis, who was otherwise healthy, had a 6 cm high-grade undifferentiated pleomorphic sarcoma resected 4 years ago from the left thigh, followed by adjuvant radiation. Surveillance chest CT now shows 15 small bilateral pulmonary metastases. MRI of the thigh is negative. CBC, creatinine, and liver function tests are all normal. The patient wishes to pursue treatment. In your discussion with her, which statement would be true about comparing the below-listed treatments to single-agent doxorubicin?
A. Doxorubicin/ifosfamide is associated with improved overall survival
B. Gemcitabine/docetaxel is associated with improved overall survival
C. Pazopanib would have less hepatotoxicity
D. Doxorubicin/ifosfamide has double the response rate
E. Gemcitabine/docetaxel has less toxicity

21. A 53-year-old female with metastatic uterine leiomyosarcoma, peritoneal and liver metastases, and no evidence of lung metastases receives gemcitabine and docetaxel treatment. The docetaxel and prednisone are stopped after 2 cycles because of significant peripheral neuropathy. Two days after the fourth cycle of gemcitabine, she presents to an emergency room with increasing cough and dyspnea. She is afebrile, WBC 5.0, normal differential. Chest x-ray shows bilateral reticulonodular infiltrates. Chest CT shows ground-glass and reticular opacities, bilaterally. Her saturated oxygen level is 88% on room air. The patient is started on oxygen and admitted to the intensive care unit. The gemcitabine is held. The next decision would be:
A. Start patient on IV heparin
B. Switch chemotherapy to doxorubicin because of lymphangitic spread
C. Start IV antibiotics and restart gemcitabine once patient is stable
D. Start patient on corticosteroids
E. Obtain a lung biopsy

22. Which of the following is characteristic of gastrointestinal stromal tumors?
A. Similar staging system as other soft tissue sarcomas
B. Rarely present with GI bleeding
C. Lung and lymph node spread is common
D. The most common GI sarcoma
E. The small intestine is the most common primary site

23. A 63-year-old woman presents with abdominal fullness and anemia. A CT scan reveals a 4-cm gastric mass. Endoscopic biopsy is consistent with a gastrointestinal stromal tumor. The patient undergoes resection, and a mutational analysis reveals an Exon 11 mutation. Which is the most important variable in helping to determine whether this patient should receive adjuvant imatinib therapy?
A. Tumor site
B. Tumor size
C. Tumor mitotic rate
D. Lymph node involvement
E. Histological GIST subtype

24. A 25-year-old man has noted abdominal fullness for 4 months with intermittent nausea. An abdominal CT scan shows a 15-cm mass arising from the fundus of the stomach with no other intraabdominal disease. Hgb is 10.0. An endoscopic biopsy is immunohistochemically positive for CD117 and DOG1, and the mitotic index is three mitoses per 50 high-power fields. The patient undergoes an RO resection (complete resection with no microscopic residual tumor). What would you relate to the patient about considering treatment with adjuvant imatinib?
A. Gastric GIST is associated with a worse prognosis.
B. Both tumor size and mitotic rate predict a response to imatinib.
C. Mutational analysis may be helpful in assessing imatinib benefit.
D. Imatinib 400 mg by mouth daily for 5 years is the standard of care.
E. Patients with the PDGFRA D842V mutation require 800 mg imatinib daily.

25. An 18-year-old woman presents with abdominal pain and fullness of 5 months' duration. The pregnancy test is negative. She has had a history of long-term gastritis. She undergoes an endoscopy, which reveals several tumor nodules, the largest of which is 3 cm in diameter. Pathology of the tumors is consistent with an epithelioid GIST, CKIT and DOG1 positive. Mutational analysis is negative for CKIT and platelet-derived growth factor receptor (PDGFR) mutations. This patient's tumor is most likely characterized as being:
A. RAS mutation positive
B. Imatinib sensitive
C. Associated with neurofibroma
D. SDHB immunohistochemistry stain negative
E. Presenting with an aggressive course with lymph node and liver metastases

26. A 64-year-old man with an 8-cm gastric GIST and three liver metastases is started on imatinib 400 mg daily. Mutational analysis reveals an Exon 11 KIT mutation. He is very anxious and asks for a CT scan to be repeated at 6 weeks. The CT scan shows no change in the size of the gastric mass, but an increase in size of the liver metastases and two new small liver lesions, all with decreased density. What is the next best step in management for this patient?
A. Continue imatinib 400 mg
B. Increase imatinib to 800 mg
C. Switch to sunitinib 37.5 mg/daily
D. Resect the gastric tumor and switch to sunitinib 37.5 mg/daily
E. Resect all disease and increase imatinib to 800 mg

27. A 65-year-old man is referred to the Medical Oncology Department after undergoing resection of a 5-cm gastric GIST. Pathology reveals a tumor that is CD117 and CD34 positive with one mitosis per 50 high-power fields, and

the margin of resection is 1 mm. Mutational analysis was sent and shows a KIT Exon 11 mutation. You would recommend:
- **A.** Imatinib 400 mg daily for 3 years
- **B.** Imatinib 800 mg daily for 3 years
- **C.** No further therapy
- **D.** Re-resection for close margin
- **E.** Radiation therapy for close margin

28. The following is characteristic of patients with Ewing sarcoma:
- **A.** More common in patients of African and Asian descent
- **B.** Associated with a 9;22 chromosomal translocation
- **C.** Classical Ewing and primitive neuroectodermal tumor (PNET) are felt to be separate tumor entities
- **D.** Rarely presents with a soft tissue mass
- **E.** Pathological response to neoadjuvant chemotherapy is predictive of survival

29. The following is true regarding classic chondrosarcoma:
- **A.** It is usually treated with surgical resection.
- **B.** It arises in predominantly young patients.
- **C.** It is more common in females.
- **D.** Vertebral body involvement is common.
- **E.** It can arise from a preexisting benign lesion (i.e., fibromatosis).

30. What factor has been shown to correlate with survival benefit regarding neoadjuvant chemotherapy for osteosarcoma?
- **A.** Patients with greater than 50% necrosis after neoadjuvant chemotherapy
- **B.** Adding ifosfamide for patients with a poor pathological response
- **C.** Addition of mifurmatide for patients with poor pathological response
- **D.** Addition of pegylated interferon for pathological good responders
- **E.** None of the above

31. An 18-year-old runner develops pain over the right lower thigh. He begins walking with a limp and is taking ibuprofen. Continuing symptoms lead the patient to an emergent-care facility. An x-ray shows an abnormality in the distal femur. He is referred to an orthopedic oncologist. An MRI shows a 6 × 5 cm cystic lesion of the left distal femur. A CT-guided core needle biopsy reveals a high-grade osteosarcoma. Bloodwork, including a CBC and a CMP, is normal. Further workup for this patient should include:
- **A.** CT scan of the chest and a bone scan
- **B.** Left inguinal sentinel node biopsy and chest CT
- **C.** CT scan of the chest, abdomen, and pelvis
- **D.** CT scan of the chest, abdomen, and pelvis and a bone scan
- **E.** PET-CT scans and brain MRI

32. An 18-year-old college student presents to the health center with shoulder pain, swelling, and a low-grade fever. Physical exam reveals a large and firm scapular mass. Blood work is significant for both the elevated erythrocyte sedimentation rate and a high lactate dehydrogenase concentration. Radiographic evaluation of the mass shows a very large permeative lucent lesion of the scapula with evidence of soft tissue involvement. Pathological examination of the patient's tumor will most likely reveal:
- **A.** Spindle cells with a chondroid component and chondroid matrix
- **B.** Spindle cells with an osteoid matrix and calcification
- **C.** Round blue tumor cells with a unique reciprocal chromosomal translocation
- **D.** Spindle cells with central round nuclei and scattered osteoclast-like giant cells
- **E.** Histiocytes, large granular eosinophils, pink cytoplasm, coffee-bean-shaped nuclei

---

ANSWERS

1. B
Ewing sarcoma is most commonly associated with an 11;22 translocation. Myxoid/round cell liposarcoma is associated with a 12;16 fusion of FUS with DDIT3. Alveolar rhabdomyosarcoma is associated with a 2;13 translocation. Synovial sarcoma (PAX3-FOX O1) with an x;18 translocation, either monophasic or biphasic, and dermatofibrosarcoma protuberans occurs with a 17;22 translocation, involving COL1A1 and PDGFB. Chromosomal translocations are the most common cytogenetic abnormality occurring in neoplasms of the soft tissue. They can be highly diagnostic for specific histological subtypes and helpful in confirming a diagnosis as well as identifying specific molecular therapeutic targets.

2. E
Radiation-induced sarcomas, until recently, were thought to have somewhat of a worse prognosis. They usually occur between 10 and 40 years after previous radiation. Common histological subtypes include osteogenic sarcoma, MFH of bone, and angiosarcoma. They are usually treated with chemotherapy, in addition to surgery. LFS, an autosomal dominant condition, is associated with an increased risk for sarcoma, gliomas, breast carcinomas, leukemia, and adrenocortical cancer.

3. D
Pediatric patients with familial retinoblastoma have a 13q deletion and are at an increased risk, later in life, for developing osteosarcoma, not only in the previous radiated field but also elsewhere.

4. A
Leukemia, osteosarcoma, breast cancer, and soft tissue sarcoma are all represented in one family. These malignancies are seen in families that have LFS, which is associated with mutations in *TP53*, a gene present on the short arm of chromosome 17 (17p13.1). The cancers noted above are hallmark cancers in LFS and typically occur before the age of 45.

5. C
The National Cancer Institute of Canada performed a randomized trial of preoperative versus postoperative radiation therapy for extremity soft tissue sarcoma. It was found that preoperative radiation therapy is associated with more wound complications. Local control and survival is the same for either preoperative or postoperative radiation therapy. Postoperative treatment results in more late tissue fibrosis and possible bone fracture. The radiation port size is smaller with preoperative treatment.

6. B and **E**

Biopsy of the primary tumor is essential for most patients with soft tissue masses. The preferred biopsy approach is generally the least invasive technique required to allow a definitive histological diagnosis and assessment of grade. In most centers, core needle biopsy provides satisfactory tissue for a diagnosis and usually provides adequate material for molecular testing. If done under CT guidance, one can obtain multiple passes in areas where there is a solid tumor component as well as necrosis. Another option would be an incisional biopsy oriented longitudinally for extremity lesions, which facilitates a definitive wide local excision and removal of the biopsy tract in situ. Care should be taken for meticulous hemostasis to prevent dissemination of tumor cells into adjacent tissue. Fine needle aspiration is helpful in confirming suspected recurrent disease, but does not usually yield enough tissue for a definitive diagnosis and/or molecular testing.

7. C

Myxoid/round cell liposarcomas are characterized by a reciprocal translocation between chromosomes 12 and 16, and they display a curious tendency to metastasize to soft tissue sites other than the lungs. Therefore, it is recommended for this specific sarcoma subtype to obtain a CT scan not only of the chest, but also of the abdomen and pelvis, and MRI of the spine.

8. D

The prevalence of lymph node metastasis in adults with most sarcomas is very low; therefore, there is no role for routine regional lymph node dissection. However, patients specifically with angiosarcoma, embryonal rhabdomyosarcoma, epithelioid sarcoma, and clear cell sarcoma have an increased incidence of lymph node metastasis and should be carefully examined for adenopathy by physical examination, imaging, and possible sentinel lymph node sampling.

9. D

Soft tissue sarcomas of the extremity usually recur locally or metastasize to the lung. It is unlikely for soft tissue sarcomas to metastasize elsewhere, with the exception of myxoid liposarcoma, which can spread to multiple nonpulmonary sites, and alveolar soft part sarcoma, which has a propensity to metastasize to the brain. The role, cost effectiveness, and feasibility of a PET scan in the staging and surveillance of soft tissue sarcomas remain to be defined; further prospective studies are needed. For low-grade soft tissue sarcomas, one usually follows the patient with chest radiograph and MRI; high-grade soft tissue sarcomas are followed with chest CT and MRI.

10. E

This retroperitoneal tumor mass is consistent with a leiomyosarcoma, based on immunohistochemical staining. The standard of treatment for a retroperitoneal leiomyosarcoma is surgical resection. There is no definitive evidence for the use of neoadjuvant chemotherapy and/or radiation. The use of imatinib is typically reserved for a GIST.

Retroperitoneal sarcomas (RPSs) are relatively uncommon, constituting 10%–15% of all soft tissue sarcomas, with the most common histologies in adults being leiomyosarcoma and liposarcoma.

Surgical resection has traditionally been the only curative approach for localized, potentially resectable RPS. However, these tumors are usually diagnosed late with a large size and anatomic complexity. A complete resection with microscopically negative margins (R0 resection) is required but not always achieved, and locoregional recurrence is common. Management by physicians experienced in the treatment of this entity is crucial. Adjunctive RT can reduce the risk of local recurrence but has not been shown to improve overall survival. Due to the complexity of treatment and potential toxicity, preoperative RT also should only be performed at centers proficient in the treatment of these sarcomas.

The European Organisation for Research and Treatment of Cancer (EORTC) is currently performing a prospective randomized phase III trial (NCT01344018, STRASS Trial) of preoperative RT and surgery versus surgery alone, which hopefully should determine the role of preoperative RT in the management of RPS.

11. C

This patient history should be cause for suspicion of a hemorrhagic thigh sarcoma. Undergoing a needle biopsy in the clinic could miss areas of a tumor and only obtain areas of hemorrhage or necrosis. It is advised that the patient undergo multiple CT-guided Tru cut core biopsies. The CT guidance allows better visualization of the mass and therefore increases the likelihood that not only necrotic and hemorrhagic areas will be biopsied but also the solid tumor area.

12. B

This is an unfortunate woman who had a morcellator myomectomy procedure. Women with symptomatic uterine fibroids may have chosen to undergo this procedure because of the benefits of shorter postoperative recovery time and reduced infection risk compared with abdominal hysterectomy and myomectomy. However, recent reports and FDA guidelines now suggest that this can carry the risk of spreading cancerous tissues, which were not detected during the initial pathological examination, namely uterine leiomyosarcoma. The patient is now presenting with bilateral pulmonary nodules, which are most consistent with metastatic leiomyosarcoma. The treatment of choice for this patient would be chemotherapy with either gemcitabine/docetaxel or a doxorubicin-containing regimen.

13. C

This is a middle-aged woman with a mass found in her thigh where an excisional procedure has been performed with positive margins. The treatment of choice, if possible, would be re-resection. Studies have shown there is residual disease in approximately 50% of patients. Following resection, the patient should receive adjuvant radiation. These patients can still be treated with a limb-sparing procedure and do not require an above-knee amputation. Adjuvant chemotherapy for soft tissue sarcoma of the extremities is still controversial and is decided on an individual patient basis, based on the patient's age, organ function and performance status, tumor size, and grade.

14. C

AIDS-associated Kaposi sarcoma (KS) is the most common malignancy occurring in patients with HIV. For those patients not already on HAART, it is indicated as the first treatment (regardless of CD4 count).

Immune reconstitution can often result in regression of KS lesions without additional treatments. For extensive cutaneous, rapidly progressive disease, and/or visceral involvement, systemic chemotherapy is indicated, liposomal doxorubicin being the treatment of choice. It is associated with a high response rate and very good tolerability; it is superior and safer compared with combination chemotherapy. For patients intolerant or refractory to liposomal doxorubicin, paclitaxel in a weekly or biweekly regimen is preferred as a second-line treatment.

15. A

Dermatofibrosarcoma protuberans (DFSP) is a rare sarcoma involving the soft tissue characterized by a 17;22 chromosomal translocation involving the COL1 A1 and PDGFB genes, causing upregulation of the PGFF beta receptor. Imatinib has activity against the PDGF beta pathway, and it has been shown to be effective in patients with advanced DFSP. Alveolar soft part sarcoma is highly vascular but is a chemoresistant histology. Responses with both sunitinib and cediranib (both potent vascular endothelial growth factor receptor [VEGFR] inhibitors) have been seen.

16. E

This is an older male with a conventional chondrosarcoma. These are usually treated with surgical resection and are resistant to standard chemotherapy. Those chondrosarcomas that are treated with chemotherapy include dedifferentiated chondrosarcoma, using a multidisciplinary approach similar to that used for osteosarcoma, as well as mesenchymal chondrosarcoma, which has a biphasic histology with cellular areas composed of small anaplastic cells reminiscent of Ewing sarcoma interspersed with islands of bland-appearing chondroid matrix. They are treated with therapy similar to Ewing sarcoma.

17. D

Synovial sarcomas are known to be sensitive to ifosfamide. Leiomyosarcomas are sensitive to doxorubicin and gemcitabine/docetaxel. Myxoid/round cell liposarcomas are treated with Adriamycin (doxorubicin), gemcitabine/docetaxel. Most recently, trabectedin has been FDA approved for both leiomyosarcoma and liposarcoma with a significant improvement in progression-free survival. Scalp angiosarcomas are sensitive to paclitaxel. Finally, alveolar cell sarcomas are chemotherapy resistant. More recently, they have been treated with Cediranib or sunitinib.

18. C

One has to be very careful when treating patients with high-dose MTX, since patients are at risk for both renal and other toxicities. Recommendations include maintaining a urine pH greater than or equal to 7.0 (alkalinizing the urine) and vigorous hydration with adequate urine output, so the drug will not precipitate in the renal tubules. Co-administration of proton pump inhibitors is associated with delayed elimination of MTX, and therefore should be avoided, if possible, during treatment. Twenty-four hours after starting MTX, the patient should begin to receive calcium leucovorin every 6 hours until the MTX level is below 0.05–0.1 μM. Glucarpidase (carboxypeptidase G2) was FDA approved in 2012 for the treatment of toxic MTX plasma concentrations (>1 μM) in patients with delayed MTX clearance due to impaired renal function. Although the indications for its use are not fully established, one should consider the use of this drug in a patient with early renal dysfunction if the serum MTX level is greater than 10 μM beyond 42–48 hours. Glucarpidase metabolizes folic acid (and leucovorin) and other chemically similar antifolates (i.e., MTX) to their inactive metabolites. A single dose can rapidly decrease MTX levels by 98% in the first 30 minutes, which, in the majority of patients, is sustained. Adverse effects are minimal. Another name for calcium leucovorin is folinic acid. One should never use this name, since it is similar to folic acid and can be confused with it. Folic acid will not rescue normal cells; it does not enter into the folic acid cycle beyond the MTX block.

19. D

This woman has high-risk features for ifosfamide-induced encephalopathy. The factors associated with increased risk for ifosfamide-induced encephalopathy include a large pelvic lesion, elevated creatinine, a low albumin, prior cisplatin treatment, and/or concomitant aprepitant use. The encephalopathy is thought to be secondary to the accumulation of chloracetaldehyde, one of the breakdown products of ifosfamide. Treatment of choice for this patient would be to stop the ifosfamide, continue IV hydration and alkalinization of the urine, and consider starting the patient on methylene blue. All patients treated with ifosfamide should have a G6PD deficiency assay performed prior to starting the drug, since the use of methylene blue can cause massive hemolysis in a G6PD-deficient patient. If the patient is G6PD deficient, one could consider treatment with either valium or thiamine. Phenobarbital is contraindicated since several reports have shown worsening of the encephalopathy.

20. D

Single-agent doxorubicin is the benchmark against which single and multiagent regimens should be tested. In the EORTC trial 62012, which randomized patients to doxorubicin single agent versus doxorubicin plus ifosfamide for advanced/metastatic soft tissue sarcoma, the doublet was associated with a doubling in response rate and increased toxicity, but it was not associated with an overall survival benefit.

The GeDDiS trial presented at ASCO 2015 randomized patients with advanced/metastatic soft tissue sarcoma to doxorubicin or gemcitabine/docetaxel. The doublet showed no benefit in progression-free or overall survival, and was associated with increased toxicity. Pazopanib, unlike doxorubicin, carries a risk of hepatotoxicity (which is occasionally life threatening). Given this risk, close monitoring of liver function tests is recommended, specifically for the first 9 weeks of treatment.

There is no overall survival benefit in metastatic soft tissue sarcoma from combination chemotherapy. Single-agent doxorubicin is still recommended for palliation and as a reference for newly designed randomized trials. Since the combination of doxorubicin and ifosfamide showed double the response rate, it should be considered for patients in the neoadjuvant setting, for tumor shrinkage requiring symptom control, and for imminently life-threatening disease. These decisions need to be made on an individual basis with the patient.

21. D

This patient has been on gemcitabine and has been taken off steroids and docetaxel for docetaxel peripheral neuropathy toxicity. The patient is now short of breath with a low oxygen saturation. She is afebrile, with a normal white blood count and no evidence of pulmonary emboli. Chest x-ray and CT findings are most consistent with gemcitabine-induced pulmonary toxicity. The treatment of choice for this patient is to stop the gemcitabine and start the patient on corticosteroids. Early recognition is important because there have been fatalities from this condition reported in the literature. Reintroduction of gemcitabine is contraindicated since this may result in fatal pulmonary toxicity.

22. D

Gastrointestinal stromal tumors are the most common GI sarcoma. They have a different staging system than other soft tissue sarcomas. Because of their vascularity, they can commonly present with GI bleeding. It is uncommon for them to spread to lung or lymph nodes. They most commonly arise in the stomach approximately 60% of the time, with the next most common site being the small intestine.

23. C

The primary determination of whether a patient should receive adjuvant therapy for a primary resected GIST is based on the tumor site, size, and mitotic rate. Tumor rupture predisposes a patient to a higher risk of recurrence. The most important factor for GIST recurrence after surgery is a high tumor mitotic rate (>5 mitoses per 50 high-power fields).

24. C

When considering adjuvant imatinib for a patient following surgical resection of a primary GIST, gastric GISTs have a somewhat better prognosis. Tumor size and mitotic rate are important in determining the use of adjuvant imatinib; however, they are not important in predicting the response. Imatinib is recommended at 400 mg for 3 years, based on long-term data from a Scandinavian study. Patients with the PDGFR D842V mutation do not respond well to imatinib. A mutational analysis can be helpful in assessing those patients who will respond to imatinib.

25. D

This describes a young woman with a succinate dehydrogenase B-deficient GIST. These tend to occur in the stomach of young female patients. Although they stain positive for CKIT and DOG1, they do not have mutations in either KIT or PDGFR. They are usually imatinib insensitive. They can present with multiple synchronous tumors within the stomach, and can spread to the lymph nodes and liver, but they are associated with an indolent course.

26. A

This male patient with a metastatic gastric GIST to the liver receiving imatinib has had CT scans performed fairly early. One does not always see a decrease in tumor size at this point in time. Following imaging of liver metastasis, one can see an increase in size but with decreased density, suggesting necrosis and a response to imatinib. In addition, smaller liver metastases, which were not seen in an earlier scan, once necrosed, can also appear with a low density. A PET scan at this time showed no FDG activity. Therefore, this patient appears to be having a response to imatinib, and one would continue this patient on 400 mg and not increase to 800 mg or switch to sunitinib.

27. C

For patients who have an initial resection of a primary GIST, the decision to recommend adjuvant imatinib is dependent on the risk of recurrence, which is based on tumor size, mitotic index, anatomic location, and the occurrence or absence of tumor rupture (spontaneous or during surgery). It is also recommended to obtain mutational analysis, since patients with a PGFRA D842V, SDH deficient, or NF-1-related tumor are usually imatinib insensitive.

There are several risk stratification models. A modification of the National Institutes of Health Consensus Criteria incorporates both site and tumor rupture, as well as size and mitotic index. An alternative to these risk stratifications systems, which classify patients into discrete categories (very low risk to very high risk), is attempting to quantify the risk of disease recurrence as a continuous variable with the use of a GIST prognostic nomogram (MSKCC website).

Most guidelines recommend adjuvant imatinib for "high risk" category patients, and those who have an estimated risk of recurrence that is greater than 30%–50%. However, each patient must be assessed individually, balancing age, performance status, and comorbid medical problems with the estimated likelihood of recurrence.

The standard of care treatment is 3 years of adjuvant imatinib at 400 mg daily, based on the SSG XVIII randomized trial of 1 year versus 3 years. There is no adjuvant data on 800 mg imatinib or the use of other tyrosine kinase inhibitors. SSG XVIII defined "high risk" as a tumor size greater than 10 cm, mitotic index greater than 10 per 50 high-power fields, or tumor size greater than 5 cm and greater than 5 mitoses per 50 high-power fields.

This patient, by consensus criteria, would be classified as low risk and by the MSKCC GIST nomogram would have a 2-year and 5-year recurrence-free survival, after surgery, of 95% and 91%, respectively. Therefore, no adjuvant imatinib would be recommended.

28. E

Ewing sarcoma is more common in Caucasians, and rare in patients of African or Asian descent. It is most commonly associated with an 11;22 chromosomal translocation. Both classical Ewing sarcoma and PNET are felt to be similar entities, and both are now classified as part of the Ewing family of tumors and treated similarly. Ewing sarcoma can commonly present with a soft tissue mass. The pathological response to neoadjuvant chemotherapy can be predictive of survival.

29. A

Chondrosarcomas are a heterogeneous group of tumors that characteristically produce a cartilage matrix with calcification and myxoid changes. Clinical behavior is dependent on grade, and treatment is predominantly surgical resection. They are the second most common primary tumor of bone and predominantly arise in older individuals (>50 years of age), with an equal distribution amongst males and females. The pelvis is most commonly affected; the femur, ribs, and humerus are other common sites. They can arise in preexisting benign lesions, such as multiple enchondromas (Ollier disease or Maffucci disease) or with multiple hereditary osteochondromas.

30. E

Neoadjuvant chemotherapy has been shown to be of benefit for patients with primary osteosarcoma. Those patients who, on histopathological review, have greater than 90% tumor necrosis appear to have an improved survival. Adding ifosfamide for patients with a poor pathological response has not been shown to be beneficial. Although approved in Europe, the addition of mifurmatide has not definitively been shown to add to improved survival, especially in those patients with a poor pathological response. Pegylated interferon in the EURAMOS Randomized Study was not shown to be of benefit for pathological good responders. A significant number of patients were unable to complete the 2 years of treatment because of toxicity.

31. A

After diagnosis of a primary osteosarcoma, further workup should include a CT scan of the chest and a bone scan. The patient is at risk for the development of lung metastases as well as skip bone lesions. It is extremely rare for osteosarcoma to involve lymph nodes or metastasize to the abdomen or brain.

32. C

This young man's history of a fast-growing tumor of the scapula, an elevated sedimentation rate and LDH, and x-rays showing a permeative lucent lesion are suggestive of a small round blue cell tumor consistent with Ewing sarcoma. Immunohistochemical staining for CD99 (mic2 antigen) and glycogen is usually positive. In order to confirm the diagnosis, one should send out tissue for chromosomal analysis. Ewing sarcoma is most often associated with a t11;22 chromosomal translocation. The treatment of choice should be aggressive chemotherapy with vincristine, adriamycin, cyclophosphamide (VAC) alternating with IE for several cycles, followed by surgical resection and then additional alternating chemotherapy with VAC/IE.

REFERENCES

Question 1

1. Knight JC, Renwick PJ, Dal Cin P, Van den Berghe H, Fletcher CD. Translocation t(12;16)(q13;p11) in myxoid liposarcoma and round cell liposarcoma: molecular and cytogenetic analysis. *Cancer Res.* 1995;55(1):24–27.

Question 2

1. Virtanen A, Pukkala E, Auvinen A. Incidence of bone and soft tissue sarcoma after radiotherapy: a cohort study of 295,712 Finnish cancer patients. *Int J Cancer.* 2006;118(4):1017–1021.
2. Gladdy RA, Qin L-X, Moraco N, et al. Do radiation-associated soft tissue sarcomas have the same prognosis as sporadic soft tissue sarcomas? *J Clin Oncol.* 2010;28(12):2064–2069.
3. Riad SR, Biau D, Holt GE, et al. The clinical and functional outcome for patients with radiation-induced soft tissue sarcoma. *Cancer.* 2012;118(10):2682–2692.

Question 3

1. Marees T, Moll AC, Imhof SM, de Boer MR, Ringens PJ, van Leeuwen FE. Risk of second malignancies in survivors of retinoblastoma: more than 40 years of follow-up. *J Natl Cancer Inst.* 2008;100:1771–1779.
2. MacCarthy A, Bayne AM, Brownbill PA, et al. Second and subsequent tumours among 1927 retinoblastoma patients diagnosed in Britain 1951–2004. *Br J Cancer.* 2013;108(12):2455–2463.
3. Kleinerman RA, Tucker MA, Tarone RE, et al. Risk of new cancers after radiotherapy in long-term survivors of retinoblastoma: an extended follow-up. *J Clin Oncol.* 2005;23:2272–2279.

Question 4

1. Li FP, Fraumeni Jr JF, Mulvihill JJ, et al. A cancer family syndrome in twenty-four kindreds. *Cancer Res.* 1988;48(18):5358–5362.
2. Malkin D. Li-Fraumeni syndrome. *Genes Cancer.* 2011;2(4):475–484.

Question 5

1. O'Sullivan B, Davis AM, Turcotte R, et al. Preoperative versus postoperative radiotherapy in soft-tissue sarcoma of the limbs: a randomised trial. *Lancet.* 2002;359:2235–2241.
2. Davis AM, O'Sullivan B, Turcotte R, et al. Late radiation morbidity following randomization to preoperative versus postoperative radiotherapy in extremity soft tissue sarcoma. *Radiother Oncol.* 2005;75:48–53.
3. Pisters PW, O'Sullivan B, Maki RG. Evidence-based recommendations for local therapy for soft tissue sarcomas. *J Clin Oncol.* 2007;25:1003–1008.

Question 6

1. Bickels J, Jelinek J, Shmookler B, Malawer MM. Biopsy of musculoskeletal tumors. In: Malawer MM, Sugarbaker PH, eds. *Musculoskeletal Cancer Surgery: Treatment of Sarcomas and Allied Diseases.* Dordrecht, The Netherlands: Kluwer Academic Publisher; 1999:37–45.

Question 7

1. Fuglø HM, Maretty-Nielsen K, Hovgaard D, Keller JØ, Safwat AA, Petersen MM. Metastatic pattern, local relapse, and survival of patients with myxoid liposarcoma: a retrospective study of 45 patients sarcoma. *Sarcoma.* 2013;2013:548628, 6 pages.

Question 8

1. Fong Y, Coit DG, Woodruff JM, Brennan M. Lymph node metastasis from soft tissue sarcoma in adults. Analysis of data from a prospective database of 1772 sarcoma patients. *Ann Surg.* 1993;217(1):72–77.

Question 9

1. Rothermundt C, Whelan JC, Dileo P, et al. What is the role of routine follow-up for localised limb soft tissue sarcomas? A retrospective analysis of 174 patients British. *J Cancer.* 2014;110:2420–2426.

Question 10

1. Pawlik TM, Pisters PW, Mikula L, et al. Long-term results of two prospective trials of preoperative external beam radiotherapy for localized intermediate- or high-grade retroperitoneal soft tissue sarcoma. *Ann Surg Oncol.* 2006;13:508–517.
2. Bonvalot S, Miceli R, Berselli M, et al. Aggressive surgery in retroperitoneal soft tissue sarcoma carried out at high-volume centers is safe and is associated with improved local control. *Ann Surg Oncol.* 2010;17:1507.
3. Transatlantic RPS. Working Group Management of Primary Retroperitoneal Sarcoma (RPS) in the Adult. A consensus approach from the Trans-Atlantic RPS Working Group. *Ann Surg Oncol.* 2015;22:256–263.

Question 11

1. Kobayashi H, Ae K, Tanizawa T, Gokita T, Motoi N, Matsumoto S. A clinicopathological analysis of soft tissue sarcoma with telangiectatic changes. *Sarcoma.* 2015;2015:740571, 5 pages.

Question 12

1. Wright JD, Tergas AI, Burke WM, et al. Uterine pathology in women undergoing minimally invasive hysterectomy using morcellation. *JAMA.* 2014;312(12):1253–1255.
2. Kho KA, Nezhat CH. Evaluating the risks of electric uterine morcellation. *JAMA.* 2014;311(9):905–906.
3. Ip PP, Cheung AN. Pathology of uterine leiomyosarcomas and smooth muscle tumours of uncertain malignant potential. *Best Pract Res Clin Obstet Gynaecol.* 2011;25:691–704.

Question 13

1. Nystrom LM, Reimer NB, Reith JD, et al. Multidisciplinary management of soft tissue sarcoma. *ScientificWorldJournal.* 2013;2013:852462, 11 pages.
   Beane JD, Yang JC, White D, Steinberg SM, Rosenberg SA, Rudloff U. Efficacy of adjuvant radiation therapy in the treatment of soft tissue sarcoma of the extremity: 20-year follow-up of a randomized prospective trial. *Ann Surg Oncol.* 2014;21:2484–2489.

Question 14

1. Lichterfeld M, Qurishi N, Hoffmann C, et al. Treatment of HIV-1-associated Kaposi's sarcoma with pegylated liposomal doxorubicin and HAART simultaneously induces effective tumor remission and CD4+ T cell recovery. *Infection.* 2005;33(3):140–147.
2. Cianfrocca M, Lee S, Von Roenn J, et al. Randomized trial of paclitaxel versus pegylated liposomal doxorubicin for advanced human immunodeficiency virus-associated Kaposi sarcoma. *Cancer.* 2010;116(16):3969–3977.
3. Cooley T, Henry D, Tonda M, Sun S, O'Connell M, Rackoff W. A randomized, double-blind study of pegylated liposomal doxorubicin for the treatment of AIDS-related Kaposi's sarcoma. *Oncologist.* 2007;12(1):114–123.
4. Lim ST, Tupule A, Espina BM, Levine AM. Weekly docetaxel is safe and effective in the treatment of advanced-stage acquired immunodeficiency syndrome-related Kaposi sarcoma. *Cancer.* 2005;103:417–421.
5. Northfelt DW, Dezube BJ, Thommes JA, et al. Pegylated-liposomal doxorubicin versus doxorubicin, bleomycin, and vincristine in the treatment of AIDS-related Kaposi's sarcoma: results of a randomized phase III clinical trial. *J Clin Oncol.* 1998;16(7):2445–2451.

Question 15

1. Rutkowski P, Van Glabbeke M, Rankin CJ. Imatinib mesylate in advanced dermatofibrosarcoma protuberans: pooled analysis of two phase II clinical trials. *J Clin Oncol.* 2010;28(10):1772–1779.
2. Stacchiotti S, Pantaleo MA, Negri T, et al. Efficacy and biological activity of Imatinib in metastatic dermatofibrosarcoma protuberans (DFSP). *Clin Cancer Res.* 2016;22(4):837–846.

Question 16

1. Gelderblom H, Hogendoorn PCW, Dijkstra SD, et al. The clinical approach towards chondrosarcoma. *Oncologist.* 2008;13:320–329.
2. Italiano A, Mir O, Cioffi A, et al. Advanced chondrosarcomas: role of chemotherapy and survival. *Ann Oncol.* 2013;24:2916–2922.
3. Cesari M, Bertoni F, Bacchini P, Mercuri M, Palmerini E, Ferrari S. Mesenchymal chondrosarcoma. An analysis of patients treated at a single institution. *Tumori.* 2007;93(5):423–427.
4. Dantonello TM, Int-Veen C, Leuschner I, et al. Mesenchymal chondrosarcoma of soft tissues and bone in children, adolescents, and young adults: experiences of the CWS and COSS study groups. *Cancer.* 2008;112(11):2424–2431.
5. Mitchell AD, Ayoub K, Mangham DC, Grimer RJ, Carter SR, Tillman RM. Experience in the treatment of dedifferentiated chondrosarcoma. *J Bone Joint Surg Br.* 2000;82(1):55–61.
6. Dickey ID, Rose PS, Fuchs B, Wold LE, et al. Dedifferentiated chondrosarcoma: the role of chemotherapy with updated outcomes. *J Bone Joint Surg Am.* 2004;86-A(11):2412–2418.

Question 17

1. Fata F, O'Reilly E, Ilson D, et al. Paclitaxel in the treatment of patients with angiosarcoma of the scalp or face. *Cancer.* 1999;86(10):2034–2037.
2. Italiano A, Cioffi A, Penel N, et al. Comparison of doxorubicin and weekly paclitaxel efficacy in metastatic angiosarcomas. *Cancer.* 2012;118(13):3330–3336.
3. Penel N, Bui BN, Bay JO, et al. Phase II trial of weekly paclitaxel for unresectable angiosarcoma: the ANGIOTAX study. *J Clin Oncol.* 2008;26(32):5269–5274.

Question 18

1. Widemann BC, Adamson PC. Understanding and managing methotrexate nephrotoxicity. *Oncologist.* 2006;11(6):694–703.
2. Buchen S, Ngampolo D, Melton RG, et al. Carboxypeptidase G$_2$ rescue in patients with methotrexate intoxication and renal failure. *Br J Cancer.* 2005;92:480–487.
3. Widemann BC, Balis FM, Kim A, et al. Glucarpidase, leucovorin, and thymidine for high-dose methotrexate-induced renal dysfunction: clinical and pharmacologic factors affecting outcome. *J Clin Oncol.* 2010;28(25):3979–3986.
4. Widemann BC, Schwartz S, Jayaprakash N, et al. Efficacy of glucarpidase (carboxypeptidase G2) in patients with acute kidney injury after high-dose methotrexate therapy. *Pharmacotherapy.* 2014;34(5):427–439.
5. Santucci R, Leveque D, Lescoute A, Kemmel V, Herbrecht R. Delayed elimination of methotrexate associated with co-administration of proton pump inhibitors. *Anticancer Res.* 2010;30:3807–3810.

Question 19

1. David KA, Picus J. Evaluating risk factors for the development of ifosfamide encephalopathy. *Am J Clin Oncol.* 2005;28(3):277–280.
2. Ho H, Yuen C. Aprepitant-associated ifosfamide neurotoxicity. *J Oncol Pharm Pract.* 2010;16:137–138.
3. Kupfer A, Aeschlimann C, Wermuth B, Cerny T. Prophylaxis and reversal of ifosfamide encephalopathy with methylene-blue. *Lancet.* 1994;343(8900):763–764.
4. Pelgrims J, De Vos F, Van den Brande J, Schrijvers D, Prové A, Vermorken JB. Methylene blue in the treatment and prevention of ifosfamide-induced encephalopathy: report of 12 cases and a review of the literature. *Br J Cancer.* 2000;82:291–294.
5. Buesa JM, Garcia-Teijido P, Losa R, Fra J. Treatment of ifosfamide encephalopathy with intravenous thiamin. *Clin Cancer Res.* 2003;9:4636.
6. Patel PN. Methylene blue for management of ifosfamide-induced encephalopathy. *Ann Pharmacother.* 2006;40(2):299–303.

Question 20

1. Judson I, Verweij J, Gelderblom H, et al. Doxorubicin alone versus intensified doxorubicin plus ifosfamide for first-line treatment of advanced or metastatic soft-tissue sarcoma: a randomised controlled phase 3 trial. *Lancet Oncol.* 2014;15:415–423.
2. Seddon BM, Whelan J, Strauss SJ, Leahy MG, et al. GeDDiS: a prospective randomised controlled phase III trial of gemcitabine and docetaxel compared with doxorubicin as first-line treatment in previously untreated advanced unresectable or metastatic soft tissue sarcomas (EudraCT 2009-014907-29). *J Clin Oncol.* 2015;33(suppl; abstr 10500).
3. Van der Graff WTA, Blay JY, Chawla SP, et al. Pazopanib for metastatic soft-tissue sarcoma (PALETTE): a randomised, double-blind, placebo-controlled phase 3 trial. *Lancet.* 2012;379(9829):1879–1886.

Question 21

1. Veltkamp SA, Meerum JM, van den Heuvel MM, van Boven HH, Schellens JH, Rodenhuis S. Severe pulmonary toxicity in patients with leiomyosarcoma after treatment with gemcitabine and docetaxel. *Invest New Drugs.* 2007;25(3):279–281.
2. Barlesi F, Villani P, Doddoli C, Gimenez C, Kleisbauer JP. Gemcitabine-induced severe pulmonary toxicity. *Fundam Clin Pharmacol.* 2004;18:85–91.
3. Vander Els NJ, Miller V. Successful treatment of gemcitabine toxicity with a brief course of oral corticosteroid therapy. *Chest.* 1998;114:1779–1781.
4. Boiselle PM, Morrin MM, Huberman MS. Gemcitabine pulmonary toxicity: CT features. *J Comput Assist Tomogr.* 2000;24:977–980.
5. Belknap SM, Kuzel TM, Yarnold PR, et al. Clinical features and correlates of gemcitabine-associated lung injury: findings from the RADAR project. *Cancer.* 2006;106:2051–2057.

Question 22

1. Joensuu H, Eriksson M, Hall KS, et al. One vs three years of adjuvant imatinib for operable gastrointestinal stromal tumor a randomized trial. *JAMA.* 2012;307(12):1265–1272.
2. Cioffi A, Maki RG. GI stromal tumors: 15 years of lessons from a rare cancer. *J Clin Oncol.* 2014;59:7344.
3. Maki R, Blay J-Y, Demetri GD, et al. A brief history of GIST: redefining the management of solid tumors. *Oncologist.* 2015;20:823–830.

Question 23

1. Joensuu H, Vehtari A, Riihimaki J, et al. Risk of recurrence of gastrointestinal stromal tumour after surgery: an analysis of pooled population-based cohorts. *Lancet Oncol.* 2012;13(3):265–274.
2. ESMO/European Sarcoma Network Working Group. Gastrointestinal stromal tumours: ESMO Clinical Practice Guidelines for diagnosis, treatment and follow-up. *Ann Oncol.* 2014;25(suppl 3):iii21–iii26.
3. De Matteo RP, Gold JS, Saran L, et al. Tumour mitotic rate, size and location independently predict recurrence after resection of primary gastrointestinal stromal tumour (GIST). *Cancer.* 2008;112:608–615.

Question 24

1. ESMO/European Sarcoma Network Working Group. Gastrointestinal stromal tumours: ESMO Clinical Practice Guidelines for diagnosis, treatment and follow-up. *Ann Oncol.* 2014;25(suppl 3):iii21–iii26.
2. Joensuu H, Eriksson M, Hall KS, et al. One vs three years of adjuvant imatinib for operable gastrointestinal stromal tumor a randomized trial. *JAMA.* 2012;307(12):1265–1272.
3. Joensuu H, Eriksson M, Hall KS, et al. Adjuvant imatinib for high-risk GI stromal tumor: analysis of a randomized trial. *J Clin Oncol (Current Abstracts).* 2016;34:244–250.

Question 25

1. Miettinen M, Wang ZF, Sarlomo-Rikala M, Osuch C, Rutkowski P, Lasota J. Succinate dehydrogenase-deficient GISTs: a clinicopathologic, immunohistochemical, and molecular genetic study of 66 gastric GISTs with predilection to young age. *Am J Surg Pathol.* 2011;35(11):1712–1721.

Question 26

1. Werewka-Macguza A, Osinski T, Chrzan R, Buczek M, Urbanik A. Characteristics of computed tomography imaging of gastrointestinal stromal tumor (GIST) and related diagnostic problems. *Pol J Radiol*. 2011;76(3):38–48.
2. Choi H, Charnsangavej C, Faria SC, et al. Correlation of computed tomography and positron emission tomography in patients with metastatic gastrointestinal stromal tumor treated at a single institution with imatinib mesylate: proposal of new computed tomography response criteria. *J Clin Oncol*. 2007;25(13):1753–1759.
3. Mabille M, Vanel D, Albiter M, et al. Follow-up of hepatic and peritoneal metastases of gastrointestinal tumors (GIST) under imatinib therapy requires different criteria of radiological evaluation (size is not everything!!!). *Eur J Radiol*. 2009;69(2):204–208.
4. Benjamin RS, Choi H, Macapinlac HA, et al. We should desist using RECIST, at least in GIST. *J Clin Oncol*. 2007;25(13):1760–1764.

Question 27

1. Corless CL, Ballman KV, Antonescu C, et al. Relation of tumor pathologic and molecular features to outcome after surgical resection of localized primary gastrointestinal stromal tumor (GIST): results of the intergroup phase III trial ACOSOG Z9001. *J Clin Oncol*. 2010;28:15s, Abstract 10006.
2. ESMO/European Sarcoma Network Working Group. Gastrointestinal stromal tumours: ESMO Clinical Practice Guidelines for diagnosis, treatment and follow-up. *Ann Oncol*. 2014;25(suppl 3):iii21–iii26.
3. Gold JS, Gonen M, Gutierrez A, et al. Development and validation of a prognostic nomogram for recurrence-free survival after complete surgical resection of localised primary gastrointestinal stromal tumour: a retrospective analysis. *Lancet Oncol*. 2009;10(11):1045–1052.
4. Chok AY, Goh BK, Koh YX, et al. Validation of the MSKCC gastrointestinal stromal tumor nomogram and comparison with other prognostication systems: single-institution experience with 289 patients. *Ann Surg Oncol*. 2015;22(11):3597–3605.

Question 28

1. Gaspar N, Hawkins DS, Dirksen U, et al. Ewing sarcoma: current management and future approaches through collaboration. *J Clin Oncol*. 2015;33(27):3036–3046.

Question 29

1. Fiorenza F, Abudu A, Grimer RJ, et al. Risk factors for survival and local control in chondrosarcoma of bone. *J Bone Joint Surg Br*. 2002;84:93–99.

Question 30

1. Isakoff MS, Bieloff SS, Meltzer P, Gorlick R. Osteosarcoma: current treatment and a collaborative pathway to success. *J Clin Oncol*. 2015;33(27):3029–3035.
2. Luetke A, Meyers PA, Lewis I, Juergens H. Osteosarcoma treatment—where do we stand? A state of the art review. *Cancer Treat Rev*. 2014;40:523–532.
3. Meyers PA, Schwartz CL, Krailo MD, et al. Osteosarcoma: the addition of muramyl tripeptide to chemotherapy improves overall survival—a report from the Children's Oncology Group. *J Clin Oncol*. 2008;26(4):633–638.

Question 31

1. Isakoff MS, Bielack SS, Meltzer P, Gorlick R. Osteosarcoma: current treatment and a collaborative pathway to success. *J Clin Oncol*. 2015;33(27):3029–3035.

Question 32

1. Gaspar N, Hawkins DS, Dirksen U, et al. Ewing sarcoma: current management and future approaches through collaboration. *J Clin Oncol*. 2015;33(27):3036–3046.

QUESTIONS

1. A 72-year-old man with no significant past medical history presents with worsening pain in his lower back. Computed tomography (CT) and bone scans show innumerable osteoblastic lesions throughout the appendicular skeleton. MRI of the spine reveals no evidence of cord compression. Prostate-specific antigen (PSA) is elevated at 107 ng/mL. Multiple attempts are made to biopsy the bone lesions, but insufficient samples are obtained for histological diagnosis. Which of the following is the next best step in management?
   A. Androgen deprivation therapy (ADT)
   B. ADT plus docetaxel
   C. Enzalutamide
   D. Abiraterone
   E. Carboplatin and paclitaxel

2. A 29-year-old man presents with worsening dyspnea on exertion and nonspecific chest discomfort. The workup includes a CT of the chest, abdomen, pelvis with intravenous (IV) contrast, which reveals mediastinal adenopathy measuring up to 3 cm in diameter, and no other suspicious lesions. Bronchoscopy with biopsy is performed, and the malignant cells obtained stain positive for OCT3/4 and SOX2. Which of the following should be included in the further evaluation of this patient?
   A. PET imaging
   B. Bone scan
   C. Testicular ultrasound, serum beta-hCG, LDH, and alpha fetoprotein (AFP)
   D. Pleural biopsy
   E. Retroperitoneal lymph node dissection

3. A 56-year-old woman with a history of a myocardial infarction requiring percutaneous coronary intervention with two drug-eluting stents 2 months ago presents with increasing abdominal girth and discomfort. A CT scan of the chest, abdomen, and pelvis with IV contrast shows diffuse peritoneal lesions. Diagnostic and therapeutic paracentesis reveals a low serum albumin-ascites gradient and positive fluid cytology for adenocarcinoma. Cells obtained from the ascitic fluid are too few for immunohistochemical analysis. CA-125 is elevated at 2300. Bilateral diagnostic mammography and breast MRI are negative. The patient is currently deemed too high of a surgical risk for any surgical interventions given her recent myocardial infarction. A colonoscopy 1 year ago was unremarkable. Which of the following is the most appropriate management?
   A. FOLFOX
   B. Carboplatin and paclitaxel
   C. Intraperitoneal cisplatin
   D. Olaparib
   E. Capecitabine

4. A 48 year old female presents with a left-sided axillary mass and no other abnormalities on physical exam. Ultrasound-guided fine needle aspiration reveals poorly differentiated adenocarcinoma. Immunohistochemical stains are positive for CK7 and negative for ER and PR. HER2/neu expression is 1+. Bilateral breast mammography, ultrasound, and MRI confirm the presence of the 1.5 cm node and do not reveal any other suspicious lesions. Positron emission tomography (PET)/CT scan shows focal uptake in the left axilla (SUVmax 15) but in no other locations. Which of the following is the next best step in management?
   A. Esophagogastroduodenoscopy, laryngoscopy, and bronchoscopy
   B. Bone scan
   C. Left modified radical mastectomy and axillary lymph node dissection
   D. Mediastinoscopy
   E. Whole body skin examination

5. A 64-year-old man with a 40-pack-year smoking history, multivessel coronary artery disease, and congestive heart failure (left ventricular ejection fraction of 30%) presents with dyspnea and nonproductive cough from a recurrent right-sided pleural effusion. Pleural fluid cytology from a thoracentesis specimen reveals epithelioid cells with positive immunohistochemical stains for CK5/6, WT1, and calretinin. CT of the chest, abdomen, and pelvis shows no other abnormalities other than the effusion. The patient is deemed not a surgical candidate due to his cardiac comorbidities. He has normal renal and hepatic function. Which of the following is the best treatment option for this patient?
   A. Carboplatin and pemetrexed
   B. Carboplatin and paclitaxel
   C. Carboplatin and gemcitabine
   D. Carboplatin and etoposide
   E. Pembrolizumab

6. A 68-year-old man is evaluated for nonspecific right upper quadrant abdominal pain. An ultrasound reveals multiple bilobar hypoechoic hepatic lesions measuring up to 4 cm in diameter. A PET-CT confirms the lesions seen on ultrasound, and they are suspicious for metastases with SUVmax up to 20, but no new lesions are identified. After two attempts, a CT-guided core liver biopsy reveals a poorly differentiated adenocarcinoma. Immunohistochemical stains are positive for CK20 and CDX-2, and negative for CK7. No viable tumor specimen remains for further analysis. Serum PSA is within normal limits. Colonoscopy and upper endoscopy are performed with no significant findings noted. What is the next best step in management?
   A. Repeat liver biopsy
   B. MRI liver
   C. FOLFOX and bevacizumab

D. Exploratory laparotomy
E. Fecal occult blood testing

7. A 57-year-old woman who has never smoked presents with a painless left-sided neck mass. Fine needle aspiration of a level 2 lymph node reveals squamous cell carcinoma that stains positive for p16 on immunohistochemistry. A PET-CT scan does not reveal the source of the primary lesion, and there is no evidence of distant metastatic disease. This malignancy should be approached most similarly to which of the following primary tumor sites?
A. Lung
B. Cervix
C. Breast
D. Esophageal
E. Head and neck

8. A 72-year-old man with a 30-pack-year smoking history presents with a 20-pound unintentional weight loss over the last 3 months. He is physically active and continues to walk 1 mile every day. PET-CT reveals multiple FDG-avid bilobar liver lesions (SUVmax 18), but no other areas of abnormal FDG uptake. Core biopsy of one of the liver lesions reveals poorly differentiated adenocarcinoma, and immunohistochemical stains are positive for TTF-1, CK7, and napsin A, and negative for chromogranin and synaptophysin. Testing for *EGFR* mutations, *ALK*, and *ROS-1* rearrangements are negative. PD-L1 staining is 0%. Brain MRI shows no abnormalities. Which of the following is the next best step in management?
A. Carboplatin, paclitaxel, and bevacizumab
B. Pembrolizumab
C. Cisplatin and etoposide
D. Gemcitabine and nab-paclitaxel
E. FOLFOX and bevacizumab

9. A 43-year-old man with history of HIV (CD4 count 160, viral load 8000, on highly active antiretroviral therapy) presents with left-sided inguinal swelling for 2 months. Core biopsy of a left inguinal node reveals poorly differentiated carcinoma, and immunohistochemical stains positive for CK5/6 and p63, and negative for CK7 and CK20. CT of the abdomen and pelvis with intravenous contrast shows no other lesions or lymphadenopathy, and physical exam of the penis, scrotum, and anus with anoscopy show no suspicious lesions. Inguinal lymph node dissection reveals a single 3.2 cm node with similar pathology and evidence of extranodal extension. Which of the following is the next best step in management?
A. Systemic chemotherapy with carboplatin and paclitaxel
B. Systemic chemotherapy with doxorubicin
C. Retroperitoneal lymph node dissection
D. Radiation therapy to the nodal basin
E. Observation

10. A 67-year-old woman with a 60-pack-year smoking history presents with a 15-pound unintentional weight loss and worsening right upper quadrant pain over the last month. CT of the chest, abdomen, and pelvis reveals multiple bilobar hepatic lesions and no other signs of malignancy. CT-guided core needle biopsy reveals poorly differentiated carcinoma cells that stain positive for synaptophysin and chromogranin on immunohistochemical analysis with a Ki67 proliferation index of 70%. A brain MRI is negative for metastatic disease, and PET-CT and octreotide scans only show the previously identified liver lesions. Which of the following is the next best step in management?

A. Octreotide
B. Everolimus
C. Temozolomide and capecitabine
D. Gemcitabine and nab-paclitaxel
E. Carboplatin/etoposide

11. A 72-year-old man without a significant past medical history presents with worsening abdominal pain and distention. Clinical exam is consistent with moderate ascites and no palpable masses. PET-CT reveals no specific findings. Diagnostic and therapeutic paracentesis reveals a low serum albumin-ascites gradient and positive fluid cytology for adenocarcinoma with positive immunohistochemical stains for CK20, CDX-2, and negative for CK7. Which of the following serum laboratory tests is most likely to be elevated in this patient?
A. CA 19-9
B. CA-125
C. PSA
D. Carcinoembryonic antigen (CEA)
E. AFP

12. A 58-year-old man with a 50-pack-year smoking history presents with an enlarged right cervical that he first noticed 2 months ago. A fine needle aspirate reveals squamous cell carcinoma. A triple endoscopy is recommended for this patient. Which of the following comprise a triple endoscopy?
A. Esophagogastroduodenoscopy, colonoscopy, and capsule endoscopy
B. Esophagogastroduodenoscopy, laryngoscopy, and bronchoscopy
C. Esophagogastroduodenoscopy, colonoscopy, and bronchoscopy
D. Diagnostic laparoscopy, thoracoscopy, and colonoscopy
E. Esophagogastroduodenoscopy, diagnostic laparoscopy, and thoracoscopy

13. A 63-year-old right-handed woman presents with worsening expressive aphasia over the last 3 weeks and a generalized headache. She is otherwise healthy without any significant past medical history. A head CT without intravenous contrast and subsequent brain MRI with and without contrast demonstrate a 3.7 cm left temporal mass with ring enhancement, T1 hypointense, T2 hyperintense, with minimal vasogenic edema and minimal central necrosis. Brain biopsy of the mass shows malignant cells that stain positive for CD45, CD20, and MUM-1. Cerebrospinal fluid cytology is negative. PET-CT does not reveal any significant findings. Which of the following is the most appropriate initial treatment for this patient?
A. Chemotherapy regimen including high-dose methotrexate 8 g/m^2 with leucovorin rescue and rituximab
B. Concurrent chemoradiation with temozolomide
C. Surgical resection of the left temporal mass
D. Whole brain radiation therapy
E. High-dose chemotherapy regimen with stem cell rescue

14. Which of the following is true regarding the use of molecular profiling in the management of patients with a carcinoma of unknown primary?
A. Molecular profiling of tumors in patients with carcinoma of unknown primary leads to a survival benefit compared with immunohistochemical analysis alone.
B. Molecular profiling has the potential to identify biomarkers with druggable targets and should be considered in patients with carcinoma of unknown primary, but more research must be performed to demonstrate a

survival benefit compared with immunohistochemical analyses alone.

C. *BRAF* mutations identified by molecular profiling respond to targeted inhibition with vemurafenib.

D. Molecular profiling platforms are Food and Drug Administration (FDA) approved for use in the diagnosis of carcinomas of unknown primary.

E. Molecular profiling is a cost-effective tool in the diagnosis of carcinomas of unknown primary.

15. What percentage of carcinomas of unknown primary are adenocarcinomas?
A. 2%–5%
B. 15%–20%
C. 40%–50%
D. 60%–70%
E. 90%–100%

ANSWERS

1. B

The patient has metastatic prostate cancer with multiple bone metastases and should be treated with combined ADT and docetaxel per the results of the CHAARTED trial, which demonstrated significant improvement in overall survival compared with ADT alone. Tissue diagnosis is typically preferable before initiating chemotherapy; however, an elevated PSA with osteoblastic lesions in an older man is consistent with a diagnosis of metastatic prostate cancer. Enzalutamide and abiraterone are approved in metastatic castrate-resistant prostate cancer only. Carboplatin and paclitaxel would be an appropriate regimen for metastatic squamous cell carcinoma of unknown primary.

2. C

This patient's clinical presentation is consistent with a stage III embryonal carcinoma, a nonseminomatous germ cell tumor, due to nonregional nodal metastatic disease. Recognition of the diagnosis of a germ cell tumor is important, as it is often curable with systemic chemotherapy despite the presence of metastatic disease. OCT3/4 and SOX2 are most commonly expressed in embryonal carcinoma. Upfront PET and bone scans are not indicated in the workup for patients with germ cell tumors (PET-CT scans can be useful later on in the evaluation of residual masses following primary chemotherapy). Pleural biopsy has no role in the evaluation of this patient. Retroperitoneal lymph node dissection is indicated in patients with nonseminomatous germ cell tumors with residual retroperitoneal masses following systemic chemotherapy.

3. B

The patient has an adenocarcinoma of unknown primary with peritoneal carcinomatosis and elevated CA-125. Given this presentation, the patient should be treated as if she has an ovarian primary. Treatment would ideally involve optimal surgical debulking with overall curative intent; however, any potential surgical intervention will have to be postponed in this patient due to a recent myocardial infarction. Thus, systemic therapy with carboplatin and paclitaxel is most appropriate at this time. FOLFOX chemotherapy would be a good choice if she had metastatic colorectal cancer, but her presentation is more consistent with ovarian cancer, and treatment for metastatic colorectal cancer with peritoneal carcinomatosis would be with palliative intent. Intraperitoneal cisplatin is only indicated for patients with optimally debulked stage II or III ovarian cancer, and is generally given in combination with intravenous cisplatin and paclitaxel. Olaparib would be indicated only after failure of multiple lines of therapy for ovarian cancer. Capecitabine would be an appropriate choice for metastatic breast cancer with peritoneal carcinomatosis.

4. C

Adenocarcinoma within an isolated axillary lymph node frequently represents occult breast cancer in women. This patient with clinical T0N1M0 disease should undergo either mastectomy with axillary lymph node dissection, or axillary lymph node dissection followed by radiation. Endoscopies may be useful in evaluating an occult primary in a cervical lymph node, but they should not be utilized in this patient. A bone scan is unlikely to reveal occult osseous metastases in the setting of a negative PET-CT. Mediastinoscopy is used to evaluate mediastinal nodal disease in patients with lung cancer and does not have a role in this scenario. Skin examination may be useful in finding a primary melanoma lesion, but it is more likely that this patient has axillary breast cancer given histology consistent with adenocarcinoma.

5. A

The patient's clinical presentation is consistent with malignant pleural mesothelioma (MPM) as evidenced by pleural fluid cytology positive for CK5/6, WT1, and calretinin. Mesothelin would also likely be positive. Diagnosis may also warrant a video-assisted thoracoscopic surgery (VATS) with pleural biopsy; however, this patient has been deemed not to be a surgical candidate. The standard of care treatment for inoperable MPM consists of platinum plus pemetrexed, with or without bevacizumab. In this patient with multiple comorbidities, carboplatin may be used instead of cisplatin, based on multiple phase II studies. Carboplatin in combination with paclitaxel, gemcitabine, or etoposide would be appropriate treatments in metastatic non-small cell lung cancer (in the absence of an actionable *EGFR* mutation and *ALK* or *ROS1* rearrangements). Pembrolizumab is indicated in untreated patients with metastatic lung adenocarcinoma with PD-L1 expression above 50% and negative or unknown *EGFR*, *ALK*, and *ROS1* status.

6. C

The patient has an adenocarcinoma of unknown primary with multiple liver metastases. Given the immunohistochemical staining pattern, the patient most likely has metastatic colorectal cancer. Thus, the patient should receive systemic chemotherapy with a fluoropyrimidine-based regimen. A repeat liver biopsy is unlikely to yield additional information. Liver MRI may help distinguish metastases from multifocal hepatocellular carcinoma, but this diagnosis is unlikely as the tumor is CK20 negative. It is unlikely that an exploratory laparotomy would reveal new diagnostic information, and it would not change the staging as metastatic disease has already been demonstrated. Fecal occult blood testing is not indicated in the setting of negative endoscopies, and metastatic small bowel adenocarcinoma would be managed similarly to metastatic colorectal cancer.

7. E

The patient's isolated p16 positive squamous cell carcinoma in a cervical lymph node most likely reflects a human papillomavirus (HPV)-associated head and neck primary tumor. Thus, management options for this patient include primary neck dissection followed by adjuvant radiation with or without chemotherapy or upfront chemoradiation followed by observation or neck dissection. Cervical and anal squamous cell carcinoma may also be HPV-associated and stain positive for p16, but there would likely be other evidence of regional lymphadenopathy. Breast, lung, and esophageal cancers are generally not associated with HPV.

8. A

The patient has multiple liver metastases from an occult lung adenocarcinoma, manifested by positive TTF-1, CK7, and napsin A staining in a patient with a heavy smoking history. As the PD-L1 expression is below 50%, first-line pembrolizumab is not indicated. Standard of care for previously untreated metastatic non-small lung cancer would thus consist of a platinum (cisplatin or carboplatin) in combination with bevacizumab and paclitaxel or pemetrexed. Chromogranin and synaptophysin stains would be positive in a patient with small cell lung cancer, in which case cisplatin and etoposide would be appropriate treatment for extensive stage disease. Gemcitabine and nab-paclitaxel or FOLFOX and bevacizumab would be appropriate regimens for patients with previously untreated metastatic pancreatic adenocarcinoma or metastatic colorectal adenocarcinoma, respectively.

9. D

The patient has squamous cell carcinoma of unknown primary, manifested by positive staining for CK5/6 and p63, and negative for CK7 and CK20. This cancer likely arose from the anogenital tract. He only has one isolated area of unilateral inguinal lymph node involvement, but extranodal extension places him at a higher risk of cancer recurrence; thus, adjuvant radiation therapy to the nodal basin should be offered. Carboplatin and paclitaxel could be an appropriate option following radiation therapy. Doxorubicin is an appropriate treatment for systemic Kaposi sarcoma, which this patient does not have. Retroperitoneal dissection may be indicated in germ cell tumors, but not in this case. Observation would be inappropriate given extranodal extension seen at the time of lymph node dissection.

10. E

The patient has metastatic poorly differentiated neuroendocrine carcinoma of unknown primary as the tumor stains positive for synaptophysin and chromogranin on immunohistochemistry. It is a high grade, aggressive tumor with a high Ki67 proliferation index of 70%. Regimens designed for extensive stage small cell lung cancer (platinum and etoposide) are generally used for treatment of this disease. Octreotide can be used in patients with unresectable or metastatic gastrointestinal neuroendocrine carcinoma or carcinoid syndrome, but would be inappropriate in this patient with aggressive small cell histology. Everolimus and temozolomide and capecitabine are options in refractory unresectable or metastatic gastrointestinal neuroendocrine carcinoma, and gemcitabine and nab-paclitaxel is a treatment option in patients with metastatic pancreatic adenocarcinoma.

11. D

This patient presents with malignant ascites and positive ascitic fluid cytology for CK20 and CDX-2, which are indicative of metastatic colorectal adenocarcinoma. Serum CEA is most commonly elevated in these patients. CA19-9 is elevated in pancreaticobiliary cancers, PSA in prostate cancer, CA125 in ovarian cancer, and AFP in hepatocellular carcinoma.

12. B

Triple endoscopy for the workup of occult head and neck squamous cell carcinoma consists of esophagogastroduodenoscopy, laryngoscopy, and bronchoscopy to differentiate squamous cell carcinoma of the esophagus, oropharynx/larynx, and lung, respectively.

13. A

The patient has a primary central nervous system lymphoma (PCNSL) as evidenced by characteristic findings on MRI and immunohistochemical staining pattern. Appropriate induction therapy consists of high-dose methotrexate (MTX) plus rituximab (temozolomide can also be included). Another induction option is MTX 3.5 g/m^2 with radiation and either vincristine, procarbazine, and cytarabine (with or without rituximab), or ifosfamide. Chemoradiation with temozolomide is appropriate for the treatment of glioblastoma multiforme following surgical resection. Surgery has no established role in the management of PCNSL in the absence of impending herniation. Whole brain radiation therapy is a viable option for patients who would not tolerate chemotherapy, and a high-dose chemotherapy regimen with stem cell rescue can be used as consolidation therapy for patients in complete remission following high-dose MTX.

14. B

Molecular profiling has become more commonplace in the clinic for use in carcinomas of unknown primary. In a single-arm prospective study, a 92-gene assay was associated with a median overall survival of 12.5 months in carcinoma of unknown primary patients treated with assay-directed therapy. However, there are no prospective randomized trials demonstrating such a survival benefit compared with immunohistochemical analysis, and no cost-effectiveness has been shown. *BRAF* V600E mutations can predict the response to single-agent vemurafenib in metastatic melanoma, but this finding does not hold true for metastatic *BRAF*-mutant colorectal cancer. There is no specific FDA approval for this technology for use in the diagnosis of carcinoma of unknown primary.

15. C

Approximately 48% of carcinomas of unknown primary are adenocarcinomas. Squamous cell carcinoma accounts for around 14%, while epithelial/unspecified and undifferentiated tumors account for 28% and 2%, respectively. In the United States, 33,770 cancers annually are classified as being from an unspecified primary site.

REFERENCES

Question 1

1. Sweeney CJ, Chen YH, Carducci M, et al. Chemohormonal therapy in metastatic hormone-sensitive prostate cancer. *N Engl J Med.* 2015;373(8):737–746.

Question 2

1. Looijenga LH, Stoop H, Biermann K. Testicular: biology and biomarkers. *Virchows Arch.* 2014;464(3):301–313.

Question 4

1. NCCN. Breast cancer version 2.2017. NCCN clinical practice guidelines in oncology. <https://www.nccn.org/professionals/physician_gls/pdf/breast.pdf>; Accessed 02.05.17.

Question 5

1. Conner JR, Hornick JL. Metastatic carcinoma of unknown primary: diagnostic approach using immunohistochemistry. *Adv Anat Pathol.* 2015;22(3):149–167.
2. NCCN. Malignant pleural mesothelioma version 1.2017. NCCN clinical practice guidelines in oncology. <https://www.nccn.org/professionals/physician_gls/pdf/mpm.pdf>; Accessed 04.05.17.

Question 7

1. Galloway TJ, Ridge JA. Management of squamous cancer metastatic to cervical nodes with an unknown primary site. *J Clin Oncol.* 2015;33(29):3328–3337.

Question 8

1. NCCN. Non-small cell lung cancer version 5.2017. NCCN clinical practice guidelines in oncology. <https://www.nccn.org/professionals/physician_gls/pdf/nscl.pdf>; Accessed 03.05.17.

Question 9

1. NCCN. Occult primary version 2.2017. NCCN clinical practice guidelines in oncology. <https://www.nccn.org/professionals/physician_gls/pdf/occult.pdf>; Accessed 04.05.17.

Question 10

1. NCCN. Neuroendocrine tumors version 2.2017. NCCN clinical practice guidelines in oncology. <https://www.nccn.org/professionals/physician_gls/pdf/neuroendocrine.pdf>; Accessed 04.05.17.

Question 12

1. Guardiola E, Chaigneau L, Villanueva C, Pivot X. Is there a role for triple endoscopy as part of staging for head and neck cancer? *Curr Opin Otolaryngol Head Neck Surg.* 2006;14(2):85–88.

2. McGuirt WF. Panendoscopy as a screening examination for simultaneous primary tumors in head and neck cancer: a prospective sequential study and review of the literature. *Laryngoscope.* 1982;92:569–576.
3. Atkinson D, Fleming S, Weaver A. Triple endoscopy: a valuable procedure in head and neck surgery. *Am J Surg.* 1982;144:416–419.

Question 13

1. NCCN. Central nervous system cancers 1.2016. NCCN clinical practice guidelines in oncology. <https://www.nccn.org/professionals/physician_gls/pdf/cns.pdf>; Accessed 05.05.17.
2. Citterio G, Reni M, Gatta G, Ferreri AJM. Primary central nervous system lymphoma. *Crit Rev Oncol Hematol.* 2017;113:97–110.

Question 14

1. Greco FA, Rubin MS, Boccia RV, et al. Molecular gene expression profiling to predict tissue of origin and direct site-specific therapy in unknown primary cancer: accuracy of tissue of origin prediction. *Oncologist.* 2010;15(5):500–506.
2. Varadhachary G. New strategies for carcinoma of unknown primary: the role of tissue-of-origin molecular profiling. *Clin Cancer Res.* 2013;19(15):4027–4033.
3. Mao M, Tian F, Mariadason JM, et al. Resistance to BRAF inhibition in BRAF-mutant colon cancer can be overcome with PI3K inhibition or demethylating agents. *Clin Cancer Res.* 2013;19(3):657–667.
4. Varadhachary GR, Raber MN. Cancer of unknown primary site. *N Engl J Med.* 2014;371(8):757–765.

Question 15

1. Mnatsakanyan E, Tung WC, Caine B, Smith-Gagen J. Cancer of unknown primary: time trends in incidence, United States. *Cancer Causes Control.* 2014;25(6):747–757.
2. American Cancer Society, Cancer Statistics Center. <https://cancerstatisticscenter.cancer.org>; 2017 Accessed 04.05.17.

Malignancies of the Central Nervous System

Fabio M. Iwamoto and Andrew B. Lassman

Primary

QUESTIONS

1. A 43-year-old woman with a history of a T2N1M0 infiltrating ductal carcinoma (ER negative, PR negative, and HER2 positive [IHC 3+]) underwent a mastectomy and chemotherapy with trastuzumab, doxorubicin, cyclophosphamide, and paclitaxel in 2012. She had been in remission for 5 years and presented with progressive headaches for 1 month, and for the last 2 days, she developed with nausea, vomiting, and blurry vision. On the exam, she has papilledema and her gait is impaired. A brain MRI with gadolinium showed a noncommunicating hydrocephalus and leptomeningeal enhancement but no brain metastases. She then underwent a lumbar puncture with opening pressure of 30 cm of water, and CSF cytology was positive for carcinoma. Which of the following is correct about intrathecal chemotherapy?
   A. Intra-CSF chemotherapy through lumbar puncture or through an Ommaya reservoir is contraindicated because of the increase intracranial pressure and hydrocephalus.
   B. Intrathecal chemotherapy with methotrexate is indicated for this specific patient because of its activity in breast cancer.
   C. Recent studies established intrathecal trastuzumab with pertuzumab as the best option in this situation.
   D. Intra-CSF chemotherapy through an Ommaya reservoir is the only acceptable way to deliver intra-CSF chemotherapy in patients with hydrocephalus.
   E. Intrathecal chemotherapy for solid tumors can provide long-term disease-free survival due to the high concentration of chemotherapy directly into the CSF.

2. A 61-year-old woman presented with progressive apathy, personality changes, and aphasia and underwent a brain MRI, which showed a large left-frontal mass originating from the dura mater but invading the brain and causing vasogenic brain edema. She underwent a craniotomy and partial tumor resection because the portion of the tumor invading the brain could not be safely resected. Pathology was compatible with a WHO grade 3 (anaplastic) meningioma. The tumor had rhabdoid fea-

tures and ≥20 mitoses per high-powered field. What is the recommended next step for this patient?
   A. Whole brain radiation
   B. Observation only
   C. Involved field radiation to the residual tumor and tumor margin
   D. Sunitinib
   E. Trabectedin

3. A 58-year-old man presented with word-finding difficulties and progressive aphasia. A brain MRI showed a 3-cm left temporal enhancing mass with necrotic component and surrounding vasogenic edema. He underwent an awake craniotomy and had an almost complete macroscopic resection of the enhancing tumor. Pathology was compatible with a glioblastoma with MGMT promoter methylation and positive for the activating mutation of EGFR caused by deletion of exons 2–7 (EGFR variant III, EGFRvIII). He underwent standard therapy with involved field radiation to the surgical bed at a total dose of 6000 cGy over 30 treatments with daily temozolomide at 75 mg/m^2 for 6 weeks. He is now 4 weeks from the end of radiation and is clinically well without any neurological deficits. His current brain MRI report describes worsening of enhancement within margins of the surgical cavity, which now measures 1.5 cm compared with less than 0.5 cm on the immediate postsurgical scan. What is the best next step for this patient?
   A. Observation only
   B. Proceed with adjuvant temozolomide and consider tumor treating fields (TTFields) with early MRI follow-up in 1–2 months
   C. Second-line therapy with Avastin
   D. Second-line therapy with erlotinib or another targeted anti-EGFR therapy
   E. Radiosurgery

4. A 55-year-old woman had a successful initial treatment of her primary CNS lymphoma with a combination of chemotherapy with high-dose methotrexate, high-dose cytarabine, rituximab, and radiation, and she has been in clinical remission for 18 months. She initially presented with right-sided hemiparesis and aphasia, but the neurological deficits resolved completely, and she continues to have no deficits on the bedside exam. For the last 2 months, however, she has progressive visual floaters and was diagnosed with uveitis by her local ophthalmologist. She was started on topical dexamethasone eyedrops since last week with partial improvement of the symptoms. What are the most likely diagnosis and the next diagnostic procedure?

A. Autoimmune uveitis triggered by her prior chemo-radiation treatment, so the patient should continue topical dexamethasone eyedrops further until complete resolution of symptoms and follow-up with her ophthalmologist

B. Early sign of CSF involvement by lymphoma, and patient should get a lumbar puncture with cytology and flow cytometry

C. Either radiation or high-dose cytarabine eye toxicity, so she should continue topical dexamethasone eyedrops and reassess with her ophthalmologist

D. Recurrent brain involvement by lymphoma and a brain MRI with gadolinium

E. Ocular involvement by lymphoma and slit lamp exam by an ophthalmologist

5. A 20-year-old man presented with progressive headaches, ataxia, and dysarthria. A brain MRI showed a 3-cm right cerebellar lesion with gadolinium enhancement and diffusion restriction. He underwent a craniotomy and gross total resection of the tumor, and pathology was compatible with a medulloblastoma (WHO grade IV). His total spine MRI with gadolinium and his CSF cytology were negative for tumor. What is the recommended treatment for this patient with standard risk medulloblastoma and a gross totally resected tumor?

A. Involved field radiation to the margins of the tumor with temozolomide

B. Involved field radiation to the margins of the tumor followed by observation

C. Craniospinal radiation with lomustine, cisplatin, and vincristine

D. Chemotherapy followed by autologous stem cell transplant

E. Chemotherapy with lomustine, cisplatin, and vincristine without radiation

6. A 60-year-old previously healthy man presented with a 1-month history of rapidly progressive short-term memory loss, personality changes, and headaches. A brain MRI showed a diffusely enhancing and diffusion restricted lesion within the splenium of the corpus callosum with surrounding vasogenic edema. A stereotactic brain biopsy showed a diffuse large B-cell lymphoma positive for MUM1 and negative for BCL-6, and CD10 and CD138. In situ hybridization for EBER-1–mRNA was negative. Extent of disease workup showed no ocular involvement by a slit-lamp exam, CSF cytology and flow cytometry were negative, and body PET-CT and bone marrow biopsy were negative. Patient was started on dexamethasone with neurological and performance status improvement. He had no history of iatrogenic immunosuppression, his serum HIV was negative, and the diagnosis was compatible with a primary central nervous system lymphoma in an immunocompetent individual. What is the best first step in treatment?

A. Brain irradiation as this is a stage I_E diffuse large B-cell lymphoma

B. R-CHOP with possible addition of lenalidomide because this is a nongerminal center diffuse large B-cell lymphoma

C. Intrathecal or intra-Ommaya methotrexate as this type of stage I_E diffuse large B-cell lymphoma does not require systemic chemotherapy

D. High-dose methotrexate in combination with other drugs such as rituximab, high-dose cytarabine, and thiotepa

E. Autologous stem cell transplant

7. A 27-year-man was diagnosed with tuberous sclerosis as a child when he presented with seizures, facial angiofibromas, cognitive impairment, and retinal and brain hamartomas. He was lost to follow-up and was admitted through the emergency room because of progressive headaches and left hemiparesis. His brain MRI showed a 5-cm diffusely enhancing lesion in the deep right cerebral hemisphere and mild hydrocephalus. Patient underwent a partial resection of the tumor. Pathology was compatible with a subependymal giant cell astrocytoma. What is the best next step for this patient?

A. Involved field radiation to the residual tumor

B. Involved field radiation with temozolomide as a radiosensitizing agent

C. Observation only

D. Lomustine, cisplatin, and vincristine

E. Everolimus

ANSWERS

1. A

The correct response is intra-CSF chemotherapy through lumbar puncture or through an Ommaya reservoir is contraindicated because of the increased intracranial pressure and hydrocephalus. Increased intracranial pressure or hydrocephalus are contraindications for intrathecal or intra-Ommaya chemotherapy, because they imply abnormal CSF flow, which compromises CSF drug distribution, treatment efficacy, and significantly increases neurotoxicity at the site of CSF injection. Intra-CSF chemotherapy is more established in certain subtypes of leukemias and lymphomas, and no randomized trial has cleared demonstrated a survival benefit in leptomeningeal metastases from solid tumors. Intrathecal trastuzumab is currently in early phase trials for HER2 positive leptomeningeal metastases, but no efficacy data are available. Leptomeningeal metastases tend to be a terminal event in metastatic cancer patients; the median survival of solid tumors leptomeningeal metastases was only 2.3 months in a large retrospective series.

2. C

The correct answer is involved field radiation to the residual tumor and tumor margin. Meningiomas are graded in the WHO classification as benign (grade I, about 80% of cases), atypical (grade II, 17% of cases), and anaplastic (grade III, 3% of cases). Malignant meningiomas are locally aggressive neoplasms with a very high rate of recurrence or progression, even after gross total resection. Distant systemic metastases are uncommon. Adjuvant focal RT is a standard component of initial management for all malignant meningiomas, regardless of the extent of resection, to improve local control and overall survival. In a series of 63 patients with anaplastic (WHO grade III) meningiomas treated with surgery and radiation, recurrence-free survival rates at 2, 5, and 10 years after initial therapy were 80%, 57%, and 40%, respectively, and overall survival rates were 82%, 61%, and 40%. There are no known medical treatments with activity against meningiomas.

3. B

The correct answer is to proceed with adjuvant temozolomide and consider TTFields with early MRI follow-up in 1–2 months. It is well known that chemoradiotherapy with temozolomide for glioblastoma patients is associated with progressive and enhancing lesions on MRI, noted immediately after the end of treatment, which are not related to tumor progression, but which are a treatment effect. This so-called pseudoprogression can occur in up to 20% of patients who have been treated with temozolomide chemoradiotherapy and can explain about half of all cases of increasing lesions after the end of this treatment. These lesions decrease in size or stabilize without additional treatments and often remain clinically asymptomatic. Pseudoprogression occurs more often in glioblastomas with methylated MGMT promoter and continuation of temozolomide and clinical confirmation of pseudoprogression may be associated with better outcomes. Moving to a second-line therapy too quickly based on first MRI post chemoradiotherapy is not recommended in this situation, especially when MRI changes are asymptomatic. The recent trial EF-14 showed that addition of TTFields to adjuvant temozolomide after chemoradiotherapy improves outcomes. Median overall survival was 20.5 months in the TTFields plus temozolomide group ($n = 196$) and 15.6 months in the temozolomide alone group ($n = 84$) (HR = 0.64, $P = 0.004$). TTFields have been FDA approved for the first-line glioblastoma therapy based on these results. There are no targeted drugs with proven activity against EGFRviii glioblastomas, and trials of EGFR tyrosine kinase inhibitors and peptide vaccine rindopepimut have been disappointing.

4. E

The correct response is ocular involvement by lymphoma and slit lamp exam by an ophthalmologist. About 30% of the recurrences of primary central nervous system (CNS) lymphoma involve the eyes. Visual floaters, uveitis, and visual loss are the most common presentations. Slit lamp is a low-power microscope combined with a high-intensity light source that can be focused as a thin beam to better exam the eye. Ocular involvement usually affects the posterior segment of the eye, including the vitreous, choroid, or retina, with subsequent development of uveitis, exudative retinal detachment, and retinal or vitreous hemorrhages. Diagnosis can be made clinically with the slit lamp in patients with known primary CNS lymphoma or by biopsy of the involved vitreous, choroid, or retina in less typical cases.

5. C

The correct answer is craniospinal radiation with lomustine, cisplatin, and vincristine. Patients older than 3 years of age at diagnosis with totally or near totally resected, nondisseminated disease (average risk) still need to undergo craniospinal radiation because of the high risk of neuroaxis tumor dissemination. Younger patients are at highest risk of severe cognitive, developmental, and endocrinological abnormalities with craniospinal radiation. Over the last few decades, craniospinal radiation doses have been reduced from 3600 cGy to 2340 cGy and chemotherapy has been added. The most commonly used regimen involves lomustine, cisplatin, and vincristine. The 5-year event-free survival and overall survival are above 80% for standard risk medulloblastoma patients treated with craniospinal radiation and chemotherapy.

6. D

The correct is answer is high-dose methotrexate in combination with other drugs such as rituximab, high-dose cytarabine, and thiotepa. Until the 1990s, primary

central nervous system lymphoma was often treated with whole brain radiation (WBRT) alone. Although this is a radiosensitive tumor, relapses were frequent, and the median survival on the RTOG 8315 trial was only 11.6 months. The addition of a high-dose methotrexate-based regimen to WBRT on the single arm RTOG 9310 trial increased the median overall survival to 36.9 months. The best combination of drugs in addition to high-dose methotrexate is not defined, but randomized trials through the IESLG showed that addition of high-dose cytarabine, rituximab, and thiotepa improved outcomes. CHOP has no role in PCNSL due to poor blood-brain barrier penetration and a negative randomized trial showing its lack of efficacy. Intra-CSF therapy has very limited penetration into the brain parenchyma disease but could be useful in patients with positive CSF. Autologous stem cell transplant is under investigation as a consolidation regimen after induction with high-dose methotrexate-based regimens.

7. E

The correct answer is the mammalian target of rapamycin (mTOR) inhibitor everolimus. Tuberous sclerosis complex is a genetic disorder leading to constitutive activation of mTOR and growth of benign tumors in several organs. In the brain, growth of subependymal giant cell astrocytomas can cause life-threatening symptoms such as hydrocephalus, requiring surgery. EXIST-1 was a double-blind, placebo-controlled, phase 3 trial, where patients (aged 0–65 years) were randomly assigned, in a 2:1 ratio to oral everolimus 4·5 mg/m² per day (titrated to achieve blood trough concentrations of 5–15 ng/mL) or placebo. In addition, 117 patients were randomly assigned to everolimus ($n=78$) or placebo ($n=39$). There were 27 (35%) patients in the everolimus group had at least 50% reduction in the volume of subependymal giant cell astrocytomas versus none in the placebo group ($P<.0001$).

REFERENCES

Question 1

1. Clarke JL, Perez HR, Jacks LM, et al. Leptomeningeal metastases in the MRI era. *Neurology*. 2010;74:1449–1454.

Question 2

1. Sughrue ME, Sanai N, Shangari G, et al. Outcome and survival following primary and repeat surgery for World Health Organization Grade III meningiomas. *J Neurosurg*. 2010;113:202–209.
2. Iwamoto FM. Comment: medical therapy for recurrent or progressive meningiomas remains elusive. *Neurology*. 2015;84:285.

Question 3

1. Brandsma D, Stalpers L, Taal W, et al. Clinical features, mechanisms, and management of pseudoprogression in malignant gliomas. *Lancet Oncol*. 2008;9:453–461.
2. Brandes AA, Franceschi E, Tosoni A, et al. MGMT promoter methylation status can predict the incidence and outcome of pseudoprogression after concomitant radiochemotherapy in newly diagnosed glioblastoma patients. *J Clin Oncol*. 2008;26:2192–2197.
3. Stupp R, Taillibert S, Kanner AA, et al. Maintenance therapy with tumor-treating fields plus temozolomide vs temozolomide alone for glioblastoma: a randomized clinical trial. *JAMA*. 2015;314:2535–2543.

Question 4

1. Grimm SA, McCannel CA, Omuro AM, et al. Primary CNS lymphoma with intraocular involvement: International PCNSL Collaborative Group Report. *Neurology*. 2008;71:1355–1360.

Question 5

1. Packer RJ, Gajjar A, Vezina G, et al. Phase III study of craniospinal radiation therapy followed by adjuvant chemotherapy for newly diagnosed average-risk medulloblastoma. *J Clin Oncol.* 2006;24:4202–4208.

Question 6

1. Nelson DF, Martz KL, Bonner H, et al. Non-Hodgkin's lymphoma of the brain: can high dose, large volume radiation therapy improve survival? Report on a prospective trial by the Radiation Therapy Oncology Group (RTOG): RTOG 8315. *Int J Radiat Oncol Biol Phys.* 1992;23:9–17.
2. DeAngelis LM, Seiferheld W, Schold SC, et al. Combination chemotherapy and radiotherapy for primary central nervous system lymphoma: Radiation Therapy Oncology Group Study 93-10. *J Clin Oncol.* 2002;20:4643–4648.
3. Citterio G, Reni M, Ferreri AJ. Present and future treatment options for primary CNS lymphoma. *Expert Opin Pharmacother.* 2015;16:2569–2579.

4. Ferreri AJ, Reni M, Foppoli M, et al. High-dose cytarabine plus high-dose methotrexate versus high-dose methotrexate alone in patients with primary CNS lymphoma: a randomised phase 2 trial. *Lancet.* 2009;374:1512–1520.
5. Mead GM, Bleehen NM, Gregor A, et al. A medical research council randomized trial in patients with primary cerebral non-Hodgkin lymphoma: cerebral radiotherapy with and without cyclophosphamide, doxorubicin, vincristine, and prednisone chemotherapy. *Cancer.* 2000;89:1359–1370.

Question 7

1. Franz DN, Belousova E, Sparagana S, et al. Efficacy and safety of everolimus for subependymal giant cell astrocytomas associated with tuberous sclerosis complex (EXIST-1): a multicentre, randomised, placebo-controlled phase 3 trial. *Lancet.* 2013;381: 125–132.

Metastatic

QUESTIONS

1. A 45-year-old woman had a seizure. Noncontrast CT of the head shows a hypodense abnormality in the right frontal lobe with small internal foci of calcification. Brain MRI shows a 3-cm lesion that is hyperintense on T2 sequences with subtle enhancement following injection of gadolinium contrast. Gross-total resection demonstrates anaplastic oligodendroglioma (World Health Organization grade III). Molecular analyses demonstrate 1p19q co-deletion, IDH1 mutation, and MGMT promoter methylation. Seizures are well controlled with levetiracetam without other signs or symptoms. Performance status is normal. What phase III supported treatment do you recommend?
   A. Observation
   B. Bevacizumab
   C. Radiotherapy (RT) before/after chemotherapy with procarbazine, lomustine (CCNU), and vincristine ("PCV")
   D. RT alone
   E. Temozolomide alone

2. A 60-year-old woman suffered a generalized convulsion (seizure) while driving. Imaging showed a heterogeneously enhancing mass in the left frontal lobe. Resection demonstrated glioblastoma (GBM). Molecular analysis demonstrated no mutation in IDH and no methylation of the MGMT promoter but high expression of PDL1. She is on phenytoin for seizures. Her performance status is normal. Which of the following do you recommend?
   A. Temozolomide
   B. Bevacizumab
   C. RT and concurrent temozolomide followed by adjuvant temozolomide and NovoTTF
   D. RT
   E. RT and temozolomide and either nivolumab or pembrolizumab

3. A 50-year-old man has a GBM that recurred after RT+ concurrent temozolomide and 3 cycles of post-RT temozolomide. Reresection 1 week ago demonstrated recurrent tumor. His Karnofsky Performance Status is 90. What do you recommend?

A. Lomustine and bevacizumab to start next week
B. Carboplatin alone
C. Observation
D. Resume temozolomide alone
E. Lomustine alone

4. A 45-year-old man has headaches leading to an MRI. There was a partially enhancing mass, subtotally resected. Histology shows WHO grade III anaplastic astrocytoma. 1p19q FISH shows no deletion of either allele, and MGMT promoter is unmethylated. His KPS is 70. What do you recommend?
   A. Bevacizumab
   B. Temozolomide
   C. RT and concurrent temozolomide followed by adjuvant temozolomide
   D. Observation
   E. Ipilimumab

5. A 50-year-old man had a seizure. Imaging shows a non-enhancing mass, 3-cm, confined to one hemisphere. Incomplete resection demonstrates a low-grade (WHO-grade II) oligodendroglioma with 1p19q co-deletion, *IDH* mutation, and *MGMT* promoter methylation. Seizures are well controlled with levetiracetam, and performance status is normal. What do you recommend?
   A. Bevacizumab
   B. 60 Gy radiotherapy followed by chemotherapy with PCV
   C. Carboplatin
   D. 54 Gy radiotherapy
   E. 54 Gy radiotherapy followed by chemotherapy with PCV

6. A 50-year-old man has lung adenocarcinoma. He is a heavy smoker, and tissue obtained at resection demonstrates no actionable mutations in EGFR, ALK, or other genes. Following systemic therapy with carboplatin and pemetrexed, he has stable disease. However, 12 months after diagnosis, he presents with word finding difficulty. Brain imaging by contrast enhanced MRI discloses one enhancing lesion near the surface of the left frontal lobe. Systemic restaging is stable without any other sites of disease outside the lungs or the brain. What do you recommend for treatment of the brain metastasis?
   A. 30 Gy of whole brain radiotherapy (WBRT)
   B. 60 Gy of WBRT
   C. Resection followed by 60 Gy of WBRT

D. Resection followed by 30 Gy of WBRT

E. Erlotinib

7. A 50-year-old man has adenocarcinoma of the right lung. He is a heavy smoker, and tissue obtained at resection demonstrates no actionable mutations in EGFR, ALK, or other genes. Following systemic therapy with carboplatin and pemetrexed, he has stable disease. However, 12 months after diagnosis, he presents with word finding difficulty. Brain imaging by contrast enhanced MRI discloses three deep enhancing lesions, each in different lobes. The largest diameter is 3 cm for 1 lesion and 2 cm for the other 2 lesions. Systemic restaging shows no new sites of extracranial metastases and improved disease in the right lung. What do you recommend for treatment of the brain metastasis?

A. Erlotinib

B. 60 Gy of WBRT

C. Stereotactic radiosurgery (SRS) to the largest lesion followed by active surveillance with contrast-enhanced every 2–3 months

D. SRS to each lesion followed by active surveillance with contrast-enhanced brain MRI scans every 2–3 months

E. PD-1 inhibitor

8. A 50-year-old women with 10 pack years of smoking history presents to the emergency department with a seizure. Brain imaging discloses three hemorrhagic lesions. The most likely source of a primary cancer is:

A. Melanoma

B. Breast

C. Colorectal

D. Non-Hodgkin lymphoma

E. Prostate

ANSWERS

1. B

The correct answer is RT before/after chemotherapy with PCV. Observation would not be appropriate for a high-grade (WHO grade III, anaplastic) glioma. 1p19q co-deletion is a diagnostic marker of oligodendroglioma histology and is rare in astrocytomas or other glioma subtypes. It is also a favorable prognostic marker regardless of treatment. Finally, it is predictive of benefit from DNA alkylator chemotherapy as demonstrated by long-term results of RTOG and EORTC phase III studies. Patients with 1p19q co-deleted anaplastic oligodendroglial tumors lived about twice as long following RT+PCV than RT alone. In RTOG 9402 survival was 14.7 versus 7.3 years ($P = .03$, hazard ratio 0.59), and in EORTC 26951 survival was not reached versus 9.3 years ($P = .0594$, hazard ratio 0.56). Although the EORTC results didn't quite reach traditional measures of statistical significance ($P < .05$), this analysis (survival in 1p19q deleted cases) was not preplanned or powered for survival, as the importance of 1p19q deletion was not elucidated until after the trial was designed. Of note, the RTOG trial used four cycles of "neoadjuvant" (pre-RT) "intensive" PCV (with higher doses of each drug and shorter cycles) and the EORTC trial used up to 6 cycles of post-RT adjuvant PCV at standard dosing. Accordingly, RT alone is inadequate. Bevacizumab prolongs progression-free survival in newly diagnosed and recurrent glioblastoma, and may have a role in other gliomas, but bevacizumab alone would not be appropriate treatment. Some investigators would advocate for chemotherapy alone and would replace PCV by temozolomide. The Phase III Intergroup Study of RT versus Temozolomide Alone versus RT with Concomitant and Adjuvant Temozolomide for Patients with 1p/19q Codeleted Anaplastic Glioma (the "CODEL" trial) led by the Alliance for Clinical Trials in Oncology (formerly the North Central Cancer Treatment Group) originally randomized patients to RT alone, RT with concurrent and adjuvant temozolomide, or temozolomide alone in an exploratory arm. After mature results from RTOG 9402 (and then EORTC 26951) became available, that trial was redesigned, and the RT arm was replaced by RT and PCV (at standard dosing).

2. C

The correct answer is RT and concurrent temozolomide followed by adjuvant temozolomide and GBM and NovoTTF. EORTC trial 22981-26981-NCIC trial CE.3 demonstrated

that RT with concurrent temozolomide followed by 6 cycles of temozolomide improved survival versus RT alone; thus, RT alone is inadequate (median survival 14.6 vs. 12.1 months, hazard ratio 0.63, $P < .001$). The 5-year follow-up also demonstrated a sustained benefit from temozolomide. Of note, PCP prophylaxis is recommended during concurrent treatment. GBM is a highly vascular tumor, but bevacizumab has not been shown to improve survival in newly diagnosed or recurrent disease. For example, two randomized studies for newly diagnosed GBM (RTOG 0825 and AVAglio) found prolonged progression-free survival (PFS) but not overall survival (OS) by adding bevacizumab to RT and TMZ for newly diagnosed GBM versus placebo. Similarly, EORTC trial 26101 found improved PFS but not OS for bevacizumab added to lomustine versus lomustine alone for recurrent GBM. Regardless, bevacizumab alone without RT or temozolomide is not supported by clinical trial data. Studies in elderly patients have suggested temozolomide alone in the context of MGMT methylation is a reasonable option, but it is not a reasonable option in younger patients such as in this case. Checkpoint and PD1 inhibitors are under investigation in various clinical trials for gliomas. Finally, a recent phase III trial also demonstrated improved PFS and OS from the addition of NovoTTF, a device that delivers low-intensity, intermediate frequency electric fields when worn on the scalp (median PFS 7.1 months vs. 4.0 months, hazard ratio 0.62, $P = .001$; median OS 20.5 months vs. 15.6 months, hazard ration 0.64, $P = .004$). However, that trial has been criticized for lacking a placebo control, and it has not gained widespread use yet. Therefore, RT and concurrent temozolomide followed by adjuvant temozolomide without NovoTTF remains the most commonly used approach.

3. A

The correct answer is lomustine. The combination of bevacizumab and lomustine was studied definitively in European Organisation for the Research and Treatment of Cancer (EORTC) trial 26101; patients were randomized to lomustine or lomustine and bevacizumab. There was improved progression-free survival from the addition of bevacizumab but not overall survival. Therefore, controversy remains whether the risks and costs of bevacizumab are warranted versus lomustine alone. Notwithstanding such controversy, bevacizumab increases the risk of surgical wound dehiscence and should be deferred until 4 weeks or more postoperatively. Carboplatin alone has limited to no efficacy in recurrent GBM. Lomustine alone is the most reasonable choice of the options presented, but has limited efficacy (median PFS ~2 months, median OS ~9 months); accordingly, a clinical trial may be preferable.

4. C

Of the options presented, treatment as a WHO grade IV GBM with RT and temozolomide is the most appropriate. There is no data to support bevacizumab alone, although small studies suggest prolonged PFS in recurrent anaplastic astrocytoma from bevacizumab. In the absence of MGMT methylation, temozolomide alone will likely have limited efficacy and is not a widely accepted treatment, although one study from the Neurooncology Working Group of the German Cancer Society (NOA-04) suggested noninferiority of primary chemotherapy followed by radiotherapy at recurrence. As a high-grade tumor, observation is not appropriate. There is no data to suggest ipilimumab monotherapy is effective in gliomas. An ongoing international trial (phase III trial on concurrent and adjuvant temozolomide chemotherapy in non-1p/19q deleted anaplastic glioma: the CATNON intergroup trial) led by the EORTC (trial 26053-22054) will definitively address the efficacy of RT and temozolomide versus RT alone for anaplastic (WHO grade III) gliomas without 1p19q codeletion.

5. E

The correct answer is 54 Gy radiotherapy followed by chemotherapy with PCV. RTOG 9802 randomized patients with low-grade gliomas who either were over 40 or had incomplete resection to RT or RT followed by PCV. The addition of PCV prolonged both PFS and OS on long-term analysis (median survival 13.3 vs. 7.8 years, hazard ratio, P = .03). The benefit was most striking in oligodendrogliomas. Therefore, RT alone is inadequate. Bevacizumab has no established role in the treatment of low-grade (WHO grade II) gliomas. Similarly, carboplatin alone is not supported by available data. As opposed to high-grade (WHO grade III–IV) gliomas that are typically treated with approximately 60 Gy of RT, low-grade (WHO grade II) gliomas are typically treated with a lower-RT dose. EORTC trial 22844 demonstrated no PFS or OS benefit in patients randomized to 59.4 Gy versus 45 Gy of RT (median OS 6.6 years in both arms). An intergroup trial similarly showed no OS benefit but increased toxicity from a 64.8 Gy versus 50.4 Gy. Therefore, 60 Gy is generally considered excessive for WHO grade II gliomas. Younger patients (under 40 years) with completely resected small tumors may have long survival and experience late toxicities from aggressive early therapy; observation, or chemotherapy alone for those patients may be reasonable, but clear randomized data is lacking as reviewed elsewhere.

6. D

The correct answer is Resection followed by 30 Gy of WBRT. WBRT is an accepted treatment for brain metastases (BMs). The Radiation Therapy Oncology Group conducted a series of trials in the 1970s–1990s, and none demonstrated a fractionation or treatment schedule clearly superior to 30–35 Gy in 10–15 fractions. The use of surgery was studied in three randomized trials in combination with WBRT versus WBRT alone. The most widely cited trial demonstrated that survival was prolonged and functional independence maintained for longer in patients with one BM who underwent resection and WBRT compared with WBRT alone (median survival 9.2 vs. 3.5 months, P = .01). In addition, functional independence was maintained for a longer

duration, and recurrence of the local BM was lower in the patients who underwent surgery. Although other trials showed conflicting results, surgery followed by WBRT is widely accepted as appropriate for patients with one resectable BM. Whether patients with two or more metastases should undergo resection is more controversial; radiosurgery is also considered an acceptable treatment and likely superior to WBRT alone for patients with one BM. Whether WBRT itself can be omitted in patients who undergo resection of (or radiosurgery treatment to) one BM is an area of controversy. In the absence of an EGFR mutation, erlotinib is not a preferred choice.

7. D

The correct answer is radiosurgery to each lesion followed by active surveillance with contrast-enhanced brain MRI scans every 2–3 months. WBRT is an accepted treatment for brain metastases (BMs). The Radiation Therapy Oncology Group conducted a series of trials in the 1970s–1990s, and none demonstrated a fractionation or treatment schedule clearly superior to 30–35 Gy in 10–15 fractions. As the lesions are deep in the brain and multiple, SRS rather than resection is reasonable. Several randomized trials compared WBRT with or without radiosurgery. The addition of SRS to WBRT may not improve survival, but it reduces the risk of recurrence at the original sites and throughout the brain. Select subsets also live longer following combination therapy. Therefore, SRS and WBRT is preferable over WBRT alone. Concerns over neurocognitive injury from WBRT led to further studies that omitted WBRT following surgery or SRS and determined whether WBRT itself can be omitted in patients who undergo resection of (or radiosurgery treatment to) 1–3 BMs is an area of controversy. Although WBRT following SRS to 1–3 BMs may not improve survival, it reduces the local rate of recurrence and the risk of new BMs developing. Some studies suggest the risk of neurocognitive deterioration from recurrent BMs is higher than from WBRT. Accordingly, SRS to each lesion followed by WBRT would also represent a reasonable choice, although that was not among the options listed. In the absence of an EGFR mutation, erlotinib is not a preferred choice. PD-1 inhibitors are being studied in the treatment of brain metastases, but they are not presently approved for that indication. Leaving two of the lesions untreated would not be appropriate.

8. A

The correct answer is melanoma. All BMs can hemorrhage. However, among the choices listed, melanoma is the most frequently hemorrhagic. Prostate metastases to the brain parenchyma are extraordinarily unusual, although prostate cancer can spread to the dura.

REFERENCES

Question 1

1. Cairncross JG, Ueki K, Zlatescu MC, et al. Specific genetic predictors of chemotherapeutic response and survival in patients with anaplastic oligodendrogliomas. *J Natl Cancer Inst*. 1998;90:1473–1479.
2. Cairncross G, Wang M, Shaw E, et al. Phase III trial of chemoradiotherapy for anaplastic oligodendroglioma: long-term results of RTOG 9402. *J Clin Oncol*. 2013;31:337–343.
3. van den Bent MJ, Brandes AA, Taphoorn MJ, et al. Adjuvant procarbazine, lomustine, and vincristine chemotherapy in newly diagnosed anaplastic oligodendroglioma: long-term follow-up of EORTC brain tumor group study 26951. *J Clin Oncol*. 2013;31(3):344–350.

Question 2

1. Stupp R, Mason WP, van den Bent MJ, et al. Radiotherapy plus concomitant and adjuvant temozolomide for glioblastoma. *N Engl J Med*. 2005;352:987–996.
2. Stupp R, Hegi ME, Mason WP, et al. Effects of radiotherapy with concomitant and adjuvant temozolomide versus radiotherapy alone on survival in glioblastoma in a randomised phase III study: 5-year analysis of the EORTC-NCIC trial. *Lancet Oncol*. 2009;10:459–466.
3. Chinot OL, Wick W, Mason W, et al. Bevacizumab plus radiotherapy–temozolomide for newly diagnosed glioblastoma. *N Engl J Med*. 2014;370:709–722.
4. Gilbert MR, Dignam JJ, Armstrong TS, et al. A randomized trial of bevacizumab for newly diagnosed glioblastoma. *N Engl J Med*. 2014;370:699–708.
5. Wick W, Brandes A, Gorlia T, et al. LB-05PHASE III trial exploring the combination of bevacizumab and lomustine in patients with first recurrence of a glioblastoma: the EORTC 26101 trial. *Neuro-Oncology*. 2015;17:v1.
6. Stupp R, Taillibert S, Kanner AA, et al. Maintenance therapy with tumor-treating fields plus temozolomide vs temozolomide alone for glioblastoma: a randomized clinical trial. *JAMA*. 2015;314:2535–2543.

Question 3

1. Wick W, Brandes A, Gorlia T, et al. LB-05PHASE III trial exploring the combination of bevacizumab and lomustine in patients with first recurrence of a glioblastoma: the EORTC 26101 trial. *Neuro-Oncology*. 2015;17:v1.

Question 4

1. Wick W, Hartmann C, Engel C, et al. NOA-04 randomized phase III trial of sequential radiochemotherapy of anaplastic glioma with procarbazine, lomustine, and vincristine or temozolomide. *J Clin Oncol*. 2009;27:5874–5880.

Question 5

1. Buckner JC, Shaw EG, Pugh SL, et al. R9802: Phase III study of radiation therapy (RT) with or without procarbazine, CCNU, and vincristine (PCV) in low-grade glioma: results by histologic subtype. *Neuro Oncol*. 2014;16:v11, abstract AT-13 (oral presentation update).
2. Karim AB, Maat B, Hatlevoll R, et al. A randomized trial on dose-response in radiation therapy of low-grade cerebral glioma: European Organization for Research and Treatment of Cancer (EORTC) Study 22844. *Int J Radiat Oncol Biol Phys*. 1996;36:549–556.
3. Shaw E, Arusell R, Scheithauer B, et al. Prospective randomized trial of low- versus high-dose radiation therapy in adults with supratentorial low-grade glioma: initial report of a North Central Cancer Treatment Group/Radiation Therapy Oncology Group/Eastern Cooperative Oncology Group study. *J Clin Oncol*. 2002;20:2267–2276.
4. Schaff LR, Lassman AB. Indications for treatment: is observation or chemotherapy alone a reasonable approach in the management of low-grade gliomas? *Semin Radiat Oncol*. 2015;25:203–209.

Question 6

1. Patchell RA, Tibbs PA, Walsh JW, et al. A randomized trial of surgery in the treatment of single metastases to the brain. *N Engl J Med*. 1990;322:494–500.
2. Mintz AH, Kestle J, Rathbone MP, et al. A randomized trial to assess the efficacy of surgery in addition to radiotherapy in patients with a single cerebral metastasis. *Cancer*. 1996;78:1470–1476.
3. Noordijk EM, Vecht CJ, Haaxma-Reiche H, et al. The choice of treatment of single brain metastasis should be based on extracranial tumor activity and age. *Int J Radiat Oncol Biol Phys*. 1994;29:711–717.
4. Andrews DW, Scott CB, Sperduto PW, et al. Whole brain radiation therapy with or without stereotactic radiosurgery boost for patients with one to three brain metastases: phase III results of the RTOG 9508 randomised trial. *Lancet*. 2004;363:1665–1672.

Question 7

1. Andrews DW, Scott CB, Sperduto PW, et al. Whole brain radiation therapy with or without stereotactic radiosurgery boost for patients with one to three brain metastases: phase III results of the RTOG 9508 randomised trial. *Lancet*. 2004;363:1665–1672.
2. Sperduto PW, Shanley R, Luo X, et al. Secondary analysis of RTOG 9508, a phase 3 randomized trial of whole-brain radiation therapy versus WBRT plus stereotactic radiosurgery in patients with 1–3 brain metastases; poststratified by the graded prognostic assessment (GPA). *Int J Radiat Oncol Biol Phys*. 2014;90:526–531.
3. Brown PD, Asher AL, Ballman KV, et al. NCCTG N0574 (Alliance): a phase III randomized trial of whole brain radiation therapy (WBRT) in addition to radiosurgery (SRS) in patients with 1 to 3 brain metastases. ASCO Meeting Abstracts. *J Clin Oncol*. 2015;33:LBA4.
4. Aoyama H, Tago M, Shirato H, for the Japanese Radiation Oncology Study Group I. Stereotactic radiosurgery with or without whole-brain radiotherapy for brain metastases: secondary analysis of the jrosg 99-1 randomized clinical trial. *JAMA Oncol*. 2015;1(4):457–464.
5. Aoyama H, Tago M, Kato N, et al. Neurocognitive function of patients with brain metastasis who received either whole brain radiotherapy plus stereotactic radiosurgery or radiosurgery alone. *Int J Radiat Oncol Biol Phys*. 2007;68:1388–1395.
6. Meyers CA, Smith JA, Bezjak A, et al. Neurocognitive function and progression in patients with brain metastases treated with whole-brain radiation and motexafin gadolinium: results of a randomized phase III trial. *J Clin Oncol*. 2004;22:157–165.
7. Li J, Bentzen SM, Renschler M, Mehta MP. Regression after whole-brain radiation therapy for brain metastases correlates with survival and improved neurocognitive function. *J Clin Oncol*. 2007;25:1260–1266.
8. DeAngelis LM, Posner JB. *Neurological Complication of Cancer*. 2nd ed. New York, NY: Oxford University Press, Inc.; 2009.

CHAPTER 32

Hereditary Cancer Syndromes

Filipa Lynce

QUESTIONS

1. Of the following syndromes, which one is associated with increased risk of renal cancer?
   A. Neurofibromatosis type 1
   B. Hereditary diffuse gastric cancer syndrome
   C. *BRCA*-associated hereditary breast and ovarian cancer
   D. Cowden syndrome
   E. Bartter syndrome

2. A 44-year-old man presents to the emergency room with acute shortness of breath. Chest X-ray reveals a right-sided pneumothorax. Physical exam is remarkable for a young male in respiratory distress with whitish papules on his nose and cheeks. During his hospitalization he has a computed tomography (CT) scan that reveals multiple pulmonary cysts and three nodules in the left kidney measuring between 1 and 2 cm each. What gene do you suspect to be involved in this syndrome?
   A. Folliculin gene, also known as the Birt-Hogg-Dube (*BHD*) gene
   B. Hamartin (*TSC1*) gene
   C. Tuberin (*TSC2*) gene
   D. Von Hippel-Lindau (*VHL*) gene
   E. Hereditary papillary renal cell carcinoma (*HPRC*) gene

3. A 32-year-old healthy-looking man presents to your office for an initial consultation. He tells you that his mother was diagnosed with colon cancer in her early 30s and his young sister was diagnosed with hepatoblastoma. His sister underwent genetic testing and was found to have a mutation in the *APC* gene. He wants to know what other cancers he is at increased risk for if he is also found to have the same mutation. All the following are correct except for:
   A. Papillary thyroid cancer
   B. Gastric carcinoma
   C. Duodenal ampullary carcinoma
   D. Medulloblastomas
   E. Melanoma

4. Based on the Amsterdam II criteria, who should undergo genetic testing for LS?
   A. A 39-year-old man diagnosed with right-sided colorectal carcinoma (CRC) and maternal aunt with endometrial cancer at the age of 48. No diagnosis of FAP.
   B. A 43-year-old woman diagnosed with cancer of the small bowel, father with CRC diagnosed at age 52, and paternal grandfather diagnosed with CRC at age 48. No diagnosis of FAP.
   C. A 53-year-old woman diagnosed with transitional cell carcinoma of the ureter, father with CRC at the age of 52, and paternal aunt diagnosed with endometrial cancer at the age of 60. No diagnosis of FAP.

   D. A 32-year-old woman diagnosed with endometrial cancer.
   E. A 33-year-old man diagnosed with CRC, has a brother diagnosed with small bowel carcinoma at 39 and a sister diagnosed with breast cancer at age 42. No diagnosis of FAP.

5. Which of the following is *not* a characteristic of Lynch-associated CRC?
   A. CRC is predominantly right sided in location.
   B. Individuals with LS are at an increased risk for synchronous and metachronous CRCs.
   C. Adenomas that evolve to Lynch-associated CRC tend to be larger and flatter and more often have high-grade dysplasia as compared with sporadic adenoma.
   D. Overall 5-year survival from CRC in Lynch is shorter than compared with sporadic CRC.
   E. It occurs at a younger age as compared with sporadic CRC.

6. A 24-year-old female presents to your office after being found to carry a *MSH2* deleterious mutation. Her older brother was recently diagnosed with a stage II right-sided CRC. Her mother was diagnosed with endometrial cancer at the age of 47. Which option is a management recommendation for unaffected individuals with Lynch syndrome (LS)?
   A. Hemicolectomy at the time of development of the first adenoma
   B. Breast magnetic resonance imaging (MRI) starting at the age 25
   C. Prophylactic hysterectomy and bilateral salpingo-oophorectomy (BSO) once childbearing age is complete and after age 40
   D. MRI of the pancreas every 3–5 years
   E. Yearly upper endoscopy with extended duodenoscopy

7. What is considered an uninformative genetic testing result?
   A. No mutation is identified after full sequencing or testing for deleterious mutations, and no mutation has been previously identified in the family.
   B. Finding of a deleterious mutation (185delAG) as part of the *BRCA* Ashkenazi Jewish 3-site Mutation panel.
   C. Finding of a *CHEK2* mutation (1100delC) in an individual without a personal history of malignancy.
   D. No mutation identified in the sister of a woman with a deleterious *VHL* mutation.
   E. Finding of a somatic *BRCA2* mutation after molecular tumor profiling.

8. Which of the following is not associated with increased risk of breast cancer?
   A. Peutz-Jeghers syndrome
   B. Hereditary diffuse gastric cancer

C. Cowden syndrome
D. FAP
E. Li Fraumeni syndrome

9. A 29-year-old woman is referred for genetic counseling after her mother was found to carry a germline deleterious *BRCA1* mutation. She undergoes genetic testing and is found to have the same mutation. She asks several questions about the risks associated with carrying this mutation and differences with *BRCA2*. Which of the following statements is correct?
   A. *BRCA2* carriers usually have earlier onset of ovarian cancer than *BRCA1* carriers.
   B. *BRCA1* carriers often develop breast cancers with characteristics similar to sporadic breast cancers, whereas *BRCA2* carriers more often develop triple negative breast cancer (TNBC).
   C. Patients with *BRCA1* mutations who develop breast cancer often have an aggressive course of the disease that is resistant to most chemotherapy agents.
   D. The lifetime risk of breast cancer in *BRCA1* carriers is estimated to be between 40% and 50%.
   E. The lifetime risk of ovarian cancer is estimated to be 40% for *BRCA1* carriers and about 15% for *BRCA2* carriers.

10. A 32-year-old nulliparous woman presents to the high-risk clinic after being found to carry a germline deleterious *BRCA2* mutation. Her mother was diagnosed with ovarian cancer at the age of 52, and her sister was diagnosed with breast cancer at 43. She asks several questions about what she can do to decrease her risk of developing breast and ovarian cancer. Which of the following statements is correct regarding management of *BRCA1/2* carriers?
   A. BSO when childbearing age is complete is associated with decreased ovarian cancer incidence but not improved all-cause and ovarian cancer mortality.
   B. Breast MRI as the sole breast imaging modality beginning at age 25 and continued annually until at least age 75.
   C. Prophylactic mastectomy should be performed in all *BRCA1/2* carriers and has been associated with improved all-cause, breast cancer, and ovarian cancer mortality.
   D. Transvaginal ultrasound and CA125 are effective screening methods for ovarian cancer in *BRCA1/2* carriers who have not undergone BSO.
   E. Discuss tamoxifen as a chemoprevention option.

11. Which of the following vignettes meets the criteria for Li-Fraumeni testing?
   A. A 14-year-old boy diagnosed with Ewing sarcoma of the left femur
   B. A 41-year-old man with soft tissue sarcoma of the right thigh and mother with breast cancer diagnosed at the age of 51
   C. A 57-year-old man diagnosed with osteosarcoma of the knee at the age of 52 and now diagnosed with adrenocortical carcinoma
   D. A 57-year-old female diagnosed with rhabdomyosarcoma of the orbit
   E. A 28-year-old female diagnosed with left breast cancer

12. A 43-year-old woman with a history of fibrocystic breast disease presents with a newly diagnosed uterine cancer. Her family history is significant for a son with autism, an aunt with breast cancer, and a sister with papillary thyroid

cancer at age 40. What gene is most likely to be mutated in this patient?
   A. *PTEN*
   B. *CDH1*
   C. *TP53*
   D. *STK11*
   E. *CHEK2*

13. A 43-year-old female diagnosed with breast cancer is referred for genetic counseling. Her mother was diagnosed with breast cancer at the age of 48, and her grandmother had ovarian cancer at the age of 42. After discussing the risks and benefits, she decides to have multigene panel testing. This testing detects a deleterious mutation in *PALB2*. Which of the following statements is correct about women with *PALB2* mutations?
   A. As compared with the general population, the risk of breast cancer is 8–9 times higher for *PALB2* carriers younger than 40 years and 6–8 times for those between 40 and 60 years of age.
   B. Women who carry a *PALB2* mutation have a risk of breast cancer equivalent to the risk seen in women who carry a *BRCA1* mutation.
   C. The absolute risk for breast cancer by age 50 for *PALB2* female mutation carriers ranged from 33% for those with no family history of breast cancer to 58% for those with two or more first-degree relatives with early-onset breast cancer.
   D. *PALB2* carriers have an increased risk for thyroid cancer.
   E. Pathogenic mutations in *PALB2* account for approximately 10% of all familial breast cancer.

14. A 41-year-old woman presents to her primary care physician with epigastric pain. She undergoes endoscopy with gastric biopsies that reveal signet ring gastric carcinoma. Her father died of metastatic gastric cancer at the age of 44. She undergoes a total gastrectomy, and lymph nodes and margins of resection are free of cancer. In addition to being referred to a medical oncologist, she is evaluated by a genetic counselor, and a germline cadherin-1 (*CDH1*) gene mutation is detected. She is at a higher risk of developing which of the following:
   A. Inflammatory breast cancer
   B. Invasive lobular breast cancer
   C. Mucinous breast cancer
   D. Ductal carcinoma in situ
   E. Metaplastic breast cancer

15. Which of the following statements regarding hereditary ovarian cancer are true? (Multiple answers are correct.)
   A. Hereditary ovarian cancer is the major cause of all ovarian neoplasms.
   B. *BRCA1* and *BRCA2* are tumor suppressor genes that play a role in the repair of DNA damage.
   C. *BRCA1* and *BRCA2* are located in chromosomes 17 and 13, respectively.
   D. Inheritance of these mutations confers a significantly increased lifetime risk for ovarian cancer.
   E. Inheritance of these mutations confers a significantly increased lifetime risk for nonserous endometrial cancer.

16. A 27-year-old healthy woman was noted to have a large abdominal mass at the time of her routine annual visit with her gynecologist. A pregnancy test was negative. A CT scan of the abdomen was performed and revealed a 13-cm mass in the midportion of the mesentery. She was

referred to a general surgeon and underwent resection of the mass and had removal of a portion of her small bowel and cecum. The pathology revealed a 13-cm desmoid tumor, and 100 adenomatous polyps were incidentally noted in the cecum. The patient has no family history of cancer. Both of her parents had recent baseline colonoscopies that were unremarkable. Which of the following statements are correct about this patient's hereditary cancer syndrome? (Multiple answers are correct.)

A. It is inherited in an autosomal dominant fashion.
B. *De novo* mutations occur in about 30% of cases.
C. Individuals with this syndrome have hundreds to thousands of adenomatous polyps.
D. Individuals with this syndrome have a 60% lifetime risk of developing CRC.
E. It is due to a germline mutation in a mismatch repair gene.

ANSWERS

1. D
Cowden syndrome is an autosomal-dominant disorder characterized by the development of multiple hamartomas and, importantly, carcinomas of the thyroid, breast, endometrium, and kidney. Germline mutations in the *PTEN* gene are found in many patients with Cowden syndrome. All the other syndromes are not associated with increased risk of renal carcinoma. Bartter syndrome is a group of similar kidney disorders that cause an imbalance of potassium, sodium, chloride, and related molecules in the body.

2. A
BHD syndrome is an inherited condition characterized by an increased risk for the development of bilateral multifocal kidney cancer and various dermatological and pulmonary lesions. This syndrome is caused by mutations in the folliculin gene, also known as the *BHD* gene. Tuberous sclerosis complex (*TSC*) is a multisystem autosomal dominant disorder that results from mutations in one of two genes, *TSC1* or *TSC2*. It is characterized by pleomorphic features involving many organ systems, including multiple benign hamartomas of the brain, eyes, heart, lung, liver, kidney, and skin. Both children and adults with *TSC* are at risk for malignant tumors, primarily in the kidneys, brain, and soft tissues. In children this is almost entirely due to the increased incidence of brain tumors and rhabdomyosarcoma. VHL disease is a heritable multisystem cancer syndrome that is associated with a germline mutation of the *VHL* tumor suppressor gene. Affected individuals are at risk of developing various benign and malignant tumors of the central nervous system (CNS), kidneys, adrenal glands, pancreas, and reproductive adnexal organs. The HPRC c-met mutations are activating mutations linked to HPRC, a familial cancer syndrome in which affected individuals are at risk for the development of type 1 papillary renal cell carcinomas.

3. E
Familial adenomatous polyposis (FAP) is an autosomal dominant disease caused by mutations in the *APC* gene located on chromosome 5. In addition to multiple polyps and colon carcinoma, patients with FAP are at risk for several extracolonic malignancies including follicular or papillary thyroid cancer, gastric carcinoma, duodenal ampullary carcinoma, and CNS tumors. Melanoma is not one of the malignancies known to be associated with FAP.

4. B
According to the Amsterdam II criteria, LS should be suspected in individuals that meet all of the following criteria (3, 2, 1 rule): 1. Three or more relatives with histologically verified LS-associated cancers (CRC, cancer of the endometrium or small bowel, transitional cell carcinoma of the ureter or renal pelvis), one of whom is a first-degree relative of the other two and in whom FAP has been excluded. 2. Two or more generations have LS-associated cancers involving at. 3. One or more cancers diagnosed before the age of 50. FAP should be excluded in the CRC case(s). Of note, aside from the cancers listed in the Amsterdam II criteria, individuals with LS are also at increased risk for cancer of the ovary, stomach, hepatobiliary system, brain (glioma), and sebaceous neoplasms.

5. D
In a multivariate analysis, the presence of microsatellite instability in patients with CRC was associated with a significant survival advantage independent of all standard prognostic factors. CRCs in LS differ from sporadic CRCs in that they are predominantly right sided in location. LS predisposes affected individuals to develop synchronous and metachronous CRCs. Approximately 7%–10% of individuals with LS have more than one cancer by the time of diagnosis, and up to 25% of patients with LS develop a metachronous CRC after partial colectomy. Although Lynch-associated CRCs evolve from adenomas, the adenomas tend to be larger, flatter, more often proximal, and more likely to have high-grade dysplasia and/or villous histology as compared with sporadic adenomas.

6. C
The most common extracolonic tumor in LS is endometrial cancer (25%–60% lifetime risk). Although lower, the lifetime risk for ovarian cancer is between 4% and 24%. Other recommendations for individuals affected with LS syndrome include colonoscopy every 1–2 years beginning at age 20–25 years, or 2–5 years prior to the earliest age of CRC diagnosis in the family, whichever comes first. It is also recommended that one consider annual neurological examination starting at 25–30 years and annual urinalysis beginning at age 30–35 years.

7. A
Interpretation of negative genetic testing results for germline mutations depends on whether a deleterious mutation has been previously identified in the family. If a deleterious mutation has been previously identified in the family, and a close relative is tested and tests negative, then this is considered a true negative (answer D). If *no* deleterious mutation has been previously identified in the family, then the results are considered to be uninformative (answer A). Answers B and C constitute

positive test results, which means that a deleterious germline mutation associated with a hereditary cancer syndrome was identified. Regarding answer E, it is not possible to know a priori whether a deleterious *BRCA2* mutation identified in a patient's cancer was inherited or arose in the course of tumor development. In this case it is necessary to do germline testing or testing of healthy tissue (e.g., skin fibroblasts) to confirm whether the finding from the molecular testing reflects an inherited mutation or is an acquired somatic mutation.

8. D

FAP is primarily associated with an increased risk of gastrointestinal cancers including cancers of the colon, stomach, small bowel, pancreas, bile duct, and hepatoblastoma. Additional cancers include papillary thyroid cancer, adrenal tumors, and medulloblastoma, but no increased risk of breast cancer. Cowden syndrome is an autosomal disease caused by alterations in the *PTEN* gene and is associated with high-risk benign and malignant tumors of the breast, endometrium, and thyroid. Peutz-Jeghers syndrome is caused in most patients by a mutation in the tumor suppressor gene *STK11* and is associated with an increased risk of breast cancer among others. In women, the lifetime risk of breast cancer is 44%–50% by age 70. Hereditary diffuse gastric cancer is associated with an increased risk of the lobular subtype of breast cancer as well as diffuse gastric cancer. The cumulative lifetime risk of breast cancer in women with *CDH1* mutations is 39%–52%. LFS is an autosomal-dominant disorder caused by germline mutations in the *TP53* gene. These mutations confer a lifetime cancer risk of 93% in women (mainly breast cancer) and 68% in men. Other characteristic cancers seen in LFS include adrenocortical tumors, sarcomas, leukemias, and CNS malignancies.

9. E

Answer A is incorrect because *BRCA2* carriers usually have a later onset of ovarian cancer than *BRCA1* carriers. Answer B is false because *BRCA1* carriers develop TNBC in 50%–75% of the cases. Answer C is incorrect given that *BRCA* status is not an independent prognostic factor. Answer D is false because the lifetime risk of breast cancer in *BRCA1* carriers is estimated to be between 50% and 85% and in *BRCA2* carriers between 40% and 70%.

10. E

Although only limited data are available on the specific use of selective estrogen receptor modulators (i.e., tamoxifen, raloxifene) in patients with *BRCA1/2* mutations, the use of these agents should be discussed with *BRCA1/2* carriers. Answer A is false because BSO when childbearing age is complete is associated with improved all-cause, ovarian cancer, and possibly breast cancer–related mortality. Answer B is false because breast MRI yearly starting at the age of 25 is recommended for *BRCA* carriers and should be alternated with yearly mammograms to start at the age of 30. Prophylactic mastectomy should be offered to *BRCA1/2* carriers. However, the decision should be based on personal preference as there are effective screening methods available. Transvaginal ultrasound and CA125 can be discussed with *BRCA1/2* carriers who have not undergone BSO; however, these have not been proven to be effective screening methods for ovarian cancer.

11. B

Answer B meets the criteria to undergo genetic testing for deleterious *TP53* mutation. LFS results from germline mutations in the *TP53* tumor suppressor gene and is characterized by a remarkable inherited cancer susceptibility disorder with a wide tumor spectrum. The Chompret criteria were developed to facilitate the clinical recognition of this syndrome and take into account the three clinical situations suggestive of LFS:

a. Familial presentation—a proband with an LFS tumor (breast cancer, STS, osteosarcoma, CNS tumor, adrenocortical carcinoma, leukemia, bronchoalveolar lung cancer) diagnosed before age 46 and one first- or second-degree relative with an LFS tumor who is younger than 56 years or with multiple tumors

b. Multiple primary tumors—two of which belong to the narrow LFS spectrum, the first of which developed before age 46

c. Rare cancers—adrenocortical carcinoma or choroid plexus carcinoma (CPC) irrespective of the family history

12. A

Cowden syndrome is an autosomal disease caused by alterations in the *PTEN* gene. It is associated with high-risk benign and malignant tumors of the breast, endometrium, and thyroid. In addition, autism and macrocephaly are associated with Cowden syndrome, as well as pathognomic mucocutaneous lesions. Mutations in the tumor suppressor gene *STK11* are often associated with Peutz-Jeghers syndrome. *CDH1* mutations are associated with hereditary diffuse gastric cancer, which is associated with an increased risk of the lobular subtype of breast cancer as well as diffuse gastric cancer. Li-Fraumeni syndrome (LFS) is an autosomal-dominant disorder caused by germline mutations in the *TP53* gene. Inherited mutations in the *CHEK2* gene have also been linked to increased risk of breast cancer.

13. A

Answer A is the correct answer. *PALB2* is a breast cancer susceptibility gene that encodes a *BRCA2* interacting protein. Women who carry a *PALB2* mutation have a risk of breast cancer equivalent to the risk of women who carry a *BRCA2* mutation and not a *BRCA1* mutation (Answer B). Answer C is incorrect because these numbers apply to the risk by age 70 and not age 50. The absolute breast cancer risk for *PALB2* female mutation carriers by 70 years of age ranged from 33% (95% CI, 25–44) for those with no family history of breast cancer to 58% (95% CI, 50–66) for those with two or more first-degree relatives with breast cancer at 50 years of age. Answer D is not correct because there is no increased risk for thyroid cancer in *PALB2* carriers. There may be an increased risk of pancreatic cancer although the absolute risk is unclear. Answer E is false; pathogenic mutations seem to account for approximately 2.4% of familial breast cancer.

14. B

Hereditary diffuse gastric cancer is characterized by a susceptibility to diffuse gastric cancer and is associated with *CDH1* germline mutations. Women with *CDH1* mutations have a 60% risk of developing lobular breast cancer by age 80.

15. B, C, D

Hereditary ovarian cancer constitutes 5%–15% of cases of ovarian cancers not the majority of all ovarian neoplasms. *BRCA1* and *BRCA2* are tumor suppressor genes that play a role in the repair of DNA damage. *BRCA1* and *BRCA2* are located in chromosomes 17 and 13, respectively. Inheritance of these mutations confers an increased lifetime risk for both ovarian and breast cancer, and these typically occur with an earlier age of onset compared with the general population. Although there has been debate about whether *BRCA1/2* mutations increase the risk for uterine cancer, the current evidence indicates no increased risk of endometrioid endometrial carcinoma but perhaps a very small absolute increased risk of serous endometrial carcinoma.

16. A, B, C

This young woman has FAP, which is due to a mutation in the tumor suppressor gene *APC*. This gene is inherited in an autosomal dominant fashion. FAP carriers have close to a 100% risk of colon cancer, which typically occurs at a very young age (median age ~35). Given the absence of a family history of cancer and the fact that both of her parents had normal colonoscopies, she most likely has a *de novo* mutation in *APC*. *De novo* mutations are thought to occur in about 30% of cases. In addition to the marked increased risk for colon cancer, these individuals also have increased risk of cancers of the small bowel, stomach, pancreas, and rarely hepatoblastomas and thyroid cancer. Gardner syndrome is an FAP subset with characteristic colon polypsis as well as extracolonic growths including desmoid tumors, osteomas, epidermoid or sebaceous cysts, fibromas, congenital hypertrophy of retinal pigment epithelium (CHRPE), and supernumerary teeth. Answer E is incorrect because mutations in mismatch repair genes are associated with LS.

Additional questions, answers, rationales, and interactive assessments available on Expert Consult.

REFERENCES

Question 1

1. Ngeow J, Stanuch K, Mester JL, Barnholtz-Sloan JS, Eng C. Second malignant neoplasms in patients with Cowden syndrome with underlying germline PTEN mutations. *J Clin Oncol.* 2014;32(17):1818–1824.
2. Liaw D, Marsh DJ, Li J, et al. Germline mutations of the PTEN gene in Cowden disease, an inherited breast and thyroid cancer syndrome. *Nat Genet.* 1997;16(1):64–67.

Question 2

1. Schmidt LS, Linehan WM. Molecular genetics and clinical features of Birt-Hogg-Dube syndrome. *Nat Rev Urol.* 2015;12(10):558–569.
2. Crino PB, Nathanson KL, Henske EP. The tuberous sclerosis complex. *N Engl J Med.* 2006;355(13):1345.
3. Narod SA, Stiller C, Lenoir GM. An estimate of the heritable fraction of childhood cancer. *Br J Cancer.* 1991;63(6):993.
4. Lonser RR, Glenn GM, Walther M, et al. Von Hippel-Lindau disease. *Lancet.* 2003;361(9374):2059–2067.
5. Zhar B, Tory K, Merino M, et al. Hereditary papillary renal cell carcinoma. *J Urol.* 1994;151(3):561.

Question 3

1. Vasen HF, Blanco I, Aktan-Collan K, et al. Revised guidelines for the clinical management of Lynch syndrome (HNPCC): recommendations by a group of European experts. *Gut.* 2013;62(6):812–823.

Question 4

1. Vasen HF, Watson P, Mecklin JP, Lynch HT. New clinical criteria for hereditary nonpolyposis colorectal cancer (HNPCC, Lynch syndrome) proposed by the International Collaborative group on HNPCC. *Gastroenterology.* 1999;116(6):1453–1456.

Question 5

1. Gryfe R, Kim H, Hsieh ET, et al. Tumor microsatellite instability and clinical outcome in young patients with colorectal cancer. *N Engl J Med.* 2000;342(2):69–77.

2. Kalady MF, McGannon E, Vogel JD, Manilich E, Fazio VW, Church JM. Risk of colorectal adenoma and carcinoma after colectomy for colorectal cancer in patients meeting Amsterdam criteria. *Ann Surg.* 2010;252:507–513.

Question 6

1. Giardiello FM, Allen JI, Axilbund JE, et al. Guidelines on genetic evaluation and management of Lynch syndrome: a consensus statement by the US Multi-Society Task Force on Colorectal Cancer. *Dis Colon Rectum.* 2014;57(8):1025–1048.
2. NCCN guidelines v2. 2016. Colorectal Cancer Screening.

Question 7

1. Robson ME, Bradbury AR, Arun B, et al. American Society of Clinical Oncology policy statement update: genetic and genomic testing for cancer susceptibility. *J Clin Oncol.* 2015;33(31):3660–3667.

Question 8

1. Waller A, Findeis S, Lee MJ. Familial adenomatous polyposis. *J Pediatr Genet.* 2016;5(2):78–83.
2. Ngeow J, Stanuch K, Mester JL, Barnholtz-Sloan JS, Eng C. Second malignant neoplasms in patients with Cowden syndrome with underlying germline PTEN mutations. *J Clin Oncol.* 2014;32(17):1818–1824.
3. Pederson HJ, Padia SA, May M, Grobmyer S. Managing patients at genetic risk of breast cancer. *Cleve Clin J Med.* 2016;83(3):199–206.

Question 9

1. Chen S, Parmigiani G. Meta-analysis of *BRCA1* and *BRCA2* penetrance. *J Clin Oncol.* 2007;25(11):1329–1333.
2. Foulkes WD. Inherited susceptibility to common cancers. *N Engl J Med.* 2008;359:2143–2153.

Question 10

1. NCCN guidelines version 1. 2017. Genetic/Familial High-Risk Assessment: Breast and Ovarian.
2. Le-Petross HT, Whitman GJ, Atchley DP, et al. Effectiveness of alternating mammography and magnetic resonance imaging for screening women with deleterious *BRCA* mutations at high risk of breast cancer. *Cancer.* 2011;117(17):3900–3907.

Question 11

1. Bougeard G, Renaux-Petel M, Flaman JM, et al. Revisiting Li-Fraumeni syndrome from TP53 mutation carriers. *J Clin Oncol.* 2015;33(21):2345–2352.

Question 12

1. Ngeow J, Stanuch K, Mester JL, Barnholtz-Sloan JS, Eng C. Second malignant neoplasms in patients with Cowden syndrome with underlying germline PTEN mutations. *J Clin Oncol.* 2014;32(17):1818–1824.

Question 13

1. Antoniou AC, Casadei S, Heikkinen T, et al. Breast-cancer risk in families with mutations in PALB2. *N Engl J Med.* 2014;371(6):497–506.

Question 14

1. Fitzgerald RC, Hardwick R, Huntsman D, et al. International Gastric Cancer Linkage Consortium. Hereditary diffuse gastric cancer: updated consensus guidelines for clinical management and directions for future research. *J Med Genet.* 2010;47(7):436.

Question 15

1. Prat J, Ribé A, Gallardo A. Hereditary ovarian cancer. *Hum Pathol.* 2005;36(8):861–870.
2. Shu CA, Pike MC, Jotwani AR. Uterine cancer after risk-reducing salpingo-oophorectomy without hysterectomy in women with BRCA mutations. *JAMA Oncol.* 2016;2(11):1434–1440.

Question 16

1. Leoz ML, Carballal S, Moreira L, Ocaña T, Balaguer F. The genetic basis of familial adenomatous polyposis and its implications for clinical practice and risk management. *Appl Clin Genet.* 2015;8:95–107.

CHAPTER

33

Coagulation

Marc J. Kahn, Alice D. Ma, Molly Weidner Manderenach, Ara Metjian, Anita Rajasekhar, Brandi Reeves, and Marc Zumberg

QUESTIONS

1. A 42-year-old woman with a 20-year history of ITP treated with prednisone, vincristine, splenectomy, and rituximab presents for a second opinion. The patient has been healthy throughout her life and has never had significant bleeding. Her physical examination is unremarkable, without bruising or petechiae. Her peripheral smear shows normal appearing RBCs with large platelets that are reduced in number. Her neutrophils are notable for blue inclusions in the cytoplasm. Her CBC is shown:

Hgb	13.2 g/dL
Hct	39.5%
WBC	7200×10^9/L
Platelet	$68,000 \times 10^9$/L

   Her disorder is most likely due to a defect in which gene?
   A. MYH9
   B. CALR
   C. ADAMTS13
   D. MPL
   E. PI3K

2. A 48-year-old woman is sent for evaluation of 6 years of thrombocytosis. The patient is otherwise healthy and has not had any bleeding or thrombotic episodes. Her physical exam is remarkable for a palpable spleen. Her CBC is shown:

Hgb	14.2 g/dL
Hct	42.6%
WBC	8400×10^9/L
Platelet	$742,000 \times 10^9$/L

   She is found to have wild type *JAK2* and *mpl*. She is bcr/abl negative. Mutations in which of the following genes is most likely to be responsible for her condition?
   A. PI3K
   B. BCL2
   C. CALR
   D. MYH9
   E. PML

3. A 63-year-old man is referred for a second opinion for treatment of chronic ITP. He was diagnosed around 1 year ago and has had transient responses to pulse dexamethasone, as well as daily oral prednisone. His past medical history is significant for oxygen dependent COPD, CAD with intermittent angina, and morbid obesity (weight 178 kg). He is not actively bleeding, and examination is otherwise unremarkable. He is currently taking 80 mg of prednisone daily.
   Labs:

Hemoglobin	13.6 g/dL
Hematocrit	44%
Platelet count	9000×10^9/L
Leukocyte count	$12,600 \times 10^9$/L
Serum creatinine	0.9 mg/dL
Serum electrolytes	Normal
Liver function tests	Mildly elevated AST and ALT
Hepatitis C antibodies	Negative
Hepatitis B surface antigen	Positive

   Administration of which of the following would be most appropriate?
   A. Rituximab
   B. Splenectomy
   C. Romiplostim
   D. Danazol
   E. Azathioprine (Imuran)

4. A 60-year-old man with a history of coronary artery disease presents with angina and is diagnosed with a non-ST-elevation myocardial infarction. He subsequently undergoes left heart catheterization with placement of a stent in the left circumflex artery. He is treated with unfractionated heparin intravenously, and his hospital course is complicated by the development of pneumonia. On the sixth day of admission, his platelet count begins to decrease. You suspect heparin-induced thrombocytopenia (HIT) with an intermediate pretest probability based on the 4T scoring system.
   Which of the following laboratory tests should be ordered first in your evaluation?
   A. Serotonin release assay
   B. Anti PF4 antibody ELISA
   C. Heparin induced platelet aggregation assay
   D. Platelet aggregation studies
   E. Platelet function assay

5. A patient is evaluated for assessment of easy bruising and nose bleeds. He states that this has been present his whole life, and that removal of his tonsils was associated with heavy bleeding. His referring physician performed preliminary laboratory testing that showed a normal PT, aPTT, and CBC results. A platelet aggregation assay is then performed that shows the following results:

Saline	3%	(>60%)
Collagen (10 µg/mL)	13%	(>60%)
Adenosine diphosphate (5 µM)	22%	(>60%)
Ristocetin (1.5 mg/mL)	86%	(>60%)
Arachidonic acid (0.5 mg/mL)	1%	(>60%)
Thromboxane A2 (1.0 µM)	11%	(>60%)

Which of the following is the most likely diagnosis?
A. Bernard-Soulier syndrome
B. Glanzmann thrombasthenia
C. An aspirin-like defect
D. Surreptitious use of clopidogrel
E. May-Hegglin anomaly

6. A 35-year-old Caucasian woman is sent for evaluation of a greater than 6-year history of refractory thrombocytopenia. A bone marrow biopsy showed normal megakaryocyte number and ploidy. Her treatment has been characterized by a failure of repeated cycles of high-dose corticosteroids, splenectomy, and rituximab. Upon review of her platelet count, the following pattern of thrombocytopenia is noted, which the patient states has typically occurred during her menses, leading to menorrhagia (Fig. 33.1).

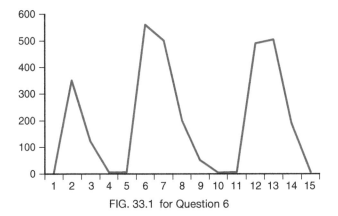

FIG. 33.1 for Question 6

Based upon these findings, you conclude that the patient has:
A. Congenital amegakaryocytic thrombocytopenia
B. Quebec platelet disorder
C. Cyclic thrombocytopenia
D. Scott syndrome
E. Hermansky-Pudlak

7. A 26-year-old woman who is at 36 weeks gestation during her first pregnancy is referred for thrombocytopenia. She has no past medical history. The only medication she takes is a multivitamin and folic acid supplement. A complete blood count (CBC) from her first trimester was normal. She has no other prior CBCs outside of pregnancy. She denies any symptoms of bleeding or bruising. On physical exam she has no petechiae, ecchymoses, or oral purpura. Her CBC today is as follows. A peripheral blood smear shows few large platelets.
Labs:

Hemoglobin	12.5 g/dL
Hematocrit	38%
Platelet count	82,000/µL
Leucocyte count	13,400/µL

Serum creatinine	0.9 mg/dL
Serum electrolytes	Normal
Liver function tests	Normal
Acute hepatitis panel	Negative
HIV panel	Negative

Which of the following is the most appropriate recommendation at this time?
A. Consider elective Cesarean section rather than vaginal delivery
B. Intravenous immunoglobulin (IVIG)
C. Prednisone
D. Observation
E. Deliver baby now

8. A 30-year-old man was referred to a hematology clinic for an incidental finding of platelet 66,000 × 10⁹/L on a routine CBC done by his PCP 6 weeks ago. The remainder of his CBC was normal. His medical history is significant for depression and anxiety. There is no family history of cytopenias or bleeding. He is on lorazepam as needed. A prior CBC 1 year ago was normal. The patient denies any current or prior bleeding symptoms but has not had any surgical challenges. He drinks approximately two beers per week. Physical exam is normal, without any signs of bleeding or bruising. His CBC in clinic today reveals:

Leukocyte count	7200 × 10⁹/L
Hemoglobin	12.0 g/dL
Hematocrit	36.0%
Platelet count	62,000 × 10⁹/L

A peripheral blood smear reveals normal leukocyte and erythrocyte morphology. There are decreased platelet numbers without clumping or schistocytes. He has an upcoming dental extraction of two wisdom teeth, scheduled next week.
What is the most appropriate next step in management?
A. Perform a bone marrow biopsy to evaluate for primary bone marrow disorder
B. Administer IVIG today in preparation for dental extraction next week
C. Start Prednisone in preparation for dental extraction next week
D. Repeat CBC at next visit in 3 months
E. Perform testing for *Helicobacter pylori* infection

9. A 22-year-old female presents to the emergency room with increased bruising on her arms and legs. She denies any other bleeding. She has no other comorbidities. She is on a multivitamin and started trimethoprim-sulfamethoxazole 5 days ago for a recently diagnosed urinary tract infection. A complete blood count (CBC) checked in the ER is as follows:

Leukocyte count	12,000/µL
Hemoglobin	11.0 g/dL
Hematocrit	33%
Platelet count	25,000/µL

Coagulation studies, creatinine, and liver function tests are normal.
She has no prior CBCs. Physical exam reveals moderate-sized ecchymoses on her arms and legs, and few scattered petechia of the lower extremities.
What is the next best course of action?
A. Perform a bone marrow biopsy to evaluate for primary bone marrow disorder
B. Stop trimethoprim-sulfamethoxazole and recheck CBC in a few days
C. Administer IVIG
D. Start prednisone

10. A 42-year-old woman with no prior medical history presents with acute onset of bruising. She is afebrile, and her physical examination is remarkable only for findings of bruising and petechiae. Laboratory values include the following (Table 33.1) and and a peripheral blood smear is shown (Fig 33.2).

TABLE 33.1 Laboratory Values: Question 10		
Laboratory Test	**Patient's Result**	**Reference Range**
Hemoglobin	8.3 g/dL	13–17.3 g/dL
Hematocrit	24.9%	39%–50.2%
White blood cell count	5200 × 10⁹/L, with normal differential	4–10 × 10⁹/L
Platelet count	10 × 10⁹/L	150–450 × 10⁹/L
Creatinine	1.2 mg/dL	0.7–1.3 mg/dL
Lactate dehydrogenase	1200 units/L	100–240 units/L
ADAMTS13 activity	<5%	>60%

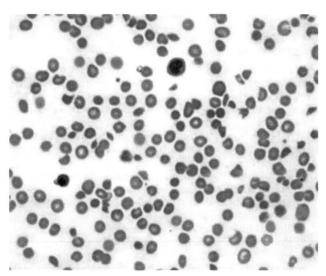

FIG. 33.2 Peripheral blood smear, John Lazarchick, ASH image bank 2001;Image # 00003.

What is the underlying etiology of this disorder?
- **A.** An abnormal von Willebrand factor with a "gain of function" leading to increased binding to the platelet receptor, glycoprotein Ib
- **B.** An acquired deficiency of a von Willebrand factor-cleaving protease
- **C.** Complement mutation resulting in complement dysregulation
- **D.** Autoantibody directed against platelet factor 4 complex

11. A 65-year-old woman with a history of coronary artery disease and severe mitral valve regurgitation is admitted for single-vessel CABG and prosthetic mitral valve replacement. Her platelet count was 400,000 × 10⁹/L preoperatively (normal 150,000–450,000 × 10⁹/L) and acutely dropped to 75,000 × 10⁹/L 10 days after surgery. She received unfractionated heparin during bypass and postoperatively for prophylaxis. Heparin platelet antibody was

drawn on postoperative day 10 and returned elevated at 1.5 relative OD (normal <0.4 relative OD), and the serotonin release assay is strongly positive. Doppler ultrasound confirms an acute right common femoral vein thrombus. She is diagnosed with heparin-induced thrombocytopenia with thrombosis (HITT). Liver function tests are normal, and her creatinine is 3 mg/dL (normal 0.4–0.9 mg/dL). Which of the following is the most appropriate treatment for this patient?
- **A.** Argatroban
- **B.** Aspirin
- **C.** Enoxaparin
- **D.** Fondaparinux
- **E.** Rivaroxaban

12. A previously healthy 25-year-old presents to the ER with delirium. His roommate confirms the patient has been experiencing fever, shaking chills, a cough productive of yellowish blood-tinged sputum, and pleuritic right chest pain for the last week. In the last day he developed epistaxis and purpura. On exam he is obtunded with crusted blood around his nares.
Labs:
PT   18 seconds (normal 11.9–15 seconds)
PTT   48 seconds (normal 23–38 seconds)
D-Dimer 6 (normal <0.46 μg/mL)
WBC   21,000 × 10⁹/L
Hematocrit 47%
Platelet 40,000 × 10⁹/L

Chest x-ray confirms a large right-sided effusion. Diagnostic pleural tap is performed and reveals pus with many diplococci. Antibiotics are ordered, and CT surgery is consulted to place a chest tube. Regarding chest tube placement and the patient's coagulopathy, what is the most appropriate course of action?
- **A.** Defer chest tube placement for 24 hours while allowing the antibiotics to become effective
- **B.** Administer 6 units of FFP, followed by the chest tube insertion
- **C.** Administer recombinant factor VIIa prior to chest tube placement
- **D.** Administer 2 units of single donor platelets prior to chest tube placement
- **E.** Place the chest tube and begin antibiotics

13. A 35-year-old man with acute promyelocytic leukemia completed induction chemotherapy 14 days ago. Immediately prior to morning rounds, he develops chills, rigors, epistaxis, purpura, hypotension, and tachypnea. Blood cultures were obtained and broad-spectrum antibiotics were administered.
Labs:
PT   17 seconds (normal 11.9–15 seconds)
PTT   45 seconds (normal 23–38 seconds)
D-Dimer 5 (normal <0.46 μg/mL)
WBC   700/μL
ANC   60/μL
Hematocrit 20%
Platelet 20,000/μL

What best predicts mortality associated with his coagulopathy?
- **A.** The degree of PT and PTT prolongation
- **B.** The development of multiorgan dysfunction syndrome (MODS)
- **C.** The presence of schistocytes on the peripheral blood smear
- **D.** The presence of underlying malignancy
- **E.** The degree of D-dimer elevation

14. An 18-year-old college freshman is referred to hematology for evaluation of thrombocytopenia found during an examination at the college infirmary for sore throat and malaise. His platelet count 2 weeks ago at the time of that visit was $52,000 \times 10^9/L$. WBC and hemoglobin were within the limits of normal. He has no prior CBCs for comparison. He has no history of easy bruising nor bleeding. He drinks two to three beers per weekend. He takes no medications. He has no siblings.

Physical examination shows a well-developed man with no palpable lymphadenopathy in the cervical, supraclavicular, axillary, or inguinal chains. There is no hepatosplenomegaly. There is no rash.

Labs:

WBC	$7500 \times 10^9/L$
Hgb	13.6 g/dL
MCV	90 fL
Platelets	$50,000 \times 10^9/L$
MPV	5.3 fL
AST	33 units/L
ALT	34 units/L

Peripheral blood smear shows no platelet clumping.
Which of the following is the most likely cause of his thrombocytopenia?
A. A mutation in WASp
B. Immune thrombocytopenia
C. Alcohol use
D. Recent viral illness

15. A 24-year-old man presents for evaluation of isolated thrombocytopenia to $120,000 \times 10^9/L$ discovered during a preemployment physical. He is otherwise in excellent health, with no recent illness. He has had a mild bleeding tendency since childhood, with larger than average ecchymoses for routine, and gum oozing after minor dental procedures. He drinks two to three beers per weekend. He takes an occasional ibuprofen for headaches but takes no other prescription medications, over-the-counter medications, or herbal supplements. His mother also has mild thrombocytopenia and has had lifelong heavy menses, resulting in iron deficiency. His maternal grandmother died from acute leukemia at age 60. DNA testing shows a RUNX1 mutation.

Two years later, he develops acute myeloid leukemia with poor-risk cytogenetics and is recommended for allogeneic stem cell transplantation. He has one brother, age 22, who is in good health and has a normal platelet count. His brother has no children and refuses to be tested for the RUNX1 mutation.
Which of the following stem cell donors is most ideal in this case?
A. 8/8 matched unrelated donor
B. Matched sibling donor
C. Cord blood donor
D. Autologous donation

16. A 63-year-old woman with Glanzmann thrombasthenia is planned for total knee arthroplasty for severe degenerative joint disease. She has never had a prior surgical intervention. She has received platelets twice in the remote past for peripartum bleeding. She previously used an oral antifibrinolytic agent to control menorrhagia, but since menopause 10 years ago, she has not used this.
CBC shows:

WBC	$7500 \times 10^9/L$
Hgb	13.6 g/dL
Platelets	$214,000 \times 10^9/L$

Which of the following is the most appropriate management during the perioperative period?
A. Platelet transfusion plus antifibrinolytic therapy
B. Antifibrinolytic therapy
C. DDAVP
D. Von Willebrand factor concentrate

17. A 67-year-old is hospitalized with a platelet count of $9,000 \times 10^9/L$. She has had no laboratory testing in over 10 years. There is no bleeding. HIV testing is nonreactive. Hepatitis testing shows hepatitis B surface antibody positive, surface antigen negative, and hepatitis C antibody negative. Bone marrow evaluation shows a slightly hypercellular marrow with increased normal-appearing megakaryocytes. Blood type is O, Rh negative.

She received IVIG 1 g/kg on days 1 and 2 and dexamethasone 40 mg PO daily × 4 days. On day 7, she has no increase in her platelet count and no bleeding symptoms. She is given rituximab 375 mg/m² on day 7. On day 12, her platelet count remains 9000/μL. She is not bleeding.
Which of the following is the next best step in management?
A. Continue the rituximab course
B. Anti-D
C. Splenectomy
D. Vincristine

18. A 13-year-old presents to your office for evaluation of thrombocytopenia, discovered during initial evaluation of heavy menses. She has a lifelong history of easy bruising with minimal trauma; she has had no surgical procedures. She does not take oral contraceptive pills. She is adopted and knows no family medical history.

WBC	$7500 \times 10^9/L$
Hgb	11.6 g/dL
MCV	78 fL
Platelets	$75,000 \times 10^9/L$
MPV	11.6 fL

Liver tests are within the limits of normal.
aPTT and PT are within the limits of normal.
Von Willebrand factor (vWF) antigen and activity levels are within the limits of normal.
Peripheral blood smear reveals macrothrombocytes and hypochromic, microcytic red blood cells. The leukocytes are normal.
Platelet aggregation testing shows normal aggregation with ADP and collagen, and absent aggregation with ristocetin.

Which of the following tests is most likely to be diagnostic?
A. Platelet flow cytometry
B. MYH9 gene mutation analysis
C. Platelet electron microscopy
D. PFA-100

19. A 55-year-old with type II heparin-induced thrombocytopenia complicated by upper extremity venous thromboembolism diagnosed by positive PF-4 antibody ELISA and positive serotonin release assay has been on argatroban for 3 days. Her platelet count has recovered from a nadir of 5500–$72,000 \times 10^9/L$ today. She feels well and has had no thrombotic or bleeding complications. Her aPTT has been stable at 60 seconds (3 times the upper limit of normal) and INR is 1.5. She would like to go home.
Which of the following is the most appropriate for ongoing management of HITT?
A. Continue argatroban infusion
B. Continue argatroban and add warfarin 10 mg PO daily
C. Continue argatroban and add warfarin 5 mg PO daily

D. Stop argatroban and begin apixaban

E. Stop argatroban and begin aspirin

20. A 40-year-old African American woman was evaluated by her primary care provider for fatigue and found to have a mild thrombocytosis to 500,000 × 10⁹/L on two occasions, spaced apart by 2 weeks. She had a normal CBC 2 years ago. Physical examination shows koilonychia. There is no hepatosplenomegaly. Labs show:

WBC	7500 × 10⁹/L
Hgb	10.6 g/dL
MCV	74 fL
RDW	16.8%
Platelets	500,000 × 10⁹/L
MPV	9.0 fL

Review of the peripheral blood smear shows hypochromic, normocytic red blood cells. The leukocytes and platelets are normal in appearance and number.

What is the next best step in the diagnosis of this patient's thrombocytosis?

A. JAK2 V617F gene mutation testing

B. CALR gene mutation testing

C. Ferritin

D. Bone marrow biopsy

21. A 27-year-old woman presented to an outside hospital fever of 38.3°C, confusion, and a petechial rash that developed over 1 day. Laboratory evaluation showed:

WBC	11,500 × 10⁹/L
ANC	8000 × 10⁹/L
Hgb	9.6 g/dL
Platelets	24,000 × 10⁹/L
Creatinine	0.99 mg/dL (0.60–1.00 mg/dL)
ALT	35 units/L (15–48 units/L)
LDH	1205 units/L (338–610)
Total bilirubin	3.3 mg/dL (0.8–1.2 mg/dL)
Indirect bilirubin	2.7 mg/dL
aPTT	28 seconds (25.7–38.8 seconds)
PT	11 seconds (9.5–12.7 seconds)
D-dimer	elevated
Blood pressure	149/92

Blood cultures are obtained. Peripheral smear is shown (Fig. 33.3).

The physician at the local hospital asks for management recommendations and requests emergent transfer for

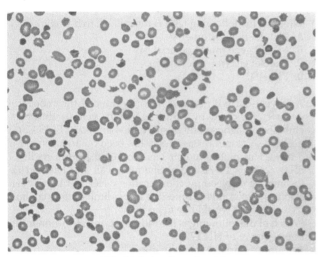

FIG. 33.3 for Question 21

initiation of plasma exchange; it is estimated that the patient will arrive in 8–10 hours.

What should be recommended as a temporizing measure in this patient while transfer is being arranged?

A. IV unfractionated heparin

B. Cryoprecipitate

C. Platelet

D. Fresh frozen plasma

22. A 60-year-old woman presents for evaluation of thrombocytosis. She was noted to have a platelet count of 650,000 × 10⁹/L with normal WBC and normal hemoglobin after initial workup of new onset of migraine headaches and burning erythematous palms by her PCP. CBC 5 years prior was normal. She is otherwise healthy. She takes ibuprofen once daily for headache, but otherwise takes no medications.

Physical examination 4 weeks later is notable for erythematous palms bilaterally. The neurologic examination is normal. There is no hepatosplenomegaly. BP is 135/78, HR 72. Pulse oximetry is 98% on room air.

Labs show:

WBC	7500 × 10⁹/L
Hgb	13.6 g/dL
MCV	90 fL
RDW	13%
Platelets	660,000 × 10⁹/L
ESR	12 mm/h
CRP	0.2 mg/dL
Ferritin	70 ng/mL
Head CT, noncontrast	no mass nor hemorrhage

JAK2 V617F PCR from peripheral blood is negative for the mutation.

PML/RAR-alpha FISH from peripheral blood is negative.

Peripheral blood smear shows thrombocytosis and no further abnormalities.

Which of the following is the next best step in the evaluation?

A. No further workup

B. CALR mutation testing

C. MPL mutation testing

D. Thrombopoietin testing

23. A 43-year-old African American woman complains of 1 year of progressive LUQ pain, early satiety, and drenching night sweats. She had no fevers nor adenopathy. She works in a chicken processing plant and has not traveled outside the United States and does not hunt. She does not drink alcohol. She has no easy bruising, peripheral neuropathy, diarrhea, constipation, foamy urine, nor rashes.

Physical examination reveals a well-nourished woman in no apparent distress. The spleen is palpable within the LLQ. The neurologic examination is normal. The cardiopulmonary examination is normal.

WBC	7600 × 10⁹/L with normal differential
Hgb	11.6 g/dL
MCV	84 (80–100 fL)
Platelets	107,000 × 10⁹/L

AST/ALT/total bilirubin is normal. Peripheral blood smear shows thrombocytopenia but is otherwise normal. CT chest/abdomen/pelvis demonstrates splenomegaly to 20 cm but no lymphadenopathy.

She has two full sisters and no children. She is not aware of any cancers or chronic medical conditions in her siblings. Her mother died during childbirth, and her father died from a myocardial infarction at the age of 67.

Bone marrow biopsy and aspiration revealed mild hypercellularity, with appropriately maturing trilineage hematopoiesis. There was no lymphoma identified by morphologic, immunohistochemical, or flow cytometric analysis. Scattered histiocytes filled with nonpolarizable debris were present throughout the marrow.

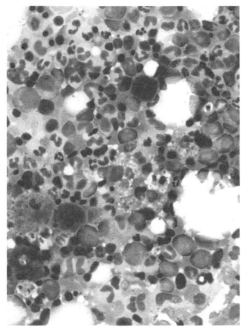

FIG. 33.4 for Question 23

What is the next best step in management?
A. Splenectomy
B. Rituximab monotherapy
C. Corticosteroids
D. Analysis for lysosomal storage diseases

24. A 65-year-old man with essential thrombocythemia presents for his biannual hematologic evaluation. He feels well and has not had any thrombotic events. He denies erythromelalgia, headaches, or epistaxis. He has no history of cardiovascular disease and denies palpitations, angina, presyncope, or syncope. He takes aspirin 81 mg daily for thrombotic prophylaxis in addition to amlodipine for hypertension. His laboratory testing today shows:

WBC	$10,500 \times 10^9/L$
Hgb	13.6 g/dL
MCV	90 fL
Platelets	$924,000 \times 10^9/L$
Creatinine	0.8 mg/dL
Potassium	6.8 mmol/L

Which of the following is the next best step in the management of his hyperkalemia?
A. Check a plasma potassium level
B. Administer furosemide
C. Administer calcium gluconate
D. Begin hydroxyurea

25. A 42-year-old man presents with fever, headaches, chest pain, and thrombocytopenia. Peripheral blood smear shows greater than five schistocytes per high power field. A hemolytic anemia is evident, and there is no evidence of DIC. His blood pressure on admission is 149/87. He takes no medications and denies herbal supplements or over-the-counter medications. ADAMTS 13 activity is less than 10%, and an inhibitor is present.

He is urgently started on corticosteroids and plasma exchange using 1.5 volumes of plasma. Over the next week, there is no improvement in his platelet count nor LDH. Which of the following is the next best step in treatment?
A. Continue current therapy
B. Administer rituximab
C. Administer bortezomib
D. Splenectomy

26. A 20-year-old college student presents for evaluation of thrombocytopenia after presenting to the college infirmary 3 weeks ago with flu-like symptoms. At that time, her WBC $6.5 \times 10^9/L$ with a normal differential, hemoglobin 14.6 g/dL, and platelet count of $80,000 \times 10^9/L$. Repeat testing in your office shows no change in the complete blood count. She has no hepatosplenomegaly on examination.

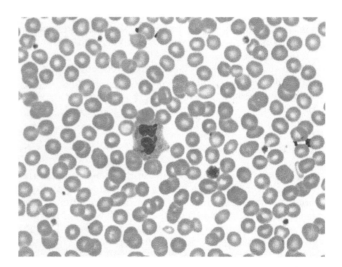

Which of the following is the next best test for evaluating her thrombocytopenia?
A. Mutation panel for *MYH9*
B. Bone marrow aspiration and biopsy
C. Platelet electron microscopy
D. Von Willebrand activity, antigen, and multimers

27. A 55-year-old woman presents for left leg pain and swelling of 1 day's duration. She had been admitted to the vascular surgery service 2 weeks prior for right tibial artery occlusion. She was treated successfully with thrombolytic therapy and unfractionated heparin and then discharged 10 days ago with an enoxaparin bridge to warfarin, along with clopidogrel. Past medical history includes diabetes, hypercholesterolemia, renal insufficiency, and tobacco use. Her enoxaparin was discontinued 4 days after discharge (6 days ago) when her INR reached 2.0. Her most recent INR checked 2 days ago was 2.4. Physical examination shows well-healing wounds from her thrombolytic procedure. Her left leg is

tense, red, and swollen to the level of the midthigh. She is afebrile with normal vital signs. Duplex ultrasonography shows extensive left leg venous thrombosis. CBC shows hemoglobin 10 g/dL, WBC $12,000 \times 10^9$/L, platelet count $165,000 \times 10^9$/L. Platelet count at discharge was $72,000 \times 10^9$/L. Creatinine is 2.8; at discharge, it was 2.2. Which of the following is the most appropriate next step in management?

A. Start fondaparinux
B. Start argatroban
C. Start unfractionated heparin
D. Test for factor V Leiden
E. Measure D-dimer

28. A 55-year-old man with cirrhosis due to hepatitis C is known to have chronic thrombocytopenia with a baseline platelet count in the $40,000 \times 10^6$/L range. He was recently diagnosed with a large cerebellar glioma requiring surgical resection, and he presents for recommendations about perioperative management of his thrombocytopenia. PMHx includes peptic ulcer disease, grade 2 esophageal varices, splenomegaly, and internal hemorrhoids. He neither drinks nor smokes. He refuses transfusion since he is a Jehovah's Witness. Ultrasound shows a spleen size of 19 cm and portal hypertension. He is treated with eltrombopag at 25 mg daily for 2 weeks, with his platelet count rising from 45,000 to $110,000 \times 10^6$/L. His surgery is scheduled for 2 days from now. The patient is planned to remain on eltrombopag for 10 days postoperatively and then taper off over the next week.
Which of the following is the most frequent risk of this medical therapy in this patient?

A. Myelofibrosis
B. Cataracts
C. Liver failure
D. Portal vein thrombosis
E. Acute myeloid leukemia

29. A 25-year-old woman presents with altered mental status and fever. She has a history of opioid abuse and was noted to have been injecting oxymorphone extended release tablets (Opana ER) for the past 6–8 weeks. Her family noted slurred speech and staggering gait and brought her to the emergency department. In the ED, vital signs were significant for T 38.5, HR 110, BP 100/55, and RR 18. She had a 2/6 systolic murmur, which increased with inspiration. Track marks are present in bilateral antecubital and forearm veins. Neurologic exam was nonfocal. Laboratory data showed Hgb 10.5, WBC 16, platelet count 33. BUN 45, Cre 2.2, T bili 2.1, LDH 775. Peripheral blood smear reveals numerous schistocytes. PT and aPTT were within reference ranges. ADAMTS13 activity level is within reference range, and no inhibitor is demonstrated.
Which of the following is the most appropriate course of action at this point?

A. Supportive care
B. Plasma infusion
C. Plasma exchange
D. Heparin
E. Corticosteroids

30. A 55-year-old woman is admitted for pinning of a pathologic hip fracture caused by metastatic breast cancer. Three days postoperatively, she develops a thrombosis of her left common femoral vein. Labs show a normal platelet count and PT/aPTT at this time. She is treated

with enoxaparin bridged to warfarin and discharged to a skilled nursing facility on postoperative day 6. Two days later (POD #8), her INR is noted to be 2.4, and her enoxaparin is discontinued. Four days later (POD #12), she develops acute chest pain and is diagnosed with an acute pulmonary embolus. Her INR is 2.8. Her CBC shows a hemoglobin of 11.2 g/dL, WBC 9600×10^6/L, and platelet count is $85,000 \times 10^3$/L.
Which is the most appropriate anticoagulant at this time?

A. Enoxaparin
B. Unfractionated heparin
C. Warfarin
D. Argatroban
E. Rivaroxaban

31. A 45-year-old woman presents for evaluation of incidentally discovered thrombocytopenia. She has a history of reflux esophagitis and anxiety. Medications include omeprazole, citalopram, and a multivitamin. She has noted no bruising, no epistaxis, no gum bleeding, and no heavy menstrual bleeding. The platelet count found on CBC evaluation drawn at her routine annual examination returns at $17,000 \times 10^9$. Hemoglobin and WBC are within reference ranges. Peripheral blood smear is as shown.
See Fig. 33.5.

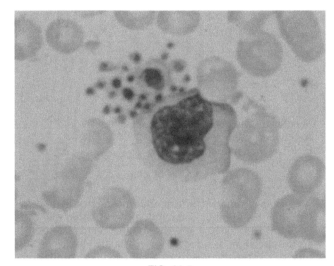

FIG. 33.5

Which of the following is the most appropriate action to take at this point?

A. Start corticosteroids
B. Start aspirin
C. Stop omeprazole
D. Stop citalopram
E. Reassurance

32. A 26-year-old pregnant woman G1P0 at 34 weeks' gestation is referred for thrombocytopenia. Her pregnancy has been uncomplicated, and she takes only a prenatal vitamin and a steroid nasal spray for seasonal allergies. Current vital signs are normal. There is no peripheral edema. Abdominal exam reveals a gravid uterus with no organomegaly, and no tenderness or guarding. Neurologic examination shows no focal abnormalities. No hyperreflexia. See Table 33.2 for laboratory values.

TABLE 33.2 Laboratory Data: Question 32

CBC

	WBC	5300 × 10⁹/L
	Hgb	10.0 g/L
	Hct	30%
	Platelets	89,000 × 10⁹/L
Serum		
	BUN	22 mg/dL
	Cre	1.1 mg/dL
	LDH	935 μ/L
	AST	97 μ/L
	ALT	122 μ/L
	T bili	1.2 mg/dL

Peripheral blood smear shows no platelet clumping, no red cell fragments. PT and aPTT are within reference ranges. Which of the following is the most appropriate next step in management?
A. Emergent delivery of the fetus
B. Recheck platelet count in 2 weeks
C. Start corticosteroids
D. Start gammaglobulin
E. Test antiplatelet antibodies

33. A 26-year-old pregnant woman G1P0 at 34 weeks' gestation is referred for thrombocytopenia. Her pregnancy has been uncomplicated, and she takes only a prenatal vitamin and a steroid nasal spray for seasonal allergies. Current vital signs show a BP of 140/90 and HR 100. There is 1+ peripheral edema. Abdominal exam reveals a gravid uterus with no organomegaly, but mild tenderness in the RUQ without guarding. Neurologic examination shows no focal abnormalities. No hyperreflexia is noted.
Peripheral blood smear shows no platelet clumping, one–two red cell fragments per high power field. PT and aPTT are within reference ranges.
Which of the following is the most appropriate next step in management?
A. Emergent delivery of the fetus
B. Recheck platelet count in 2 weeks
C. Start corticosteroids
D. Start gammaglobulin
E. Test antiplatelet antibodies

34. A 72-year-old woman with ischemic cardiomyopathy underwent placement of a continuous flow left ventricular assist device 6 months ago. She is maintained on clopidogrel and warfarin. Her last INR was 2.5 three days ago. She has not been on any new medications. Her diet remains stable. She presents with angina, fatigue, and black tarry stools for 2 weeks. On exam, she is pale and has scattered ecchymoses. Her initial labs show the following:

Hgb	6 g/dL
Hct	18%
Platelet count	144,000/μL
INR	2.9
aPTT	36 seconds

How should the patient be treated at this time?
A. Fresh frozen plasma
B. Four-factor prothrombin complex concentrate
C. Platelet transfusion
D. Recombinant activated factor VII
E. Red cell transfusion

35. A 71-year-old woman with a 20-year history of atrial fibrillation and a recently diagnosed outpatient pneumonia presents with a 2-hour history of bruising and hematemesis. She has been maintained on warfarin with a target INR of 2.5 and was recently treated with erythromycin. On exam her pulse is 120, with a blood pressure of 80/50. She has scattered ecchymosis on her extremities. Her current INR is 12.7.
In addition to stopping warfarin and giving vitamin K, which of the following should be given to stop her bleeding?
A. Fresh frozen plasma
B. Prothrombin complex concentrate
C. Amino caproic acid
D. Factor VIIa

36. A 32-year-old woman with a 10-year history of allergic rhinitis, depression, and Hashimoto thyroiditis presents to the emergency department 2 hours after vomiting blood. The patient has been compliant with her medications that include nasal fluticasone, fexofenadine, paroxetine, levothyroxine, and norgestrel. On exam, her pulse is 90 with a blood pressure of 110/70. She appears comfortable.
Which of the following drugs increased her risk for hematemesis?
A. Fluticasone
B. Fexofenadine
C. Paroxetine
D. Levothyroxine
E. Norgestrel

37. A 42-year-old woman is brought into the emergency room 1 hour after being found unconscious in a highway rest stop in western North Carolina. The patient's blood pressure is 60/40, pulse is 128, temp is 101°F, and RR is 14. She is minimally responsive and has bleeding gums and a large ecchymosis on her right calf that is oozing blood. Her laboratory studies include:

Hgb	11 g/dL
HCT	33%
WBC	18,200/μL
Platelet	67,000/μL
INR	3.1
aPTT	57 seconds
fibrinogen	80 mg/dL
FSP	40 mg/mL

In addition to providing hemodynamic support, which of the following would be most effective at correcting her coagulopathy?
A. Factor VIIa
B. Fresh frozen plasma
C. Tranexamic acid
D. Prothrombin complex concentrate
E. Polyvalent crotalid antivenin

38. A 45-year-old woman presented with a 2-year history of painful bruises on the lower extremities that were typically preceded by itching in the area of the subsequent

bruise. These lesions appeared sporadically every 2 months. She had a history of depression for 6 years and had been diagnosed with chronic fatigue syndrome. She takes no medications, including over-the-counter drugs. On exam, she was noted to have a few slightly tender ecchymosis on her thighs and legs. There was no bleeding from mucosal surfaces and no petechiae. CBC, including platelet count, PFA-100, PT, aPTT, and ANA, have all been normal.

What is the most appropriate next step in management?

A. Platelet function tests

B. Platelet electron microscopy

C. Psychiatric referral

D. Reptilase time

E. Platelet ADP/ATP ratio

39. A 22-year-old woman complains of menorrhagia for most of her postadolescent life. She has had one one successful pregnancy 2 years prior, complicated by postpartum hemorrhage necessitating transfusion. Her family history is remarkable for a maternal aunt who died during childbirth from bleeding. On exam, she has scattered ecchymosis without a history of trauma. These are mostly on her extremities. Her laboratory studies are shown:

Hgb	9.2 g/dL
Hct	27.4%
Platelets	$477,000 \times 10^9$/L
INR	1.8
aPTT	47 seconds
Mixing study	Correction of aPTT
Factor V	20%
Factor VII	95%
Factor VIII	10%
Factor IX	94%
Factor X	97%
Factor XI	103%

What is her most likely diagnosis?

A. Type 2N von Willebrand disease

B. Vitamin K deficiency

C. Liver disease

D. Factor V and VIII combined deficiency

E. Lupus anticoagulant

40. A 12-year-old girl presents for evaluation of easy bruisability, present throughout most of her life. She was the product of a normal gestation and delivery and has been otherwise healthy. On exam she has multiple bruises of her extremities, some as large as 6 cm. Her laboratory studies are as follows:

Hgb	10.2 g/dL
Hct	30%
Platelets	269,000/μL
INR	1.0
aPTT	28 seconds
PFA-100	Closure time > 300 sec

Platelet aggregation studies:
  Decreased primary response to ADP, collagen, epinephrine. Normal response to ristocetin.

What is her most likely diagnosis?

A. Glanzmann thrombasthenia

B. Bernard-Soulier

C. Grey platelet syndrome

D. Delta storage pool disease

E. Scott syndrome

41. A 23-year-old woman with von Willebrand disease (vWD), she thinks is type IIb presents to establish care. She has experienced nosebleeds as a child and experiences heavy menstrual bleeding, as well as prolonged bleeding after minor procedures. She is not aware of her prior treatments and has no records to provide today. It is decided to obtain prior records and repeat laboratory studies to confirm the diagnosis. Which of the following would be most consistent with the diagnosis of type IIb vWD?

A. Decrease in all von Willebrand factor multimers

B. vWF:Ristocetin cofactor: vWF antigen (vWF:RCo: vWF Ag) ratio of 0.4

C. Thrombocytosis

D. Decreased aggregation on ristocetin-induced platelet aggregation (RIPA) assay

E. Lack of aggregation to all agonists except ristocetin on platelet aggregation

42. A 45-year-old woman of Ashkenazi Jewish descent is sent for perioperative recommendations prior to a planned total hip arthroplasty. She notes that she had excessive bleeding after a cholecystectomy, appendectomy, and after extraction of her wisdom teeth. She describes both her mother and sister as "bleeders." She has never had prior hematologic evaluation.

Laboratory results:

CBC	Normal
PT	12 seconds
INR	1
aPTT	51 seconds
aPTT 1:1 dilution	35 seconds
Fibrinogen	Normal
Thrombin time (TT)	Normal
Factor VIII activity	82%
Factor IX activity	91%

Based on the most likely diagnosis, which of the following would you recommend for pre- and perioperative support?

A. Fresh frozen plasma (FFP)

B. Cryoprecipitate

C. Recombinant factor VIII concentrate

D. Platelets

E. Recombinant vWF

43. A 48-year-old female with an elevated aPTT is referred for preoperative consultation. She presented to the emergency room earlier this morning with abdominal pain and was subsequently diagnosed with appendicitis. An appendectomy is scheduled for later in the afternoon.

She reports no personal or family history of excessive bleeding. She has had a prior uncomplicated cholecystectomy, partial mastectomy, and wisdom teeth extraction. She denies any recent bleeding or bruising.

Lab results:

CBC	Normal
PT	12 seconds
aPTT	65 seconds
aPTT 1:1 dilution	49 seconds
Fibrinogen	Normal
TT	Normal
Factor VIII activity	82%
Factor IX activity	91%
Factor XI activity	78%

Which is the most appropriate recommendation?

A. Cancellation of surgery

B. Await results of factor XII activity

C. Await results of factor VIII inhibitor (Bethesda) assay
D. Proceed with surgery
E. Await results of lupus anticoagulant

44. A 55-year-old man presents to the emergency room with melena and is found to have a hemodynamically significant GI bleed. His only prior medical history is MGUS with an IgG kappa M-spike of 0.5 g/dL.

In the last 6 months he has noted increased bruising, bleeding while shaving, and two spontaneous nosebleeds. Two weeks ago a CBC was unremarkable as were kidney and liver function tests. He had no bleeding with previous wisdom tooth extraction. He takes no prescribed or over-the-counter medications.

Labs drawn in the ED include:

CBC	Normal except for hemoglobin of 8.3 g/dL
PT	12 seconds
aPTT	33 seconds
Fibrinogen	Normal
TT	Normal
PFA	Greater than 300 seconds with ADP and collagen

Further diagnostic testing is not immediately available. In addition to endoscopy and consideration of PRBC transfusion, which of the following interventions would be most successful in controlling bleeding?
A. Factor VIII
B. Platelets
C. Recombinant factor VIIa
D. Fresh frozen plasma
E. Intravenous immunoglobulin

45. A 34-year-old man with mild hemophilia B (baseline levels around 10%) presents to the ED after an automobile accident. He is found to have a psoas muscle hematoma, but no other bleeding. You decide to provide recombinant factor IX replacement, targeting peak levels of 80%. His current weight is 100 kg.

A factor IX level is not available at this time, but his aPTT is prolonged to 52 seconds and corrects to normal at 35 seconds on 1:1 dilution with normal donor plasma.

Which is the most appropriate recommendation at this time?
A. Recombinant factor IX 4200 units
B. NovoSeven 9 mg
C. FEIBA (Factor eight inhibitor bypass activity) 5000 units
D. Recombinant factor IX 8400 units
E. Recombinant factor IX 12,000 units

46. A 28-year-old woman had an urgent and complicated vaginal delivery. Within a few hours of surgery she develops respiratory distress, hypotension, and intractable vaginal bleeding that does not respond to uterine massage, pitocin, or other obstetric measures. An amniotic fluid embolism is suspected.

A thromboelastogram (TEG) is obtained for evaluation of bleeding (see Fig. 33.6). A normal tracing is shown on top of her results as a comparison.

Her TEG tracing (bottom) is most consistent with:
A. Anticoagulant effect
B. Fibrinolysis
C. Thrombotic state
D. Decreased or dysfunctional platelets
E. Coagulopathy

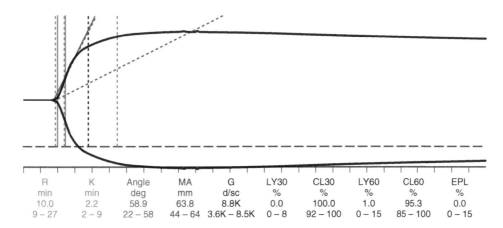

R min	K min	Angle deg	MA mm	G d/sc	LY30 %	CL30 %	LY60 %	CL60 %	EPL %
10.0	2.2	58.9	63.8	8.8K	0.0	100.0	1.0	95.3	0.0
9 – 27	2 – 9	22 – 58	44 – 64	3.6K – 8.5K	0 – 8	92 – 100	0 – 15	85 – 100	0 – 15

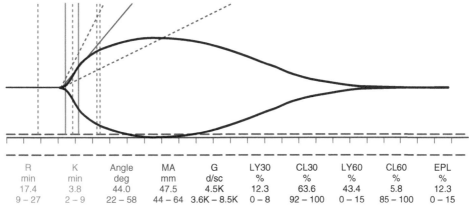

R min	K min	Angle deg	MA mm	G d/sc	LY30 %	CL30 %	LY60 %	CL60 %	EPL %
17.4	3.8	44.0	47.5	4.5K	12.3	63.6	43.4	5.8	12.3
9 – 27	2 – 9	22 – 58	44 – 64	3.6K – 8.5K	0 – 8	92 – 100	0 – 15	85 – 100	0 – 15

FIG. 33.6 for Question 46

47. A 40-year-old man with hemophilia A with a native factor VIII level less than 1% is transported to the emergency room following a motor vehicle accident. CT of the head confirms intraventricular hemorrhage. A routine clinic appointment 2 weeks prior to the results of his annual Bethesda assay revealed a factor VIII inhibitor of 10 Bethesda units.

Which medication would be most appropriate in this setting?

A. Humate-P
B. Porcine factor VIII
C. FEIBA
D. Recombinant factor VIII
E. DDAVP

48. A 48-year-old man with a past medical history of well-controlled systemic lupus erythematosus, antiphospholipid antibody syndrome (APLS) on chronic anticoagulation, and HTN underwent an uncomplicated cholecystectomy. In the next 96 hours he develops progressive renal failure, altered mental status, and a left lower extremity diagnosed DVT. He is started on high-dose steroids and anticoagulation without improvement.

Labs show moderate thrombocytopenia and severe renal failure. A lupus anticoagulant is detected by dilute Russell viper venom time (DRVVT). ELISA for PF4-heparin antibodies is negative, and ADMATS-13 is normal. A kidney biopsy shows microthrombi in the small vessels.

Which of the following therapies should be initiated next?

A. Eculizumab
B. Rituximab
C. Pulse dexamethasone
D. Therapeutic plasma exchange
E. Direct thrombin inhibitor

49. A 73-year-old African American woman with a history of rheumatoid arthritis is referred for evaluation of continued postoperative bleeding. She was admitted after falling on her left arm and developing compartment syndrome. She underwent a fasciotomy that was complicated by two additional returns to the operating room for continued bleeding. Her medical records note numerous prior operations, including hysterectomy and coronary artery bypass grafting without any hemorrhagic complications. You note the following laboratory evaluation that has been performed:

WBC	$22,600 \times 10^9/L$
Hemoglobin	10.5 g/dL
Hematocrit	30.8%
MCV	95 fL
Platelets	$345,000 \times 10^9/L$
ANC	$11,900 \times 10^9/L$
ALC	$9800 \times 10^9/L$
PT	11.1 sec
APTT	64.1 sec
vWF:Ag	370%
vWF:RCo	333%
FVIII	1%
BU	57.6 µ/L

6-months prior: PT 11.4 sec, aPTT 29.5 sec

She is diagnosed with acquired hemophilia and is immediately started on bypassing therapy to treat her active bleeding. Which of the following should also be recommended at this time?

A. Continued treatment with bypassing therapy alone
B. Prednisone
C. Cyclophosphamide

D. Rituximab
E. Prednisone + Cyclophosphamide

50. A 29-year-old Caucasian woman is referred for a consultation for possible von Willebrand disease and the need for a punch biopsy to evaluate for an abnormal pigmented lesion on her back. Her history is remarkable for prolonged bleeding following a tonsillectomy, excessive bruising after wisdom teeth extraction, and menorrhagia. While she has not been definitively diagnosed with vWD, she reports that her mother and aunt carry this diagnosis. She is currently on combined oral contraceptive therapy to treat her menorrhagia and symptoms of endometriosis. The following laboratory tests are sent and show the following:

WBC	$4500 \times 10^9/L$
Hemoglobin	9.8 g/dL
Hematocrit	30.6%
MCV	72 fL
Platelets	$329,000 \times 10^9/L$
vWF:Ag	39%
vWF:RCo	42%
FVIII	52%

As part of her preoperative consultation, which of the following recommendations is most appropriate?

A. Preoperative trial of DDAVP
B. DDAVP, 0.3 µg/kg, IV
C. ε-aminocaproic acid
D. vWF:FVIII concentrates
E. Recombinant vWF

51. A 34-year-old Caucasian woman admitted for possible preterm labor on the Labor and Delivery floor. She is noted to have a history of thrombocytopenia. She is G4P3 and in her 32nd week of gestation.

Her history is significant for long-standing thrombocytopenia, even when she has not been pregnant, although pregnancy has worsened the measured platelet count. She relates a long history of easy bruising, with her wisdom teeth extraction being complicated by prolonged bleeding. The patient reveals that with G2 and G3, she was repeatedly treated with steroids and IVIg, which were ineffective in raising her platelet count. Review of her platelet counts reveals that she has normal platelet counts on occasion (peak of 176), with a nadir of $22,000 \times 10^9/L$ documented with G3. A number of laboratory tests have been performed over the years, which have not elucidated the cause of her thrombocytopenia. In passing, she mentions that for while it was thought that she might have von Willebrand disease, but this was "ruled out" when her platelet count decreased following the administration of DDAVP.

Which of following tests would most likely lead to the correct diagnosis?

A. Flow cytometry for gpIB/IX/V expression
B. Ristocetin-induced platelet aggregation (RIPA)
C. Staining neutrophils for nonmuscular myosin heavy chain IIA (NMMHC-IIA)
D. Platelet autoantibodies
E. ADAMTS13 activity

52. A 67-year-old man with history of diabetes mellitus-II, hypertension, tobacco use, and ischemic cardiomyopathy is in the cardiothoracic ICU when an urgent consultation is requested. There is no history of postoperative or spontaneous bleeding. His cardiac function has progressively declined to the point where medical therapy alone is no longer effective. While awaiting a heart transplant, he has decompensated further, resulting in his placement on extracorporeal membranous oxygenation (ECMO), followed by implantation of a continuous flow left ventricular assist device. The patient remained in guarded condition for several days afterwards and is being maintained on an unfractionated heparin drip and single-agent antiplatelet therapy with aspirin. On postoperative day #9, he developed hemodynamic instability, followed thereafter by the presence of melenic stools. A hemoglobin from early morning labs was noted to be 10.7 g/dL and is now measured at 6.1 g/dL. His heparin is stopped, and an urgent EGD shows the presence of arteriovenous malformations that are laser photocoagulated.

In addition to the possible role of anticoagulation and antithrombotic therapy, what other testing should be performed?

A. Platelet aggregometry
B. Thrombin time
C. Heparin/PF4 antibody ELISA, followed by serotonin release assay
D. von Willebrand panel, including multimer analysis

53. An 18-year-old man with severe FVIII deficiency is evaluated in clinic. Until age 17, he lived in India, where he had no access to clotting factor. Since being in the United States, he has been on twice to thrice weekly prophylaxis with rFVIII, but this has been complicated by access and compliance issues. He presents urgently to the hematology clinic for a left knee bleed that has not responded to therapy. While his infusions logs are spotty, it is noted that in the last 4 days, despite regular infusions of rFVIII, his symptoms have persisted, if not worsened. There have been no changes to his medications since he was last seen 6 months previously for a routine clinic visit. His parents are able to demonstrate proper technique, their supply of recombinant FVIII has not expired, and this appears to have been stored correctly.

Which of the following is the most appropriate next step in management?

A. Check CBC to evaluate for thrombocytopenia
B. Check for the presence of an inhibitor
C. Increase dose of recombinant FVIII
D. Switch to plasma-derived factor VIII
E. Prescribe tranexamic acid

54. A 21-year-old man with severe hemophilia B presents to the ER for severe gluteal hematoma. He has recently moved here from Mexico, where he had no access to clotting factor.

His diagnosis was made in the United States 3 months ago. He has a known family history of a bleeding disorder. He was given a dose of rFIX for a right knee bleed, without any adverse events. There had been one prior episode of a left buttock hematoma, which occurred when he fell down on a step, which was treated with a single-dose of rFIX. Most recently, he developed another lump in his left buttock and presented for evaluation. Immediately following completion of the infusion, the ER nurse noted "red-splotches" and that he started wheezing shortly thereafter. Hematology is consulted.

Based upon this history, which of the following is the most likely explanation for the reaction?

A. Development of an inhibitor
B. Improper infusion technique

C. Allergy to the diluent
D. Bacterial contamination of the rFIX vial
E. Use of an expired product

55. A 19-year-old man with autism and severe hemophilia B is known to have developed an inhibitor. His bleeds are felt to be adequately controlled by infusions of rFVIIa, and it is noted that his inhibitor titer has decayed to 0.0 BU. However, his parents do not feel that the on-demand use of rFVIIa is adequate, as they wish to use rFIX in a prophylactic regimen. As a result of their online research, during a scheduled clinic visit, they inquire about the role of immune tolerance therapy (ITT) to eradicate Justin's inhibitor. The risks and benefits of embarking upon this course, which include the lower rates of success with ITT, recurrence of his inhibitor to FIX, costs, and possible need for central access, are discussed.

Which of the following is another important possible complication of ITT?

A. Pulmonary fibrosis from immune complex deposition
B. Heart failure
C. Transaminitis leading to liver failure
D. Nephrotic syndrome
E. ANA-negative polyarthritis

56. A 64-year-old woman with a past medical history of diabetes mellitus-II, hypertension, and obesity is scheduled for a left total knee replacement. She is currently in the preoperative holding area, and hematology is urgently consulted. She has undergone a right total knee replacement with this orthopedic surgeon in the past with good results, prompting her to have the left knee replaced. During her preoperative visit with anesthesia the week prior, routine labs were sent, which included a PT and aPTT. This was remarkable for an aPTT of **117** seconds (26.8–37.1). However, this appeared to have been overlooked, and when she arrived for her operation, this was noted and rechecked, yielding another aPTT of 121 seconds (26.8–37.1).

It is recommended that surgery be delayed until the patient can be evaluated. Testing is recommended and shows:

WBC	6200×10^9/L
Hemoglobin	12.5 g/dL
Hematocrit	36%
MCV	95 fL
Platelets	$345,000 \times 10^9$/L
PT	11.1 seconds (INR 1)
aPTT	119
aPTT Mix	
	0 minutes 35.7 seconds
	60 minutes 35.3 seconds
FVIII	97%
FIX	105%
FXI	83%
FXII	6% (48%–151%)

Which of the following is the most appropriate recommendation?

A. Proceed without any additional interventions
B. Infusion of FFP, bolus of 30 mL/kg, followed by 10 mL/kg every 12 hours
C. An intermediate purity vWF:FVIII concentrate, dosed at 50 units/kg
D. rFVIIa, initial bolus of 30 μg/kg, followed by 15 μg/kg every 4 hours
E. Four-factor prothrombin complex concentrate, 2500 units 30 minutes prior to surgery

57. A consultation is requested for a patient is a 54-year-old homeless man, with a past history of schizophrenia and alcohol abuse. He was found unresponsive in the middle of a sidewalk and was initially thought to be the victim of assault. As a result, he was brought in by EMS as a Level 1 trauma, wherein his clothes were removed and revealed ecchymoses, particularly on his legs. This prompted a closer physical examination and revealed the appearance of "petechiae" along his hair follicles, as well as gingival swelling, leading the medical student to suspect leukemic infiltration. "Palpable purpura" is noted when the blood pressure cuff is removed. Hematology is consulted.

Laboratory testing showed the following:

WBC	$12,900 \times 10^9$/L
Hemoglobin	9.8 g/dL
Hematocrit	28.4%
MCV	104 fL
Platelets	$98,000 \times 10^9$/L

Review of the peripheral smear shows no blasts, mild anisocytosis with moderate target cells, without evidence for fragmentation. No platelet clumping is observed.

PT	14.1 sec
INR	1.3
aPTT	35.8 sec
Fibrinogen	226 g/dL
FVIII	298%

Based upon the available history, physical examination, and laboratory data, which test should be performed next?
A. Ethanol level
B. Ascorbic acid level
C. Methylmalonic acid level
D. PT mixing study
E. Bone marrow biopsy

58. A consultation is urgently called to evaluate a 74-year-old man on the orthopedic service. His past medical history is remarkable for hypertension, diabetes mellitus, nonischemic cardiomyopathy, and atrial fibrillation, for which he has been maintained on therapeutic anticoagulation with warfarin. He had been admitted for an elective right total hip arthroplasty, following which he resumed anticoagulation with warfarin at his home dose. Prior to his discharge to rehabilitation, he developed a fever and was noted to have erythema of the surgical site. He was started on piperacillin/tazobactam and gentamicin, but the following day purulent discharge was noted to be coming from the wound. He remains febrile and is now tachycardic and hypotensive. He is to be taken urgently to the OR for probable removal of the prosthesis. The standard preoperative labs are remarkable for the following:

PT	>120 seconds (9.5–13.2)
INR	>10
aPTT	>120 seconds (26.8–37.1)

Which of the following is the most appropriate next step in management?
A. Vitamin K, 10 mg PO
B. Vitamin K, 10 mg IV
C. Fresh frozen plasma, 4 units
D. Vitamin K (10 mg IV) + fresh frozen plasma (4 units)
E. A four-factor prothrombin complex concentrate (50 IU FIX/kg)
F. A four-factor prothrombin complex concentrate (50 IU FIX/kg) + vitamin K 10 mg

59. A 63-year-old woman with ischemic cardiomyopathy was admitted for worsening heart failure symptoms, ultimately requiring intubation and placement of an intraaortic balloon pump (IABP). With aggressive diuresis and optimization of her inotropic agents, she required less support, allowing for extubation, with her IABP to be discontinued after shift change. However, she suddenly developed a severe headache with photophobia and meningeal signs. A stat head CT showed the presence of a subarachnoid hemorrhage, felt to be due to a ruptured aneurysm. Neurosurgery is ready to take her to the OR for coil embolization of the aneurysm and another one noted nearby. However, they cannot do so until the effect of her heparinization for the IABP is reversed. An urgent hematology consult is requested.

Which of the following is the most appropriate recommendation?
A. Vitamin K, 10 mg IV
B. Fresh frozen plasma, 4 units IV
C. Cryoprecipitate, 10 units IV
D. Protamine sulfate, 1 mg/100 units heparin IV
E. Recombinant FVIIa, 90 μg/kg

60. A 21-year-old college student presents to the University Student Health Care Center with a several-year history of heavy menstrual bleeding. She was recently diagnosed with iron deficiency anemia. She has had a long history of intermittent epistaxis but otherwise no major bleeding or bruising. She is only on iron supplementation. Based on the following data (Table 33.3), what is the most likely etiology of the bleeding problem?

TABLE 33.3 Laboratory Values: Question 60

	Patient Result	Reference Interval
Platelet count	$175,000 \times 10^9$/L	150 K–450 K $\times 10^9$/L
PT	10.5 s	9–13.8 s
PTT	34 s	28–38 s
vWF antigen	20 IU/dL	50%–200%
Ristocetin cofactor activity (vWF activity)	20 IU/dL	51%–215%
von Willebrand multimers	All multimers present but in decreased concentrations	Normal

What is the most likely type of coagulopathy in this patient?
A. Type 1 von Willebrand disease
B. Type 2A von Willebrand disease
C. Type 2B von Willebrand disease
D. Type 2M von Willebrand disease
E. Type 3 von Willebrand disease

61. A 14-year-old girl recently presented to her pediatrician for heavy menstrual bleeding. As a child she experienced frequent bruising and a knee hemarthrosis after falling off her bicycle. Her FMHx is significant for a paternal uncle who was diagnosed with mild hemophilia but poorly responds to FVIII boluses. The patient's laboratory values are shown in Table 33.4.

TABLE 33.4 Laboratory Values: Question 61

	Patient Result	Reference Interval
Platelet count	$220,000 \times 10^9$/L	$150,000$–$450,000 \times 10^9$/L
PT	11.5 seconds	9–13.8 seconds
PTT	45 seconds	28–38 seconds
vWF antigen	42 IU/dL	50–200%
Ristocetin cofactor activity (vWF activity)	40 IU/dL	51–215%
von Willebrand multimers	Normal	Normal

The most likely etiology of this patient's bleeding disorder is:
  A. Mild quantitative deficiency of vWF
  B. Carrier of FVIII mutation
  C. Mutation in the factor VIII binding site of vWF
  D. Mutation in vWF leading to abnormal synthesis or packing of vWF

62. A 25-year-old woman is referred for evaluation of epistaxis and easy bruising that she has had for several years. She denies any fevers, chills, night sweats, or weight loss. She has no other comorbidities. There is no family history of bleeding disorders. Physical exam is notable for dried blood at the nares and petechiae on her feet. The patient's platelet count is $58,000 \times 10^9$/L. A CBC from 5 years ago revealed a platelet count of $56,000 \times 10^9$/L. PTT and PT are normal. Peripheral blood smear is shown (see Fig. 33.7). Platelet aggregation studies reveal normal platelet aggregation in the presence of adenosine diphosphate (ADP), arachidonic acid (AA), epinephrine, and collagen, but decreased aggregation with ristocetin. What is the most likely diagnosis?
  A. Type 1 von Willebrand disease
  B. Hemophilia A carrier
  C. Glanzmann thrombasthenia
  D. Bernard-Soulier syndrome

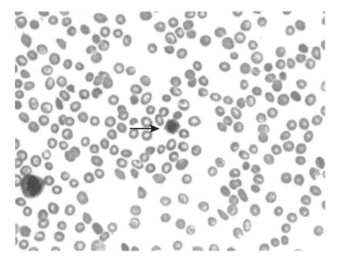

FIG. 33.7 Peripheral blood smear.

63. A 42-year-old woman presents with a history of recurrent miscarriages and a bleeding disorder diagnosed at the age of four in Peru. She does not speak English and cannot give a detailed history of how her prior bleeding episodes were treated. She can relay that she has had a long history of easy bruising, heavy menstrual cycles, and subcutaneous hematomas. As a child she had umbilical stump bleeding and one spontaneous intracranial hemorrhage. Today her CBC is normal, PT is 12 seconds (reference interval: 9–13.8 seconds), and aPTT is 28 seconds (normal 28–38 seconds). A thrombin time is 12 seconds (normal 10–15 seconds). D-dimer and fibrin split products are normal. She is on no medications. What is the most likely diagnosis?
  A. Disseminated intravascular coagulation (DIC)
  B. Hemophilia A or hemophilia B
  C. Fibrinogen deficiency or dysfibrinogenemia
  D. Factor XIII deficiency

64. A 45-year-old male of Ashkenazi Jewish descent is sent for perioperative recommendations prior to a planned total hip arthroplasty. He notes that he had excessive bleeding previously after a cholecystectomy, appendectomy, and after wisdom teeth extraction. Family history is significant for "easy bleeders" in the family. His laboratory results are shown in Table 33.5.

TABLE 33.5 Laboratory Values: Question 64

	Patient Result	Reference Interval
Complete blood count	Normal	Normal
PT	12 s	11–15 s
PTT	51 s	29–36 s
PTT 1:1 mix	35 s	29–36 s
von Willebrand studies	Normal	Normal
FVIII and FIX activity	>75%	60%–120%

Which of the following is the most appropriate product to administer preoperatively?
  A. DDAVP
  B. Fresh frozen plasma
  C. Cryoprecipitate
  D. Recombinant FVIIa

65. A 43-year-old woman is referred for evaluation of a prolonged aPTT detected on preoperative screening. The aPTT was repeated a week later and confirmed. She is scheduled to undergo an abdominal hysterectomy for fibroid uterus next week. She has no prior personal or family history of bleeding. She is on no medications. Her physical exam is normal. Laboratory values are shown in Table 33.6.

TABLE 33.6 Laboratory Values: Question 65

	Patient Result	Reference Interval
Complete blood count	normal	normal
PT	13 seconds	11–15 seconds
PTT	>120 seconds	29–36 seconds
PTT 1:1 mix	35 seconds	29–36 seconds
FVIII, FIX, XI activity	>75%	60–120%
FXII activity	12%	60–120%

Which of the following is the most appropriate treatment for her abnormal aPTT prior to surgery?
A. Recombinant FVIIa
B. Prothrombin complex concentrate
C. No treatment
D. Antifibrinolytic
E. Fresh frozen plasma
F. Cryoprecipitate

66. A 79-year-old man with a history of hypertension and severe aortic stenosis (mean gradient >40 mm Hg) presents with melena. An esophagogastroduodenoscopy (EGD) reveals arteriovenous malformations in the small bowel. He also reports a 3-month history of increased bruising and epistaxis. He has no personal or family history of bleeding. The only medication he takes is an antihypertensive. You initiate a coagulopathy workup.
Which of the following laboratory results shown in Table 33.7 is most likely to be found in this patient?

TABLE 33.7 Question 66					
Answer	**A**	**B**	**C**	**D**	**E**
Platelet count	Normal	Low	Low	Normal	Normal
vW activity cofactor (ristocetin activity)	20	20	20	20	20
vW antigen	20	20	80	80	80
vW multimers	Loss of HMWM	Uniform decrease in all multimers	Absent multimers	Loss of HMWM	Uniform decrease in all multimers

67. A 56-year-old woman is admitted for acute chest pain. She is found to have an acute myocardial infarction by EKG and laboratory findings. She undergoes emergent coronary artery angioplasty. Intraoperatively she received unfractionated heparin. Postprocedurally she is placed on Abciximab. Approximately 8 hours later she develops epistaxis, hematuria, and bleeding at her central venous catheter site. Her laboratory values are as follows (Table 33.8):

TABLE 33.8 Laboratory Values: Question 67		
	Prior to Angioplasty	**8 Hours After Angioplasty**
Platelet count	195,000 × 10⁹/L	12,000 × 10⁹/L
Hemoglobin	12.5 g/dL	10 g/dL
PTT	32 s	29–36 s
PT	13 s	11–15 s
Thrombin time		
Anti-PF4/heparin antibody testing by ELISA	Not checked	OD < 0.4 (reference range <0.4)

PF4: platelet factor 4; ELISA: enzyme-linked immunosorbent assay; OD: optical density

Which of the following most accurately describes the mechanism leading to this drug-induced thrombocytopenia?
A. Drug-dependent platelet antibodies
B. Formation of immune complexes
C. Fab-binding monoclonal antibodies
D. Drug-induced autoantibody formation

68. A 27-year-old man with severe FVIII deficiency (native factor VIII <1%) has been treated with "on-demand" plasma-derived FVIII concentrate for the last 1½ years since moving to this country from Ethiopia. He has only required two doses his entire life: once for circumcision and once for a knee hemarthrosis. Over the last 2 months he and his wife have noticed increased spontaneous joint bleeding with minor activity. He has had two ankle bleeds last month, which resolved with two doses of FVIII concentrate each. This morning he developed a spontaneous knee bleed, and after taking one dose of FVIII concentrate 25 u/kg this morning, his FVIII activity is 70% in clinic.
Which of the following should be recommended at this point?
A. Continue with "on demand" therapy and increase dose to 30 units/kg
B. Switch to recombinant FVIII concentrate
C. Start FVIII "prophylaxis" 3 times a week
D. Check for an FVIII alloantibody development

69. An otherwise healthy 18-year-old man presents with a swollen, tender knee 12 hours following trauma. He has a history of bleeding with mild trauma from a young age. He has no signs or symptoms of liver disease or vitamin K deficiency. His laboratory results are shown in Table 33.9.

TABLE 33.9 Laboratory Values: Question 69		
	Patient Result	**Reference Interval**
Complete blood count	Normal	Normal
PT	16 s	11–15 s
PTT	40 s	29–36 s
PTT 1:1 mix	34 s	29–36 s
PT 1:1 mix	12 s	11–15 s
Thrombin time	19 s	10–15 s

Which of the following is the best recommendation for treatment of the patient's bleeding?
A. FVIII/vWF concentrate
B. Cryoprecipitate
C. Fresh frozen plasma (FFP)
D. DDAVP
E. Recombinant FVIIa

70. A 63-year-old woman with a history of systemic lupus erythematosus (SLE) presents with a spontaneous intracranial hemorrhage and severe subcutaneous hematomas over her chest and upper and lower extremities. She has no prior personal or family history of bleeding. She takes Plaquenil for SLE. On exam she has left-sided hemiparesis. A CT-angiogram of her head reveals a moderate sized R parietal lobe hemorrhage without any evidence of aneurysm. Her laboratory values are shown in Table 33.10.

TABLE 33.10 Laboratory Values: Question 70

	Patient Result	Reference Interval
Complete blood count	Normal	Normal
PT	16 s	11–15 s
PTT	40 s	29–36 s
PTT 1:1 mix	34 s	29–36 s
PT 1:1 mix	12 s	11–15 s
Thrombin time	19 s	10–15 s

Which of the following is the most appropriate treatment at this time?
A. Recombinant human FVIII concentrate
B. FVIII/VWF concentrate
C. Recombinant FVIIa (rFVIIa)
D. Rituximab
E. Cryoprecipitate

71. An 18-year-old male with mild hemophilia A (native factor VIII activity = 15%) is scheduled for two teeth extractions in 3 weeks. They are not impacted. He is not on prophylaxis with FVIII concentrates and has only had one bleed related to circumcision at birth. He is not on any medications. He weighs 60 kg. He has had a prior intravenous DDAVP challenge, with increase in FVIII activity by threefold.
Which of the following is the most appropriate treatment prior to his dental surgery?
A. DDAVP 150 µg intranasally
B. DDAVP 40 µg spray intranasally
C. Recombinant FVIII concentrate 3000 units intravenously
D. Recombinant FVIII concentrate 6000 units intravenously

72. A 58-year-old man with a history of type I von Willebrand disease plans to have two teeth extracted in 1 week. He has utilized epsilon aminocaproic acid (Amicar) following previous dental extractions with adequate control of bleeding. Which statement best describes the mechanism of action of epsilon aminocaproic acid?
A. It binds the lysine binding site on plasminogen preventing binding of plasminogen and TPA to fibrin.
B. It acts as a cofactor for the posttranslational gamma-carboxylation of factors II, VII, IX, and X.
C. It cleaves plasminogen to plasmin on fibrin surface.
D. It potentiates the action of antithrombin III.

73. A 35-year-old woman with a history of heavy menstrual bleeding who is currently 38 weeks pregnant presents to labor and delivery for evaluation of consistent contractions. She is deemed to be in active labor and anesthesia requests a CBC and coagulation studies prior to placing an epidural.
Labs:
WBC $10,200 \times 10^9/L$
Hematocrit   31%
Platelet $220,000 \times 10^9/L$
PT   17.9 sec
INR   1.5
PTT   24 sec

What is the most appropriate laboratory study to order next?
A. PT 1:1 mix
B. PTT 1:1 mix
C. Thrombin time
D. Factor XII

E. Factor IX
F. Factor VII

74. A 4-year-old is evaluated in the clinic for a possible bleeding disorder. He bruises spontaneously and has experienced recurring epistaxis and gingival bleeding since birth. He was last evaluated in the ER for an episode of epistaxis requiring admission and PRBC transfusion. His parents are distant cousins.
Labs:
vWF antigen   85 IU/dL
vWF ristocetin cofactor 90 IU/dL
Platelet count $175,000 \times 10^9/L$
MPV   7.7 fL
Which of the following is the most likely diagnosis?
A. Glanzmann thrombasthenia
B. von Willebrand disease type 2B
C. Bernard-Soulier syndrome
D. von Willebrand disease type 1
E. Hermansky Pudlak syndrome

75. A 30-day-old boy is transported by ambulance to the ER for evaluation of a seizure witnessed by his parents. On exam, minor bruising is present; however, it is not suspicious for physical abuse. His parents indicate he experienced umbilical stump bleeding after detachment of the umbilical cord. CT confirms intracranial hemorrhage. His parents deny any family history of bleeding. Prothrombin time, partial thromboplastin time, and thrombin time are within normal limits. Which of the following is the most likely diagnosis?
A. Factor VII deficiency
B. Factor VIII deficiency
C. Factor IX deficiency
D. Factor X deficiency
E. Factor XIII deficiency

76. A 42-year-old man with moderate hemophilia A treated with on-demand factor VIII replacement therapy presents with progressive left knee swelling × 2 days not improved with factor VIII self-administration of 50 units/kg q 8 hours. His FVIII activity level is 2% 2 hours after his most recent dose of FVIII. An inhibitor is found. He is started on FEIBA 75 units/kg every 8 hours.
Which of the following is best followed to guide FEIBA therapy?
A. Control of bleeding symptoms
B. Correction of aPTT
C. FVIII activity level
D. FVIII inhibitor titer

77. A 79-year-old man with a history of hypertension presents with new onset of severe left arm pain and swelling secondary to compartment syndrome from an intramuscular hematoma. Laboratory evaluation shows WBC $6800 \times 10^9/L$, normal differential, hemoglobin 8.4 g/dL, MCV 90 fL, RDW 16.4, platelets $154,000 \times 10^9/L$. PT 10.3 seconds (9.5–12.7 seconds) and aPTT prolonged at 68 seconds. The aPTT corrects to 48 seconds (30–40 seconds) with a 1:1 mixing study; an inhibitory pattern is found. FVIII activity is less than 1%.
He has no prior bleeding history. His only medications are metoprolol and aspirin. He needs to proceed to the operating room for urgent fasciotomy due to the compartment syndrome.
What is the best strategy to achieve hemostasis?
A. Recombinant human factor VIII
B. Plasma-derived human factor VIII
C. Recombinant porcine factor VIII
D. Plasmapheresis
E. Desmopressin

78. A 67-year-old man is referred for evaluation of a prolonged aPTT and PT found on screening laboratory testing for impending colonoscopy. He complains of 2 years of diarrhea and a 40-pound weight loss and worsening dyspnea on exertion. He takes no medications. He denies any history of abnormal bleeding, though he has noted easy bruising over the last 3 months.

WBC	7000×10^9/L with normal differential
Hgb	10.4 g/dL
MCV	99 fL
Platelets	$383,000 \times 10^9$/L
aPTT	52.6 seconds
1:1 mixing study	40.3 seconds
PT	19.7 seconds (INR 1.7)
FII	77% (77–131)
FV	176% (72–153)
FVIII	244% (54–161)
FX	16% (73–146)

Amyloidosis is suspected. A bone marrow biopsy shows 8% lambda-restricted plasma cells; Congo red staining is negative for amyloid deposition. Bilateral axillary adenopathy is found, and he is planned for excisional lymph node biopsy for further evaluation.
What is the best management strategy for his underlying coagulopathy?
A. Proceed urgently and administer recombinant FVIIa
B. Proceed urgently and administer prothrombin complex concentrate
C. Proceed after pharmacokinetic study with prothrombin complex concentrate
D. Proceed after pharmacokinetic study of rFVIIa

79. A 65-year-old man with mild hemophilia A (baseline FVIII activity level of 8%) with paroxysmal atrial fibrillation is referred for consideration of secondary stroke prophylaxis with anticoagulation. He has had two transient ischemic attacks in the last year, has medication-controlled hypertension, and diabetes mellitus type 2. He has mild arthropathy involving the left knee and ankle, but otherwise no target joints. He has had only a few bleeding episodes in his lifetime, each secondary to trauma.

WBC	7600×10^9/L
Hgb	14.5 g/dL
Platelets	$300,000 \times 10^9$/L
Creatinine	0.89 mg/dL (0.60–1.00 mg/dL)
AST/ALT	normal
FVIII activity	8% (50%–150%)
Bethesda inhibitor	none detected

Which of the strategies shown in Table 33.11 would provide the best secondary stroke prevention while mitigating bleeding risk?

TABLE 33.11 Answer Options: Question 79

	Clotting Factor Replacement to Keep FVIII >30%	Other
A	No	Warfarin, INR 1.5–2.0
B	No	Aspirin
C	No	Aspirin
D	Yes	Warfarin, INR 2.0–3.0
E	Yes	Warfarin, INR 1.5–2.0

80. A 54-year-old woman presents for presurgical evaluation. She has a history of soft tissue bleeding in childhood and was told that she was a lyonized carrier of hemophilia A, with low FVIII activity levels. She is planned to undergo an open laparotomy for staging of ovarian cancer.
She has four full siblings, a sister who has experienced menorrhagia and three brothers, one of whom has had hemarthroses and soft tissue bleeds. All have low FVIII activity levels of 12% to 45%. Her mother has a history of menorrhagia but no soft tissue or joint bleeding. Her father has had postoperative bleeding after a knee replacement. Her paternal uncle has a history of mild hemophilia A, with a FVIII activity of 10%.
The patient has laboratory testing that shows a FVIII activity level of 24%, with a normal vWF antigen and activity level. Blood type is O+.
Which of the following is the next best step in evaluation of her low FVIII activity level?
A. DDAVP trial
B. von Willebrand: FVIII binding assay
C. von Willebrand multimer analysis
D. Platelet aggregation studies
E. Whole FVIII gene sequencing

81. A 31-year-old G1P0 with severe type 1 von Willebrand disease presents in active labor at 38 weeks gestation while on vacation to visit her family. She has been under the care of a high-risk obstetrician during her pregnancy and has not had any complications. Your hospital does not have the ability to rapidly determine vWF antigen or activity levels. Her CBC is normal. The patient tells you that her baseline vWF activity level is "10%" and that she has had levels of "56% to 70%" throughout her pregnancy.
What is the next best step in the management of this patient's imminent delivery?
A. Administer DDAVP
B. Administer 1 unit of platelets
C. Administer an antifibrinolytic
D. Transfer to a tertiary referral center when the baby is safely delivered

82. A 68-year-old with type 1 von Willebrand disease presents with a recent diagnosis of nephrolithiasis after the onset of abdominal pain and gross hematuria. Of late, he has also noted some melena and epistaxis. His hemoglobin has not changed from baseline values. He has had a colonoscopy 2 weeks ago that was of good preparative quality and did not show any polyps or masses. His vWF activity level is 15%. He has previously responded well to DDAVP. He is not taking aspirin or NSAIDs.
Which of the following is the best treatment option for the vWF-associated mucocutaneous bleeding in this male patient?
A. Tranexamic acid
B. Aminocaproic acid
C. DDAVP
D. FFP

83. Which of the laboratory parameters shown in Table 33.12 best fits those of a patient with coagulopathy secondary to liver disease?

84. A 25-year-old woman presents with severe anemia. She has had a lifelong history of easy bruising. She has heavy menstrual bleeding, with periods lasting 9 days

TABLE 33.12 Answer Options: Question 83

	PT (Seconds) (9.6–12.6)	aPTT (Seconds) (26.0–37.3)	FII (50%–150%)	FV (72%–153%)	FIX (50%–150%)	FVIII (54%–161%)	Fibrinogen (mg/dL) (208–409)
A	Increased	Increased	Decreased	Decreased	Decreased	Increased	Decreased
B	Increased	Normal	Decreased	Normal	Decreased	Normal	Normal
C	Increased	Normal-increased	Decreased	Decreased	Decreased	Decreased	Decreased
D	Normal	Increased	Normal	Normal	Normal	Decreased	Normal

monthly, 6 days of which are heavy, requiring the use of both an extra plus tampon and an overnight pad, both changed every 1 to 2 hours. She had excessive bleeding when her four wisdom teeth were extracted. She awoke the next morning with a pillow soaked with blood and required packing and stitching. Her mother and two older sisters also have heavy menstrual bleeding, and her mother required a hysterectomy at age 26 for bleeding. The hysterectomy was complicated by the development of a postoperative hematoma. Neither of the patient's three brothers bleeds abnormally, and the maternal grandfather and uncles were all likewise without bleeding symptoms. The patient has felt weak and fatigued, and recent laboratory studies have shown a CBC with hemoglobin of 5.6 g/dL, normal WBC, and platelets of 560,000 × 10⁹/L. MCV is 68 fL. The PFA-100 shows closure times of 280 seconds in the collagen/epinephrine cartridge and 180 seconds in the collagen/ADP cartridge. PT/INR are within reference ranges. aPTT is 72 seconds and corrects fully with 1:1 mixing. Which of the following is the most likely diagnosis?
A. Essential thrombocytosis
B. Factor XI deficiency
C. Factor XII deficiency
D. Hemophilia B
E. von Willebrand disease

85. A 55-year-old man with severe hemophilia A presents to the emergency department with headache and vomiting after falling and hitting his head on stone steps. He normally self-administers 2000 units of recombinant factor VIII for treatment of hemarthroses. The patient has normal vital signs and is noted to have a large temporoparietal hematoma of his scalp. Pupils are symmetric and reactive. His weight is 80 kg.
Which is the most appropriate step to take in the management of this patient?
A. Administer recombinant factor VIII, 2400 units
B. Administer recombinant factor VIII, 4000 units
C. Measure factor VIII level
D. Perform head CT
E. Perform head MRI

86. A 75-year-old woman presents with severe hematuria and a right forearm hematoma. She has never had abnormal bleeding with her prior surgeries, including cesarean section × 2, cholecystectomy, hysterectomy, and bilateral cataract extractions. Her family history is negative for bleeding disorders. Physical examination is significant for multiple ecchymoses over all extremities and the left flank. There is a taut right forearm with large hematoma. The right fingers are cool, with delayed capillary refill and some paresthesias. Laboratory data show Hgb 9.2 g/dL, normal MCV, platelet count, and WBC. PT is 12.5 seconds, aPTT 72 seconds. aPTT 1:1

mix is 42 seconds immediate and 64 seconds after 1 hour incubation at 37°C.
Therapy with recombinant activated FVII is recommended. Which of the following measurements is the best way to follow the hemostatic efficacy of this therapy?
A. aPTT
B. CBC and urinalysis
C. FVII activity
D. FVIII activity
E. PT

87. A 55-year-old man with mild hemophilia A and a baseline FVIII level of 12% to 15% presents with flank pain and gross hematuria. PMHx is otherwise notable for a history of renal calculi. He denies fever. Physical examination shows a man, rocking in pain. He is afebrile, and tachycardic to 110 bpm. The urinalysis shows 4+ blood, no organisms, and no WBCs. The electrolytes, BUN, and creatinine are normal.
Which of the following agents is currently contraindicated in this patient?
A. Cryoprecipitate
B. Desmopressin
C. Epsilon aminocaproic acid
D. Plasma-derived fVIII
E. Recombinant fVIII

88. A 35-year-old woman presents for evaluation of bleeding management with upcoming surgery to correct a deviated nasal septum. She has been told she has von Willebrand disease. She bled abnormally with wisdom tooth extraction requiring transfusion and has had a severe muscle hematoma following a skiing accident when she landed on an ice block with her left thigh. She had heavy menstrual bleeding requiring oral contraceptive pills starting at age 14.
The laboratory studies show vWF antigen of 55% (nL 50–150) and vWF activity of 22%. (nL 50–150). The FVIII activity level is 82%. The CBC shows Hgb 11.5 g/dL, platelets 120,000 × 10⁹/L. The WBC and differential are normal.
Which of the following represents the best therapy to recommend preoperatively?
A. Cryoprecipitate
B. Desmopressin
C. Epsilon aminocaproic acid
D. Intermediate purity FVIII
E. Recombinant FVIII

89. A 65-year-old man with severe congestive heart failure had a continuous flow left ventricular assist device implanted 4 months ago. Since that time, he has had recurrent episodes of GI bleeding requiring transfusions every 2 to 3 weeks. Multiple endoscopies show the presence of arteriovenous malformations. He has never had abnormal bleeding before and in fact had undergone multiple

surgeries and tooth extractions done without unusual bleeding before implantation of his cardiac device. There is no family history of abnormal bleeding.

Which option in Table 33.13 is the most likely pattern of vWF antigen and vWF activity for this patient?

TABLE 33.13 Answer Options: Question 89

	vWF Antigen	vWF Activity
A	20	20
B	90	20
C	<10	<10
D	100	100
E	250	250

90. A 55-year-old woman with a history of smoldering myeloma presents with new onset severe bruising and hematoma formation. There is no personal or family history of abnormal bleeding. She has not had any therapy for her myeloma. She is on no medications.

Initial evaluation reveals normal CBC, PT of 12.5 seconds, aPTT 60 seconds, and 1:1 aPTT mix is 28 seconds.

Which of the following laboratory test is most likely to lead to the correct diagnosis?
   A. Factor VIII activity
   B. Factor VIII Bethesda titer
   C. Factor X activity
   D. Lupus inhibitor screen
   E. von Willebrand activity

91. A 45-year-old nursing assistant presents with massive GI bleeding. Past medical history is significant for degenerative joint disease, depression, and anxiety. Personal and family history are negative for known bleeding diathesis. Medications include paroxetine, extra-strength acetaminophen, and celecoxib. Physical examination reveals an anxious, ill-appearing woman, suffering hematemesis and melena. She is afebrile. BP 90/48, HR 130, and RR 20. Abdomen soft, lungs clear, and CV tachycardic. Laboratory data show a hemoglobin of 7.2 g/dL, Hct 22%, WBC 13,000 × 10^9/L, and platelets 390,000 × 10^9/L. PT 72 seconds, INR 14.8, and aPTT 63 seconds. 1:1 mixing completely corrects the PT and aPTT. Factor activity levels are as follows: II 7%, V, 92%, VII less than 1%, IX 3%, and X 9%. Warfarin level 0. She is treated with vitamin K and four-factor prothrombin complex concentrate, with complete resolution of bleeding and correction of clotting times over the course of 3 days. Endoscopy shows no definitive source of bleeding. She returns with recurrent bleeding and similar prolongation of PT and aPTT, as well as coagulation factor activity levels 5 days after discharge from the hospital.

Which of the following diagnostic tests is most likely to lead to the correct diagnosis?
   A. Acetaminophen level
   B. Hepatic ultrasound
   C. Vitamin K level
   D. Superwarfarin level
   E. Warfarin level

92. A 55-year-old man presents with bruising and dyspnea. He has noted progressive ankle swelling and has developed increased abdominal girth. Physical examination

shows muffled heart sounds, decreased breath sounds at the bases bilaterally, and ascites is present. There is 4+ pedal edema to the upper thighs. Large bruises at all phases of healing are present over the thighs, calves, shins, and buttocks. Laboratory data show Hgb 11.4 g/dL, Hct 34%, normal WBC, and platelet count. PT is 22 seconds, aPTT 45 seconds. and TCT is 11 seconds. 1:1 mixing completely corrects the PT and aPTT abnormalities.

He excretes 4 g of urinary protein in 24 hours. SPE and immunofixation shows a monoclonal IgG lambda of 0.5 g/L. Bone marrow biopsy shows 3% monoclonal plasma cells and pinkish material, which gives apple green birefringence on Congo red staining.

What is the most likely diagnosis?
   A. Acquired von Willebrand disease
   B. Dysfibrinogenemia
   C. Factor VIII inhibitor
   D. Factor X deficiency
   E. Factor X inhibitor

93. A 62-year-old man with a history of mild hemophilia A is known to have a baseline FVIII activity level of 15%. He has been treated with cryoprecipitate for tonsillectomy and with DDAVP for wisdom tooth removal in the past. He undergoes left knee replacement and is treated with recombinant FVIII preoperatively and for 2 weeks postoperatively. He does well and is undergoing physical therapy without difficulty. He presents with a significant upper GI bleed 32 days after his procedure. The hemoglobin value is 11.9, 2 g lower than baseline. Platelet count and WBC are normal. PT is normal. Factor VIII activity level is less than 1%.

Which of the following is the most appropriate agent to administer now?
   A. Cryoprecipitate
   B. DDAVP
   C. Plasma derived factor VIII
   D. Recombinant activated factor VII
   E. Recombinant factor VIII

94. A 33-year-old woman presents for evaluation of abnormal bleeding following sinus surgery. She is known to have a low factor VIII activity level of 18% and was pretreated with desmopressin 0.3 µg/kg given 30 minutes preoperatively. She did well initially but then was noted to have significant bleeding later that afternoon, about 6 hours postoperatively. Her factor VIII activity level at the time of bleeding is 18%. A DDAVP trial was performed prior to surgery, showing her fVIII activity level rose to 96% 1 hour after 0.3 µg/kg DDAVP. There is no family history of any bleeding disorder. vWF antigen and activity levels are both above 100%. Factor VIII genotyping shows no mutations in the factor VIII gene.

Which of the following tests is the most likely to yield the correct diagnosis?
   A. Factor VIII inhibitor titer
   B. Platelet aggregation with low-dose ristocetin
   C. VWF propeptide levels
   D. VWF FVIII binding assay
   E. VWF collagen binding assay

95. A 66-year-old man with atrial fibrillation for 20 years and mild dementia for the past 2 years is brought in by his daughter with multiple bruises on his extremities and epistaxis. The patient has been treated with dabigatran and atenolol, and has confused his medications. On exam, his BP is 110/70; pulse is 98 and irregular. He has large ecchymosis on his upper and lower extremities, bright red

blood per nares, and bleeding gums. His laboratory studies are shown:

Hgb   12.7 g/dL
Hct   38%
aPTT   89 seconds

Which of the following would best control his coagulopathy?
A. Four-component prothrombin complex concentrate
B. Fresh frozen plasma
C. Cryoprecipitate
D. Idarucizumab
E. Rituximab

96. A 65-year-old woman with a 20-year history of atrial fibrillation managed with dabigatran for the past 2 years presents with acute appendicitis necessitating surgical intervention. She reports her last dose of dabigatran was 6 hours prior to surgery. Her physical examination is remarkable for a temperature of 102°F, pulse of 110, and guarding and rebound in her left lower quadrant.
Which of the following tests would best predict her level of anticoagulation?
A. Prothrombin time
B. Activated partial thromboplastin time
C. Activated clotting time
D. Reptilase time
E. Dilute thrombin time

97. A 27-year-old woman presents with pain and swelling in her left leg 24 hours after beginning clomiphene for infertility. The patient has been otherwise healthy and currently takes no other medications. She has no family history of thrombosis. On exam she has a left thigh that is 4 cm larger than the right. She has edema in her ankle, and all pulses are intact. She is not currently pregnant. A duplex ultrasound confirms the presence of an acute DVT. On further evaluation, she is found to be heterozygous for the prothrombin 20210 mutation.
How should she be managed?
A. Enoxaparin for 5 days with warfarin indefinitely
B. Enoxaparin for 5 days with warfarin for 3 months
C. Warfarin indefinitely
D. Warfarin for 3 months
E. tPA

98. A 35-year-old woman presents with a prolonged aPTT (49 seconds) on screening at a wellness clinic. She was subsequently found to have a lupus anticoagulant and IgG anticardiolipin antibodies at a moderately positive titer (40), with antibodies to beta 2 glycoprotein1. She has no family or personal history of thrombosis or miscarriage. She has no rheumatologic disorder and does not smoke or take oral contraceptives. She is not pregnant and does not plan on becoming pregnant.
How should she be managed?
A. No anticoagulation
B. Low-dose aspirin
C. Warfarin with target INR 2.0–3.0
D. Warfarin with target INR 2.5–3.5
E. Rivaroxaban

99. A 25-year-old woman is found to be heterozygous for the MTHFR C677T mutation while being evaluated due to a DVT and PE that occurred in her sister. The patient is healthy, takes no medications, and is not pregnant. She has never had a thrombotic episode. She eats a normal diet. Further evaluation revealed a serum homocysteine

level of 15 μm/L that was top normal for the laboratory in which it was tested. The remainder of her workup for thrombophilia was unremarkable.
How should she be managed?
A. Warfarin to INR 2.0–3.0
B. Low-dose aspirin
C. Prophylactic dose enoxaparin
D. B vitamin and folate supplementation
E. No further intervention

100. A 27-year-old woman at 33 weeks gestation presents to the emergency room with crampy abdominal pain and bleeding. She is found to have fetal demise in utero. The obstetrician suspects antiphospholipid antibody syndrome and begins the appropriate laboratory evaluation.
Which of the following laboratory studies would support the diagnosis of antiphospholipid antibody syndrome?
A. Mildly elevated anti beta 2 glycoprotein IgM
B. Prolonged aPTT
C. Prolonged DRVVT
D. Mildly elevated anti-B2 glycoprotein IgG
E. Mildly elevated anticardiolipin IgG

101. A 54-year-old woman with no prior medical history develops abdominal pain and is found to have ascites. AST and ALT are markedly elevated. Thrombosis of the main hepatic vein is noted on abdominal imaging. Anticoagulation has been started and thrombolysis is being considered. Thrombophilia testing is pursued.
Laboratory studies are as follows:
Hemoglobin   15.3.g/dL
Hematocrit: 46%
Platelet count   469,000 × 10⁹/L
Leucocyte count   12,600 × 10⁹/L
MCV   78 fL
Serum creatinine   0.9 mg/dL
Serum electrolytes   Normal
Liver function tests Markedly elevated AST and ALT

Which of the following tests would be most likely to diagnose the condition predisposing to hepatic vein thrombosis in this patient?
A. JAK2 mutation
B. PNH testing
C. Antiphospholipid antibodies
D. Antithrombin III
E. Factor V Leiden

102. A healthy 23-year-old woman is pregnant with her first child. She has no prior medical or surgical history. Her sister recently developed a left lower extremity DVT while on estrogen-containing contraceptives and was found to be heterozygous for the prothrombin gene mutation (P20210). Screening was performed in the presented patient, and she is also found to be heterozygous for the prothrombin gene mutation (P20210).
You recommend:
A. No anticoagulation, but close clinical surveillance
B. Antepartum and postpartum prophylaxis with LMWH
C. Postpartum prophylaxis with LMWH
D. Antepartum and postpartum treatment doses of LMWH
E. Antepartum prophylaxis and postpartum treatment doses of LMWH

103. A 54-year-old man was recently diagnosed with a provoked popliteal RLE DVT at the end of a prolonged hospital course for cellulitis. His past medical history

consists of ischemic cardiomyopathy with an EF of 40%, chronic kidney disease with a CrCl of 40 mL/min, and hypertension on metoprolol. His appetite is poor, and he is frequently on and off antibiotics. He is otherwise ready to go home today and is anxious for discharge. He would like to avoid injectable medications and to be discharged as soon as possible. He is currently on no medications that would interact with warfarin or any of the new oral anticoagulants.

Which of the following anticoagulants do you recommend?

A. Warfarin
B. Apixiban
C. Dabigatran
D. Edoxaban
E. Fondaparinux

104. A 53-year-old woman is seen for an assessment of her right popliteal DVT. She had been in her usual state of health, which was characterized by gastroesophageal reflux disease, obesity, and tobacco use, when she developed right calf pain and tenderness that progressed over the course of 4 days. Approximately 4 months prior, she had been started on oral contraceptive therapy, as she started to exhibits symptoms of heavy menstrual bleeding, which she explains as, "They thought I was going through menopause."

She presented to an urgent care, where a pleasant, nontoxic-appearing 53-year-old woman was observed. Her vital signs were within normal range, with a BMI measured at 41.3 kg/m², and an erythematous and swollen right leg. A D-dimer was performed and noted to be markedly elevated, prompting her referral to the emergency room. Once there, an ultrasound was performed that showed the presence of a right popliteal DVT extending into the trifurcation. She was instructed to stop her estrogens and therapeutic anticoagulation with a low-molecular-weight heparin was initiated. Due to issues with her insurance, she was bridged to warfarin, which she has remained upon for the last 4 months without any hemorrhagic complications. Review of the entirety of her PT/INR values show that she has remained within the therapeutic range.

Which of the following should be recommended?

A. Stop therapeutic anticoagulation
B. Continue warfarin, at a target INR of 2.5, range 2.0–3.0 for a total of 6 months
C. Reduce dose of warfarin to an INR range to 1.5–2.0
D. Start apixaban, 2.5 mg BID
E. Start rivaroxaban 20 mg daily

105. The patient is a 39-year-old woman, with no significant past medical history and on no medications, developed vague right upper quadrant pain over the course of a week. Her symptoms progressed to include malaise, anorexia, abdominal distention, and scleral icterus. She presented to the emergency room, where marked transaminitis and hyperbilirubinemia was noted. She was admitted to medicine, where a full workup ensued, including Doppler ultrasound of her liver. This was significant for hepatic vein thrombosis in the absence of collateral formation, prompting initiation of therapeutic anticoagulation with unfractionated heparin. Hematology is called for a hypercoagulable evaluation.

Which of the following is the most appropriate test to send?

A. Antiphospholipid antibodies
B. Antithrombin activity

C. JAK2 V617F
D. Protein C activity
E. Protein S activity

106. A 56-year-old man is admitted for additional treatment of a pulmonary embolism. He was in his usual state of good, having recently flown from Munich to Chicago, when he developed progressive right-sided pleuritic chest pain over the course of 2 days. He presented to the ER, where a CT angiogram showed the presence of extensive right main and upper lobar pulmonary artery thrombus, with opacities in the right upper lung concerning for infarction, with radiographic findings of right heart strain. The patient is admitted to the MICU, where an emergent transthoracic echocardiogram showed no evidence of right heart failure, with normal right ventricular pressures. Two sets of Troponin-I are negative for cardiac injury, and he remains hemodynamically stable, requiring only 2 L of supplemental oxygen via nasal cannula. At the same time, bilateral lower extremity ultrasound is performed, showing occlusive thrombus from the left common femoral to popliteal vein, becoming nonocclusive in the trifurcation and extending into one of the paired tibial veins.

Which of the following is the most appropriate management at this time?

A. Initiation of therapeutic anticoagulation with low-molecular-weight heparin
B. Unfractionated heparin with dual antiplatelet therapy
C. Administration of tissue type plasminogen activator, 100 mg IV, over 2 hours
D. Placement of a permanent IVC filter
E. Placement of a retrievable IVC filter

107. A 58-year-old man has been sent for a consultation from the cardiovascular surgery clinic. His past medical history is significant for: rheumatic fever as a child; hypertension; chronic kidney disease stage 2; and coronary artery disease, with a history of a non-ST elevation MI 8 months ago.

During his admission for the NSTEMI, the patient underwent a left heart catheterization with the use of a gpIIb/IIIa inhibitor, followed by treatment with unfractionated heparin. This showed diffuse coronary artery disease that was not amenable to percutaneous intervention and severe mitral stenosis. Following his procedure, the platelet count was observed to have dramatically declined to a nadir of 53,000 × 10⁹/L. As part of his evaluation, testing was sent to evaluate for the presence of heparin/PF4 antibodies, which showed a level of 0.863 OD (<0.400). A serotonin release assay was ordered, but was not collected. He was empirically placed on a bivalirudin infusion and bridged to warfarin after his platelet count remained greater than 150 for 2 days, which he remained upon since that time.

While there have been no hemorrhagic complications from the use of his warfarin, he has developed progressive dyspnea on exertion and was sent to the cardiovascular surgery clinic for an evaluation for mitral valve replacement. Given his comorbidities, it was not felt that he was an appropriate candidate for either a percutaneous or minimally invasive laparoscopic approach for repair of his valve. It was recommended that he undergo an open mitral valve replacement with a mechanical valve on bypass. Due to his history, Mr. Thomas has been sent to the Hematology Clinic for recommendations regarding his use of warfarin and his prior exposure to heparin.

As his planned surgical date is a month away, which of the following is the most appropriate recommendation:
A. Stop warfarin
B. Continue warfarin at a target INR of 2.5, range 2.0–3.0
C. Continue warfarin at a target INR of 3.0, range 2.5–3.5
D. Transition to the use of an oral direct thrombin inhibitor following surgery, given his sensitivity to heparin

108. In addition to the recommendations regarding the previously listed patient's oral anticoagulation in question 107, hematology is also asked to provide recommendations regarding the possible use of heparin while he is on cardio-pulmonary bypass. At that clinic visit, a repeat heparin/PF4 ELISA was sent and showed a level of 0.278 OD.
Which of the following is the most appropriate recommendation?
A. Use of bivalirudin while on bypass and continuing postoperatively as a bridge to warfarin, at a target INR of 2.5, range 2.0–3.0
B. Use of unfractionated heparin while on bypass, followed by bivalirudin as a bridge toward therapeutic anticoagulation with warfarin
C. Use of unfractionated heparin while on bypass, followed by enoxaparin as a bridge toward therapeutic anticoagulation with warfarin
D. Use of unfractionated heparin while on bypass, followed by an unfractionated heparin drip as a bridge toward therapeutic anticoagulation with warfarin

109. A 43-year-old woman was diagnosed with a left leg DVT 4 months ago. She was seen at her local ER and started on rivaroxaban, 15 mg twice daily for 21 days, followed by 20 mg daily, which she has remained upon without any hemorrhagic complications. Due to a reported family history of thrombosis, she underwent a thrombophilia evaluation through her primary care physician, which showed the following results:

Antithrombin activity	104%
Protein C activity	>150%
Protein S activity	>150%
Lupus anticoagulant	Detected (not detected)
APCR	Positive (negative)
ACA and anti-B2GP1 IgA/ IgG/IgM	Negative
Factor V Leiden	Negative
PTG20210A	Negative

What is the most likely interpretation for these results?
A. She has antiphospholipid syndrome.
B. She has factor V Leiden.
C. She has antiphospholipid syndrome and factor V Leiden.
D. The elevated levels of Protein C and S counterbalance the presence of the lupus anticoagulant.
E. Interference from the effect of rivaroxaban.

110. A 36-year-old woman who currently at 36-week gestation. She was admitted early in her second trimester for dehydration from severe hyperemesis gravidarum, which required the placement of a left arm PICC line. This was complicated by a left basilic vein thrombosis, for which the line was pulled after a week, and she was treated with low-molecular-weight heparin for another week. She was recently seen at a regularly scheduled obstetric visit, where her history of thrombosis was reviewed.

The patient is aware that the third trimester and postpartum period are periods of increased thrombotic risk, which prompted a thrombophilia evaluation. This showed the following:

Antithrombin activity	87%
Protein C activity	93%
Protein S activity	42% (52–136)
Factor V Leiden	Negative
PTG20210A	Negative
MTHFR	Negative
Homocysteine	12.8
Lupus anticoagulant	Not detected
ACA and anti-B2GP1 IgA/IgG/IgM	Negative

Which of the following is the most appropriate recommendation?
A. No treatment is required
B. Start enoxaparin, 40 mg daily
C. Start enoxaparin, 1 mg/kg BID immediately, and continue until 6 weeks postpartum
D. Start enoxaparin, 1 mg/kg BID immediately, and continue until 6 weeks postpartum, followed by bridging to therapeutic dosing of warfarin

111. A 68-year-old woman is referred to the Orthopedic Clinic for further treatment options for a painful left knee. Despite an attempt at weight loss and intraarticular steroid injections, it is felt that she has failed conservative management. As such, a left total knee arthroplasty is recommended. She is then evaluated in the anesthesia preoperative clinic, where routine labs are drawn, showing the following:

WBC	8700×10^9/L
Hemoglobin	12.4 g/dL
Hematocrit	37.2%
MCV	92 fL
Platelets	$217,000 \times 10^9$/L
PT	11.9 sec
aPTT	58.9 sec

She is then sent to the Hematology Clinic for additional evaluation and treatment. During her visit, it is noted that there is no prior history of thrombosis or recurrent pregnancy loss. She has undergone tonsillectomy as a child, and the vaginal delivery of three children, without any hemorrhagic complications. She denies alopecia, photosensitivity, oral ulcers, kidney disease, or any other arthralgias. Additional testing shows the following:

aPTT	61.3 seconds (26.8–37.1)
aPTT Mix	0 minute 48.3 seconds (<37.1)
aPTT Mix	60 minutes 53 seconds (<37.1)
DRVVT screen	1.39 (<1.2)
DRVV confirm	1.33 (<1.2)
Hexagonal phase neutralization	1.29 (<1.2)
ACA and anti-B2GP1 IgA/IgG/IgM negative	
FVIII	137%
FIX	89%
FXI	104%

Based upon her testing, which of the following recommendation is most appropriate?
A. Enoxaparin, 40 mg/day for 10–14 days following her knee replacement
B. Enoxaparin, 1 mg/kg BID, as a bridge to warfarin, at a target INR of 2.5, range 2.0–3.0

C. Enoxaparin, 1 mg/kg BID, as a bridge to warfarin, at a target INR of 3.0, range 2.5–3.5

D. Enoxaparin, 1 mg/kg BID, as a bridge to warfarin, at a target INR of 2.5, range 2.0–3.0, plus aspirin 81 mg/day

E. Enoxaparin, 1 mg/kg BID, as a bridge to warfarin, at a target INR of 2.5, range 2.0–3.0, aspirin 81 mg/day, and hydroxychloroquine 200 mg daily

112. A 25-year-old man who presents to hematology clinic for a second opinion regarding his DVT/PE management. His history is remarkable for an idiopathic right popliteal DVT, for which he was started on warfarin following a standard course of low-molecular-weight heparin. Four months into his treatment, his course was complicated by an episode of hematemesis. He noted increased bruising over his usual baseline during his treatment with warfarin, leading to discontinuation of his anticoagulation. He then developed sudden onset dyspnea and right-sided pleuritic chest pain a week after discharge, and was found to have a PE. He is admitted and started on apixaban 10 mg twice daily. A limited thrombophilia evaluation is sent, and shows the following:

Antithrombin activity (thrombin-based)	102%
Factor V Leiden	Negative
PTG20210A	Negative
Thrombin time	32.1 sec
ACA and anti-B2GP1 IgA/IgG/IgM	Negative
FVIII	256%

Which of the following is the most appropriate recommendation at this time?
A. No further workup indicated
B. Sequencing of *F8* to determine cause of elevated level
C. Reptilase time
D. Lupus anticoagulant panel
E. Protein C and S activities, clot-based

113. A 34-year-old woman has been on combined oral contraceptive therapy for 7 years following the birth of her second child. She recently injured her ankle in a skiing accident, for which she was placed in a cast. Two weeks later, she was noted to have sustained thrombosis of one of her paired tibial veins and a peroneal vein. No proximal DVT was noted. She was started on enoxaparin, but her OB/gyn was concerned for thrombophilia to explain the thrombosis, as she had been on estrogens for years without any prior problems. This was significant for showing heterozygosity for the C677T mutation in *MTHFR*. The OB/gyn has recommended stopping her estrogen, started folate/B-vitamin supplementation, and indefinite anticoagulation. In addition, she has been sent to hematology for evaluation and treatment of her inherited thrombophilia.

Which of the following is the most appropriate recommendation at this time?
A. Transition to warfarin, target INR of 2.5, range 2.0–3.0
B. Transition to a direct oral anticoagulant
C. Transition to an oral agent and continuation of her vitamin supplementation
D. Stop the enoxaparin and vitamin supplementation

114. A 49-year-old man undergoes scheduled coronary artery bypass graft surgery and is currently at postoperative day 8. Hematology is consulted for persistent thrombocytopenia. His physical examination reveals a swollen, red, tender right thigh. He has no signs of bleeding or bruising. He is not febrile. Laboratory values are shown in Table 33.14.

TABLE 33.14 Laboratory Values: Question 114

Laboratory Test	Patient's Result Preoperatively	Patient's Results POD #8	Reference Range
Hemoglobin	13.7 g/dL	11.0 g/dL	12–16 g/dL
Hematocrit	41%	33%	35%–48%
White blood cell count	7900 × 10⁹/L, with normal differential	112,000 × 10⁹/L, with normal differential	4000–10,000 × 10⁹/L
Platelet count	195,000 × 10⁹/L	36,000 × 10⁹/L	150,000–450,000 × 10⁹/L
Prothrombin time (PT)	12.7 s	13.0 s	11–15 s
Activated partial thromboplastin time (aPTT)	29 s	31 s	29–36 s
Fibrinogen	Not available	200 mg/dL	150–450 mg/dL

Which of the following is the most important next step?
A. Request heparin-associated antibody testing
B. Start Prednisone 1 mg/kg daily
C. Discontinue all heparin and start nonheparin anticoagulation
D. Give platelet transfusion

115. A 35-year-old woman develops an acute superficial femoral vein thrombosis 3 days after undergoing a hysterectomy for uterine fibroids. She has no prior personal or family history of thrombosis. She is initially started on weight-based low-molecular-weight heparin and transitioned to a direct oral anticoagulant of discharge. She comes to see you in clinic 2 weeks later for recommendations on length of anticoagulation. Her physical exam and laboratory results are normal.

What is the most appropriate recommendation for duration of anticoagulation?
A. 1.5 months
B. 3 months
C. 6 months
D. 12 months
E. Indefinite

116. A 32-year-old Caucasian woman develops a 4 days after a colectomy for ulcerative colitis. She is started on unfractionated heparin and is transitioned to warfarin. She has no family or personal history of venous thrombosis (VTE). On exam her vital signs are stable and the left leg is swollen, red, and tender. Laboratory values revealed on postoperative day 9 are shown in Table 33.15. She is referred to you for recommendations on the length of anticoagulation.

TABLE 33.15 Laboratory Values: Question 116

Laboratory Test	Patient's Results	Reference Range
Hemoglobin	11.7 g/dL	12–16 g/dL
Hematocrit	34%	35%–48%
White blood cell count	10,000 × 10⁹/L, with normal differential	4000–10,000 × 10⁹/L
Platelet count	185,000 × 10⁹/L	150–450 × 10⁹/L
International normalized ratio (INR)	2.6	0.8–1.2
Protein C activity	20 IU/dL	65–135 IU/dL
Protein S activity	25 IU/dL	65–135 IU/dL
Factor V Leiden (FVL)	Heterozygous	No mutations
Prothrombin 20210 mutation	No mutations	No mutations

Which of the following is the most appropriate recommendation for the duration of anticoagulation?
A. 3 months anticoagulation for provoked PE
B. 12 months anticoagulation for provoked PE
C. Indefinite anticoagulation due to protein C and protein S deficiency
D. Indefinite anticoagulation due to FVL heterozygosity

117. A 78-year-old man is referred to the hematology clinic by his gastroenterologist, who has scheduled a screening colonoscopy for the patient in 2 weeks. The patient is on warfarin for a history of atrial fibrillation with a CHADS score of 4. Today the international normalized ratio (INR) is 2.8 (goal, 2.0–3.0). He is not on an antiplatelet agent.
Which of the following is the best recommendation for perioperative management of warfarin?
A. Continue the current dose of warfarin and proceed with surgery.
B. Stop the warfarin now; when the INR is less than 2.0, start therapeutic doses of low-molecular-weight heparin (LMWH), with the last dose given 24 hours before surgery.
C. Stop the warfarin 5 days before surgery; recheck the INR the morning of surgery, and if it is less than 2.0, proceed with surgery. Postoperatively restart home dose of warfarin.
D. Stop the warfarin 5 days before surgery; start therapeutic doses of LMWH and warfarin 12–24 hours after surgery.

118. A 64-year-old man is admitted for scheduled total hip arthroplasty for severe osteoarthritis. He has no personal or family history of venous thromboembolism (VTE). There is no evidence of bleeding.
Which of the following is the most appropriate recommendation for VTE prophylaxis?
A. Intermittent pneumatic compression devices (IPCD) alone
B. IPCD plus pharmacologic prophylaxis
C. Inferior vena cava filter plus IPCD
D. Inferior vena cava filter plus pharmacologic prophylaxis
E. No prophylaxis necessary

119. A 63-year-old woman presents to the emergency room at 1 pm with altered mental status, headaches, and mild weakness on the left side of her body. A CT scan of her brain reveals an acute moderate-sized intracranial hemorrhage without evidence of shift or herniation. She is on apixaban for atrial fibrillation, and her last dose was at 9 am this morning. On exam she is alert to person only and has 4/5 left hemibody paresis. Her laboratory results are shown in Table 33.16.

TABLE 33.16 Laboratory Values: Question 119

Laboratory Test	Patient's Results	Reference Range
Hemoglobin	10.7 g/dL	12–16 g/dL
Hematocrit	32.5%	35%–48%
White blood cell count	11,000 × 10⁹/L, with normal differential	4000–10,000 × 10⁹/L
Platelet count	205,000 × 10⁹/L	150–450 × 10⁹/L
International normalized ratio (INR)	1.9	0.8–1.2
PTT	39	29–36 s
Antifactor Xa activity (by chromogenic assay)	Detectable	Undetectable

Which of the following should be recommended at this time?
A. Fresh frozen plasma
B. Protamine
C. Idarucizumab
D. Four-factor prothrombin complex concentrate
E. Andexanet

120. A 42-year-old woman with valvular atrial fibrillation was placed on warfarin 6 years ago. She has a history of aortic valve replacement with a mechanical valve 10 years prior. Her INRs has been in range 65% of the time. She has had no bleeding complications. Laboratory results are notable for a serum creatinine is 1.4 mg/dL (creatinine clearance 54 mL/min). On exam she is noted to be in atrial fibrillation. She comes to you to discuss switching to a direct oral anticoagulant.
Which of the following is the most appropriate recommendation at this point?
A. Switch to apixaban
B. Switch to dabigatran
C. Switch to rivaroxaban
D. Continue coumadin

121. A 78-year-old man is on apixaban for nonvalvular atrial fibrillation (CHADS score 3 based on age, hypertension, and diabetes). He needs semielective resection of a complex thigh mass. The surgery is thought to be of high bleeding risk due to vascular involvement of the mass. He is on no other medications. His physical exam is notable for atrial fibrillation and an enlarged right thigh that is tender on palpation. Laboratory results reveal a creatinine clearance of 52 mL/min.
Which of the following is the most appropriate preoperative recommendation for his anticoagulation?
A. Hold apixaban 12 hours preoperatively
B. Hold apixaban 24 hours preoperatively
C. Hold apixaban 72 hours preoperatively
D. Transition to low-molecular-weight heparin bridging preoperatively

122. A 24-year-old female with h/o symptomatic right iliofemoral deep vein thrombosis (DVT) diagnosed at age 22 while on drospirenone/ethinyl estradiol oral contraceptive is now 8 weeks pregnant with her first child. She received 3 months of therapeutic anticoagulation for treatment of her prior DVT. Thrombophilia workup was negative. She has no family history of VTE.

You recommend the following for VTE prophylaxis during this pregnancy:
A. Antepartum and 6 weeks postpartum therapeutic anticoagulation with LMWH
B. Antepartum and 6 weeks postpartum prophylaxis with LMWH
C. Clinical surveillance
D. 6 weeks of postpartum prophylaxis

123. A 26-year-old man with history of intravenous drug use is admitted for endocarditis. He has a peripherally inserted central catheter (PICC) for intravenous antibiotics. One week after the PICC is inserted, he develops acute right upper extremity swelling and pain. A Doppler ultrasound confirms a right upper extremity deep vein thrombosis. He is started on low-molecular-weight heparin (LMWH). The infectious disease consult service recommends 8 weeks of intravenous antibiotics. He has had no bleeding side effects from LMWH. He has no prior personal or family history of venous thromboembolism. On exam his right upper arm is swollen, red, and tender, without signs of limb ischemia.

You recommend:
A. Immediate removal of PICC and treatment of DVT for a total of 3 months of anticoagulation
B. Removal of PICC in 8 weeks when intravenous antibiotics have been completed and discontinuation of anticoagulation at that time
C. Immediate removal of PICC and treatment of DVT for a total of 1 month of anticoagulation
D. Immediate removal of PICC and thrombolysis of acute upper extremity DVT followed by 3 months of anticoagulation

124. A 90-year-old man with chronic atrial fibrillation was on warfarin for 25 years and ASA 81 mg QD for stroke and systemic embolism prevention. Four months ago he was switched to dabigatran. One week ago he fell and sustained head trauma. His family brings him to the emergency room for gradual decline in mental status over the last 72 hours. In the emergency room he is found to have bilateral subacute subdural hematomas. His last dose of dabigatran was 24 hours ago. Today his creatinine is 1.4 mg/dL and platelets are 195,000 × 10⁹/L.
What is the best lab to exclude a clinically relevant dabigatran level in this bleeding patient?
A. Activated Partial thromboplastin time (aPTT)
B. Prothrombin time (PT)
C. Thrombin time (TT)
D. Antifactor Xa activity

125. A 24-year-old woman presents to the emergency room with acute onset L sided hemiplegia and facial droop that began approximately 3 hours ago. She is found to have an acute right middle cerebral artery stroke. She does not receive intravenous tissue plasminogen activator (tPA) because of mild thrombocytopenia of 105,000 × 10⁹/L and her delayed presentation to the ER outside of the therapeutic window if tPA. She has no other past medical history, although she has had mild chronic

thrombocytopenia for 5 years (range 98,000 × 10⁹/L–125 × 10⁹/L) that has never been worked up. She also has a history of one second trimester miscarriage last year. Her stroke workup, including an EKG, bubble echocardiogram, and carotid Doppler ultrasounds, has been negative. Laboratory results are shown in Table 33.17.

TABLE 33.17 Laboratory Values: Question 125

Laboratory Test	Patient's Results	Reference Range
Hemoglobin	12.5 g/dL	12–16 g/dL
Hematocrit	37.5%	35%–48%
White blood cell count	4000 × 10⁹/L, with normal differential	4.0–10 × 10⁹/L
Platelet count	105 × 10⁹/L	150–450 × 10⁹/L
International normalized ratio (INR)	1.0	0.8–1.2
PTT	45	29–36 s

Which of the following tests is most likely to abnormal in this patient?
A. Antithrombin deficiency
B. Lupus anticoagulant
C. Prothrombin 20210 gene mutation
D. Factor V Leiden mutation
E. JAK2 V617F mutation

126. A 17-year-old high school student is diagnosed with a right lower-extremity deep vein thrombosis 1 week after a left ankle fracture he sustained while playing soccer. He has no prior history of thrombosis. His mom was diagnosed with combined heterozygosity for prothrombin 20210 gene mutation and factor V Leiden after she developed a pulmonary embolism as a teenager on oral contraceptives. The patient's father has a history of heterozygous factor V Leiden. The patient's hypercoagulable workup revealed homozygosity for factor V Leiden. He is started on the direct oral anticoagulant Rivaroxaban.
What is the mechanism by which factor V Leiden increases the risk of venous thromboembolism?
A. A gain of function mutation that leads to enhanced activity of activated protein C
B. A deficiency of a natural anticoagulant
C. A mutation in a clotting factor leading to resistance to cleavage by activated protein C
D. Disruption of annexin V shield on membranes
E. Enhanced binding of factor V to phospholipid

127. A 22-year-old woman who is 6 weeks postpartum presents to the emergency room with gradual worsening fatigue, confusion, and decreased urine output. She has had no symptoms of infection such as diarrhea, cough, fever, or dysuria. In the emergency room, she is afebrile but her blood pressure is 170/100 mm Hg. On exam she is alert to person and place but not to time. She has mild tenderness on palpation of abdomen. There are no signs of bleeding or bruising. Laboratory results are shown in Table 33.18. A peripheral blood smear is shown (Fig. 33.8).
The patient is initiated on emergent therapeutic plasma exchange (TPE). However, after 5 days of TPE, her renal function continues to worsen and she is started on hemodialysis.

TABLE 33.18 Laboratory Values: Question 127

Laboratory Test	Patient's Postpartum Day 1	Patient's Results Today	Reference Range
Hemoglobin	10.8 g/dL	8.6 g/dL	12–16 g/dL
Hematocrit	32.40%	25.8%	35%–48%
White blood cell count	5.2 × 10⁹/L, with normal differential	9.9 × 10⁹/L, with normal differential	4–10 × 10⁹/L
Platelet count	198 × 10⁹/L	87 × 10⁹/L	150–450 × 10⁹/L
Creatinine	1.2 mg/dL	4.6 mg/dL	0.7–1.3 mg/dL
Lactate dehydrogenase	N/A	1200 units/L	100–240 units/L
ADAMTS13 activity	N/A	57%	>60%
Aspartate transaminase (AST)	32 units/L	36 units/L	0–37 units/L
Alanine transaminase (ALT)	29 units/L	39 units/L	0–41 units/L
Total bilirubin	0.9 mg/dL	1.6 mg/dL	0.0–1.0 mg/dL
Direct bilirubin	0.1 mg/dL	0.2 mg/dL	0.0–0.2 mg/dL
Alkaline phosphatase	65 units/L	69 units/L	35–129 units/L
Prothrombin time (PT)	12.7 s	13.0 s	11–15 s
Activated partial thromboplastin time (aPTT)	29 s	31 s	29–36 s

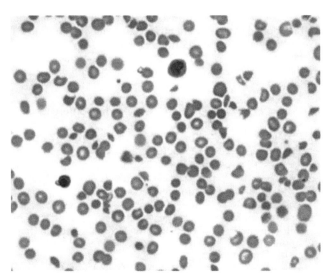

FIG. 33.8 Peripheral blood smear, John Lazarchick, ASH image bank 2001;Image # 00003.

What is best treatment to initiate at this time?
A. Prednisone 1 mg/kg daily
B. Monoclonal antibody that inhibits terminal complement
C. Platelet transfusion
D. Anti-CD20 monoclonal antibody

128. A 52-year-old obese female is admitted for a newly diagnosed deep vein thrombosis (DVT) in the left lower extremity. She is initiated on enoxaparin twice-daily and warfarin 15 mg once daily. She discharged the next day. Due to a high copayment for the enoxaparin, the patient decides to only fill her prescription for warfarin. She presents to the emergency room 6 days later with painful ecchymosis of the lateral surface of the right thigh that had progressed to necrosis with eschar formation within 48 hours at home. Her international normalized ratio (INR) on re-presentation was 1.7. She was immediately started on therapeutic unfractionated heparin and the warfarin was stopped. Histopathologic findings on skin biopsy revealed epidermal necrosis with evidence of fibrin deposits in the postcapillary venules, absence of arteriolar thrombosis, and lack of vascular or perivascular inflammation.
Which of the following most accurately represents the etiology of this patient's skin condition?
A. Protein C deficiency
B. Antiphospholipid antibodies
C. Rapid inactivation of factor II, VII, IX, and X
D. Calciphylaxis
E. Heparin-induced thrombocytopenia

129. A 70-year-old woman with metastatic colon cancer presents to the emergency room with severe shortness of breath. She is receiving chemotherapy for her colon cancer, and her last treatment was about 2 weeks ago. She is short of breath on exam and has some difficulty speaking in full sentences. Her oxygen saturation is 88% on room air, and her blood pressure is 90/60 mm Hg. CT of the chest confirms the presence of a large saddle pulmonary embolus.
Which of the following is the most appropriate therapy at this point?
A. Warfarin
B. tPA
C. Dabigatran
D. Apixaban
E. Aspirin

130. A 75-year-old man with coronary artery disease, chronic renal insufficiency (baseline creatinine 2.5), and diabetes mellitus is diagnosed with atrial fibrillation.
Which of the following is the most appropriate anticoagulant to choose?
A. Rivaroxaban
B. Fondaparinux
C. Enoxaparin
D. Warfarin
E. Unfractionated heparin

131. A 65-year-old man with a history of hepatitis C cirrhosis is diagnosed with portal vein thrombosis on screening ultrasound. His hepatitis C was previously treated; however, he did not respond to antiviral therapy. No lesions suspicious for hepatocellular carcinoma were identified on the ultrasound. He denies worsening abdominal pain or distention, and his laboratory values are unchanged. You review the ultrasound with the

radiologist who is unable to determine the chronicity of the clot.

What is the most appropriate management at this time?

A. Warfarin for 3 months
B. Warfarin indefinitely
C. Aspirin
D. Thrombolytic therapy
E. Observation

132. A 55-year-old man is diagnosed with a provoked DVT of the right popliteal vein after undergoing surgery for a fractured femur sustained in a motor vehicle accident. During his hospital stay, a thrombophilia workup is sent. He is found to be heterozygous for the prothrombin 20210 mutation. He presents to hematology clinic for recommendations regarding the duration of anticoagulation.

What is the most appropriate recommendation?

A. Indefinite anticoagulation
B. Anticoagulation for 3 months
C. Anticoagulation for 3 months followed by aspirin
D. Anticoagulation for 6 months
E. Anticoagulation for 6 months followed by aspirin

133. A 35-year-old otherwise healthy woman is 22 weeks pregnant with her first child. She is referred for anticoagulation recommendations. Her past medical history is negative for VTE; however, her father developed an unprovoked pulmonary embolism several years ago, prompting an evaluation for thrombophilia. The patient was also tested at that time and found to be homozygous for factor V Leiden mutation. What is the most appropriate recommendation regarding VTE prophylaxis for this patient?

A. No prophylaxis
B. Antepartum prophylaxis now until delivery
C. Postpartum prophylaxis for 3 weeks
D. Postpartum prophylaxis for 6 weeks
E. Antepartum prophylaxis followed by postpartum prophylaxis for 6 weeks

134. A patient with polycythemia vera (hematocrit is 68%) is evaluated with a new proximal leg DVT. Baseline PT testing is elevated (INR 1.4), and aPTT is normal. The patient has no history of bleeding diathesis; platelet count has been $500,000 \times 10^9$/L. His only medications are hydroxyurea and aspirin. Liver tests are normal.

Which is the best course of action at this point?

A. Repeat the PT/INR with less citrate
B. Perform PT mixing study
C. Ristocetin cofactor activity assay
D. Measure FXa activity

135. A 56-year-old woman presents to the hematology clinic after recently being found to have unprovoked bilateral lower extremity DVTs. She requests an evaluation for occult malignancy. Her clinical breast examination, mammography, screening colonoscopy, and PAP smears are up to date. She has never smoked. She has no history of prior VTE and no family history of VTE. She has no history of malignancy in her family. A chest x-ray showed no nodules or masses.

Regarding further cancer screening, which of the following is the best recommendation?

A. CT abdomen/pelvis
B. CA-125 and CA 19-9
C. CT abdomen/pelvis and CA-125 and CA 19-9
D. No additional screening

136. A 54-year-old woman presents for guidance 1 week after her first DVT of the proximal right leg provoked by cholecystectomy. Her right leg swelling is improving but has not resolved. She joined an online VTE support group who recommended the use of elastic compression stockings to prevent chronic postthrombotic syndrome. She obtained over-the-knee stockings with 30–40 mm Hg graded compression, but finds them unbearable.

Which of the following is the most appropriate recommendation concerning prevention of postthrombotic syndrome at this time?

A. Reinforce use of 30–40 mm Hg compression stockings
B. Prescribe 20–30 mm Hg compression stockings
C. Prescribe 10–20 mm Hg compression stockings
D. Discontinue use of compression stockings

137. A 30-year-old woman presents with the acute onset of abdominal pain and jaundice. Evaluation shows obstruction in the portal venous outflow tract consistent with Budd-Chiari syndrome. CT scan of the abdomen and pelvis reveals no masses and no cirrhotic changes.

She has no history of prior thrombotic events and no underlying liver dysfunction. Testing for hepatitis B and C are negative. Anticardiolipin and anti-beta 2 glycoprotein antibodies are negative. She has no hereditary thrombophilia identified, with normal testing for FV Leiden mutation and prothrombin gene mutation. She has two sisters, one brother, and a large extended family—none with a history of thrombosis. She has no history of hematuria.

She smokes one pack of cigarettes per day. She does not use oral contraceptives. She is not pregnant.

CBC shows:

WBC	$10,400 \times 10^9$/L with a normal differential
Hgb	13.7 g/dL
MCV	90 fL
Platelets	$190,000 \times 10^9$/L

Which of the following is the next best test to understand the etiology of her portal vein thrombosis?

A. Bone marrow biopsy
B. PNH testing
C. Liver biopsy
D. JAK2 V617F mutation from peripheral blood

138. A 78-year-old woman presents to the ED with the acute onset of headache and hemiparesis. Noncontrast head CT shows a large intracerebral hemorrhage.

Her medications include dabigatran, simvastatin, and metoprolol. Her accompanying family member is uncertain when the patient last took medications.

Labs show:

WBC	$11,400 \times 10^9$/L with normal differential
Hgb	11.6 g/dL
Platelets	$352,000 \times 10^9$/L
Creatinine	1.34 mg/dL (0.60–1.00 mg/dL)
AST	34 units/L (14–38 units/L)
ALT	43 units/L (15–48 units/L)

PT and aPTT are within the limits of normal.

In addition to a neurosurgery consultation, which of the following which of the following is the best step in management?

A. Recombinant FVIIa
B. Activated prothrombin complex concentrate
C. No hemostatic agent advised
D. Idarucizumab
E. Four-factor prothrombin complex concentrate

139. A 50-year-old woman presents for evaluation of a painful "cord" in her medial thigh. A lower extremity duplex Doppler ultrasound shows a clot in the greater saphenous vein, measuring 6 cm. She has no history of malignancy and takes no medications. She has never had a prior venous thromboembolism. She is otherwise healthy and lives independently. Her renal and hepatic function are normal.

    Which of the following is the most appropriate recommendation?

    A. Observation with repeat ultrasound in 1 week
    B. Rivaroxaban, 15 mg PO BID × 2 weeks followed by 20 mg PO daily × 3 months
    C. Fondaparinux, 2.5 mg sq × 45 days
    D. NSAIDs and warm compresses

140. A 54-year-old man is 15 days status post cholecystectomy for symptomatic cholelithiasis. He undergoes repeat chest CT scan ordered for follow-up of a pulmonary nodule noted 6 months previously. The CT identifies a possible left lower lobe subsegmental pulmonary embolism. The previously seen pulmonary nodule is no longer present. He has felt well, without complaint of dyspnea or leg pain. He has no prior history of thrombosis. He is up to date on age and gender-appropriate cancer screening. His kidney and hepatic function are normal. D-dimer testing is normal (no elevation). Bilateral lower extremity Doppler ultrasound shows no clot.

    Which of the following is the best recommendation for management of the incidentally noted subsegmental pulmonary embolism?

    A. Observation
    B. Fondaparinux
    C. Aspirin
    D. Rivaroxaban
    E. Enoxaparin bridge to warfarin

141. A 66-year-old man with colon cancer receiving FOLFIRI chemotherapy develops pain and swelling in his right arm. He is found to have a thrombosis of the right subclavian vein. He has a port in his right chest for chemotherapy administration; it is still functional. His renal and hepatic functions are normal, and his ECOG performance status is 1.

    Labs show:
    WBC $10,600 \times 10^9/L$
    Hgb   10.6 g/dL
    Platelets $145,000 \times 10^9/L$

    Which of the following is the most appropriate recommendation?

    A. Remove the catheter and administer LMWH × 3–6 months
    B. Leave the catheter in place and administer LMWH × 3–6 months and as long as the catheter is in place
    C. Remove the catheter and give no anticoagulation
    D. Leave the catheter and administer alteplase

142. A 48-year-old woman is admitted to the neurology service for management of a cerebral sinus thrombosis found during evaluation of persistent headaches and papilledema. The CT scan shows a small associated intracerebral hemorrhage.

    Which of the following is the most appropriate recommendation for management?

    A. Observation
    B. IV unfractionated heparin
    C. Aspirin
    D. Systemic thrombolysis

143. A 62-year-old woman with a history of recurrent venous thromboembolism presents for consideration of changing her anticoagulation from warfarin to a direct oral anticoagulant due to fluctuating INR values, typically in the mildly supratherapeutic range. She has tried to maintain a steady level of vitamin K in her diet, although does admit difficulty in following dietary guidelines. Her BMI is 45. She has renal dysfunction, with estimated creatinine clearance of 20 mL/min. Which of the following do you recommend regarding management of her anticoagulation?

    A. Continue warfarin, administer vitamin K 100 μg PO daily
    B. Change to LMWH
    C. Change to dabigatran
    D. Change to fondaparinux

144. A 35-year-old man presents with acute left common femoral vein thrombosis after leg swelling of 1 day's duration. He has no medical problems, takes no medications, and denies prior surgery, trauma, or immobility. He is treated with warfarin after an enoxaparin bridge and has had no trouble maintaining his INR in the therapeutic range in the 3 months he has been anticoagulated. He is referred for further management. There is no prior personal or family history of thrombosis. He is a nonsmoker and nondrinker. He is nonobese.

    Which of the following is the most appropriate measure at this time?

    A. Check D-dimer and stop anticoagulation if negative
    B. Check for inherited thrombophilia and stop anticoagulation if negative
    C. Continue anticoagulation indefinitely
    D. Repeat ultrasound of leg and stop anticoagulation if clot has resolved
    E. Stop anticoagulation now

145. A 35-year-old man presents with acute left common femoral vein thrombosis after leg swelling of 1 day's duration, 1 week after undergoing surgery on his left ankle. He has no other medical problems and takes no medications currently. He is treated with warfarin after an enoxaparin bridge and has had no trouble maintaining his INR in the therapeutic range in the 3 months he has been anticoagulated. He is referred for further management. There is no prior personal or family history of thrombosis. He is a nonsmoker and nondrinker. He is nonobese.

    Which of the following is the most appropriate measure at this time?

    A. Check D-dimer and stop anticoagulation if negative
    B. Check for inherited thrombophilia and stop anticoagulation if negative
    C. Continue anticoagulation indefinitely
    D. Repeat ultrasound of leg and stop anticoagulation if clot has resolved
    E. Stop anticoagulation now

146. A 45-year-old woman known to be heterozygous for factor V Leiden undergoes liver transplantation for cirrhosis from a donor negative for factor V Leiden. Six months after her transplantation, her hypercoagulable evaluation is performed. Which of the options in Table 33.19 is the most likely set of results?

TABLE 33.19 Answer Options: Question 146

	Factor V Leiden	APC Resistance
A	Negative	Negative
B	Negative	Positive
C	Positive	Negative
D	Positive	Positive

147. A 55-year-old woman with a history of varicose veins is diagnosed with a thrombosis in her right superficial femoral vein following a vein stripping procedure on the left leg. Which of the following is the most appropriate course of action at this time?
   A. Apixaban for at least 3 months
   B. Enoxaparin for 4 weeks
   C. Fondaparinux for 1 week
   D. No anticoagulation
   E. Rivaroxaban indefinitely

148. In which of the following patients would an IVC filter be most indicated?
   A. A 25-year-old woman with morbid obesity without thrombotic history prior to undergoing bariatric surgery.
   B. A 35-year-old woman with a saddle pulmonary embolus and residual femoral vein clot on the left.
   C. A 45-year-old man who suffers a PE 1 day after starting unfractionated heparin. His aPTT was subtherapeutic cbc.
   D. A 55-year-old man with a DVT 1 day after craniotomy for removal of a glioblastoma.
   E. A 65-year-old woman with a history of subdural hematoma 3 years ago, now with acute DVT and PE.

ANSWERS

1. A

There are many causes of thrombocytopenia distinct from ITP. Reviewing the peripheral smear can be helpful in identifying disorders leading to thrombocytopenia. The constellation of macrothrombocytopenia and Döhle bodies raises the possibility of the May-Hegglin anomaly, a congenital disorder due to mutations in the nonmuscle myosin heavy chain gene (MYH9). May-Hegglin is typically a benign disorder that does not require treatment. CALR mutations have been associated with JAK2 wild-type myeloproliferative neoplasms. ADAMTS13 levels are reduced in TTP. Mutations in MPL may lead to thrombocytosis. PI3Ks are a family of enzymes responsible for cell growth, proliferation, and differentiation.

2. C

Mutations in calreticulin (CALR) have recently been described in patients with essential thrombocytosis or primary myelofibrosis who do not have JAK2 V617F or MPL mutations. Such patients appear to have better thrombosis-free survival than those patients with mutated JAK2. BCL2 overexpression is associated with follicular lymphomas. PI3K is an enzyme responsible for cellular processes. MYH9 is mutated in macrothrombocytopenic conditions such as May-Hegglin. PML is fused with RAR-alpha in acute promyelocytic leukemia.

3. C

Although the majority of adults with ITP respond to steroids, most will relapse after steroids are tapered or stopped. Many second-line options for chronic ITP exist and the choice of therapy should be based on patient comorbidities and preference. Splenectomy, rituximab, and TPO receptor agonists are all considered reasonable second-line therapies for chronic ITP. This patient's morbid obesity, CAD with angina, as well as oxygen-dependent COPD make him a suboptimal surgical candidate (choice B). Based on his liver function tests and hepatitis studies he likely has chronic hepatitis B, and therefore rituximab would not be an optimal choice, due to the risk or hepatitis B reactivation. Romiplostim, a thrombopoietin receptor agonist, is FDA approved for second-line therapy of ITP with an expected response rate of 60%–80% and would be a reasonable, albeit unlikely curative, option (choice C). Many other drugs including danazol and azathioprine have been used in chronic ITP, but response rates are generally less than 20%, and use is typically reserved to those refractory to the aforementioned second-line therapies.

4. B

HIT antibody testing should only be performed in those patients with an intermediate to high suspicion of HIT. Two types of tests utilized for the diagnosis of HIT include enzyme immunoassays for the antiplatelet factor 4 (PF4)/heparin antibodies and functional assays such as the serotonin release assay (SRA) and heparin-induced platelet aggregation assay. Sensitivity of the enzyme immunoassay is high (close to 99%); therefore clinically insignificant antibodies may be detected. Functional assays such as SRA or heparin-induced platelet aggregation assay are performed to confirm the diagnosis of HIT in the setting of a positive enzyme immunoassay. Thus answer B is the appropriate first step in the laboratory evaluation of HIT in this case scenario. Answers D and E are incorrect, as the platelet function assay and platelet aggregation tests are utilized to measure platelet adhesion and aggregation and has no role in the diagnosis of HIT.

5. B

Glanzmann thrombasthenia is an autosomal recessive disorder with normal coagulation laboratory testing and platelet count. It is caused by defects, either qualitative or quantitative, in the receptor for fibrinogen on platelets, glycoprotein IIb/IIIa, a.k.a., $\alpha_{2b}\beta_3$ in the integrin nomenclature. The hallmark diagnostic finding is the failure for platelets to aggregate in response to platelet agonists, such as collagen, arachidonic acid, or ADP. The response of platelets to ristocetin is preserved.[1]

Bernard-Soulier is another autosomal recessive platelet disorder that presents with lifelong bleeding that is caused by defects in the platelet receptor complex, glycoprotein Ib/IX/V.[2] Since this receptor binds to ristocetin, which causes platelet *agglutination*, as opposed to *aggregation*, on platelet aggregation testing only the response to ristocetin is impaired, with the response to all other platelet agonists intact. In addition, it is characterized by a *macrothrombocytopenia*, further differentiating it from Glanzmann thrombasthenia.

Platelets from patients who have ingested aspirin or who have an aspirin-like defect, will not respond to arachidonic acid. Arachidonic acid is eventually converted into thromboxane A2 (TXA2), which leads to platelet aggregation. Aspirin irreversibly inhibits cyclooxygenase-1 and -2, which is the first step in TXA2 synthesis. The addition of TXA2 bypasses this block and leads to normal platelet aggregation, confirming the presence of either aspirin or an aspirin-like defect. Platelet responses to collagen, ADP, and TXA2 would still expected to be normal.

Clopidogrel, along with similar agents such as prasugrel, ticagrelor, and ticlopdine, inhibit the ADP-receptor on platelets, P2Y$_{12}$. Thus, only a blunted response to ADP in a platelet aggregation assay would be expected.

The May-Hegglin anomaly is an *MYH9*-related disorder, and is characterized by a *macrothrombocytopenia* and Döhle-like bodies in neutrophils, along with the variable presence of sensorineural hearing loss, glomerular disease, and/or cataracts. Response to platelet aggregation is typically preserved.[3]

6. C

Cyclic thrombocytopenia is characterized by intermittent oscillations in the platelet count, which range from marked thrombocytopenia and, commonly, thrombocytosis. It is frequently misdiagnosed as ITP, with affected patients commonly receiving a number of treatments for ITP that are frequently ineffective. While the precise mechanism(s) for cyclic thrombocytopenia remain(s) unknown, a hormonal effect is noted, as affected women typically experience nadir platelet counts with their menstrual cycles.

Congenital amegakaryocytic thrombocytopenia presents early in infancy with marked thrombocytopenia and, later, bone marrow failure. It is caused by defects in the thrombopoietin receptor, *c-mpl*.

Quebec platelet disorder is a very rare genetic disease that can manifest with a mild thrombocytopenia, although platelet counts can be normal, and occurs without thrombocytosis. It is associated with postsurgical bleeding, although affected patients can have many other bleeding symptoms. It is caused by a duplication of the urokinase plasminogen activator gene, *PLAU*. It is treated with the use of antifibrinolytics, such as ε-aminocaproic acid or tranexamic acid.

Scott syndrome is another very rare platelet disorder that is characterized by an inability of platelets to translocate phosphatidylserine to the platelet surface. This leads to a severe hemorrhagic phenotype that is associated with completely normal coagulation testing and normal platelet counts. The only known treatment is with platelet transfusions.

Hermansky-Pudlak is an autosomal recessive disease that is associated with easy bleeding and following procedures. Extrahematologic manifestations include oculocutaneous albinism and pulmonary fibrosis. Platelet counts are normal in patients with this disease.

7. D

Thrombocytopenia occurs in up to 10% of women during pregnancy. The prevalence of a platelet count of less than $100,000 \times 10^9/L$ is observed in only 1% of pregnant women. Causes of thrombocytopenia during pregnancy may or may not be pregnancy-specific. The most common cause of thrombocytopenia during pregnancy is gestational thrombocytopenia (GT), which accounts for 70%–80% of cases. The mechanism of GT is unknown, but accelerated clearance and hemodilution may play a role. GT commonly occurs during the second or third trimester and is associated with a platelet count greater than 70,000/µL. No special management is required, and thrombocytopenia resolves within 6 weeks postpartum. GT is not associated with neonatal thrombocytopenia. This patient's clinical picture is most consistent with GT, and therefore no treatment is indicated. The mode of delivery should be based on obstetric indications. Prednisone and IVIG are first-line therapies for immune mediated thrombocytopenia in pregnancy. ITP usually presents earlier in gestation and with lower platelet counts. Treatment for ITP is indicated for clinically relevant bleeding or platelet count less than 30,000/µL. Other rare causes of thrombocytopenia in pregnancy include severe preeclampsia, HELLP syndrome, and acute fatty liver of pregnancy. The treatment for these conditions after 34 weeks gestation is delivery and supportive care.

8. D

The patient has a mild non-life-threatening thrombocytopenia that has been stable over 6 weeks. He is asymptomatic. Given a prior normal CBC 1 year ago and current isolated thrombocytopenia, this patient likely has immune thrombocytopenia (ITP). Therapy consists of treating and preventing bleeding episodes. The decision to treat ITP should be based on an individual patient's symptoms, bleeding risk (based on prior bleeding episodes and other risk factors for bleeding), potential side effects from treatment, and upcoming surgeries/procedures. In adults, treatment may be indicated in the absence of bleeding if the platelet count is very low ($<30,000 \times 10^9/L$). For this patient, the degree of thrombocytopenia he has should not put him at increased risk for bleeding for minor surgeries like upcoming wisdom tooth extraction. Therefore no treatment is indicated at this time. Instead, a conservative approach with follow-up of her platelet count should be sufficient. *Helicobacter pylori* infection is rarely associated with ITP, most frequently in patients from endemic areas such as Japan and parts of Europe. In this setting, without specific symptoms associated with *H. pylori* infection, testing would be of low yield. More extensive testing such as a bone marrow biopsy is generally not indicated in young, otherwise asymptomatic patients with isolated mild thrombocytopenia.

9. B

Drug-induced thrombocytopenic pupura (DITP) should be considered in any patient with acute onset thrombocytopenia. Many mechanisms of DITP exist. In the case of sulfonamide antibiotics, an antibody is produced that binds to normal platelets only in the presence of the sensitizing drug. The diagnosis is suspected by establishing that the candidate drug preceded the thrombocytopenia, withdrawing the drug results in complete and sustained recovery of platelet count, and when other causes of thrombocytopenia are ruled out. Typically 5–7 days of exposure is needed to produce sensitization in a patient given the drug for the first time. A detailed medication history (prescription and over-the-counter medications) should be elicited when evaluating such patients. Negative antibody testing does not rule out the diagnosis. Many patients do not require targeted therapy other than stopping the offending drug. For patients with severe thrombocytopenia or "wet purpura," platelet transfusions should be considered. Corticosteroids are often given, but there is no role in DITP, unlike idiopathic ITP. Once the offending drug is confirmed, patients should permanently avoid exposure to the drug. Recovery of platelet count begins in 1–2 days and is usually complete by 1 week.

10. B

This patient has TTP based on labs and a peripheral blood smear with schistocytes that reveal thrombotic microangiopathy. The diagnosis of TTP is secured by the pathognomonic low ADAMTS 13 activity of less than 5% due to either a congenital or acquired deficiency of this von Willebrand factor-cleaving protease. Lack of ADAMTS13 leads to unusually large von Willebrand multimers and the risk of platelet thrombi in microvasculature with high shear stress. An ADAMTS13 activity less than 5% is not seen with other thrombotic microangiopathies such as atypical hemolytic uremic syndrome, which is caused by complement dysregulation. Further, aHUS can be distinguished from TTP based on the degree of renal insufficiency, with the former leading to more pronounced dysfunction. Type 2B von Willebrand disease is characterized by a "gain of function mutation," leading to increased binding of the vWF to platelets with resultant thrombocytopenia from increased clearance. However, type 2B vWB is typically not associated with this degree of thrombocytopenia and renal insufficiency or hemolysis. Heparin-induced thrombocytopenia is caused by autoantibodies directed against platelet factor 4 in complex with heparin, which this patient is not on.

11. A

Argatroban is a nonheparin anticoagulant, which is cleared by the liver and is FDA approved for the treatment of heparin-induced thrombocytopenia (HIT) with or without thrombosis. Enoxaparin is a low-molecular-weight heparin, and all heparin products should be avoided in patients diagnosed with HIT. In addition, enoxaparin is contraindicated in patients with severe renal failure. While fondaparinux may be used in the treatment of HIT, this patient's renal dysfunction precludes its use. Aspirin does not provide adequate anticoagulation, and rivaroxaban has not been studied in the setting of HIT.

12. E

The most appropriate consideration in a patient with DIC is to treat the underlying cause; thus placement of the chest tube and initiation of antibiotics is the most appropriate course of action for this patient. Deferring chest tube placement would likely result in worsening of the empyema, and there is no role for platelet, FFP, or factor VIIa infusion.

13. B

Multi-organ dysfunction syndrome (MODS) is a complication of DIC as a result of microvascular thrombosis. It has a high mortality rate and is the primary cause of death among patients experiencing processes that initiate DIC. At autopsy, most or all target organs are found to be damaged or rendered ineffective by thromboses and hemorrhage occurring more often in the microvasculature. The heart and kidneys fail while liver function test results deteriorate at an alarming rate. Cardiogenic

shock with circulatory collapse additionally causes shock liver. Over 35 years ago, Mant and King showed that 85% of patients with acute, severe DIC expired, and most expired, in their opinion, from the underlying disease and not from DIC itself. The presence of malignancy alone, schistocytes on the peripheral blood smear, or degree of PT, PTT, or D-dimer abnormality do not directly correlate with mortality in patients with DIC.

14. A

Any male with thrombocytopenia and small platelets should be evaluated for WASp expression and gene mutations. X-linked thrombocytopenia is a mild variant of WAS that presents with congenital thrombocytopenia that is sometimes intermittent. XLT generally follows a benign disease course, although carries an increased risk for severe life-threatening infections, cancer, serious hemorrhage, and autoimmunity.

15. A

Familial RUNX1 follows an autosomal dominant inheritance pattern, thus offspring of an affected parent have a 50% chance of carrying the mutation. Familial RUNX1 mutation carriers may be asymptomatic and have normal platelet counts. Allogeneic stem cell transplantation from a donor with somatic RUNX1 mutation can result in more myeloid or lymphoid malignancies, and affected individuals should be excluded as donors.

16. A

Glanzmann thrombasthenia results from a defect in the platelet surface Gp IIb/IIIa receptor leading to a defect in platelet aggregation. In patients with no platelet alloimmunization, administration of platelets plus antifibrinolytic therapy is highly effective at achieving hemostasis in the perioperative period. Since patients with Glanzmann thrombasthenia have a defective Gp IIb/IIIa receptor, which is responsible for binding von Willebrand factor and fibrinogen, neither administration of von Willebrand factor concentrate nor DDAVP would be expected to lead to reliable hemostasis. Further, while antifibrinolytics may be used to help lessen minor physiologic bleeding, they are not expected to result in adequate primary hemostasis after a major surgical intervention such as a total knee arthroplasty.

17. A

Initial responses with rituximab are expected in 7–56 days. Adding another agent such as an immune modulatory agent (i.e., cyclosporine) or TPO-mimetic is reasonable while awaiting response to rituximab. Vincristine can be associated with significant peripheral neuropathy and constipation, and should not be used in this early setting. Anti-D use requires the patient to be Rh positive. Splenectomy is a reasonable consideration; however, she is not bleeding, and there has not been a sufficient trial of rituximab that has already been initiated.

18. A

Bernard-Soulier syndrome is a macrothrombocytopenia with a primary defect in hemostasis caused by reduced levels and/or dysfunctional platelet receptor GPIb leading to reduced adhesion. The platelets characteristically do not aggregate with ristocetin. MYH9 related disorders also have macrothrombocytopenia; however, the lack of platelet aggregation with ristocetin is characteristic of Bernard-Soulier. Bernard-Soulier platelets may appear abnormal by electron microscopy; however, the ultrastructural changes are not diagnostic of the syndrome. The PFA-100 is a good screening test for platelet dysfunction, but is not diagnostic.

19. A

Do not begin warfarin until platelets have recovered to normal levels AND stable anticoagulation is achieved with another anticoagulant such as argatroban. Warfarin is expected to initially cause a decrease in protein C levels, resulting in an initially prothrombotic state. When warfarin is started, it is suggested that initial dosing be less than 5 mg so as not to drop the protein C levels precipitously. Argatroban will increase the PT/INR; formulas exist to correct for this to determine the increased PT/INR due to warfarin alone. Correction of the underlying thrombocytopenia typically occurs rapidly within 7 days. The direct oral anticoagulants have not been studied in HIT and are not advised for routine use in the treatment of HIT. Aspirin has not been proven to be of benefit in HIT.

20. C

Iron deficiency is a common cause of thrombocytosis. Unless masked polycythemia vera or myelofibrosis is suspected from the clinical history and examination (e.g., history of erythromelalgia, migraines, aquagenic pruritus, abdominal vein thrombosis, splenomegaly), thrombocytosis is likely to be due to secondary causes. Bone marrow biopsy would be indicated in the case of anemia refractory to iron replacement, to evaluate for an underlying myelodysplastic or myeloproliferative process.

21. D

Thrombotic thrombocytopenic purpura (TTP) is a thrombotic microangiopathy caused by severely reduced activity of the von Willebrand factor-cleaving protease ADAMTS13. TTP is a medical emergency that is almost always fatal if appropriate treatment is not initiated promptly. TTP is thought to be caused by an acquired inhibitor of the ADAMTS13. As such, the goals of treatment are (1) replacement of ADAMTS13 and (2) removal of the inhibitor. To date, this is best achieved with therapeutic plasma exchange and high-dose corticosteroids. Not all patients have ready access to a center capable of initiating plasma exchange. If a significant delay (i.e., >6 hours) is expected, the administration of FFP can be used as a temporizing measure, with the thought that it is providing some level of ADAMTS13 replacement.

22. B

In a patient with persistent thrombocytosis and no evidence of a secondary cause (normal iron stores, no evidence of inflammation, history not suggestive of an underlying malignancy), a primary etiology (myeloproliferative neoplasm) should be evaluated. While 60% of ET patients have the JAK2 V617F mutation, in those JAK2 negative cases, more than half will have a mutation in CALR Exon 9. Patients with CALR mutations often present with isolated thrombocytosis. MPL mutations are present in only about 5% of ET cases. Thrombopoietin testing has not proven reliable to distinguish reactive from autonomous causes of thrombocytosis.

23. D

Niemann-Pick type B is a pan-ethnic disorder resulting from a deficiency of acid sphingomyelinase and

resulting in histiocytic accumulation of lipids, resulting in a "foamy" histiocyte appearance. It can present in adulthood with splenomegaly and thrombocytopenia secondary to sequestration. Splenectomy should be used cautiously in these diseases, as histiocytic build-up may thereafter develop in other organs such as the liver. The thrombocytopenia in this case was not related to ITP nor a lymphoma. Neither corticosteroids nor rituximab are a valid treatment for Niemann-Pick type B disease.

24. A

In patients with thrombocytosis or leukocytosis, the increased cellular components may leak intracellular contents into the serum fraction after blood collection, thereby causing a pseudohyperkalemia on plasma potassium testing. In order to test for "true" hyperkalemia, the test should be repeated using plasma. Beginning hydroxyurea will lower the platelet count, thereby preventing pseudohyperkalemia. However, it is not appropriate to begin this agent solely for the purpose of preventing pseudohyperkalemia. Similarly, it is not necessary to administer furosemide or calcium gluconate if the potassium is not truly elevated.

25. B

Thrombotic thrombocytopenic purpura (TTP), which is caused by an inhibitor to ADAMTS13, a von Willebrand factor-cleaving protease, should respond to corticosteroids + plasma exchange within 4–7 days. The presence of such an inhibitor in this case strongly favors the diagnosis of TTP rather than an alternative explanation. In such cases of refractory TTP, rituximab is expected to be of clinical benefit in most cases, often within 2 weeks of administration. Twice daily plasma exchange has also been proposed, although there is less data on this option. Splenectomy may be of use, but with the significant associated morbidity, rituximab would be the first choice. There are case reports to demonstrate the efficacy of bortezomib; however, there are no trials of this agent in refractory TTP.

26. A

This patient's peripheral blood smear demonstrates the characteristic Döhle-like bodies and macrothrombocyte associated with May-Hegglin related disorders. This group of disorders have variable presentations that can include a platelet-type bleeding diathesis, sensorineural hearing loss, cataracts, and renal failure.

The platelet electron microscopy may be abnormal in the giant platelets of May-Hegglin related disorders. However, the neutrophilic inclusions strongly suggest the diagnosis and genetic testing should be confirmatory.

27. B

This patient has delayed heparin-induced thrombocytopenia with thrombosis (HIT/T). Antibodies in patients with HIT form against complexes of heparin and PF4 (platelet factor 4) and lead to drops in platelet counts of 50% or more. Paradoxically, HIT patients may go on to develop arterial or venous thrombosis. HIT is reported to occur in up to 1% of individuals who have been treated with unfractionated heparin. While classic HIT occurs 5–10 days after start of heparin therapy, HIT may also occur after heparin cessation. Delayed-onset HIT should be considered when a patient presents with thrombosis with or without thrombocytopenia up to 3 weeks after the end of heparin therapy.

Patients with HIT/T should be treated with a direct thrombin inhibitor such as argatroban. While certain patients may be treated with fondaparinux, this patient has worsening renal insufficiency, and thus a renally cleared anticoagulant such as fondaparinux would not be appropriate therapy. Patients with HIT should not receive further heparin therapy. The patient's thrombosis was caused by HIT, and thus further hypercoagulable testing would not be useful. Lastly, a D-dimer would add nothing to the management of this patient, who has already been diagnosed with thrombosis and is recently postop.

28. D

Eltrombopag is a small molecule agonist of the TPO receptor and is indicated for treatment of immune thrombocytopenia, aplastic anemia, and hepatitis C-associated thrombocytopenia requiring interferon therapy. Eltrombopag has also been used to raise platelet counts in patients with cirrhosis and thrombocytopenia prior to invasive procedures. In this latter group, however, an increased rate of portal vein thrombosis was noted, necessitating early termination of the study. Hepatic laboratory abnormalities (increased serum alanine aminotransferase, aspartate aminotransferase, and bilirubin) are frequent (up to 10% in the EXTEND study), usually mild, and reversible with drug discontinuation; moreover, they are infrequently associated with clinically significant symptoms. At the current time, no available data show an increased risk of either development or progression of hematologic malignancies or cataracts with either short- or long-term treatment. Development of myelofibrosis is reversible with drug discontinuation and may be more related to the increased megakaryocyte load in ITP patients, rather than other patient populations.

29. A

In 2013, the CDC issued a bulletin reporting a TTP-like illness in 15 patients who had crushed the oral narcotic Opana ER and injected it intravenously. Twelve patients were treated with plasma exchange. All patients recovered. Miller and colleagues subsequently reported 18 cases of thrombotic microangiopathy in 15 patients, all of who were treated with supportive care only for infections and renal dysfunction. All recovered without the use of plasma exchange. This TTP-like illness induced by IV Opana use does not appear to require plasma exchange for recovery. Plasma infusions, corticosteroids, and anticoagulation do not appear to be required for recovery of this illness.

30. D

The patient has developed a new thrombosis while therapeutic on warfarin anticoagulation. This could certainly be a warfarin failure due to malignancy (in which case we might change her warfarin back to long-term enoxaparin or other low-molecular-weight heparin), but notably, the patient has thrombocytopenia in conjunction with the thrombosis. The thrombocytopenia was noted 9 days after starting therapy with low-molecular-weight heparin. There are no other potential causes of thrombocytopenia, and this gives the patient a 4T score of 8—putting her at very high probability of having heparin-induced thrombocytopenia. The best treatment at this time is argatroban. Heparin or LMWH is contraindicated. The patient has already clotted through therapeutic warfarin. Rivaroxaban is indicated neither for HITT nor for cancer associated

malignancy, and would also not be the correct answer. A reasonable choice might be fondaparinux, but this was not given as an option.

31. E

Pseudothrombocytopenia occurs in certain individuals who make a substance, which leads to platelet clumping in the presence of EDTA anticoagulation. The clumping can be seen on examination of the peripheral blood smear. The clumped platelets are not recognized as individual platelets by the Coulter counter, and the platelet count is thus falsely depressed. In many cases, rechecking the platelet count on blood drawn into a citrate-anticoagulated tube may lead to a more accurate platelet count by blocking the platelet clumping. The thrombocytopenia is artifactual, and does not need therapy, so treatment with corticosteroids would not be indicated. The platelet clumping occurs only in vitro, so antiplatelet agents are also not indicated. Stopping medications will not necessarily have an effect on this benign condition. Patients should be reassured about this condition and counseled about informing future health care providers about their spurious laboratory values.

32. B

Thrombocytopenia during pregnancy is a common finding. Gestational thrombocytopenia is the most common cause of a low platelet count in a pregnant woman. It is most common during the third trimester and does not cause a platelet count of below $50,000 \times 10^9/L$. When the platelet count falls below, then ITP should be suspected. Barring that, treatment with corticosteroids of gammaglobulin is not indicated. There is no thrombotic microangiopathy (TTP, eclampsia, or HELLP) necessitating emergent delivery of the fetus. Once thrombocytopenia is identified, careful platelet monitoring is warranted. Antiplatelet antibody titers will not aid in the diagnosis.

33. A

Thrombocytopenia during pregnancy is a common finding. This patient has thrombocytopenia complicated by microangiopathic hemolytic anemia, with elevated liver enzymes, and this comprises the HELLP syndrome (Hemolysis, Elevated Liver enzymes, and Low Platelets). The treatment for HELLP in a woman whose fetus is of sufficient gestational age to survive outside the uterus is emergent delivery. There is no role for corticosteroids or gammaglobulin, unlike in ITP, and antiplatelet antibody titers will not aid in the diagnosis.

34. E

Nearly all patients who receive a continuous-flow LVAD develop an acquired type 2 von Willebrand disease thought secondary to shearing of high-molecular-weight von Willebrand multimers. Forty percent of these patients develop bleeding, usually from arteriovenous malformations of the GI tract. Optimal therapy for these patients has not been determined. Lowering the dose or stopping the warfarin or stopping the antiplatelet agent has not been effective in preventing recurrent bleeding episodes, and may lead to in-pump thrombosis, which requires device replacement. Neither plasma nor PCCs are indicated at this level of INR. Recombinant VIIa is not indicated in this situation and may lead to thrombosis. The platelet count and function in this situation is not compromised enough to require platelet transfusion. However, the patient is severely anemic and having angina, and requires immediate red cell transfusion to improve her oxygen carrying capacity.

35. B

A recent study comparing fresh frozen plasma with a four-component pcc in patients who require reversal of warfarin found superiority of the four-component pcc both in time to correction of INR and volume of solution infused. Amino caproic acid is useful for superficial bleeding, as it is an antifibrinolytic. Factor VIIa is only approved in the treatment of inhibitors, and off-label use is associated with morbidity.

36. C

Selective serotonin reuptake inhibitors (SSRIs) have been associated with an increased risk for GI bleeding, most likely due to their effects on platelets that normally take up serotonin in their granules. In addition, concomitant use of NSAIDs and SSRIs increase the bleeding risk due to the fact that some SSRIs inhibit p450, which helps metabolize certain NSAIDs. A recent metaanalysis confirmed the increased risk of GI bleed in patients taking SSRIs. Fluticasone, fexofenadine, and levothyroxine do not increase the risk for bleeding. Progestins such as norgestrel increase the risk for thrombosis.

37. E

Three of the four venomous snakes in the United States belong to the subfamily of crotalids that include rattlesnakes, copperheads, and water moccasins. The fourth poisonous snake in the United States, the coral snake, is a viper. Western North Carolina is home to both copperheads and timber rattlesnakes. Crotalid envenomation causes diffuse defibrination, as is shown in the labs for this patient. In addition to supportive care, trivalent crotalid antivenom should be administered to critically ill patients. If administered within 2 hours of the bite, survival is more than 99%. Factor VIIa is indicated in the treatment of hemophilia patients with inhibitors. Fresh frozen plasma would not reverse defibrination. PCCs are indicated in the rapid reversal of warfarin.

38. C

Psychogenic purpura, also known as Diamond-Gardner syndrome, is a disorder characterized by painful bruising in areas accessible by the patient's hands. Bruises are typically preceded by itching or burning, and the patients are more frequently female and typically have an underlying psychiatric diagnosis. Sometimes, the lesions have overlying bleeding. Psychogenic purpura can be distinguished from a more severe disorder by the location of the lesions that are restricted to accessible regions of the body, absence of laboratory abnormalities, and symptom complex. The disorder does not require intensive laboratory investigation.

39. D

Combined factor V and factor VIII deficiency is a rare autosomal recessive bleeding disorder due to mutations in either LMAN1 or MCFD2, which encode proteins responsible for transport of Factor V and Factor VIII proteins from the endoplasmic reticulum to the Golgi. Such patients typically present with moderate bleeding, as the presence of two defects does not appear to produce more bleeding than a single deficiency. In premenopausal women, menorrhagia and postpartum hemorrhage are common. Soft tissue hematomas are also common. Bleeding episodes are best treated with fresh frozen plasma as a source of factor V and factor VIII concentrates. Type 2N von Willebrand disease would not have a low factor V level. Vitamin K deficiency would have a low factor VII level and normal factor V levels. Liver disease would have a low factor VII level and low levels of nearly all coagulation factors except for factor VIII. Patients with lupus anticoagulants have an aPTT that does not correct with mixing, and these patients do not typically bleed.

40. A

Glanzmann thrombasthenia is a congenital qualitative platelet disorder characterized by deficiency of glycoprotein IIb/IIIa on the platelet surface. Glanzmann thrombasthenia is typically a moderate bleeding disorder characterized by mucocutaneous bleeding. Platelet aggregation studies confirm absence of primary aggregation to all agents except for ristocetin. The diagnosis can be confirmed by flow cytometry. Bernard-Soulier is another congenital platelet disorder where the platelets aggregate normally to all agents, except for ristocetin, as this is a disorder in the GP Ib/IX/V complex. Gray platelet syndrome and delta storage pool disease are characterized by abnormal secondary response in platelet aggregation studies. Scott syndrome is a platelet membrane defect leading to impaired thrombin generation. Platelet aggregation studies are normal in this disorder.

41. B

Type 2b von Willebrand disease accounts for less than 5% of all cases of vWD. The disease is due to a gain of function mutation in the A1 domain in the vWF protein, which subsequently results in increased binding to glycoprotein Ibα on platelets. This subsequently leads to increased clearance and loss of high-molecular-weight vWF multimers. In type 2b and type 2a vWD, there is a disproportionate decrease in the Ristocetin cofactor activity as compared with the level of von Willebrand antigen (vWF:RCO:vWF Ag; choice B). In type 2b vWD there is also a decrease in only the high-molecular-weight von Willebrand factor multimers due to increased binding of larger multimers to platelet glycoproteins, rather than a decrease in all vWF multimers (choice A). Thrombocytopenia is seen in 40% of cases of type 2b vWD due to increased clearance and sequestration of small platelet aggregates that are formed (choice C). RIPA is increased as the abnormal vWF binds to platelets at lower concentration of ristocetin as compared with normal vWF, leading to aggregation of platelets to low dose ristocetin, which is unique to type 2b vWD (choice D). The pattern described in choice E would be consistent with Glanzmann thrombasthenia and not vWD.

42. A

The patient presented in this vignette is of Ashkenazi Jewish heritage, has a positive bleeding history, as well as an elevated aPTT that corrects on a 1:1 dilution, suggesting a factor deficiency in the intrinsic pathway. Factors VIII and IX are normal, thereby making factor XI deficiency (Hemophilia C) the most likely diagnosis. Deficiencies in factor XII and contact factors such as prekallikrein or high-molecular-weight kininogen could lead to an elevated aPTT, but would not lead to bleeding. Of the choices listed, only FFP would have utility in treating FXI deficiency (choice A). In Europe, but not the

United States, a factor XI concentrate is available. Cryoprecipitate would be effective in fibrinogen deficiency or dysfunction, as well as in hemophilia A or vWD when specific products are not available (choice B). Recombinant factor VIII would be indicated in hemophilia A (choice C), which has been ruled out based on the normal factor VIII activity. Platelet transfusion would only be effective if the bleeding was due to thrombocytopenia or due to dysfunctional platelets and as adjunct treatment in factor V deficiency, as factor V can be found in platelet granules, but would not be effective in factor XI deficiency (choice D). Recombinant von Willebrand factor is approved for the treatment of von Willebrand disease (choice E).

43. D

The aPTT is an in vitro assay used to monitor heparin therapy and to evaluate for bleeding disorders. Many conditions that do not cause bleeding can prolong the aPTT, including a lupus anticoagulant, factor XII deficiency (choice B), and deficiency of contact factors. The best predictor of operative bleeding is a patient's prior bleeding history in the face of hemostatic challenges, which was quite benign in this patient. Given that hemophilia A, B, and C have been ruled out, a lupus anticoagulant is the most likely diagnosis. The lack of correction of the aPTT on 1:1 dilution with fresh frozen plasma is also supportive and also serves to rule out factor XII deficiency. As a lupus anticoagulant is typically not associated with bleeding, it would be safe to proceed with surgery (choice D). When faced with an unexpected elevated aPTT, the most important thing is to rule out a deficiency or acquired inhibitor to factor VIII, which has been done in this case by the normal factor VIII assay, and thus a factor VIII inhibitor assay would not be indicated (choice C). Hemophilia B or C had also been ruled out, and the semi urgent surgery should proceed as planned (choice A). The prolongation of the aPTT in this case is most likely secondary to a lupus anticoagulant, and while labs should be sent to evaluate this, there is no reason to delay surgery while waiting results (choice E).

44. E

This 55-year-old male with known MGUS has an acquired bleeding disorder. His initial evaluation reveals a defect in primary hemostasis, but no obvious coagulopathy or defects in fibrinogen function. Given the known association between MGUS and acquired vWD, this diagnosis should be strongly and further testing pursued. Of the choices listed, IVIg (choice E) would be indicated for treatment of bleeding in patients with acquired vWD secondary to a paraproteinemia. DDAVP could also be considered, but it is often ineffective and was not listed as a choice. Factor VIII infusion would not be effective, as hemophilia A is unlikely with a normal aPTT (choice A). Despite the abnormal PFA, platelet transfusion is unlikely to be helpful as the defect in acquired vWD is due to a lack of vWF and ability to bind platelets to the endothelium (choice B). FFP is not indicated as there is no evidence of a factor deficiency or fibrinogen deficit (choices C and D). Recombinant factor VIIa is not indicated for this situation.

45. D

This patient has mild hemophilia B and needs immediate replacement therapy for his psoas muscle bleed. His current level is 10%, and you plan to dose him to a target of 80%. Based on the fact that it takes two units of factor IX (as opposed to 1 unit for factor VIII) to raise the level in 1 mL of plasma from 0% to 100%, the following formula can be used to approximate the proper dosing: **Dose of factor IX = weight (kg) × (desired % increase).** As the recovery is not as great with recombinant factor IX, this dose is usually multiplied by 1.2–1.4, depending on the product. Thus in this patient the dose would be $100 \times (80-10) \times$ approx. $1.2 = 8400$ units (choice D). Choices B and C would only be appropriate if there was evidence of an inhibitor, which is rare with hemophilia B and made even less likely in this case where the aPTT corrects on 1:1 dilution. The dosing in choices A and E are incorrect. Note that dosing for factor VIII is **weight (kg) × (desired % increase) × 0.5.** Thus the dosing for factor VIII is typically half that for factor IX products.

46. B

The thromboelastogram (TEG) is a real-time assessment of the viscoelastic clot strength in whole blood. TEG has gained increasing popularity in bleeding with trauma, liver transplantation, cardiovascular surgery, and has been increasingly used in the evaluation of a variety of bleeding disorders. The initial part of the tracing (R and K) reflect the initial phases of coagulation (choices A and E). The alpha or angle reflects the kinetics of clot formation and is often affected by platelet count or dysfunction (choice D). The MA and Lysis (Ly) at 30 minutes reflect clot strength. In this tracing clot formation is normal, but the tracing shows the clot strength decreasing over time as would be seen with fibrinolysis as might be seen with an amniotic fluid embolism (choice B). Besides treating the underlying condition, treatment would be aimed at replacing fibrinogen with cryoprecipitate. The reference by Whiting provided later should serve as an excellent reference on this topic.

47. C

FEIBA is FDA approved for the treatment of bleeding in hemophilia A or B in the presence of an inhibitor. rVIIa would also be a reasonable treatment option. Porcine factor VIII (Obizur) has recently been approved for acquired, but not congenital hemophilia A. As the inhibitor titer is greater than 5 BU, a bypass agent is acquired rather than escalated doses of factor VIII replacement. Humate-P is indicated for patients with von Willebrand disease who are not predicted to respond to DDAVP. DDAVP can be considered in patients with mild hemophilia A undergoing minor procedures; however, it would not be appropriate in severe hemophilia or in patients with an inhibitor as in this case.

48. D

A small subset of patients of with APLS will develop widespread multiorgan thrombotic disease termed catastrophic antiphospholipid syndrome (CAPS). The diagnosis should be highly suspected in a patient with known APLS who develops failure of three or more organs within a week without other obvious cause and with a biopsy confirming microthrombus in at least one organ. Surgery has been described to incite CAPS in patients with previously well-controlled APLS. Mortality is high, with CAPS often reaching 50%. Steroids and anticoagulation are standard therapies. Although not investigated in large randomized trials, therapeutic plasma exchange has generally been recommended as first line therapy and should be strongly considered in this case (choice D). Eculizumab and Rituximab have been shown to be effective in resistant disease in small trials, but are not yet recommended as first line therapy (choices A and B). Pulse dexamethasone would unlikely offer additional benefit as compared with high dose prednisone (choice C). A direct thrombin inhibitor would be considered if HIT was the likely diagnosis, but would not be indicated for CAPS (choice E).

49. E

Due to the increased mortality of elderly patients with acquired FVIII inhibitors, it is recommended that an attempt be made to eradicate the inhibitor. While there have not been any direct head-to-head trials comparing these regimens, data from the European Acquired Haemophilia Registry (EACH2) showed that patients were more likely to achieve a stable complete remission (defined by an undetectable inhibitor and FVIII >70 IU/dL) with this regimen, compared with single-agent steroids or cytotoxics, such as cyclophosphamide.[5]

Although rituximab is widely used due to its relatively low toxicity profile, the observed time for its effect to be realized and lower remission rates makes this less effective than steroids and cyclophosphamide.

While there are case reports of spontaneous remissions in patients with acquired hemophilia, this is rather uncommon. As noted previously, it is recommended in the elderly to make an attempt to eradicate the inhibitor.

50. A

In any patient with the diagnosis of vWD, prior to the initial use of DDAVP for either bleeding or procedures, the response to DDAVP should be determined. This is based upon the observation that many patients with vWD do not respond fully to DDAVP.

If the patient is noted to be responsive to DDAVP, then a dose of 0.3 µg/kg should be administered immediately prior to her procedure. For minor procedures such as this, the intranasal formulation can be given, which should be the 1.5 mg/mL concentration. A generic form of intranasal DDAVP should be avoided, as this is a dilute concentration (0.1 mg/mL), and is used for the treatment of diabetes insipidus and enuresis.

While the use of either vWF:FVIII concentrates or rvWF would be reasonable if a patient was unresponsive to DDAVP, given the minor nature of the procedure, this would not the first choice of prophylaxis against bleeding prior to her procedure.

Although the use of ε-aminocaproic acid or tranexamic acid is very effective in patients with vWD, this is typically limited to areas with increased rates of fibrinolysis, such as the oral, nasopharyngeal mucosa, or genital tract.

51. B

Based upon the history provided, the most likely cause for the patient's intermittent thrombocytopenia is the presence of type 2B von Willebrand disease. This is characterized in part by an exacerbation of thrombocytopenia with pregnancy and DDAVP administration. Type 2B vWD is caused by a gain of function mutation in the 2A domain of vWF that leads to spontaneous platelet binding, leading to thrombocytopenia and loss of high-molecular-weight multimers of vWF. Type 2A vWD shows the loss of high-molecular-weight vWF multimers but not the thrombocytopenia. While sequencing of

VWF typically shows a mutation in exon 28, the RIPA, which should show an increased response at lower doses of ristocetin, is typically performed first. While the role of DDAVP in the treatment of type 2B vWD is controversial, it has been noted to decrease the platelet count further.

Flow cytometry for gpIB/IX/V expression is performed to test for Bernard-Soulier syndrome. Given the history of normal platelet counts, this is not the cause for the patient's thrombocytopenia, as these patients have a lifelong and constant thrombocytopenia.

Staining neutrophils for NMMHC-IIA is a screening test for the *MYH9*-related disorders, such as the May-Hegglin anomaly. If there is abnormal localization, characterized by a co-localization with inclusion bodies, this is diagnostic of an *MYH9* disorder. While there may be a range of platelet counts, like Bernard-Soulier, normal platelet counts are not observed, and this is not typically associated with a hemorrhagic phenotype.

While antibody-mediated destruction of platelets has long been considered to be one of the main causes of ITP, due to the low sensitivity and specificity of platelet antibody testing, this is not recommended in the evaluation of a patient with thrombocytopenia. Furthermore, the reported lack of response to IVIG and steroids casts doubt on an immune-mediated cause of this patient's thrombocytopenia.

In any pregnant patient presenting with thrombocytopenia, attention should be paid toward potentially fatal consumptive disorders, such as preeclampsia, HELLP, or TTP. While TTP can present in pregnancy, it would not be expected for someone to have recurrent events and survive without treatment. As there is no history of therapeutic plasma exchange, testing for ADAMTS13 deficiency, which would be seen in TTP, is not the correct option.

52. D

Patients who have a ventricular device placed are at an increased risk for bleeding, not only from the use of anticoagulants and/or antiplatelet agents, but from acquired von Willebrand disease. In a significant number of LVAD patients, loss of high-molecular-weight multimers of vWF is noted. This is felt to be due to the increased shear and pressures through the device.

Platelet aggregometry would be expected to be abnormal, not only due to the presence of aspirin, but from the presence of a ventricular assist device. This would not be expected to offer any worthwhile information.

A thrombin time would likewise be expected to be abnormal due to the recent use of heparin and would not provide any useful information.

Although the patient was on heparin, there is no history of thrombocytopenia or thrombosis. Testing for heparin/PF4 antibodies in the postbypass setting could yield a false-positive result.

53. B

In a person with hemophilia who no longer responds to therapy, the presence of an inhibitor must be suspected and evaluated immediately.

While the use of antiplatelet therapy or new onset thrombocytopenia remains possible, this is not supported by the history and is a less likely cause.

Prior to increasing the dose of his infusions or switching to a different product, the presence of an inhibitor needs to be evaluated. It is not likely that a weight increase over the course of 6–12 months would account for his lack of response to therapy.

The use of fibrinolytic inhibitors is very useful in sites of increased fibrinolytic activity. However, in a patient with a joint bleed and suspected inhibitor, this intervention is not likely to benefit the patient.

54. A

Even though he has received rFIX in the past without incident, the development of inhibitors in patients with hemophilia B is typically characterized by marked allergic reactions, including anaphylaxis. As a result, it has been recommended that the initial doses of replacement FIX be administered in a monitored environment.

The remaining choices are not likely to cause allergic type reactions.

55. D

As noted previously, immune tolerance therapy (ITT) for inhibitors in hemophilia B are fraught with more complications than ITT in hemophilia A. This includes the development of nephrotic range proteinuria during ITT, so that regular measurements of renal function and urine protein are recommended.

The other mentioned effects have not been noted.

56. A

The patient has factor XII deficiency, which despite the markedly elevated aPTT, is not associated with any hemorrhagic manifestations. In addition, deficiencies of high-molecular-weight kininogen and prekallikrein, which also have prolonged aPTT levels, are devoid of bleeding manifestations. As such, there is no indication for any replacement therapy.

57. B

This patient represents a typical presentation for vitamin C deficiency, although anyone with a diet devoid of citrus or vitamin C intake is at risk for developing scurvy. While there are numerous manifestations of scurvy, such as weakness, fatigue, anorexia, and myalgias, the hemorrhagic symptoms are often pronounced. This can be characterized by widespread ecchymoses, with a predilection for the legs, perifollicular hemorrhages (that can be confused for petechia), gingival swelling and bleeding, as well as increased vascular fragility, which can lead to a misdiagnosis of palpable purpura or vasculitis.

While there is a history for alcohol abuse, with the macrocytosis and thrombocytopenia supporting the effects of long-term use, regardless of the measured level, ethanol would not explain his findings.

Similarly, the likely marginal diet and macrocytosis can increase the risk for vitamin B12 deficiency. However, this would not lead to hemorrhagic manifestations.

The prolonged PT is due to a combination of liver disease from ethanol abuse and poor nutrition.

Although the patient has a macrocytosis and thrombocytopenia, a primary hematologic disorder such as myelodysplasia would not lead to his physical examination findings.

58. F

Use of a four-factor PCC is indicated, as this will allow rapid reversal of the effect of warfarin in a patient with a history of heart failure. Co-administration with vitamin K

is recommended to allow for the resynthesis of the vitamin K dependent clotting factors.

Given the urgency of the need for reversal of the anticoagulant effect, administration of vitamin K alone would not provide adequate hemostasis in time, regardless of the mode of administration. While FFP will replace the necessary coagulation factors, the volume that is needed for restoration of hemostasis would be prohibitive in a patient with a history of cardiomyopathy, particularly as repeated infusions of FFP are typically required.

59. D

Protamine is a positively charged compound that directly binds to heparin, neutralizing it. It may even be able to remove it from antithrombin, further eliminating its anticoagulant effect. For every 100 units of heparin that has been administered in the last 30–60 minutes, 1 mg of protamine is given. The maximum dose should be 50 mg.

The remaining options would have no role in the urgent/emergent reversal of heparin.

60. A

This patient has type 1 vWD, which is a mild quantitative deficiency of vWF characterized by mucocutaneous bleeding. Type 1 vWD is characterized by a von Willebrand activity:antigen ratio of greater than 0.5–0.7. Further, since type 1 vWD is a quantitative deficiency, all von Willebrand multimers are present but simply in decreased amounts. In contrast, patients with type 2 vWD have a qualitative deficiency of vWF. All type 2 vWD subtypes (type 2A, 2B, 2M) except for 2N have a vWF activity:antigen ratio of less than 0.5–0.7 due to the dysfunctional von Willebrand protein. Multimers are variably present depending on the subtype. Type 2A is characterized by a preferential loss of intermediate- and high-molecular weight vWF multimers. In type 2B vWD there is a gain-of-function mutation in vWF that leads to enhanced binding of vWF to its platelet receptor glycoprotein 1b. This increased binding leads to rapid clearance of the vWF-platelet complex and resultant thrombocytopenia and loss of high-molecular-weight multimers. Type 3 vWD is due to a complete quantitative deficiency of vWF, and therefore patients have significantly reduced von Willebrand activity and von Willebrand antigen levels, as well as absent multimers.

61. C

This patient has a history of both mucocutaneous bleeding and hemarthrosis that could be consistent with hemophilia. In addition, she has a family history of "hemophilia." However, hemophilia is an X-linked disorder passed down on the maternal side. Further, her paternal uncle does not respond well to FVIII concentrates, which is likely due to his misdiagnosis as a hemophilic. The patient and probably her uncle have type 2N vWD, which is due to a rare mutation in the factor VIII binding site of vWF. This leads to accelerated clearance of unbound FVIII and therefore severely low FVIII activity. Type 2N patients can have mildly low or normal vWF activity and antigen levels if they have inherited a type 1 allele, along with the type 2N allele. Von Willebrand multimers are typically normal. Patients are often misdiagnosed as having hemophilia. The definitive diagnosis is made by measuring the vWF:FVIII binding capacity (which is low) and can then be confirmed by genetic testing.

62. D

The patient described has bleeding consistent with primary hemostasis defect (i.e., platelet-type bleeding). Her laboratory markers reveal normal aPTT and PT, further making secondary coagulation defects less likely (e.g., hemophilia). While thrombocytopenia can be seen in type 2B von Willebrand disease (vWD), type 1 vWD does not present with thrombocytopenia. Glanzmann thrombasthenia is a congenital qualitative platelet disorder due to a mutation in the GP IIb/IIa receptor that leads to defective platelet aggregation. Bernard-Soulier syndrome is both a qualitative and quantitative platelet disorder characterized by defective GP 1b/IX platelet receptor and "giant" platelets, which are also decreased in number. Platelet aggregation studies in Glanzmann thrombasthenia reveal absent aggregation in the presence of ADP, AA, epinephrine, and collagen, but normal agglutination with ristocetin. In contrast, platelet aggregation studies in Bernard-Soulier patients show normal platelet aggregation in the presence of all stimulants but decreased agglutination in the presence of ristocetin. Since both Glanzmann thrombasthenia and Bernard-Soulier are inherited in an autosomal recessive pattern, family history may not be apparent. Therefore this clinical presentation and laboratory findings are most consistent with Bernard-Soulier syndrome.

63. D

The patient has no signs of an underlying disorder that would cause DIC. Her D-dimer is normal. Hemophilia A and B are characterized by a prolonged PTT and usually affect males, as they are X-linked disorders (although female carriers can have bleeding symptoms). Fibrinogen disorders, either quantitative or qualitative, can present with similar symptoms, as in this patient, but are characterized by a prolonged aPTT, PT, and thrombin time. This patient has FXIII deficiency, a rare bleeding disorder with an estimated prevalence of 1 in 2 million. Diagnosis can be challenging as initial screening labs are normal (aPTT, PT, and thrombin time). Relying on increased clot solubility in 5 M urea, dilute monochloroacetic acid, or acetic acid can lead to underdiagnosis as this test only detects activity levels less than 5%. The diagnosis of FXIII deficiency is made by checking FXIII activity; more specific tests such as molecular analysis should be used for confirmation. Umbilical stump bleeding and intracranial hemorrhage are hallmarks of FXIII deficiency. Women with FXIII deficiency are particularly at risk for miscarriages. Consequently, prophylaxis is often used during pregnancy to prevent fetal loss. Treatment includes FXIII concentrate and, if unavailable, cryoprecipitate, which has a higher concentration of FXIII than fresh frozen plasma.

64. B

This patient has FXI deficiency; a disorder that is prevalent in the Ashkenazi Jewish population. The phenotype is heterogeneous and does not correlate with FXI activity. Instead, prior history of bleeding is the best predictor of future bleeding. This patient has had bleeding complications with prior surgeries and therefore should receive replacement therapy prior to the upcoming total hip arthroplasty. The diagnosis of FXI deficiency is suspected by a prolonged aPTT, normal PT, and normal thrombin time. The diagnosis is confirmed by checking FXI activity. Treatment is based on antifibrinolytic agents (especially if surgery or bleeding in an area of high fibrinolytic activity), fresh frozen plasma, and FXI concentrate. Currently there are no FXI concentrates available in the United States.

65. C

This patient likely has FXII or Hageman factor deficiency, which causes prolonged coagulation in vitro without the presence of prolonged clinical bleeding in vivo. For this reason, FXII is not thought to play a critical role in in vivo hemostasis. Due to the lack of clinical manifestations from FXII deficiency, it is often diagnosed incidentally on blood work drawn preoperatively or routine clinic visits. The aPTT in XII deficiency patients is often markedly prolonged well beyond what is expected in hemophilia A, hemophilia B, or FXI deficiency. Patients are not at increased risk of bleeding with surgery and therefore can proceed without any preoperative treatment once the diagnosis is confirmed by checking FXII activity levels.

66. D

Heyde syndrome is described as an association between aortic stenosis and gastrointestinal bleeding, usually due to angiodysplastic sites. The underlying pathophysiology is the loss of hemostatically active high-molecular-weight von Willebrand multimers (HMWM) due to enhanced cleavage by ADAMTS13, when blood flow across a stenotic valve alters the conformation of HMWM. This rare acquired form of vWD has similar laboratory findings as congenital type IIA vWD. Therefore in Heyde syndrome the abnormal laboratory findings would include a low vW activity, low vW antigen, and absence of HMWM due to the previously described pathophysiology. The activity:antigen ratio is less than 0.7. The platelet count, PT, PTT (if FVIII activity is normal), and thrombin time should be normal.

The pattern in column B is reflective of a patient with type 1. Column E is what would be seen in a 2M patient. Columns A and C do not exist.

67. C

This patient's immunologic assay for heparin/PF4 antibodies was negative, therefore ruling out heparin-induced thrombocytopenia. Instead, the cause of her drug-induced thrombocytopenia is abciximab, a chimeric (human-murine) Fab fragment that is specific for platelet GPIIb/IIIa. Abciximab blocks binding of fibrinogen to GPIIb/IIIa. Thrombocytopenia can occur in 12% of patients on recurrent exposure and up to 2% of patients on first exposure due to naturally occurring antibodies that recognize the murine component of this drug. More common mechanisms of drug-induced immune thrombocytopenia include drug-dependent platelet antibodies (e.g., quinine), hapten-induced antibodies (e.g., penicillin), fiban-dependent antibodies (e.g., tirofiban and eptifibatide), drug-independent platelet autoantibodies (e.g., gold, procainamide, sulfonamides), and formation of immune complexes (e.g., unfractionated heparin).

68. C

This man needs a prophylactic regimen of FVIII concentrates, which has been shown convincingly to prevent joint disease compared with an on demand regimen in severe hemophilia (the Joint Outcomes Study). Continuing with on demand therapy will lead to higher rates of joint damage as detected on MRI, and clinical joint and total hemorrhages. There is no data that switching from plasma-derived to recombinant FVIII concentrates will prevent spontaneous or trauma-related bleeding compared with plasma-derived FVIII concentrates in this patient. While development of a FVIII inhibitor is always a consideration when bleeding pattern has changed, this patient still responds to one to two doses of FVIII concentrate, and his FVIII recovery is adequate after receiving one dose of FVIII concentrate this morning. This would be unlikely if the patient had a FVIII inhibitor.

69. B

This patient has a hypo- or dysfibrinogenemia based on his bleeding history, prolonged PTT/PT that correct on mixing studies, and prolonged thrombin time. Other causes of a prolonged thrombin time include disseminated intravascular coagulation, anticoagulants that inhibit thrombin such as heparin or direct thrombin inhibitors, or acquired antibodies to thrombin. Cryoprecipitate contains higher concentrations of fibrinogen than FFP and is a preferred treatment in fibrinogen disorders. Fibrinogen concentrate would also be a correct option for management. FVIII/vWF concentrate is used in the treatment of von Willebrand disease. DDVP is used in the treatment of mild hemophilia A. rVIIa is used for treatment of hemophilia with inhibitors or for congenital FVII deficiency.

70. C

This patient has no prior history of bleeding and now presents with life-threatening bleeding. This clinical history combined with a prolonged PTT that does not completely correct on 1:1 mixing study should raise the flag for an acquired FVIII autoantibody. While uncommon (1 in a million), this disease is associated with a high mortality between 8% and 22%. Approximately 50% of cases are associated with a predisposing condition such as an autoimmune disease, pregnancy, underlying hematologic malignancy or solid tumor, infections, or use of certain medications. Interestingly the bleeding pattern is different than that of congenital hemophilia patients with acquired alloantibodies, presenting with subcutaneous, mucosal, gastrointestinal, and CNS hemorrhages, rather than hemarthrosis. The treatment of an acquired FVIII inhibitor is twofold: treatment of the underlying bleed and treatment to eradicate the inhibitor. In cases of life-threatening bleeding, bypassing agents such as rFVIIa or prothrombin complex concentrates should be used to stop bleeding, as even large dose FVIII concentrates will not be effective. Treatment directed at eradicating the underlying inhibitor typically includes immunosuppressive agents (e.g., steroids, cyclophosphamide, rituximab, cyclosporine, or vincristine). While these agents should be started concurrently with bypassing agents, response in inhibitor titers may take weeks, and therefore the best first-line treatment remains bypassing agents for treatment of a life-threatening bleed.

71. A

This patient with mild hemophilia A has had a successful prior desmopressin or DDAVP challenge (increase in baseline FVIII activity by two- to threefold with DDAVP). Since he is having minor dental surgery and the target peak FVIII activity is 30%–50%, DDAVP should suffice for preoperative management. Caution should be used in choosing the right dose of DDAVP

for hemophilia patients. A low concentration formulation of intranasal DDAVP of 0.1 mg/mL (vs. 1.5 mg/mL used in hemophilia or von Willebrand disease) is available for the treatment of diabetes insipidus and primary nocturnal enuresis. This formulation is not effective for the treatment of hemophilia A or von Willebrand disease. DDAVP should be used whenever possible to avoid the high cost and minimize the exogenous FVIII concentrate exposure and thus risk of inhibitor development. As an adjunct to DDAVP, the patient can also be treated postoperatively with an oral antifibrinolytic such as tranexamic acid or aminocaproic acid for 3–5 days. Antifibrinolytics are particularly useful in the prevention of mucous membrane bleeding of the nose, oropharynx, and genitourinary tract, because secretions from these sites naturally contain fibrinolytic enzymes.

72. A

Amicar binds to the lysine binding site on plasminogen preventing the binding of plasminogen and TPA to fibrin, thus stabilizing the clot. Vitamin K acts as a cofactor for the posttranslational modification of factors II, VII, IX, X, and protein C and S. Thrombolytic agents such as tPA cleave plasminogen to plasmin, and heparin potentiates the action of antithrombin III.

73. F

This patient has an isolated prolonged PT and a history of menorrhagia. When the PT is only 2 second prolonged, it will likely correct on 1:1 mixing, even if there is a mild inhibitor present. However, an isolated prolongation of a PT with a normal aPTT and a history of bleeding are consistent with factor VII deficiency. The clinical phenotypes of factor VII deficient individuals range from asymptomatic to severe characterized by life-threatening and disabling symptoms. In females, menorrhagia affects approximately two-thirds of individuals. The PTT 1:1 mix would not be helpful as the PTT was normal. The thrombin time reflects the conversion of fibrinogen to fibrin and is typically prolonged as a result of unfractionated heparin exposure, elevated D-dimer/fibrin split products, or acquired or congenital deficiencies of fibrinogen, none of which are consistent with this patient's history. Deficiency in factor XIII or IX would result in an isolated prolonged PTT, which is not the case in this patient.

74. A

Glanzmann thrombasthenia is an autosomal recessive disorder of platelet receptor GPIIb/IIIa. Symptoms may manifest after birth and are characterized by mucocutaneous bleeding and spontaneous bruising. The most common manifestations include recurring epistaxis and gingival bleeding. The platelet count is typically normal, and platelet morphology on peripheral smear is normal. Bernard-Soulier syndrome is associated with thrombocytopenia and increased mean platelet volume (MPV), and platelet aggregation studies respond to all agonists except for ristocetin. Von Willebrand studies are normal, ruling out von Willebrand disease type 1 and 2B. Platelet aggregation studies in Hermansky-Pudlak syndrome may be normal or may show reduced aggregation to collagen and normal aggregation to adenosine diphosphate (ADP) and ristocetin.

75. E

The incidence of factor XIII deficiency is 1 in 2 million and is inherited in an autosomal recessive pattern.

Intracranial hemorrhage is the major cause of death in untreated individuals. Delayed-type umbilical stump bleeding is a classic finding and usually represents the first clinical sign of FXIII deficiency. Patients may also develop muscle and soft tissue bleeding. Factor XIII deficiency is treated with FFP infusions or recombinant factor XIII to prevent bleeding episodes, particularly ICH. Factor XIII deficiency does not cause prolongation of the PT, PTT, or TT. Factor VII deficiency would cause prolongation of the PT; factor VIII and IX deficiency would prolong the PTT, and factor X deficiency would prolong both.

76. A

The goal of treatment should be improvement in bleeding symptoms, not targeting an activity level nor correction of aPTT. Doses of FEIBA required to correct the aPTT are associated with an increased thrombotic risk.

77. C

This patient presents with an acquired hemophilia A, as evidenced by the FVIII activity of less than 1% with an inhibitor and in the absence of prior bleeding history or factor replacement use. The same inhibitor that is causing his own FVIII activity level to be low is also expected to affect human FVIII replacement products (regardless whether plasma-derived or recombinant), thereby rendering them ineffective. Recent studies have shown that a recombinant porcine-derived FVIII product can provide excellent hemostasis in such cases and allow one to monitor FVIII activity levels.

78. C

Baseline FX levels are not predictive of bleeding risk in AL amyloidosis patients with FX deficiency. Factor X replacement therapy should ideally be guided by individual pharmacokinetic response, given the variability in peak and tail levels after factor replacement therapy in these patients. Prothrombin complex concentrate, which contains FX, is the replacement therapy of choice.

79. D

Patients with hemophilia are not immune to cardiovascular events. In fact, given the advances in clotting factor replacement over the last decades, many patients with hemophilia are living well beyond age 60 and are facing issues on how to best manage underlying cardiovascular risk. Just as in patients without hemophilia, nonvalvular atrial fibrillation poses a risk for thromboembolism, which can be stratified based upon underlying risk factors using the CHADS-2 or CHADS2-Vasc scoring system. This patient has a CHADS-2 score of 4, corresponding to an 11%/year risk of stroke. Given this high risk, he can be considered for prophylaxis for stroke prevention. Aspirin has not been effective in preventing stroke in high-risk patients and is therefore not the best option in this case. Similarly, using warfarin to target a subtherapeutic INR has not been shown effective. A reasonable approach would therefore include warfarin targeting an INR of 2.0–3.0 or a direct oral anticoagulant, as was recently put forward by an expert consensus panel. There remains debate about the use of direct oral anticoagulants in the setting of hemophilia. While they have been shown effective to reduce stroke risk in atrial fibrillation and have short half-lives, the current lack of reversal agent and monitoring target may make warfarin more ideal in the hemophilic population.

80. B

This patient has what appears to be an autosomal rather than an X-linked disorder, making hemophilia A carrier status less likely. Type 2 N von Willebrand disease can mimic the phenotype of mild hemophilia A, with soft tissue and joint bleeds. The disorder is inherited in an autosomal recessive fashion as compared with hemophilia A, which is inherited in a sex-linked recessive fashion, and therefore affects men and women equally. In the plasma, FVIII is protected from degradation by vWF. In type 2N vWD, von Willebrand factor is unable to bind FVIII, thereby leading to a decreased half-life of FVIII in the plasma. Because 2N VWD arises from a point mutation in vWF, affecting only the FVIII binding site, vWF antigen and activity and multimeric analysis remains normal. When one does genetic analysis of hemophilia A, one starts with testing for the intron 22 mutation, which is present in about one-third of individuals, so whole gene sequencing would not be the correct answer. Platelet aggregation studies would not be abnormal in any disorder affecting FVIII levels.

81. D

Type 1 von Willebrand disease manifests with low levels of von Willebrand activity and antigen levels. These levels are impacted positively by estrogen and subsequently rise with pregnancy. Postpartum levels drop precipitously and reach baseline levels by 3 weeks. While this patient likely does not require administration of DDAVP or vWF replacement since her prepartum vWF levels are greater than 50 IU/L, she may require administration of replacement products in the postpartum period in order to prevent postpartum hemorrhage. As type I vWD is autosomal dominant, the baby is also at risk of having vWD, and forceps and vacuum extraction are relatively contraindicated.

82. C

The ureters contain a high amount of fibrinolytic activity due to an abundant supply of urokinase. Inhibiting fibrinolytic activity with agents such as tranexamic acid or aminocaproic acid in patients with gross hematuria can therefore allow blood clots to form within the ureters, and therefore use of antifibrinolytic agents is cautioned in patients with known hematuria.

83. A

Nearly all clotting factors are synthesized in the liver, with the exception of FVIII, which is at least in part synthesized in endothelial cells. Because of this, in the coagulopathy of liver disease, there will be deficiencies in all clotting factors, except FVIII. In disseminated intravascular coagulation (such as in line C), there is a general consumption of clotting factors with increased PT and decrease in all clotting factors, including FVIII. In vitamin K deficiency (B), only the vitamin K-dependent factors will be reduced (II, VII, IX, X, C, and S) and the PT will be prolonged.

84. B

This patient appears to have a congenital bleeding disorder inherited in an autosomal rather than an X-linked fashion, thus making hemophilia A or B less likely. The aPTT is quite prolonged and corrects with 1:1 mixing, suggesting there is a factor deficiency. While deficiency of factor XII can cause aPTT prolongation to this degree, it is not associated with a hemorrhagic tendency. Factor XI deficiency leads to a bleeding pattern more characterized by mucocutaneous bleeding, including heavy menstrual bleeding and postsurgical bleeding. While this history is consistent with von Willebrand disease, the patient's aPTT is too high for a patient with this disorder. The prolonged PFA-100 is a red herring, since this test is prolonged in patients with both anemia (hemoglobin <10 g/dL) or thrombocytopenia (platelet counts <100,000 × 10^9/L). While essential thrombocytosis can be associated with both platelet dysfunction as well as an acquired von Willebrand disease, this patient's elevated platelet count is reactive because of bleeding and iron deficiency.

85. B

This patient has hemophilia A and has suffered head trauma. The patient should receive factor VIII emergently, and this should precede any imaging. In addition, patients with suspected intracranial hemorrhage should be given factor VIII sufficient to raise the FVIII level to 100%. Since each unit of administered FVIII will raise the patient's factor VIII level by 2%, raising the current patient's factor VIII level from a baseline, which we presume to be less than 1% (by definition, since he is known to have severe hemophilia A), we must administer 50 units per kg, or 4000 units. Home treatment of hemarthroses, by contrast, requires raising the FVIII level to only 30%–50%, so giving the patient his home dose would significantly underdose him for a suspected head bleed. Measuring a baseline FVIII level would take too long—treat first—test later. And imaging with either CT (preferred for suspected head bleed) or MRI should be deferred until factor VIII is administered.

86. B

This patient has acquired hemophilia, as evidenced by the absence of prior personal or family history of bleeding. She has a normal PT, but a prolonged aPTT. The prolongation does not fully correct with 1:1 mixing (though the number does shorten, it does not return to the normal range), and incubation leads to re-prolongation of the aPTT. These lab findings are pathognomonic of acquired hemophilia. rVIIa is approved for treatment of acquired hemophilia. When given in therapeutic doses, rVIIa can bind to the surface of activated (not resting) platelets, where it can substitute for the fVIIIa/IXa complex to generate fXa from fX. Administration of rfVIIa can lead to shortening of the PT and aPTT, but these effects are seen at doses far smaller than therapeutic doses, so following standard coagulation assays is not helpful. In addition, measuring fVII activity level is also not helpful, since measurement of the fVII activity does NOT correlate with the Xase activity on the surface of platelets. Lastly, rVIIa administration does not affect fVIII activity levels. The hemostatic effect is thus measured with crude measures, such as the dimensions of the hematoma, the degree of hematuria, and the measurement of the hemoglobin level.

87. C

Hemophilia A can be treated with either plasma derived or recombinant fVIII. Desmopressin can also be used in mild hemophilia A, leading to release of preformed stores of FVIII from endothelial cells. Cryoprecipitate also contains factor VIII, in addition to von Willebrand factor, and can be used for hemostatic use in cases when there are no other options available, but its use carries the risk of nonpurified blood product transfusion, including TRALI and infectious

transmission. Antifibrinolytic agents (epsilon aminocaproic acid and tranexamic acid) are useful adjuncts for treatment of bleeding on mucosal surfaces, but their use is absolutely contraindicated in upper pole urinary bleeding, potentially leading to ureteral obstruction by clotted blood and resultant hydronephrosis.

88. D

The patient has a history of von Willebrand disease. She has a mismatch between vWF activity and antigen of less than 0.5, suggestive of a type 2 VWD. Though antigen levels are within normal range, this may have been driven up by use of oral contraceptive agents, which can cause elevations in vWF levels. Type 2B vWD is associated with thrombocytopenia and is due to a "gain of function" mutation, leading to a vWF molecule with an increased affinity for platelets, leading to inappropriate platelet binding and clearance. Notably, patients with type 2B vWD should not receive treatment with desmopressin, since it leads to release of this abnormally sticky vWF, with exacerbation of thrombocytopenia. Again, cryoprecipitate can be used but is inferior to purified, virally inactivated von Willebrand factor concentrates. While antifibrinolytic treatment with either amino-caproic acid or tranexamic acid would be useful adjunctive therapy, they should not be used as sole therapy for a patient with a type 2 vWD having surgery on a mucocutaneous surface involving the airway. Recombinant factor VIII contains no vWF and would not be appropriate treatment for type 2B vWD. Intermediate purity factor VIII concentrates have large quantities of vWF along with fVIII are virally inactivated and would be the treatment of choice.

89. B

Severe cardiac aortic valvular disease has long been associated with development of gastrointestinal arteriovenous malformations. This syndrome, known as Heyde syndrome, is now known to be due to shear destruction of the high-molecular-weight multimers of von Willebrand factor. This same pathophysiology underlies the bleeding seen in patients with continuous flow left ventricular assist devices and is a problematic management problem. The pattern of vWF antigen and activity will be of a type 2 pattern, with activity much lower than antigen.

90. E

Acquired VWD is one of the bleeding disorders associated with plasma cell dyscrasias. It is caused by binding and clearance of von Willebrand factor by the monoclonal paraprotein. vWF levels tend to be severely depressed, as is factor VIII. Because the cause of the low fVIII is decreased survival due to low/absent vWF levels, the aPTT will be prolonged and will fully correct with 1:1 mix (as opposed to an autoantibody to fVIII as in acquired hemophilia). Factor X deficiency can result from amyloidosis, another plasma cell dyscrasia, but this factor deficiency leads to prolongation of both the PT as well as the aPTT. A lupus inhibitor would prolong the aPTT, but not correct with 1:1 mixing and not lead to bleeding.

91. D

Munchhausen syndrome manifesting as ingestion of superwarfarins is a well-described clinical entity. Superwarfarins are rodenticides that act as warfarin does (inhibition of vitamin K recycling) to lead to coagulopathy, but differ from warfarin in their extreme lipophilic nature, leading to prolonged half-life. Patients present with bleeding and deficiency of the vitamin-K dependent clotting factors. They can respond initially to administration of vitamin K, but because of the very prolonged half-life of the superwarfarins, the patients rapidly relapse without prolonged therapy. Assays for warfarin and the many different superwarfarins are performed with HPLC and are individualized and do not cross-react with each other, so a negative warfarin level does not mean that a superwarfarin is not present. A superwarfarin panel is offered at many commercial laboratories. Normal levels of factor V (or any other vitamin K-dependent clotting factor) suggest that liver failure is not the cause of the coagulopathy, and thus acetaminophen overdose or Budd-Chiari syndrome are less likely potential diagnoses.

92. D
The patient has systemic amyloidosis based on a monoclonal paraprotein and positive Congo red staining on bone marrow biopsy. The patient has a prolonged PT and aPTT, both of which correct with mixing, suggesting a deficiency of a clotting factor in the common pathway (i.e., either fibrinogen, factor II, V, or X). Amyloidosis is known to be associated with acquired factor X deficiency. The mechanism is felt to be binding of factor X to the amyloid protein leading to accelerated clearance. There is not an inhibitor to factor X (as evidenced by the fact that the 1:1 mixing completely corrects the abnormalities). Acquired VWD can be associated with a plasma cell dyscrasia, but does not prolong the PT. A dysfibrinogenemia usually prolongs the TCT and is less associated with plasma cell dyscrasias.

93. D
Patients with hemophilia A are at risk for developing inhibitors to factor VIII, which are neutralizing alloantibodies to FVIII activity. Such inhibitors develop in about 30% of patients with severe hemophilia A (baseline factor VIII of <1%) and generally occur in childhood within the first 20–100 exposure days. Patients with mild hemophilia have factor VIII levels ranging between 5% and 25% at baseline, and thus mild hemophiliacs bleed only with surgery or trauma. Patients with mild hemophilia are exposed to less factor VIII, and thus when they do develop an inhibitor, they do so at a later age. This patient has developed an inhibitor, as evidenced by a factor VIII activity that is now undetectable (i.e., <1%). Thus factor VIII administration is likely to be ineffective, as is cryoprecipitate or DDAVP. Recombinant activated factor VII is approved for treatment of bleeding episodes in patients with hemophilia and inhibitors.

94. D
This woman has low levels of FVIII that initially rise, but then fall too quickly after DDAVP. This suggests a shortened FVIII half-life that is characteristic of the Normandy type (2N) of vWD. In this disorder, there is a mutation in the FVIII binding site of vWF. The standard vWF antigen and activity assays are normal, and the FVIII level is low due to accelerated clearance. It can be diagnosed by sequencing the D domain of the vWF gene (the fVIII binding site) or by doing assays of the ability of the patient's vWF to bid FVIII. It is inherited in an autosomal recessive fashion.

Low factor VIII levels in a woman can be caused by extreme lyonization of a female carrier of the gene for hemophilia A, but we are told this woman's FVIII genotype was normal. FVIII inhibitors block function and do not shorten half-life. Abnormal sensitivity to low dose ristocetin is a hallmark of type 2B, not type 2N vWD. vWF propeptide levels that are higher than the vWF antigen levels are a hallmark of type 1 Vicenza vWD, characterized by shortened half-life of vWF, not FVIII. The collagen binding assay is another functional assay for vWF that would not add to this patient's diagnostic evaluation.

95. D
Idarucizumab is a humanized monoclonal antibody that binds dabigatran with an affinity 350 times that of thrombin. As a consequence, idarucizumab binds both dabigatran and dabigatran-bound thrombin, and has shown significant efficacy in reversing the effects of dabigatran. In one study, 100% of the patients studied had full reversal with the administration of idarucizumab. Four-component pccs are useful in reversing warfarin as is fresh frozen plasma. Cryoprecipitate does not contain thrombin and would not reverse dabigatran. Rituximab is sometimes useful in treating hemophilia patients with inhibitors, but would not be effective in this setting.

96. E
Information regarding the level of anticoagulation may be important, such as in the scenario presented where imminent surgery is needed in a patient on dabigatran. Unfortunately, common coagulation tests (PT, aPTT, ACT) are inadequate, especially in lower plasma levels of the drug. As such, the PT, aPTT, and activated clotting times are typically normal in the setting of therapeutic levels of dabigatran. The reptilase time is useful in diagnosing a dysfibrinogenemia but is not helpful in monitoring patients on dabigatran. The dilute thrombin time is able to accurately predict therapeutic and subtherapeutic dabigatran serum concentrations over a wide range in a linear fashion.

97. B
The patient has a DVT that was provoked by the administration of clomifene for infertility. Patients with a provoked DVT have a lower risk of recurrence than those with an unprovoked DVT. Other factors that decrease the risk for recurrence include female gender, absence of an underlying malignancy, and younger age. Heterozygosity for the prothrombin mutation does not appear to be a risk factor for recurrent thrombosis. As such, the patient should be managed with short-term anticoagulation with enoxaparin followed by warfarin. Warfarin alone would be unacceptable, as the duration to anticoagulation with warfarin is several days, and warfarin will deplete protein C before it exerts its full anticoagulant effect. TPA is limited to patients with life- or limb-threatening thrombosis, and even then, the data on safety and efficacy are not clear.

98. A
A prospective randomized double-blind study comparing low-dose aspirin with placebo for the prevention of thrombosis in patients with antiphospholipid antibodies found that aspirin was no more effective than placebo in the primary prevention of thrombotic events in patients

who did not have SLE. There is similarly no evidence that warfarin is indicated to prevent thrombosis in patients with APL antibodies with a low risk of thrombosis. Rivaroxaban has not been adequately studied in the primary prevention of thrombosis in patients with asymptomatic antiphospholipid antibodies.

99. E

The C677T mutation in the MTHFR gene is common, found in more than 35% of the US population. Patients with this mutation may have modest elevations in serum homocysteine levels. Metaanalyses show no correlation with thrombosis in United States patients where grains are supplemented with folate. Although B vitamin and folate supplementation may lower serum homocysteine levels, there is little evidence that such supplementation will lower the risk for thrombosis. As such, the MTHFR mutation should not be part of routine thrombophilia screening and should not be treated if detected.

100. C

Classification criteria for the antiphospholipid antibody syndrome include both clinical and laboratory criteria. Clinical criteria include either vascular thrombosis or pregnancy morbidity. Laboratory criteria includes the presence of a lupus anticoagulant, anticardiolipin IgG and/or IgM present in medium or high titer (>40 MPL), and/or anti-B2 glycoprotein IgG and/or IgM present in titer greater than 99th percentile. Of importance to meet the diagnostic criteria for APLS, there must be sustained abnormalities on two or more occasions at least 12 weeks apart. The dilute Russell viper venom time (DRVVT) is one of multiple tests used to detect a lupus anticoagulant. An elevated aPTT may be suggestive of a lupus anticoagulant, but is nonspecific and may be caused by many etiologies.

101. A

The Budd-Chiari syndrome is due to thrombosis of the hepatic veins and/or intrahepatic or suprahepatic IVC. An underlying disorder can be identified in over 80% of the cases of Budd-Chiari syndrome. As many as 50% of cases may be due to an underlying chronic myeloproliferative disorder, and JAK2 (V617F) testing is recommended in any case where an obvious etiology is not identified. The women presented in this vignette had microcytosis in the setting of an elevated hemoglobin/hematocrit, platelet count, and white count making previously undiagnosed polycythemia very likely. A JAK2 mutation can be identified in more than 90% of cases of polycythemia vera (Answer A). PNH, antiphospholipid antibody syndrome, AT-3 deficiency, and factor V Leiden have all been identified as causes of hepatic vein thrombosis, but would be less likely in this case given the laboratory findings supporting the diagnosis of polycythemia vera (choices B–E).

102. C

The American College of Physicians has produced evidence-based guidelines for anticoagulation in many clinical situations, including for pregnant women with thrombophilia, but no prior thrombotic history. In pregnant women with a weak thrombophilic mutation, such as heterozygosity for the prothrombin gene mutation, and no prior or family history, only clinical surveillance is recommended (choice A). In pregnant women with no prior

thrombotic history, but a positive family history, postpartum prophylaxis is recommended (choice C). In pregnant women known to be homozygous for the factor V Leiden or prothrombin 20210 mutation with a family history of thrombosis, antepartum prophylaxis with postpartum prophylaxis or intermediate dose anticoagulation has been recommended (choices B and E). Treatment doses of anticoagulation antepartum and postpartum are generally not recommended in the absence of prior thrombosis (choice D).

103. B

The choice of a proper anticoagulant is very complex and depends on patient factors, patient preferences, as well as health care and social constraints. This patient has a complex history and multiple comorbidities, including poor appetite, heart failure, and CKD. In addition, he is requesting prompt discharge and no injectable anticoagulants. Apixiban would be the best of the choices listed, as it has the least renal clearance and is approved as initial therapy for VTE without need for an initial parenteral agent (choice B). Warfarin use would be difficult with his poor diet and frequent antibiotic use (choice A). The FDA approved indications for dabigatran and edoxaban require treatment with a parenteral anticoagulant for 5–7 days prior to their introduction, based on the design of clinical trials leading to approval. Thus in this patient who requests discharge as soon as possible, neither of these agents would be the best choice (choices C and D). In addition, dabigatran has significant renal clearance and therefore would again not be the best choice. Fondaparinux is an injectable agent and is also cleared renally, so would not be the best choice in this case (choice E).

104. A

Based upon her history, this patient's thrombotic event was clearly provoked by the initiation of exogenous estrogens, further exacerbated by her age, morbid obesity, and use of tobacco. As a result, only 3 months of therapeutic anticoagulation is indicated. There is no indication for continuing with warfarin or transitioning to another anticoagulant.

While the PREVENT trial, which used an INR range of 1.5–2.0, showed a reduction of recurrent venous thrombosis without an increase of bleeding, a larger and somewhat better designed study (ELATE) showed a higher rate of recurrence with no decrease in hemorrhage in the lower INR range cohort versus standard range. Thus the lower INR range is accompanied by the same risks as standard therapy, but without the benefits.

The use of a low-dose direct oral anticoagulant for the prevention of recurrent venous thromboembolism is (currently) FDA-approved in patients with idiopathic VTE. As her DVT was clearly provoked, there is no indication for continued treatment.

105. C

In general, there is a very limited utility in performing thrombophilia evaluations, particularly in the in-patient and acute setting. However, there are particular instances where a deliberate evaluation for underlying thrombophilia may be useful. Specifically, in a patient with an abdominal vein thrombosis in the absence of other overt provocative events (surgery, injury, malignancy, etc.), testing for the presence of the JAK2 V617F mutation is indicated, as this is commonly found. It is not uncommon for thrombotic manifestations to precede the development of polycythemia or thrombocytosis. The other hypercoagulable states are much less frequently associated with the Budd-Chiari syndrome and can be falsely positive if the patient is on anticoagulation or has just had a recent thrombosis.

106. A

While the use of unfractionated heparin would be acceptable, concurrent administration with antiplatelet therapy is not indicated. Since the patient is without any objective finding of either hemodynamic compromise or severe limb dysfunction, the use of thrombolytics is not warranted. As for the placement of a filter, there is no contraindication to anticoagulation. In addition, while the presence of a DVT in the setting of "submassive" PE has been used as a justification for filter placement, in a randomized prospective clinical trial, compared with anticoagulation alone, placement of a retrievable inferior vena cava filter for 3 months in addition to anticoagulation provided no benefit in terms of pulmonary embolism recurrence or mortality in patients presenting acute symptomatic pulmonary embolism.

107. A

While it is unclear if this was truly a case of heparin-induced thrombocytopenia, given the lack of reported thrombosis, only 4 weeks of anticoagulation is recommended, with 3 months in total if there was a thrombosis. As such, the patient has received more than an adequate course of anticoagulation. For this reason there is no indication to either continue or transition to a higher target/range of warfarin, regardless of what type of valve he is to receive, especially as this will have to stopped prior to surgery.

The use of any direct oral anticoagulant is contraindicated in patients with mechanical heart valves. It was observed in the RE-ALIGN trial that the use of dabigatran led to a higher rate of bleeding and thrombosis, leading to the trial's early discontinuation.

108. B

Since the measured heparin/PF4 antibody has decayed to normal, the *short-term* use of heparin for cardiac surgery is recommended. It has been observed that the intraoperative use of heparin is associated with a low risk of HIT, but can increase if used postoperatively. As warfarin will be necessary, bridging with an alternative agent is necessary. Therefore the postoperative use of heparin or enoxaparin would not be recommended.

While some centers will use a direct thrombin inhibitor for anticoagulation while on bypass, the recommended INR target is 3.0, range 2.5–3.5, for a mechanical mitral valve.

109. E

While the direct oral anticoagulants are characterized by the lack of need of monitoring their anticoagulant effect, nonetheless, all of these agents exert an effect on many tests of hemostasis. Specifically in this case, the elevated values of protein C and S can be seen in clot-based assays, whereas LA panels that employ the use of the chromogenic Xa-based assays are particularly affected by the presence of an oral Xa-inhibitor.

Even though a lupus anticoagulant is "present," (1) the presence of rivaroxaban confounds this diagnosis, and (2) the presence of an antiphospholipid antibody, such as a lupus anticoagulant, must be present after 12 weeks.

The presence of a lupus anticoagulant can lead to a positive APCR assay, in the absence of factor V Leiden. However, this would not account for the elevated protein C and S levels, and as noted previously, it is far more likely that an effect from rivaroxaban is being observed.

110. A

Among the many changes that occur in pregnancy, it is well established that protein S activity levels fall below normal by the first trimester, with the majority of pregnant patients having below normal levels by the third trimester. Thus there are no indications to provide any additional anticoagulation now or in the postpartum period. She had a line-associated superficial vein thrombosis that does not require further anticoagulation, either therapeutically or prophylactically.

111. A

This is the standard recommendation for postoperative thromboprophylaxis following a total knee replacement.

The patient has a lupus anticoagulant, as there is (1) the prolongation of a phospholipid dependent clotting assay; (2) this is not overcome with mixing; (3) it shows phospholipid dependence; and (4) there is no specific factor inhibitor. However, she does not fulfill the criteria for antiphospholipid syndrome, as there are no clinical criteria to accompany the LA, such as recurrent pregnancy loss or documented thrombosis. As such, the empiric initiation of any treatment, be it an anticoagulant, antithrombotic, or antirheumatic therapy, is not indicated.

112. C

The abnormal thrombin time is indicative of either a thrombin inhibitor (such as heparin or dabigatran, not the oral Xa-inhibitors such as apixaban) or a disorder of fibrinogen. In the case of a patient with both thrombotic and hemorrhagic manifestations, the presence of a dysfibrinogenemia should be suspected. Reptilase is snake venom that is insensitive to the presence of heparin, and the reptilase time is abnormal in the setting of a dysfibrinogenemia. If the reptilase assay is abnormal, this is highly suggestive of a dysfibrinogenemia, following which a fibrinogen antigen:activity ratio should be obtained.

While an elevated FVIII level is observed and has been associated with thrombotic events, it is also an acute phase reactant. Furthermore, there are no known *F8* sequence changes that are associated with elevated levels.

Performing a lupus anticoagulant evaluation, as well as clot-based protein C and S assays, are bound to be confounded by the presence of apixaban, and should not be performed.

113. D

With respect to the heterozygosity for the MTHFR C677T polymorphism, at best, it can be said there is conflicting data on its relevance to thrombosis. However, it is widely felt that there is no relation of this polymorphism to cardiovascular events, is not associated with venous thrombosis, and that supplementation with folate/B6 compounds does nothing to alter future events. Her thrombosis was distal and provoked, which provides no justification for prolonged anticoagulation.

114. C

Heparin-induced thrombocytopenia (HIT) is a unique cause of thrombocytopenia that is associated with thrombosis rather than bleeding. HIT should be considered for patients who have been exposed to heparin in the previous 100 days and in whom thrombocytopenia has developed, especially thrombocytopenia associated with thrombosis, as is suggested by this patient's leg exam. The pathophysiology of HIT is characterized by autoantibodies that develop against complexes of platelet factor 4 (PF4) with heparin. HIT generally occurs 5–10 days after heparin exposure, but can occur within 24 hours if there is a history of recent (<30 days) heparin exposure. The likelihood of HIT can be calculated using the 4T score. This patient has a high pretest probability based on a platelet count of at least $20 \times 10^9/\text{L}$ and a 50% decline from baseline, clear onset of 5–10 days, and no apparent other cause for the thrombocytopenia. If he is diagnosed with a DVT based on his leg symptoms, this would further increase the likelihood of HIT. The first and most important management step is discontinuation of all heparin products, including intravenous or subcutaneous forms or flushes. While heparin-associated antibody testing (initially using the immunologic assay and subsequently the functional assay to confirm the diagnosis) can help confirm the diagnosis, the results can take several days to return. In the meantime, appropriate management should not be withheld. Oral steroids such as prednisone is used for patients suspected of having immune thrombocytopenia, but does not have a role in the management of HIT. Platelet transfusions are a relative contraindicated in HIT, and their use is debated.

115. B

This patient has a clearly provoked venous thromboembolism (VTE), the major risk factor being pelvic surgery. VTE recurrence risk is highly dependent on the scenario in which the VTE occurred. Patients with a provoked VTE (e.g., by surgery, trauma, prolonged immobility) should be treated with 3 months of anticoagulation, since the recurrence risk is very low compared with unprovoked VTE (recurrence risk is ~1%–7% compared with 20% at 2 years). Studies have shown that treatment for less than 3 months leads to increased recurrence rates after stopping anticoagulation. Conversely, treatment for periods longer than 3 months (e.g., 6 months, 12 months, 24 months) does not decrease the recurrence risk once anticoagulation is stopped. Since male patients with an unprovoked VTE (or those with provoked VTE due to a persistent risk factor such as cancer) have a high risk of VTE recurrence, these patients should be offered indefinite anticoagulation. The duration of anticoagulation for female patients with a first unprovoked VTE is still controversial.

116. A

Thrombophilia testing is not indicated in adult patients with a clearly provoked VTE (e.g., VTE after surgery, trauma, or prolonged immobility). Thrombophilia testing can result in harm if the duration of anticoagulation is inappropriately prolonged—for example, when a patient is mislabeled as having a thrombophilia. Further, negative thrombophilia testing could be misinterpreted to suggest a patient dies not have a risk of recurrent thrombosis leading to premature cessation of anticoagulation. Finally, thrombophilia testing is expensive. For VTE occurring in the setting of a major transient risk factor, such as this patient, thrombophilia testing should not impact decisions on length of anticoagulant therapy. Instead, this patient should receive 3 months of anticoagulation due to the provoked nature of this VTE. The patient does not have protein S or protein C deficiency; rather, she has low protein C and protein S activities, as expected on warfarin therapy. This highlights the fact that if thrombophilia testing is undertaken, clinicians must be aware of scenarios in which thrombophilia results may be inaccurate or misleading. Heterozygous FVL mutation does not significantly increase the risk of VTE recurrence and therefore should not impact length of anticoagulation in this patient.

117. C

This patient has a CHADS$_2$ score (for atrial fibrillation risk of stroke) of 5 (age of at least 75 years, diabetes, hypertension, and history of stroke), which places him at high risk for recurrent thromboembolic event. At the same time, he is undergoing a colonoscopy, which has a low risk of bleeding. Until recently, most patients in this scenario were thought to benefit from bridging anticoagulation perioperatively by minimizing the risk of thromboembolism without increasing the risk of perioperative bleeding. The recent BRIDGE trial evaluated the need for bridging anticoagulation with LMWH in patients with atrial fibrillation that required warfarin interruption for a procedure or surgery. Patients were randomized to receive LMWH bridging or no bridging. LMWH or matching placebo was administered 3 days before the procedure until 24 hours before the procedure and then for 5–10 days after the procedure. Warfarin treatment was stopped 5 days before the procedure and was resumed within 24 hours after the procedure. This study found that forgoing bridging anticoagulation was noninferior to perioperative bridging with LMWH for the prevention of arterial thromboembolism and decreased the risk of major bleeding.

118. B

Patients undergoing certain orthopedic procedures such as total hip arthroplasty, total knee arthroplasty, or hip fracture surgery are at increased risk for VTE. The 2012 American College of Chest Physicians (ACCP) guidelines recommend pharmacologic prophylaxis (Grade 1B) in addition to mechanical prophylaxis in the form of IPCD (Grade 2C). Inferior vena cava filters are being used increasingly for primary prophylaxis in patients at high risk for VTE (e.g., major trauma, orthopedic surgery, bariatric surgery, and cancer). However, this practice is not supported by high-level evidence, is costly, and is potentially harmful to the patient. Furthermore, although these filters are inserted for temporary prophylaxis in this setting, the filter is seldom removed in these patients. The only indication for inferior vena cava filters that has received universal agreement by leading medical professional societies is for patients with acute venous thromboembolism and contraindication to anticoagulation.

119. D

This patient is on the anticoagulant apixaban, a direct oral factor Xa inhibitor. In patients with life-threatening bleeding such as CNS bleeding, patients on this medication should be treated with a bypassing agent such as prothrombin complex concentrates or recombinant FVIIa. Since apixaban does not deplete but rather inhibits factor

Xa, replacing factor Xa with fresh frozen plasma is not expected to provide hemostasis. Protamine is used for complete reversal of unfractionated heparin or partial reversal of low-molecular-weight heparin. Currently, only one true reversal agent is FDA approved for the direct oral anticoagulants. Idarucizumab is a humanized monoclonal antibody fragment whose target is the direct thrombin inhibitor dabigatran. It is anticipated that andexanet will be approved by the FDA for reversal of apixaban and rivaroxaban, but as of September 2017, there are no FDA approved reversal agents for the direct oral factor Xa inhibitors.

120. D

The direct oral anticoagulants have been studied and approved in nonvalvular atrial fibrillation and therefore are not indicated for anticoagulation in patients with valvular atrial fibrillation. Further, a recent Phase II study (RE-ALIGN) evaluating the efficacy and safety of dabigatran in mechanical heart valves was terminated prematurely due to increased rates of thromboembolic and bleeding complications compared with warfarin. Therefore as yet, the direct oral anticoagulants should not be used in patients with mechanical heart valves. With an acceptable time in therapeutic range with warfarin and no bleeding complications on warfarin, this patient should remain on warfarin.

121. C

Apixaban approximately 25% renally cleared. The half-life of apixaban is 8–13 hours and prolonged further in renal impairment. Recommendations for cessation of the direct oral anticoagulants preoperatively are based on the patient's renal function and the risk of bleeding with surgery. In this patient with mild renal insufficiency undergoing a surgery with high risk of bleeding, experts recommend stopping apixaban 72 hours prior to surgery. Because he has had no prior stroke or embolic event, does not have a known cardiac thrombus, and his CHADS2 score is less than 4, bridging anticoagulation is not required. The recent BRIDGE trial evaluated the need for bridging anticoagulation with LMWH in patients with atrial fibrillation that required warfarin interruption for a procedure or surgery. Patients were randomized to receive LMWH bridging or no bridging. LMWH or matching placebo was administered 3 days before the procedure until 24 hours before the procedure and then for 5–10 days after the procedure. Warfarin treatment was stopped 5 days before the procedure and was resumed within 24 hours after the procedure. This study found that forgoing bridging anticoagulation was noninferior to perioperative bridging with LMWH for the prevention of arterial thromboembolism and decreased the risk of major bleeding.

122. B

This patient is moderate risk for recurrent VTE during pregnancy since her first VTE was in the setting of estrogen therapy. The ACCP 2012 guidelines recommend that in patients at moderate risk for recurrent VTE (pregnancy- or estrogen-related) antepartum prophylactic- or intermediate-dose LMWH rather than clinical surveillance be used (GRADE 2C). Further, since the postpartum period is the highest risk for VTE recurrence, 6 weeks of prophylactic- or intermediate-dose LWMH is recommended over no postpartum prophylaxis (GRADE 2B). Since this patient does not have an acute VTE, there is no current indication for therapeutic anticoagulation.

123. B

This patient has an upper extremity DVT provoked by an indwelling central catheter. The 2012 ACCP Guidelines recommend that for patients with catheter-associated UEDVT and ongoing need for the catheter that is functional (in this case intravenous antibiotics for endocarditis), the catheter should not be removed (GRADE 2C). Patients with proximal UEDVT, regardless of whether catheter-associated or whether catheter is removed, should receive a standard course of anticoagulation (i.e., 3 months). Since this is a provoked UEDVT and the catheter will be removed by 3 months, extended therapeutic anticoagulation beyond 3 months is not indicated (GRADE 1B). Finally, in patients with acute UEDVT that involves the axillary or more proximal veins, anticoagulant therapy alone over thrombolysis is recommended (Grade 2C).

124. C

Unlike warfarin, the DOACs do not require regular monitoring. However, in specific circumstances (e.g., in this patient with life-threatening bleeding), an accurate laboratory test for determining anticoagulant presence would be desired. Dabigatran is a direct oral antifactor IIa (thrombin) inhibitor. It is approved for prevention of stroke and systemic embolism in patients with nonvalvular atrial fibrillation among other indications. In patients with life-threatening bleeding, the TT is the best test for qualitative measurement of drug activity. The TT exquisitely sensitive to dabigatran levels and therefore should not be used for quantification of drug concentration. However, a normal TT excludes the presence of clinically relevant drug levels, which would be helpful in this case scenario, should the patient require emergent neurosurgery. A higher degree of linearity exists between the dilute TT with plasma dabigatran concentration across a wide range of levels; however, this test is not readily available at most institutions. The aPTT exhibits a linear dose-response relationship with dabigatran levels up to 200–300 ng/mL, but flattens out at higher concentrations, thereby precluding quantitative measurement. Further, since commercial aPTT reagents differ in their sensitivity to dabigatran, the aPTT may not be prolonged, despite the presence "therapeutic" dabigatran levels (which to date have not been defined) if an insensitive reagent is used. The PT is less sensitive to dabigatran levels than the aPTT and may not be prolonged even with supratherapeutic levels of dabigatran. Since dabigatran is an antifactor IIa inhibitor, an anti-Xa activity would not be helpful.

125. B

This young patient with a cryptogenic stroke likely has antiphospholipid syndrome (APLS), a highly thrombophilic condition associated with both venous and arterial thrombosis. The laboratory diagnosis of APLS requires on two separate occasions at least 12 weeks apart either (1) moderately to highly positive immunoglobulin G (IgG) or immunoglobulin M (IgM) anti-β2 glycoprotein antibodies, (2) moderately to highly positive IgG or IgM anticardiolipin antibodies, or (3) positive lupus anticoagulant. The prolonged PTT and chronic mild thrombocytopenia also is associated with APLS. Antiphospholipid antibodies also predispose to obstetric complications. The other thrombophilias listed are typically associated with venous not arterial thrombosis. Treatment of APLS patients with a cerebral vascular accident consists of either warfarin or aspirin therapy. The JAK2 mutation would be unlikely in the presence of thrombocytopenia and a slightly low hemoglobin, as in this case.

126. C

Factor V Leiden refers to a mutation in factor V that leads to resistance to activated protein C inactivation. This patient inherited one copy of the factor V Leiden allele from each parent and thus has homozygous factor V Leiden (FVL). The prevalence of homozygous FVL is in 0.1% of Caucasians. FVL homozygosity increases the risk of incident VTE by approximately 18-fold. The risk for VTE is multiplicative with other risk factors for thrombosis. Protein C, protein S, and antithrombin deficiency are a result of a congenital or acquired deficiency in these natural anticoagulants. Disruption of annexin V shield on membranes is one mechanism of fetal loss attributed to antiphospholipid antibodies in antiphospholipid syndrome.

127. B

Thrombotic microangiopathy (TMA) and thrombocytopenia in a postpartum woman should trigger an investigation for the following syndromes: (1) hemolysis, elevated liver function tests, low platelets (HELLP) syndrome; (2) thrombotic thrombocytopenic purpura (TTP); and (3) complement-mediated TMA (C-TMA). This patient had normal liver function tests on presentation, making HELLP syndrome less likely. An ADAMTS 13 activity greater than 5%–10% rules out TTP. C-TMA (also known as atypical hemolytic uremic syndrome) is caused by a dysregulation of the alternative complement pathway, due to an underlying mutation in the complement regulatory proteins. C-TMA is usually triggered by infection, although pregnancy and more typically the postpartum state are common triggering events in women. This patient has several presenting features of atypical hemolytic uremic syndrome including hypertension and significant acute kidney injury in addition to the classic features of TMA and thrombocytopenia. Atypical hemolytic uremic syndrome can sometimes be distinguished from TTP based on more moderate thrombocytopenia and TMA, more severe renal injury, and inadequate response to TPE. In this patient whose clinical course worsened despite TPE, the monoclonal antibody against terminal complement, eculizumab, should be initiated promptly. Platelet transfusion, prednisone, and the anti-CD20 antibody rituximab are not indicated in this patient with atypical hemolytic uremic syndrome.

128. A

Warfarin inhibits the activation of vitamin K–dependent clotting factors II, VII, IX, and X and the anticoagulant proteins C and S. In this patient with an acute DVT, warfarin was started with bridging therapy, namely enoxaparin. However, upon discharge, the patient stopped taking enoxaparin and was solely on a high starting dose of warfarin therapy. The patient then presented with signs of warfarin skin necrosis, which usually occurs 3 to 5 days after drug therapy is begun. In one-third of cases, warfarin necrosis occurs in patients with an underlying, innate, and previously unknown deficiency of protein C.

The breasts, buttocks, abdomen, and thighs are more susceptible probably due to reduced blood supply in adipose tissue. The pathophysiology of warfarin skin necrosis is due to depletion of the natural anticoagulant protein C before the inactivation of other

vitamin-K- dependent procoagulant clotting factors with longer half-lives. This imbalance leads to a paradoxical hypercoagulable milieu in which fibrin clots in microvasculature of the skin. Treatment consists of stopping warfarin and in some cases using fresh frozen plasma or vitamin K to reverse the effects of warfarin. Therapeutic anticoagulation with a parenteral agent should be initiated promptly. Cautious reintroduction of warfarin can be attempted in combination with therapeutic bridging. Calciphylaxis and heparin skin necrosis can produce the same results on skin biopsy, but do not fit this clinical scenario.

129. B

This patient qualifies for thrombolytic therapy given the degree of clot burden as well as clinical symptoms to include hypoxia and hypotension. Of the medications listed, only tPA works by activating plasminogen to induce plasmin action on fibrin and ultimately degrade the clot. Warfarin is contraindicated in the acute setting without co-administration of an immediately acting anticoagulant such as unfractionated heparin or low-molecular-weight heparin. Dabigatran and apixaban could be considered following treatment with a parenteral anticoagulant; current guidelines recommend initial treatment with parenteral anticoagulation in patients with acute PE. Thus aspirin would not be adequate therapy in this setting as well.

130. D

Rivaroxaban, fondaparinux, and enoxaparin are renally cleared; thus in this patient with chronic renal insufficiency, these medications are relatively contraindicated. Warfarin would be the most appropriate choice. Unfractionated heparin would not be appropriate, as it is primarily administered IV and subcutaneous doses would be quite large to provide therapeutic efficacy.

131. E

This patient has developed an asymptomatic portal vein thrombosis secondary to his known cirrhosis. Risk factors for portal vein thrombosis include slow blood flow, hypercoagulability, and vessel wall damage, all of which occur in patients with advanced cirrhosis. Given that this patient was asymptomatic and the portal vein thrombosis was incidentally found, anticoagulation nor thrombolytic therapy are indicated. There is also no role for aspirin in this setting.

132. B

Heterozygosity for the prothrombin 20210 mutation confers a threefold increased risk of first time VTE. However, heterozygosity for the prothrombin 20210 mutation is not associated with an increased risk of recurrence of VTE. Given this, treatment decisions on duration of anticoagulation are not based on the presence of this mutation. This patient clearly had a provoked DVT; thus 3 months of anticoagulation is recommended.

133. E

For pregnant women with no prior history of VTE who are homozygous either for factor V Leiden mutation or the prothrombin 20210A mutation and have a positive family history for VTE, antepartum prophylaxis with LMWH and postpartum prophylaxis for 6 weeks with LMWH or vitamin K antagonists for a target INR 2–3 is recommended. This patient has an increased risk of developing VTE, given her known thrombophilia, family history of VTE, and pregnancy; thus no prophylaxis, antepartum prophylaxis only, or postpartum prophylaxis only is not appropriate.

134. A

The PT assay is based on a standard measure of one part citrate:nine parts whole blood. In polycythemic patients with a hematocrit of more than 55%, there is less plasma volume per same volume of whole blood, which can lead to an increased PT due to over citrating the sample. As such, the lab should be alerted of the hematocrit and can adjust the amount of citrate within the tube to maintain the 1:9 ratio.

135. D

The SOME trial randomized patients with unprovoked VTE to undergo evaluation with limited cancer screening (routine screening for breast, cervical or prostate cancer) plus chest X-ray with or without CT abdomen/pelvis. The overall incidence of developing a malignancy in this group was 3.9%, and there was no difference in cancer detection between the two screening strategies. Therefore it is NOT recommended to have CT abdomen/pelvis to evaluate for occult malignancy in the absence of symptoms. A prognostication strategy to identify those at highest risk of developing malignancy after unprovoked VTE is under investigation.

136. D

In a large randomized controlled trial, compression stockings did not prevent chronic postthrombotic syndrome. While they may help mitigate the symptoms of acute DVT (reduction in swelling/pain), their long-term utility has not been proven.

137. D

Myeloproliferative neoplasms (MPN), in particular polycythemia vera and essential thrombocythemia, are found in 8% of all splanchnic vein thrombosis, but in about 40% of cases when cancer and cirrhosis are not present. About 20% of cases will not have the characteristically elevated blood counts at the time of splanchnic vein thrombosis; however, approximately 50% of those will develop overt MPN over time. Testing for the JAK2 V617F mutation from peripheral blood is reliable to detect underlying MPN. Bone marrow biopsy results can be negative in as many as 20% of cases where JAK2 mutations are detected and there exists heterogeneity in interpreting MPN bone marrow biopsies.

138. D

The PT and aPTT may be normal despite therapeutic levels of dabigatran. In cases where dabigatran is associated with life-threatening hemorrhage, its specific reversal agent, idarucizumab, should be used. Idarucizumab will bind to and inhibit dabigatran within minutes of administration.

139. C

Superficial thrombophlebitis of greater than 5 cm in length or close to the junction of the deep venous system may benefit from prophylactic anticoagulation.

The greater saphenous vein belongs to the superficial venous system. In patients with superficial venous thrombosis, a randomized controlled trial using fondaparinux

2.5 mg sq for 45 days resulted in symptomatic improvement. The ACCP has recommended initiation of prophylactic fondaparinux in the case of superficial vein thrombosis greater than 5 cm in length.

140. A

This male patient presents with an incidentally discovered subsegmental pulmonary embolism 15 days after surgery. He has no prior history of thrombosis and no apparent risk factors for recurrence. His lower extremity Doppler ultrasound is negative, as is his D-dimer. The ACCP 2016 guidelines suggest observation rather than treatment in such cases, given the questionable validity of the diagnosis of subsegmental PE and low risk of recurrence.

141. B

In cases of catheter-associated DVT where the catheter remains functional and necessary, the ISTH recommends leaving the catheter in place and administering anticoagulation for at least 3 months and for as long as the catheter is in place.

142. B

It is thought that the etiology of cerebral hemorrhage associated with cerebral sinus thrombosis is elevated pressures from the thrombosis. Anticoagulation in this setting generally does not exacerbate hemorrhage. Systemic thrombolysis in this setting has been associated with significant mortality and is not recommended. Antiplatelet agents have not been well studied in this condition.

143. A

This patient has significant renal dysfunction and obesity in the context of recurrent VTE necessitating long-term anticoagulation. She has had a history of mildly supratherapeutic INRs on warfarin. Her morbid obesity and low renal function make changing to LMWH, fondaparinux, or dabigatran unattractive options. Continuing warfarin is likely the safest option. Some studies suggest benefit from the addition of daily low-dose vitamin K supplementation to patients who have fluctuating INRs secondary to inconsistent vitamin K intake.

144. C

Men who have an unprovoked venous thromboembolism have a 20% risk of recurrence, as compared with women, who have a 6% risk of recurrence, and it is therefore recommended that men who suffer an unprovoked VTE receive anticoagulation indefinitely. While a negative D-dimer can predict those who are at lower risk for recurrence, the reduction in risk conferred by a negative D-dimer is insufficient to recommend this course in men. The role of inherited thrombophilias in recurrent VTE is felt to be low, so a negative workup would not allow for discontinuation of anticoagulation. The presence of residual clot does increase the risk for recurrence, but a negative ultrasound does not protect against recurrence in a man.

145. E

This patient has a venous thrombosis that is provoked by surgery, which is a transient risk factor. His risk for recurrent clot is low, and therefore 3 months of anticoagulation is sufficient. He does not need thrombophilia testing, D-dimer testing, or repeat ultrasound.

146. C

The factor V Leiden gene encodes a protein in which the arginine at positive 506 is changed to a glutamine, thus abolishing the major cleave/inactivation site for activated protein C. Factor V protein is made in the liver, but the genotypic testing is done on peripheral blood cells. After a liver transplantation, FVL genotypic testing will remain positive, since the bone marrow cells retain their original DNA. However, the factor V protein will now be wild type, since the new liver will be making normal factor V from the donor factor V gene.

147. A

The superficial femoral vein, despite is unfortunate name, is a part of the deep venous system of the leg. A clot in the SFV is therefore a deep venous thrombosis and must therefore be treated as a DVT, with at least 3 months of anticoagulation. Indefinite anticoagulation is not indicated for a provoked DVT. A superficial venous clot does not necessitate full anticoagulation and might be with warm soaks and nonsteroidal antiinflammatory agents.

148. D

The American College of Chest Physicians guidelines on antithrombotic therapy evaluated the appropriate indications for placement of IV filters. They recommend IVC filter placement for patients with PE or proximal DVT and contraindications to anticoagulation (such as recent intracranial surgery, as in the patient in D, but NOT a remote history of subdural hematoma, as in the patient in E). Patients who suffer recurrent thrombosis, despite therapeutic anticoagulation represent another group of patients in which IVC filter placement is recommended. In patients undergoing routine abdominal or pelvic surgery, routine use of IVC filters is not recommended. Patients with large PE and residual clot are considered for IVC filter placement, but their routine use is not recommended.

REFERENCES

Question 1

1. Landi D, Lockhart E, Miller SE, et al. Report of a young girl with MYH9 mutation and review of the literature. *J Pediatr Hematol Oncol.* 2012;34:538–540.

Question 2

1. Yang Y, Wang X, Wang C, Quin Y. A meta-analysis comparing clinical characteristics and outcomes in CALR-mutated and JAK@V617F essential thrombocythaemia. *Int J Hematol.* 2015;101:165–172.

Question 3

1. Mitchell WB, Bussel JB. Thrombopoietin receptor agonists: a critical review. *Semin Hematol.* 2015;52(1):46–52.
2. Neunert C, Lim W, Crowther M, Cohen A, Solberg Jr L, Crowther MA. American Society of Hematology. The American Society of Hematology 2011 evidence-based practice guideline for immune thrombocytopenia. *Blood.* 2011;117(16):4190–4207.

Question 4

1. Warkentin TE, Greinacher A, Gruel Y, Aster RH, Chong BH. scientific and standardization committee of the international society on thrombosis and haemostasis. Laboratory testing for heparin-induced thrombocytopenia: a conceptual framework and implications for diagnosis. *J Thromb Haemost.* 2011;9(12):2498–2500.

Question 5

1. Nurden AT, Fiore M, Nurden P, Pillois X. Glanzmann thrombasthenia: a review of ITGA2B and ITGB3 defects with emphasis on variants, phenotypic variability, and mouse models. *Blood.* 2011; 118:5996–6005.
2. Andrews RK, Berndt MC. Bernard-Soulier syndrome: an update. *Semin Thromb Hemost.* 2013;39:656–662.
3. Althaus K, Greinacher A. MYH-9 Related Platelet Disorders: Strategies for Management and Diagnosis. *Transfus Med Hemother.* 2010;37:260–267.

Question 6

1. Go RS. Idiopathic cyclic thrombocytopenia. *Blood Rev.* 2005;19:53–59.
2. Gernsheimer T, James AH, Stasi R. How I treat thrombocytopenia in pregnancy. *Blood.* 2013;121(1):38–47.

Question 7

1. Neunert CE, Lim W, Crowther M, et al. The American Society of Hematology 2011 evidence-based practice guideline for immune thrombocytopenia. *Blood.* 2011;117:4190–4207.
2. Neunert CE. Current management of immune thrombocytopenia. *Hematology Am Soc Hematol Educ Program.* 2013;2013: 276–282.
3. Matzdorff A, Neufeld EJ, Roganovic J. To treat or not to treat—from guidelines to individualized patient management. *Semin Hematol.* 2013;50:S12–S17.

Question 8

1. Aster RH, Bougie DW. Drug-induced immune thrombocytopenia. *N Engl J Med.* 2007;357:580–587.

Question 9

1. George JN, Nester CM. Syndromes of thrombotic microangiopathy. *N Engl J Med.* 2014;371:654–566.
2. Sadler EJ. Von Willebrand factor, ADAMTS13, and thrombotic thrombocytopenic purpura. *Blood.* 2008;112:11–18.

Question 10

1. Lee GM, Arepally GM. Heparin-induced thrombocytopenia. *Hematology Am Soc Hematol Educ Program.* 2013;2013:668–674.

Question 11

1. Levi M, Toh CH, Tachil J, et al. Guidelines for the diagnosis and management of disseminated intravascular coagulation. British Committee for Standards in Haematology. *Br J Haematol.* 2009;145:24–33.
2. Wada H, Thachil J, Di Nisio M, et al. Guidance for diagnosis and treatment of disseminated intravascular coagulation from harmonization of the recommendations from three guidelines. *J Thromb Haemost.* 2013;11:761–767.

Question 12

1. Mandernach M, Kitchens CS. Disseminated intravascular coagulation. In: Kitchens CS, Kessler CM, Konkle B, eds. *Consultative Hemostasis and Thrombosis.* 3rd ed. Philadelphia: Elsevier Saunders; 2013.
2. Mant MJ, King EG. Severe acute DIC. *Am J Med.* 1979;67:557–563.

Question 13

1. Albert MH, Bittner TC, Nonoyama S, et al. X-linked thrombocytopenia (XLT) due to WAS mutations: clinical characteristics, long-term outcome, and treatment options. *Blood.* 2010;115(16): 3231–3238.

Question 14

1. Owen CJ, Toze CL, Koochin A, et al. Five new pedigrees with inherited RUNX1 mutations causing familial platelet disorder with propensity to myeloid malignancy. *Blood.* 2008;112(12):4639–4645.

Question 15

1. Poon M-C. d'Oiron R, Zotz RB, Bindslev N, Di Minno MND, Di Minno G. The international, prospective Glanzmann Thrombasthenia Registry: treatment and outcomes in surgical intervention. *Haematologica*. 2015;100(8):1038–1044.

Question 16

1. Ghanima W, Godeau B, Cines DB, Bussel JB. How I treat immune thrombocytopenia: the choice between splenectomy or a medical therapy as a second-line treatment. *Blood*. 2012;120(5):960–969.
2. Neunert C, Lim W, Crowther M, Cohen A, Solberg Jr L, Crowther MA. The American Society of Hematology 2011 evidence-based practice guideline for immune thrombocytopenia. *Blood*. 2011;117(16):4190–4207.

Question 17

1. Maldonado JE, Gilchrist GS, Brigden LP, Bowie EJ. Ultrastructure of platelets in Bernard-Soulier syndrome. *Mayo Clin Proc*. 1975;50(7):402–406.
2. Andrews RK, Berndt MC. Bernard-Soulier syndrome: an update. *Semin Thromb Hemost*. 2013;39(6):656–662.
3. Rabbolini DJ, Morel-Kopp MC, Stevenson W, Ward CM. Inherited macrothrombocytopenias. *Semin Thromb Hemost*. 2014;40(7):774–784.

Question 18

1. Greinacher A. CLINICAL PRACTICE. Heparin-induced thrombocytopenia. *N Engl J Med*. 2015;373(3):252–261.

Question 19

1. Tefferi A, Ho TC, Ahmann GJ, Katzmann JA, Greipp PR. Plasma interleukin-6 and C-reactive protein levels in reactive versus clonal thrombocytosis. *Am J Med*. 1994;97(4):374–378.

Question 20

1. Novitzky N, Jacobs P, Rosenstrauch W. The treatment of thrombotic thrombocytopenic purpura: plasma infusion or exchange? *Br J Haematol*. 1994;87(2):317–320.
2. Coppo P, Bussel A, Charrier S, et al. High-dose plasma infusion versus plasma exchange as early treatment of thrombotic thrombocytopenic purpura/hemolytic-uremic syndrome. *Medicine (Baltimore)*. 2003; 82(1):27.

Question 21

1. Cerutti A, Custodi P, Duranti M, Noris P, Balduini CL. Thrombopoietin levels in patients with primary and reactive thrombocytosis. *Br J Haematol*. 1997;99(2):281–284.
2. Klampfl T, Gisslinger H, Harutyunyan AS, et al. Somatic mutations of calreticulin in myeloproliferative neoplasms. *N Engl J Med*. 2013;369(25):2379–2390.
3. Nangalia J, Massie CE, Baxter EJ, et al. Somatic CALR mutations in myeloproliferative neoplasms with nonmutated JAK2. *N Engl J Med*. 2013;369(25):2391–2405.

Question 22

1. McGovern MM, Lippa N, Bagiella E, Schuchman EH, Desnick RJ, Wasserstein MP. Morbidity and mortality in type B Niemann-Pick disease. *Genet Med*. 2013;15(8):618–623.
2. Villarrubia J, Velasco-Rodriguez D, Piris-Villaespesa M, Caro M, Mendez G, Valles A. Type B Niemann-Pick disease. *Br J Haematol*. 2016;172(6):840.

Question 23

1. Smellie WS. Spurious hyperkalaemia. *BMJ*. 2007;334(7595): 693–695.

Question 24

1. Sayani FA, Abrams CS. How I treat refractory thrombotic thrombocytopenic purpura. *Blood*. 2015;125(25):3860–3867.

Question 25

1. Savoia A, Pecci A. MYH9-related disorders. Gene Reviews [Internet] http://www.ncbi.nlm.nih.gov/books/NBK2689/.
2. Mhawech P, Saleem A. Inherited giant platelet disorders. Classification and literature review. *Am J Clin Pathol*. 2000;113(2):176.

Question 26

1. Greinacher A. Heparin-induced thrombocytopenia. *N Engl J Med*. 2015;373(3):252–261.
2. Rice L, Attisha WK, Drexler A, Francis JL. Delayed-onset heparin-induced thrombocytopenia. *Ann Intern Med*. 2002;136(3): 210–215.

Question 27

1. Afdhal NH1, Giannini EG, Tayyab G, et al. Eltrombopag before procedures in patients with cirrhosis and thrombocytopenia. *N Engl J Med*. 2012;367(8):716–724.
2. Merli P, Strocchio L, Vinti L, Palumbo G, Locatelli F. Eltrombopag for treatment of thrombocytopenia-associated disorders. *Expert Opin Pharmacother*. 2015;16(14):2243–2256.

Question 28

1. Centers for Disease Control and Prevention (CDC). Thrombotic thrombocytopenic purpura (TTP)-like illness associated with intravenous Opana ER abuse—Tennessee, 2012. *MMWR Morb Mortal Wkly Rep*. 2013;62(1):1–4.
2. Miller PJ1, Farland AM, Knovich MA, Batt KM, Owen J. Successful treatment of intravenously abused oral Opana ER-induced thrombotic microangiopathy without plasma exchange. *Am J Hematol*. 2014;89(7):695–697.

Question 29

1. Greinacher A. CLINICAL PRACTICE. Heparin-induced thrombocytopenia. *N Engl J Med*. 2015;373(3):252–261.

Question 30

1. Berkman N, Michaeli Y, Or R, Eldor A. EDTA-dependent pseudo-thrombocytopenia: a clinical study of 18 patients and a review of the literature. *Am J Hematol*. 1991;36:195–201.

Question 31

1. Gernsheimer TB. Thrombocytopenia in pregnancy: is this immune thrombocytopenia or...? *Hematology Am Soc Hematol Educ Program*. 2012;2012:198–202.

Question 32

1. Gernsheimer TB. Thrombocytopenia in pregnancy: is this immune thrombocytopenia or...? *Hematology Am Soc Hematol Educ Program*. 2012;2012:198–202.

Question 33

1. Meyer AL, Malehsa D, Budde U, et al. Acquired von Willebrand syndrome in patients with a centrifugal or axial continuous flow left ventricular assist device. *JACC Heart Fail*. 2014;2:141–145.

Question 34

1. Goldstein JN, Refaai MA, Milling TJ, et al. Four-factor prothrombin complex concentrate versus plasma for rapid vitamin K antagonist reversal in patients needing urgent surgical of invasive interventions: a phase 3b open-label, non-inferiority randomized trial. *Lancet*. 2015;385:2077–2087.

Question 35

1. Bahuva R, Yee J, Gupta S, Atreja A. SSRI and risk of gastrointestinal bleed: more than what meets the eye. *Am J Gastroenterol*. 2015;110:346.

Question 36

1. Anz AW, Schweppe M, Halvorson J, et al. Management of venomous snakebite injury to the extremities. *J Am Acad Orthop Surg*. 2010;18:749–759.

Question 37

1. Sotirou E, Apalla Z, Apalla K, Panagiotidou D. Care report: psychogenic purpura. *Psychosomatics*. 2010;51:274–275.

Question 38

1. Zhang B, McGee B, Yamaika JS, et al. Combined deficiency of factor V and factor VIII is due to mutations in either LMAN1 or MCFD2. *Blood*. 2006;107:1903–1907.

Question 39

1. Nurden AT, Nurden P. Inherited disorders of platelet function: selected updates. *J Thromb Haemost.* 2015;13(suppl 1):S2–S9.

Question 40

1. Tosetto A, Castaman G. How I treat type 2 variant forms of von Willebrand disease. *Blood.* 2015;125(6):907–914.
2. Mikhail S, Aldin ES, Streiff M, Zeidan A. An update on type 2B von Willebrand disease. *Expert Rev Hematol.* 2014;7(2):217–231.

Question 42

1. Duga S, Salomon O. Congenital factor XI deficiency: an update. *Semin Thromb Hemost.* 2013;39(6):621–631.
2. Duga S, Salomon O. Factor XI deficiency. *Semin Thromb Hemost.* 2009;35(4):416–425.

Question 43

1. Kitchens CS. To bleed or not to bleed? Is that the question for the PTT? *J Thromb Haemost.* 2005;3(12):2607–2611.
2. Kitchens CS. Prolonged activated partial thromboplastin time of unknown etiology: a prospective study of 100 consecutive cases referred for consultation. *Am J Hematol.* 1988;27(1):38–45.

Question 44

1. Federici AB, Budde U, Castaman G, Rand JH, Tiede A. Current diagnostic and therapeutic approaches to patients with acquired von Willebrand syndrome: a 2013 update. *Semin Thromb Hemost.* 2013;39(2):191–201.
2. Tiede A, Rand JH, Budde U, Ganser A, Federici AB. How I treat the acquired von Willebrand syndrome. *Blood.* 2011;117(25):6777–6785.

Question 45

1. Franchini M, Frattini F, Crestani S, Sissa C, Bonfanti C. Treatment of hemophilia B: focus on recombinant factor IX. *Biologics.* 2013;7: 33–38.

Question 46

1. Whiting D, DiNardo JA. TEG and ROTEM: technology and clinical applications. *Am J Hematol.* 2014;89(2):228–232.
2. Ekelund K, Hanke G, Stensballe J, Wikkelsøe A, Albrechtsen CK, Afshari A. Hemostatic resuscitation in postpartum hemorrhage—a supplement to surgery. *Acta Obstet Gynecol Scand.* 2015;94(7):680–692.

Question 47

1. Erkan D, Cervera R, Asherson RA. Catastrophic antiphospholipid syndrome: where do we stand? *Arthritis Rheum.* 2003;48(12):3320.
2. Bucciarelli S, Espinosa G, Cervera R, et al. Mortality in the catastrophic antiphospholipid syndrome: causes of death and prognostic factors in a series of 250 patients. *Arthritis Rheum.* 2006; 54(8):2568.

Question 48

1. Collins P, Baudo F, Knoebl P, et al. Immunosuppression for acquired hemophilia A: results from the European Acquired Haemophilia Registry (EACH2). *Blood.* 2012;120:47–55.

Question 49

1. Federici AB, Mazurier C, Berntorp E, et al. Biologic response to desmopressin in patients with severe type 1 and type 2 von Willebrand disease: results of a multicenter European study. *Blood.* 2004;103:2032–2038.

Question 50

1. Mikhail S, Aldin ES, Streiff M, Zeidan A. An update on type 2B von Willebrand disease. *Expert Rev Hematol.* 2014;7(2):217–231.

Question 52

1. Josephson N. The hemophilias and their clinical management. *Hematology Am Soc Hematol Educ Program.* 2013;2013:261–267.

Question 53

1. Franchini M. Current management of hemophilia B: recommendations, complications and emerging issues. *Expert Rev Hematol.* 2014;7(5):573–581.

Question 54

1. Franchini M. Current management of hemophilia B: recommendations, complications and emerging issues. *Expert Rev Hematol.* 2014;7(5):573–581S.

Question 55

1. Renné T, Gailani D. Role of Factor XII in hemostasis and thrombosis: clinical implications. *Expert Rev Cardiovasc Ther.* 2007;5(4): 733–741.

Question 56

1. Singh S, Richards SJ, Lykins M, Pfister G, McClain CJ. An underdiagnosed ailment: scurvy in a tertiary care academic center. *Am J Med Sci.* 2015;349(4):372–373.

Question 57

1. Yates SG, Sarode R. New strategies for effective treatment of vitamin K antagonist-associated bleeding. *J Thromb Haemost.* 2015;13(suppl 1):S180–S186.
2. Kearon C, Akl EA, Comerota AJ, et al. Antithrombotic therapy for VTE disease: antithrombotic therapy and prevention of thrombosis, 9th ed: American College of Chest Physicians Evidence-Based Clinical Practice Guidelines. *Chest.* 2012;141:e419S– e494S.

Question 58

1. Sokolowska E, Kalaska B, Miklosz J, Mogielnicki A. The toxicology of heparin reversal with protamine: past, present and future. *Expert Opin Drug Metab Toxicol.* 2016;6:1–13.
2. Kearon C, Akl EA, Comerota AJ, et al. Antithrombotic therapy for VTE disease: antithrombotic therapy and prevention of thrombosis, 9th ed: American College of Chest Physicians Evidence-Based Clinical Practice Guidelines. *Chest.* 2012;141:e419S– e494S.

Question 59

1. Ng C, Motto DG, Di Paola J. Diagnostic approach to von Willebrand disease. *Blood.* 2015;125:2029–2037.

Question 60

1. Ng C, Motto DG, Di Paola J. Diagnostic approach to von Willebrand disease. *Blood.* 2015;125:2029–2037.
2. The National Heart. *Lung, and Blood Institute. The Diagnosis, Evaluation, and Management of Von Willebrand Disease.* Bethesda: National Institutes of Health Publication; 2007:08–5832. Available at: http://www.nhlbi.nih.-gov/guidelines/vwd.

Question 61

1. Simon D, Kunicki T, Nugent D. Platelet function defects. *Hemophilia.* 2008;14:1240–1249.

Question 62

1. Palla R, Peyvandi F, Shapiro AD. Rare bleeding disorders: diagnosis and treatment. *Blood.* 2015;125:2052–2061.
2. Schroeder V, Kohler HP. Factor XIII deficiency: an update. *Semin Thromb Hemost.* 2013;39:632–641.

Question 63

1. Palla R, Peyvandi F, Shapiro AD. Rare bleeding disorders: diagnosis and treatment. *Blood.* 2015;125:2052–2061.
2. Duga S, Salomon O. FXI deficiency. *Semin Thromb Hemost.* 2009;35:416–425.

Question 64

1. Stavrou E, Schmaier AH, Factor XII: what does it contribute to our understanding of physiology and pathophysiology of hemostasis & thrombosis. *Thromb Res.* 2010;125:210–215.

Question 65

1. Loscalzo J. From clinical observation to mechanism—Heyde's syndrome. *N Engl J Med.* 2012;367:1954–1956.
2. Tiede A. Diagnosis and treatment of acquired von Willebrand syndrome. *Thromb Res.* 2012;130(suppl 2):S2–S6.

Question 66

1. Arnold DM, Nazi I, Warkentin TE, et al. Approach to the diagnosis and management of drug-induced immune thrombocytopenia. *Transfus Med Rev.* 2013;27:137–145.
2. George JN, Aster RH. Drug-induced thrombocytopenia: pathogenesis, evaluation, and management. *Hematology Am Soc Hematol Educ Prog.* 2009:153–158. http://dx.doi.org/10.1182/asheducation-2009.1.153.

Question 67

1. Manco-Johnson MJ, Abshire TC, Shapiro AD, et al. Prophylaxis versus episodic treatment to prevent joint disease in boys with severe hemophilia. *N Engl J Med.* 2007;357:535–544.

Question 68

1. Palla R, Peyvandi F, Shapiro AD. Rare bleeding disorders: diagnosis and treatment. *Blood.* 2015;125:2052–2061.

Question 69

1. Franchini M, Lippi G. Acquired factor VIII inhibitors. *Blood.* 2008;112:250–255.
2. Huthe-Kuhne A, Baudo F, Ingerslev J, et al. International recommendations on the diagnosis and treatment of patients with acquired hemophilia A. *Hematologica.* 2009;94:566–575.

Question 70

1. Peerlinck K, Jacquemin M. Mild hemophilia: a disease with many faces and many unexpected pitfalls. *Haemophilia.* 2010;16:100–106.
2. Treatment of Hemophilia A and B. National Hemophilia Foundation. Available at: http://www.hemophilia.org.

Question 71

1. Garcia D, Baglin T, Weitz J, et al. Parenteral anticoagulants. Antithrombotic therapy and prevention of thrombosis, 9th ed: American College of Chest Physicians evidence-based clinical practice guidelines. *Chest.* 2012;141(suppl 2):e24S–e43S.
2. Van Galen KP, Engelen ET, Mauser-Bunschoten EP, et al. Antifibrinolytic therapy for preventing oral bleeding in patients with haemophilia or von Willebrand disease undergoing minor oral surgery or dental extractions. *Cochrane Database Syst Rev.* 2015;12:CD011385.

Question 72

1. Mariani G, Bernardi F. Factor VII deficiency. *Semin Thromb Hemost.* 2009;35(4):400–406.

Question 73

1. Hayward CP. Diagnostic approach to platelet function disorders. *Transfus Apher Sci.* 2008;38(1):65–76.
2. Solh T, Botsford A, Solh M. Glansmann's thrombasthenia: pathogenesis, diagnosis, and current and emerging treatment options. *J Blood Med.* 2015;6:219–227.

Question 74

1. Tahlan A, Ahluwalia J. Factor XIII: congenital deficiency factor XIII, acquired deficiency, factor XIIIa subunit, and factor XIII B subunit. *Arch Pathol Lab Med.* 2014;138(2):278–281.

Question 75

1. Aledort LM. Factor VIII inhibitor bypassing activity (FEIBA)—addressing safety issues. *Haemophilia.* 2008;14(1):39–43.

Question 76

1. Gomperts E. Recombinant B domain deleted porcine factor VIII for the treatment of bleeding episodes in adults with acquired hemophilia A. *Expert Rev Hematol.* 2015;8(4):427–432.
2. Kruse-Jarres R, St-Louis J, Greist A, et al. Efficacy and safety of OBI-1, an antihaemophilic factor VIII (recombinant), porcine sequence, in subjects with acquired haemophilia A. *Haemophilia.* 2015;21(2):162–170.

Question 77

1. Lim MY, McCarthy T, Chen SL, Rollins-Raval MA, Ma AD. Importance of pharmacokinetic studies in the management of acquired factor X deficiency. *Eur J Haematol.* 2016;96(1):60–64.

Question 78

1. Ferraris VA, Boral LI, Cohen AJ, Smyth SS, White 2nd GC. Consensus review of the treatment of cardiovascular disease in people with hemophilia A and B. *Cardiol Rev.* 2015;23(2):53–68.
2. Schutgens RE, Klamroth R, Pabinger I, Dolan G. Management of atrial fibrillation in people with haemophilia—a consensus view by the ADVANCE Working Group. *Haemophilia.* 2014;20(6):e417–e420.

Question 79

1. James AH, Konkle BA, Kouides P, et al. Postpartum von Willebrand factor levels in women with and without von Willebrand disease and implications for prophylaxis. *Haemophilia.* 2015;21(1):81–87.

Question 80

1. Wymenga LF, van der Boon WJ. Obstruction of the renal pelvis due to an insoluble blood clot after epsilon-aminocaproic acid therapy: resolution with intraureteral streptokinase instillations. *J Urol.* 1998;159(2):490–492. http://www.amicar.org/prescribing-information/.

Question 81

1. Caldwell SH, Hoffman M, Lisman T. Coagulation disorders and hemostasis in liver disease: pathophysiology and critical assessment of current management. *Hepatology.* 2006;44(4):1039–1046.

Question 82

1. Duga S, Salomon O. Congenital factor XI deficiency: an update. *Semin Thromb Hemost.* 2013;39:621–631.
2. Favaloro EJ. Clinical utility of the PFA-100. *Semin Thromb Hemost.* 2008;34:709–733.

Question 83

1. WFH Guidelines for the Management of Hemophilia. Available at http://www.wfh.org/en/resources/wfh-treatment-guidelines

Question 84

1. Hoffman M, Dargaud Y. Mechanisms and monitoring of bypassing agent therapy. *J Thromb Haemost.* 2012;10(8):1478–1485.

Question 85

1. Manjunath G, Fozailoff A, Mitcheson D, Sarnak MJ. Epsilon-aminocaproic acid and renal complications: case report and review of the literature. *Clin Nephrol.* 2002;58(1):63–67.

Question 86

1. Neff AT, Sidonio Jr RF. Management of VWD. *Hematology Am Soc Hematol Educ Program.* 2014;2014(1):536–541.

Question 87

1. Loscalzo J. From clinical observation to mechanism—Heyde's syndrome. *N Engl J Med.* 2012;367(20):1954–1956.
2. Hudzik B, Kaczmarski J, Pacholewicz J, et al. Von Willebrand factor in patients on mechanical circulatory support—a double-edged sword between bleeding and thrombosis. *Kardiochir Torakochirurgia Pol.* 2015;12(3):233–237.

Question 88

1. Coppola A, Tufano A, Di Capua M, Franchini M. Bleeding and thrombosis in multiple myeloma and related plasma cell disorders. *Semin Thromb Hemost.* 2011;37(8):929–945.

Question 89

1. King N, Tran MH. Long-acting anticoagulant rodenticide (superwarfarin) poisoning: a review of its historical development, epidemiology, and clinical management. *Transfus Med Rev.* 2015;29:250–258.

Question 90
1. Thompson CA, Kyle R, Gertz M, et al. Systemic AL amyloidosis with acquired factor X deficiency: a study of perioperative bleeding risk and treatment outcomes in 60 patients. *Am J Hematol.* 2010;85:171–173.

Question 91
1. Kempton CL, White 2nd GC. How we treat a hemophilia A patient with a factor VIII inhibitor. *Blood.* 2009;113:11–17.

Question 92
1. Bolton-Maggs PH, Lillicrap D, Goudemand J, Berntorp E. von Willebrand disease update: diagnostic and treatment dilemmas. *Haemophilia.* 2008;14(suppl 3):56–61.

Question 93
1. Pollack CV, Reilly PA, Eikelboom J, et al. Idarucizumab for dabigatran reversal. *NEJM.* 2015;373:511–520.

Question 94
1. Hawes EM, Dean AM, Funk-Adcock D, et al. Performance of coagulation tests in patients on therapeutic doses of dabigatran: a cross-sectional pharmacodynamics study based on peak and trough plasma levels. *J Thromb Haemost.* 2013;11:1493–1502.

Question 95
1. Marchiori A, Mosena LM, Prins MH, Prandoni P. The risk of recurrent venous thromboembolism among heterozygous carriers of factor V Leiden or prothrombin G201210A mutation. A systemic review. *Haematologica.* 2007;92:1107–1114.

Question 96
1. Erkan D, Harrison MJ, Levy R, et al. Aspirin for primary thrombosis prevention in the antiphospholipid syndrome: a randomized double-blind placebo-controlled trial in asymptomatic antiphospholipid antibody-positive individuals. *Arthritis Rheum.* 2007;56: 2382–2391.

Question 97
1. DenHeijer M, Lewington S, Clark R. Homocysteine, MTHFR and risk of venous thrombosis: a meta-analysis of published epidemiologic studies. *J Thromb Haemost.* 2005;3:292–299.

Question 98
1. Miyakis S, Lockshin MD, Atsumi T, et al. International consensus statement on an update of the classification criteria for definite antiphospholipid syndrome (APS). *J Thromb Haemost.* 2006;4(2):295–306.

Question 99
1. Smalberg JH, Arends LR, Valla DC, Kiladjian JJ, Janssen HL, Leebeek FW. Myeloproliferative neoplasms in Budd-Chiari syndrome and portal vein thrombosis: a meta-analysis. *Blood.* 2012;120(25):4921–4928.
2. Yonal I, Pinarbası B, Hindilerden F, et al. The clinical significance of JAK2V617F mutation for Philadelphia-negative chronic myeloproliferative neoplasms in patients with splanchnic vein thrombosis. *J Thromb Thrombolysis.* 2012;34(3):388–396.

Question 100
1. Bates SM, Greer IA, Middeldorp S, et al. VTE, thrombophilia, antithrombotic therapy, and pregnancy: antithrombotic therapy and prevention of thrombosis, 9th ed: American College of Chest Physicians Evidence-Based Clinical Practice Guidelines. *Chest.* 2012;141(2 suppl):e691S–e736S.
2. Robertson L, Wu O, Langhorne P, et al. Thrombosis: Risk and Economic Assessment of Thrombophilia Screening (TREATS) Study. Thrombophilia in pregnancy: a systematic review. *Br J Haematol.* 2006;132:171–196.
3. Brill-Edwards P, Ginsberg JS, Gent M, et al. Safety of withholding heparin in pregnant women with a history of venous thromboembolism. Recurrence of clot in this pregnancy study. *N Engl J Med.* 2000;343:1439–1444.

Question 101
1. Schulman S. Treatment of venous thromboembolism with new oral anticoagulants according to patient risk. *Semin Thromb Hemost.* 2015;41(2):160–165.
2. Randhawa J, Thiruchelvam N, Ghobrial M, et al. Practical recommendations on incorporating new oral anticoagulants into routine practice. *Clin Adv Hematol Oncol.* 2014;12(10):675–683.

Question 102
1. Ridker PM, Goldhaber SZ, Danielson E, et al. Long-term, low-intensity warfarin therapy for the prevention of recurrent venous thromboembolism. *N Engl J Med.* 2003;348:1425–1434.
2. Kearon C, Ginsberg JS, Kovacs MJ, et al. Comparison of low-intensity warfarin therapy with conventional-intensity warfarin therapy for long-term prevention of recurrent venous thromboembolism. *N Engl J Med.* 2003;349:631–639.

Question 103
1. Smalberg JH, Koehler E, Darwish Murad S, et al. The JAK2 46/1 haplotype in Budd-Chiari syndrome and portal vein thrombosis. *Blood.* 2011;117(15):3968–3973.

Question 104
1. Kearon C, Akl EA, Comerota AJ, et al. Antithrombotic therapy for VTE disease: antithrombotic therapy and prevention of thrombosis, 9th ed: American College of Chest Physicians Evidence-Based Clinical Practice Guidelines. *Chest.* 2012;141:e419S–e494S.

Question 105
1. Linkins LA, Dans AL, Moores LK, et al. Treatment and prevention of heparin-induced thrombocytopenia: antithrombotic therapy and prevention of thrombosis, 9th ed: American College of Chest Physicians Evidence-Based Clinical Practice Guidelines. *Chest.* 2012;141:e495S–e530S.
2. Eikelboom JW, Connolly SJ, Brueckmann M, et al. Dabigatran versus warfarin in patients with mechanical heart valves. *N Engl J Med.* 2013;369:1206–1214.

Question 106
1. Linkins LA, Dans AL, Moores LK, et al. Treatment and prevention of heparin-induced thrombocytopenia: antithrombotic therapy and prevention of thrombosis, 9th ed: American College of Chest Physicians Evidence-Based Clinical Practice Guidelines. *Chest.* 2012;141:e495S–e530S.
2. Warkentin TE, Sheppard JA. Serological investigation of patients with a previous history of heparin-induced thrombocytopenia who are reexposed to heparin. *Blood.* 2014;123:2485–2493.

Question 107
1. Asmis LM, Alberio L, Angelillo-Scherrer A, et al. Rivaroxaban: Quantification by anti-FXa assay and influence on coagulation tests: a study in 9 Swiss laboratories. *Thromb Res.* 2012;129:492–498.
2. Miyakis S, Lockshin MD, Atsumi T, et al. International consensus statement on an update of the classification criteria for definite antiphospholipid syndrome (APS). *J Thromb Haemost.* 2006;4: 295–306.

Question 108
1. Szecsi PB, Jorgensen M, Klajnbard A, Andersen MR, Colov NP, Stender S. Haemostatic reference intervals in pregnancy. *Thromb Haemost.* 2010;103:718–727.

Question 109
1. Falck-Ytter Y, Francis CW, Johanson NA, et al. Prevention of VTE in orthopedic surgery patients: antithrombotic therapy and prevention of thrombosis, 9th ed: American College of Chest Physicians Evidence-Based Clinical Practice Guidelines. *Chest.* 2012;141:e278S–e325S.
2. Brandt JT, Triplett DA, Alving B, Scharrer I. Criteria for the diagnosis of lupus anticoagulants: an update. On behalf of the Subcommittee on Lupus Anticoagulant/Antiphospholipid Antibody of the Scientific and Standardisation Committee of the ISTH. *Thromb Haemost.* 1995;74:1185–1190.

Question 110

1. Casini A, Blondon M, Lebreton A, et al. Natural history of patients with congenital dysfibrinogenemia. *Blood*. 2015;125:553–561.
2. Cunningham MT, Brandt JT, Laposata M, Olson JD. Laboratory diagnosis of dysfibrinogenemia. *Arch Pathol Lab Med*. 2002;126: 499–505.
3. Mansvelt EP, Laffan M, McVey JH, Tuddenham EG. Analysis of the F8 gene in individuals with high plasma factor VIII: C levels and associated venous thrombosis. *Thromb Haemost*. 1998;80: 561–565.

Question 111

1. Bezemer ID, Doggen CJ, Vos HL, Rosendaal FR. No association between the common MTHFR 677C->T polymorphism and venous thrombosis: results from the MEGA study. *Arch Intern Med*. 2007;167:497–501.
2. Lonn E, Yusuf S, Arnold MJ, et al. Homocysteine lowering with folic acid and B vitamins in vascular disease. *N Engl J Med*. 2006;354:1567–1577.

Question 112

1. Cuker A. Clinical and laboratory diagnosis of heparin-induced thrombocytopenia: an integrated approach. *Semin Thromb Hemost*. 2014;40:106–114.
2. Warkentin TE. How I diagnose and manage HIT. *Hematology Am Soc Hematol Educ Program*. 2011;2011:143–149.

Question 113

1. Baglin T, Ludddington R, Brown K, et al. Incidence of recurrent venous thromboembolism in relation to clinical and thrombophilic risk factors: prospective cohort study. *Lancet*. 2003;362: 523–526.
2. Boutitie F, Pinede L, Schulman S, et al. Influence of preceding length of anticoagulation treatment and initial presentation of venous thromboembolism on risk of recurrence after stopping treatment: analysis of individual participants' data from seven trials. *BMJ*. 2011;342:d3036.
3. Kearon C, Akl E, Comerota A, et al. Antithrombotic therapy for VTE disease: antithrombotic therapy and prevention of thrombosis, 9th ed: American College of Chest Physicians Evidence-Based Clinical Practical Guidelines. *Chest*. 2012;141: e419S–e494S.

Question 114

1. Christiansen SC, Cannegieter SC, Koser T, et al. Thrombophilia, clinical factors, and recurrent venous thrombotic events. *JAMA*. 2005;293:2353–2361.
2. Kearon C, Akl E, Comerota A, et al. Antithrombotic therapy for VTE disease: antithrombotic therapy and prevention of thrombosis, 9th ed: American College of Chest Physicians Evidence-Based Clinical Practical Guidelines. *Chest*. 2012;141: e419S–e494S.

Question 115

1. Douketis JD, Spyropoulos AC, Spencer FA, et al. Perioperative management of antithrombotic therapy: antithrombotic therapy and prevention of thrombosis, 9th ed: American College of Chest Physicians Evidence-Based Clinical Practice Guidelines. *Chest*. 2012;141(suppl 2):e326S–e350S.
2. Spyropolous AC, Douketis JD. How I treat anticoagulated patients undergoing an elective procedure or surgery. *Blood*. 2012;120:2954–2962.
3. Douketis JD, Spyropoulos AC, Kaatz S, et al. Perioperative bridging anticoagulation in patients with atrial fibrillation. *N Engl J Med*. 2015;373:823–833.

Question 116

1. Falck-Ytter Y, Francis CW, Johanson NA, et al. Prevention of VTE in orthopedic surgical patients: antithrombotic therapy and prevention of thrombosis, 9th ed: American College of Chest Physicians Evidence-Based Clinical Practice Guidelines. *Chest*. 2012;141(suppl 2):e228S–e325S.

Question 117

1. Siegal DM. Managing target-specific oral anticoagulant associated bleeding including an update on pharmacologic reversal agents. *J Thromb Thrombolysis*. 2015;39:395–402.

Question 118

1. Eikelboom JW, Connolly SJ, Bruekmann M, et al. Dabigatran versus Warfarin in patient with mechanical heart valves. *N Engl J Med*. 2013;369:1206–1214.
2. Connolly SJ, Ezekowitz MD, Yusuf S, et al. Dabigatran versus Warfarin in patient with atrial fibrillation. *N Engl J Med*. 2009;361: 1139–1151.
3. Patel MR, Mahaffey KW, Garg J, et al. Rivaroxaban versus Warfarin in nonvalvular atrial fibrillation. *N Engl J Med*. 2011;365:883–891.
4. Granger CB, Alexander JH, McMurray JJV, et al. Apixaban versus Warfarin in patient with atrial fibrillation. *N Engl J Med*. 2011;365:981–982.
5. Giugliano RP, Ruff CT, Braunwald E, et al. Edoxaban versus Warafrin in patients with atrial fibrillation. *N Engl J Med*. 2013;369: 2093–2104.

Question 119

1. Spyropoulos A, Douketis J. How I treat anticoagulated patients undergoing an elective procedure or surgery. *Blood*. 2012;120: 2954–2962.
2. Douketis J, Spyropoulos A, Spencer F, et al. Perioperative management of antithrombotic therapy. Antithrombotic therapy and prevention of thrombosis, 9th ed: American College of Chest Physicians Evidence-Based Clinical Practice Guidelines. *Chest*. 2012;141(suppl 2):e326S–3350S.
3. Connolly D, Spyropoulos AC. Practical issues, limitations, and periprocedural management of then NOACs. *J Thromb Thrombolysis*. 2013;36:212–222.
4. Douketis JD, Spyropoulos AC, Kaatz S, et al. Perioperative bridging anticoagulation in patients with atrial fibrillation. *N Engl J Med*. 2015;373:823–833.

Question 120

1. Bates SM, Greer IA, Middledorp S, et al. VTE, Thrombophilia, Antithrombotic Therapy, and Pregnancy. Antithrombotic therapy and prevention of thrombosis, 9th ed: American College of Chest Physicians Evidence-Based Clinical Practice Guidelines. *Chest*. 2012;141:e691S–e736S.

Question 121

1. Kearon C, Akl E, Comerota A, et al. Antithrombotic therapy for VTE disease: antithrombotic therapy and prevention of thrombosis, 9th ed: American College of Chest Physicians Evidence-Based Clinical Practical Guidelines. *Chest*. 2012;141:e419S–e494S.

Question 122

1. Cuker A, Siegal D. Monitoring and reversal of direct oral anticoagulants. *Hematology Am Soc Hematol Educ Program*. 2015;1:117–124.
2. Van Ryn J, Stangier J, Haertter S, et al. Dabigatran etexilate—a novel, reversible, oral direct thrombin inhibitor: Interpretation of coagulation assays and reversal of anticoagulant activity. *Thromb Haemost*. 2010;103:1116–1127.

Question 123

1. Lim W. Antiphospholipid Syndrome. *Hematology Am Soc Hematol Educ Program*. 2013;2013:675–680.
2. Ruiz-Irastorza G, Crowther M, Branch W, et al. Antiphospholipid Syndrome. *Lancet*. 2010;376:1498–1509.
3. Ruiz-Irastorza G, Cuadrado MJ, Ruiz-Arruza I, et al. Evidence-based recommendations for the prevention and long-term management of thrombosis in antiphospholipid antibody positive patients: report of a task force at the 13th International Congress on antiphospholipid antibodies. *Lupus*. 2011;20:206–218.

Question 124

1. Moll S. Thrombophilia: clinical-practical aspects. *J Thromb Thrombolysis*. 2015;39:367–378.

2. Baglin R, Gray E, Greaves M, et al. Clinical guidelines for testing for heritable thrombophilia. *BJH*. 2010;149:209–220.

Question 125

1. George JN, Nester CM, McIntosh JJ. Syndromes of thrombotic microangiopathy associated with pregnancy. *Hematology Am Soc Hematol Educ Program*. 2015;2015:644–648.
2. Loirat C, Frémeaux-Bacchi V. Atypical hemolytic uremic syndrome. *Orphanet J Rare Dis*. 2011;6:60.

Question 126

1. Kakagia DD, Papanas N, Karadimas E, et al. Warfarin-induced skin necrosis. *Ann Dermatol*. 2014;26:96–98.

Question 127

1. Kearon C, Akl E, Comerota A, et al. Antithrombotic therapy for VTE disease. Antithrombotic therapy and prevention of thrombosis, 9th ed: American College of Chest Physicians evidence-based clinical practice guidelines. *Chest*. 2012;141(suppl 2):e419s–e494s.

Question 128

1. Weitz J. New oral anticoagulants: a view from the laboratory. *Am J Hematol*. 2012;87(suppl 1):S133–S136.

Question 129

1. Kearon C, Akl EA, Comerota AJ, et al. Antithrombotic therapy for VTE disease. Antithrombotic therapy and prevention of thrombosis, 9th edition: American College of Chest Physicians Evidence-Based Clinical Practice Guidelines. *Chest*. 2012;141(suppl 2): e419s–e494s.
2. Primignani M, Tosetti G, La Mura V. Therapeutic and clinical aspects of portal vein thrombosis in patients with cirrhosis. *World J Hepatol*. 2015;7(29):2906–2912.

Question 130

1. Kearon C, Akl EA, Comerota AJ, et al. Antithrombotic therapy for VTE disease. Antithrombotic therapy and prevention of thrombosis, 9th ed: American College of Chest Physicians Evidence-Based Clinical Practice Guidelines. *Chest*. 2012;141(suppl 2):e419s–e494s.
2. Segal JB, Brotman DJ, Necochea AJ, et al. Predictive value of factor V Leiden and prothrombin G20210A in adults with VTE and in family members of those with a mutation: a systematic review. *JAMA*. 2009;301:2472–2485.

Question 131

1. Bates S, Greer I, Middeldorp S, et al. VTE, thrombophilia, antithrombotic therapy, and pregnancy. Antithrombotic therapy and prevention of thrombosis, 9th ed: American College of Chest Physicians evidence-based clinical practice guidelines. *Chest*. 2012;141(suppl 2):e691s–e736s.

Question 132

1. Spaet TH. Case 20-1979: false prolongation of prothrombin time in polycythemia. *N Engl J Med*. 1979;301(9):503.

Question 133

1. Carrier M, Lazo-Langner A, Shivakumar S, et al. Screening for occult cancer in unprovoked venous thromboembolism. *N Engl J Med*. 2015;373(8):697–704.
2. Ihaddadene R, Corsi DJ, Lazo-Langner A, et al. Risk factors predictive of occult cancer detection in patients with unprovoked venous thromboembolism. *Blood*. 2016;127:2035–2037.

Question 134

1. Berntsen CF, Kristiansen A, Akl EA, et al. Compression stockings for preventing the post-thrombotic syndrome in patients with deep vein thrombosis. *Am J Med*. 2016;129(4):447.e1–e447.e20.
2. Kahn SR, Shapiro S, Wells PS, et al. Compression stockings to prevent post-thrombotic syndrome: a randomised placebo-controlled trial. *Lancet*. 2014;383(9920):880–888.

3. Kearon C, Akl EA, Ornelas J, et al. Antithrombotic therapy for VTE disease: chest guideline and expert panel report. *Chest*. 2016;149(2):315–352.

Question 135

1. Ageno W, Riva N, Schulman S, et al. Antithrombotic treatment of splanchnic vein thrombosis: results of an international registry. *Sem Thromb Hemost*. 2014;40(1):99–105.
2. Thatipelli MR, McBane RD, Hodge DO, Wysokinski WE. Survival and recurrence in patients with splanchnic vein thromboses. *Clin Gastroenterol Hepatol*. 2010;8(2):200–205.
3. Smalberg JH, Arends LR, Valla DC, Kiladjian JJ, Janssen HL, Leebeek FW. Myeloproliferative neoplasms in Budd-Chiari syndrome and portal vein thrombosis: a meta-analysis. *Blood*. 2012;120(25):4921–4928.

Question 136

1. Eikelboom JW, Quinlan DJ, van Ryn J, Weitz JI. Idarucizumab: the antidote for reversal of dabigatran. *Circulation*. 2015;132(25):2412–2422.
2. Pollack Jr CV, Reilly PA, Eikelboom J, et al. Idarucizumab for Dabigatran Reversal. *N Engl J Med*. 2015;373(6):511–520.
3. Hawes EM, Deal AM, Funk-Adcock D, et al. Performance of coagulation tests in patients on therapeutic doses of dabigatran: a cross-sectional pharmacodynamic study based on peak and trough plasma levels. *J Thromb Haemost*. 2013;11(8):1493–1502.

Question 137

1. Decousus H, Prandoni P, Mismetti P, et al. Fondaparinux for the treatment of superficial-vein thrombosis in the legs. *N Engl J Med*. 2010;363(13):1222–1232.
2. Di Nisio M, Wichers IM, Middeldorp S. Treatment for superficial thrombophlebitis of the leg. *Cochrane Database Syst Rev*. 2013;4:Cd004982.
3. Kearon C, Akl EA, Comerota AJ, et al. Antithrombotic therapy for VTE disease: antithrombotic therapy and prevention of thrombosis, 9th ed: American College of Chest Physicians Evidence-Based Clinical Practice Guidelines. *Chest*. 2012;141(suppl 2):e419S–e494S.

Question 138

1. Kearon C, Akl EA, Ornelas J, et al. Antithrombotic therapy for VTE disease: chest guideline and expert panel report. *Chest*. 2016;149(2):315–352.

Question 139

1. Zwicker JI, Connolly G, Carrier M, Kamphuisen PW, Lee AY. Catheter-associated deep vein thrombosis of the upper extremity in cancer patients: guidance from the SSC of the ISTH. *J Thromb Haemost*. 2014;12(5):796–800.

Question 140

1. Thorell SE, Parry-Jones AR, Punter M, Hurford R, Thachil J. Cerebral venous thrombosis-a primer for the haematologist. *Blood Rev*. 2015;29(1):45–50.

Question 141

1. Mahtani KR, Heneghan CJ, Nunan D, Roberts NW. Vitamin K for improved anticoagulation control in patients receiving warfarin. *Cochrane Database Syst Rev*. 2014;5:Cd009917.

Question 142

1. Kyrle PA, Minar E, Bialonczyk C, et al. The risk of recurrent venous thromboembolism in men and women. *N Engl J Med*. 2004;350:2558–2563.
2. Prandoni P, Barbar S, Milan M, et al. Optimal duration of anticoagulation. Provoked versus unprovoked VTE and role of adjunctive thrombophilia and imaging tests. *Thromb Haemost*. 2015;113:1210–1215.
3. Kearon C, Spencer FA, O'Keeffe D, et al. D-dimer testing to select patients with a first unprovoked venous thromboembolism who can stop anticoagulant therapy: a cohort study. *Ann Intern Med*. 2015;162(1):27–34.

Question 143

1. Prandoni P, Barbar S, Milan M, et al. Optimal duration of anticoagulation. Provoked versus unprovoked VTE and role of adjunctive thrombophilia and imaging tests. *Thromb Haemost*. 2015;113:1210–1215.

Question 145

1. Nasr H, Scriven JM. Superficial thrombophlebitis (superficial venous thrombosis). *BMJ*. 2015;350. h2039.

Question 146

1. Strobel J, Ringwald J, Zimmermann R, Eckstein R. Thromboembolic risk assessment in a phenotypically cured factor-V-Leiden carrier after orthotopic liver transplantation. *Clin Lab*. 2010; 56(5–6):245–247.

Question 147

Nasr H, Scriven JM. Superficial thrombophlebitis (superficial venous thrombosis). *BMJ*. 2015;350. http://dx.doi.org/10.1136/bmj.h2039. h2039.

Question 148

1. Guyatt GH, Akl EA, Crowther M, et al. Antithrombotic therapy and prevention of thrombosis, 9th ed: American College of Chest Physicians Evidence-Based Clinical Practice Guidelines. *Chest*. 2012;141(suppl 2):7S–47S.

CHAPTER
34

Hematopoietic System Disorders

Marc J. Kahn, Marc Zumberg, Ara Metjian, Anita Rajasekhar, Brandi Reeves, Molly Weidener Mandernach, and Alice D. Ma

QUESTIONS

1. A 28-year-old man is referred with the diagnosis of hereditary coproporphyria for definitive therapy. The patient was well until 8 years ago when he began to hear voices. At that time, he dropped out of college and became homeless. At times he believed he was under demonic possession. The patient is brought in by his parents. They state he is having an acute attack characterized by altered mentation and abdominal pain. He is disheveled and unkempt. BP is 120/70, pulse 110, temperature 99°F. He is thin, has no organomegaly, and his skin exam is unremarkable. His laboratory studies are as follows:

Hgb	14.0 g/dL
Hct	42%
WBC	5800 × 10⁹/L
Platelet	187,000 × 10⁹/L

His parents have the following labs that were collected during the patient's recent hospitalization for an acute porphyric attack:

24-hour urine:
| PBG | Normal |
| ALA | Normal |

Porphyrin screen is normal except for mild elevation of coproporphyrin to 4 µg/dL (normal 1–2 µg/dL).
How should he be managed?
A. Intravenous 10% dextrose
B. Hematin
C. Propranolol
D. Referral to psychiatrist

2. A 45-year-old man with a 20-year history of rheumatoid arthritis and HTN presents with a history of anemia of unknown cause. He is asymptomatic. There is no family history of blood diseases. His physical exam shows BP of 120/70, pulse 72, temperature 99°F. He has conjunctival pallor, a prominent S4 on cardiac exam, and rheumatoid changes in his hands. His laboratory studies show:

Hgb	8.7 g/dL
Hct	26%
MCV	82 fL
Platelets	422,000 × 10⁹/L
Creatinine	1.0 mg/dL
Fe	45 µg/dL
TIBC	220 µg/dL
Ferritin	565 ng/mL

How should he be managed?
A. Oral FeSO₄
B. Ferumoxytol
C. Erythropoietin
D. Methylprednisolone
E. No treatment

3. A 39-year-old previously healthy woman is admitted to the hospital for an acute illness and anemia of 2 days' duration. The patient returned from a camping trip 2 days prior and initially noted a painful erythematous and dark lesion on her shin, presumed secondary to minor trauma. She now reports fever, fatigue, nausea, and vomiting. She has a temperature of 101°F, pulse 112, and BP of 105/68. Her skin exam is significant for a large lesion on her shin that measures 4 × 5 cm and is necrotic and painful. She has scattered petechiae on her extremities. Her laboratory studies show:

Hgb	8.2 g/dL
Hct	25%
Platelets	20,000 × 10⁹/L
WBC	13,500 × 10⁹/L
Tbili	4.2 mg/dL
Direct	0.3 mg/dL
Smear	Decreased platelets. Rare schistocytes

What is the most likely diagnosis?
A. Loxoscelism
B. MRSA cellulitis
C. Rhus dermatitis
D. Pyoderma gangrenosum
E. Lyme disease

4. A 62-year-old man with a 10-year history of CAD who underwent CABG and mechanical mitral valve replacement 3 years prior presents with worsening anemia. His physical exam is significant for slight scleral icterus and crisp mechanical valve sounds without murmur. He has trace pedal edema. His medications include warfarin, metoprolol, and simvastatin. An ECHO is read as normal. His labs are as follows:

Hgb	7.7 g/dL
Hct	22%
Platelets	150,000 × 10⁹/L
WBC	8200 × 10⁹/L
Retic	240,000 × 10⁹/L
Tbili	3.2 mg/dL
Direct	0.2 mg/dL
Smear	3–5 schistocytes per HPF

What is the most likely diagnosis?
A. TTP
B. Cold agglutinin disease

C. Valve hemolysis
D. Warm antibody hemolytic anemia
E. DIC

5. A 48-year-old African-American man is referred for several months of unexplained hemolysis. He has an unremarkable family and past history. He was diagnosed with lower extremity cellulitis 2 months prior, which was treated intermittently with oral antibiotics. His labs are as follows:

	Baseline	New
Hgb	14.9 g/dL	9.7 g/dL
Hct	45%	29%
Platelet	420,000 × 10⁹/L	375,000 × 10⁹/L
Tbili	1.0 mg/dL	4.2 mg/dL
LDH	100 U/L	479 U/L

Coombs direct and indirect NEGATIVE.
CD55/CD59/FLAER NEGATIVE.

Hgb EP	98% Hgb A, 2% Hgb A2
G6PD	Normal
PBS	Normal

What is the most likely diagnosis?
A. G6PD deficiency
B. PNH
C. Cold agglutinin disease
D. Warm antibody hemolytic anemia
E. Paroxysmal cold hemoglobinuria

6. A 26-year-old woman presents with several months' history of pancytopenia. She denies any past medical history. On exam, she weighs 91 pounds and is 5′9″. She has significant pallor. The remainder of her exam is normal. Her laboratory studies are as follows:

Hgb	6.7 g/dL
Hct	20%
Platelets	27,000/mm³
WBC	2700/mm³

Her bone marrow shows severe hypoplasia of all hematopoietic marrow elements, an absence of fat, and a diffuse accumulation of acellular pink material throughout her marrow.
What is the most likely diagnosis?
A. Aplastic anemia
B. Serous atrophy
C. Myelodysplasia
D. Metastatic tumor
E. Myelofibrosis

7. A 67-year-old man with a 12-year history of type 2 diabetes treated with metformin and glipizide presents to his primary care physician with a 6-month history of anemia. His physical examination is unremarkable. His laboratory studies are as follows:

Hgb	8.1 g/dL
Hct	24%
MCV	107 fL
Platelets	147,000 × 10⁹/L
WBC	3800 × 10⁹/L
Serum methyl malonate	Elevated

In addition to giving supplemental oral cobalamin, how should he be managed?
A. Perform Schilling test
B. Check antiparietal cell antibodies

C. Check intrinsic factor antibodies
D. Supplement calcium
E. Stop glipizide

8. A 48-year-old man is being evaluated for an anemia that he has had throughout his life. His past medical history is significant for a cholecystectomy for gallstones performed 3 years prior. His first cousin has also had a cholecystectomy. His physical exam is significant for morbid obesity. He has mild scleral icterus. His laboratory findings are as follows:

Hgb	10.2 g/dL
Hct	30%
Tbili	4.2 mg/dL
Direct	0.3 mg/dL
LDH	420 U/L
Peripheral smear	Scattered spherocytes

What is the most appropriate test to confirm the diagnosis?
A. Osmotic fragility
B. Eosin-5-maleimide
C. Protein 4.1 analysis
D. CD55/59
E. Spectrin analysis

9. A 32-year-old woman with an unremarkable past medical history presents with a 9-month history of anemia. She takes a variety of over-the-counter supplements. Except for frequent viral URIs, she has been healthy. She is placed on oral iron, and despite compliance, her laboratory studies continue to show iron deficiency. Her physical exam is significant only for mild pallor. Her laboratory studies are as follows:

Hgb	8.2 g/dL
Hct	24%
MCV	62 fL
Ferritin	11 ng/mL

Which of the following over-the-counter products is most likely causing her findings?
A. Saw palmetto
B. Black cohosh
C. Alpha lipoic acid
D. Coenzyme Q10
E. Zinc
F. Calcium

10. A 53-year-old man dependent on dialysis for 6 years presents with a 7-month history of refractory anemia. The patient had been on hemodialysis for presumed hypertensive nephropathy. He had been treated with supplemental erythropoietin and darbepoetin that allowed him to maintain a hemoglobin (Hgb) of 10.5 g/dL prior to 7 months ago. Since then, his Hgb has remained in the 7.0 g/dL range despite increasing doses of erythropoietin. His laboratory studies are as follows:

Hgb	7.0 g/dL
Hct	21%
Cr	4.7 mg/dL
Iron	150 μg/dL
Ferritin	652 ng/mL
TIBC	270 μg/dL

What other hormone should be checked in evaluation of his persistent anemia?
A. TSH
B. PTH
C. FSH

D. LH

E. GnRH

11. A 32-year-old woman has had a history of normocytic anemia since birth. The patient is healthy without complaints. She is only taking oral contraceptives. She has a strong family history of anemia of unclear etiology. Her physical exam is unremarkable. She has had normal iron studies, normal B12 and folate, and her blood smear has been reviewed as normal. Her most recent laboratory studies are as follows:

Hgb	11.7 g/dL
Hct	35%
MCV	90 fL
WBC	6200/mm^3
Platelet	354,000/mm^3

Which test should be ordered to assess hemoglobin oxygen affinity?
A. Hgb electrophoresis
B. p50
C. Pulse oximetry
D. Carboxyhemoglobin
E. Eosin 5-maleimide

12. An 18-year-old college student presented with altered mental status, confusion, and hypotension after a party following final examinations. Her physical exam showed BP 80/50, pulse 118, temperature 99°F. The remainder of her exam was only significant for delirium. Her laboratory studies were as follows:

Hgb	8.7 g/dL
Hct	26%
MCV	110 fL
WBC	2700 × 10^9/L
Platelets	34,000 × 10^9/L
Marrow	Megaloblastic changes, hypocellular

Inhalation of which of the following could cause her findings?
A. Toluene
B. Amyl nitrate
C. Cocaine
D. Marijuana
E. Nitrous oxide

13. A 42-year-old woman is being evaluated for microcytic anemia, which has been present since early childhood. The patient is currently asymptomatic. Her mother reports being told she was anemic during childbirth. Her BP is 110/70 and pulse 72. Her physical exam is otherwise unremarkable. Her laboratory studies are shown:

Hgb	10.0 g/dL
Hct	30%
MCV	65 fL
RBC count	5900 × 10^9/L

What is the most likely diagnosis?
A. Iron deficiency
B. Beta thalassemia minor
C. Hgb SC
D. Sideroblastic anemia
E. Lead poisoning

14. A 62-year-old man with a 15-year history of CLL that has not required treatment presents to the emergency department with a 2-day history of worsening yellow skin and eyes. The patient reports feeling increased fatigue and has not had his usual exercise tolerance, which he partially blames on the changing seasons and earlier sunsets. His BP is 135/70, pulse 110, RR 18/min, and temperature 98°F. He has markedly icteric sclera and skin, and large cervical lymph nodes that have not changed in size. His laboratory studies are shown:

Hgb	7.8 g/dL
Hct	23%
WBC	26,000 × 10^9/L
Platelet	136,000 × 10^9/L
Tbili	11.5 mg/dL
Direct bili	2.2 mg/dL
Peripheral smear	Clumped red cells throughout slide

How is his anemia best managed?
A. Glucocorticoids
B. IVIg
C. Plasmapheresis
D. Splenectomy
E. Rituximab

15. A 32-year-old woman with a 12-year history of ulcerative colitis and severe iron deficiency of 2 years' duration presents to the office. Her inflammatory bowel disease has been complicated by bleeding and perirectal abscesses. She has tried oral iron replacement in the past, but has stopped due to worsening GI complaints and lack of efficacy. She is a stay home single mother and would like to minimize hospital visits. Her laboratory studies are shown:

Hgb	5.2 g/dL
Hct	15%
MCV	62 fL
Ferritin	0.5 ng/mL

Which iron preparation has the highest rate of anaphylaxis?
A. Ferrous sulfate
B. Ferric carboxymaltose
C. Iron sucrose
D. Iron dextran
E. Ferumoxytol

16. A 27-year-old man with a prior history of treated syphilis presents with a 2-day history of jaundice and lethargy. He has noticed a yellowing of his skin and conjunctivae over the prior 48 hours. He had been unable to play hockey or work at his job as a meat cutter on the day of presentation. On exam, scleral icterus and yellow skin are noted. He has no organomegaly or lymphadenopathy. His laboratory studies are as follows:

Hgb	7.8 g/dL
Hct	23%
Tbili	12 mg/dL
Reticulocyte	8.2%
Absolute reticulocyte count	400,000 × 10^9/L
Coombs	Negative

Which of the following tests would be most helpful in establishing a diagnosis?
A. Eosin 5′ maleimide
B. Pyruvate kinase
C. Donath Landsteiner antibody
D. ANA
E. Sucrose hemolysis test

17. A 6-month-old boy was brought to the emergency room several hours after his mother noticed cyanosis and a blue tint on his mucous membranes. The patient was the product of normal gestation and delivery and weighed 3350 g. He was noted to have diaper rash on exam, in addition to having cyanotic skin and mucous membranes. His oxygen saturation on pulse oximetry was 97%. His mother had been treating his diaper rash with benzocaine and resorcinol cream.
How should he be managed?
A. 100% oxygen
B. Inhaled nitrous oxide
C. Intravenous methylene blue
D. Intravenous quinine

18. An 18-year-old man from Thailand presents for an evaluation of chronic anemia. The patient has been told he has been anemic since age 5 and has family members who are also anemic. He has not required a transfusion. His BP is 105/70 and pulse 88. He has pale conjunctivae. He has an enlarged liver and spleen. His laboratory studies are as follows:

Hgb	6.0 g/dL
Hct	18%
MCV	67 fL
RDW	27%
Hgb F	42%
Hgb E	58%

What is the most likely diagnosis?
A. Hgb E trait
B. Homozygous Hgb E
C. Hgb E/beta^0-thalassemia
D. Hgb SE
E. Hgb CE

19. A 28-year-old woman presents with 24 hours of bruising and icteric sclera. The patient has a sister and aunt who died of acute kidney failure. She has had an unremarkable past medical history and is only taking an oral contraceptive. She feels well. Her BP is 110/70, pulse 98, and temperature 100°F. Her physical exam is only significant for icteric sclera, petechiae on her lower extremities, and several bruises on her forearms that are over 2 cm. Her laboratory studies are shown:

Hgb	6.7 g/dL
Hct	20%
WBC	6700 × 10^9/L
Platelets	8000 × 10^9/L
Creatinine	4.6 mg/dL
ADAMTS13	60%
ADAMTS13 inhibitor	Negative
Peripheral smear	Thrombocytopenia and fragmented red blood cells

How should she be managed?
A. Plasmapheresis
B. Eculizumab
C. Rituximab
D. Glucocorticoids
E. IVIg

20. A 22-year-old healthy woman is referred for evaluation of increased iron saturation found during a workup for mild anemia. The patient is a college student who was feeling fatigued for several weeks and went to the student health service where her hemoglobin was found to be mildly reduced. Her physical exam is unremarkable. Her laboratory studies are shown:

Hgb	11.7 g/dL
Hct	36%
Iron	120 µg/dL
Transferrin sat	55%
Ferritin	310 ng/mL

Testing for mutations in HFE reveals homozygosity for the H63D mutation.
How should she be managed?
A. Phlebotomy
B. Careful observation
C. Liver biopsy
D. Deferoxamine
E. Deferasirox

21. A 42-year-old man is being evaluated for progressive neuropsychiatric deterioration, choreatic movement disorder, and myopathy of 1 year's duration. He has had an uncle and grandfather who died of presumed Huntington disease before a genetic test was available. He has tested negative for the disorder. His exam is significant for choreoathetotic movements of the upper torso. He is unable to remember any of three items at 5 minutes. He appears depressed. Review of his peripheral smear reveals acanthocytes.
Which of the following antigens is most likely absent on his red cells?
A. Rh
B. Lewis
C. Duffy
D. Kell
E. Kidd

22. A 68-year-old man presents for evaluation of erythrocytosis present for the past 6 months. The patient has a 30-year history of hypertension treated to an ACE-inhibitor and diuretic. He is currently asymptomatic. His BP is 140/75, pulse 80, and temperature 99°F. He has a barely palpable spleen. His laboratory studies are shown:

Hgb	19.6 g/dL
Hct	60%
WBC	12,300 × 10^9/L
Platelets	450,000 × 10^9/L
JAK2	Wild type
Erythropoietin	14.5 mIU/mL

What test should be ordered next?
A. Red cell mass
B. Red cell survival time
C. Bone marrow biopsy
D. CT of abdomen
E. Flow cytometry of peripheral blood

23. A 48-year-old woman is being evaluated for hyperferritinemia found during evaluation of transaminitis 2 weeks earlier. The patient is adopted so no family history is available. Her exam is unremarkable. Her laboratory studies are shown:

Hgb	12.0 g/dL
Hct	36%
Iron	60 µg/dL
Transferrin sat	32%
Ferritin	1200 µg/L
AST	60 U/L
ALT	65 U/L

This most likely reflects which genetic abnormality?
A. Homozygosity for HFE C282Y
B. Homozygosity for HFE H63D

C. HJV mutation
D. SLC40A1 mutation

24. A 42-year-old man presents for evaluation of anemia that has been present since birth. He has required blood transfusions throughout his life despite lack of obvious bleeding. He has not been responsive to oral iron and has only been partially responsive to intravenous iron preparations. On exam, he is pale with a BP of 120/70 and pulse of 100. He has no organomegaly and is guaiac negative. His laboratory studies are as follows:

Hgb	7.0 g/dL
Hct	21%
MCV	67 fL
Iron	15 µg/dL
Ferritin	0.5 µg/L

Which of the following is the most likely diagnosis?
A. Ferroportin disease
B. Variegate porphyria
C. Mutation in TMPRSS 6
D. Hemojuvelin mutation
E. Coproporphyria

25. A 41-year-old man with sickle cell (SS) disease and frequent vasoocclusive crisis (two per month) presents with worsening lower extremity swelling for the past 3 weeks. The patient has been compliant with hydroxyurea and folic acid. He is currently pain free. Her reports decreased exercise tolerance for the past 5 months. His BP is 120/70, pulse 90, temperature 98°F, and respirations 20. He has a loud P2 on cardiac auscultation, an inspiratory S3, and clear lung fields. He has 3+ peripheral edema in his lower extremities. A chest x-ray is normal.
Which of the following is most likely responsible for his physical exam findings?
A. Pulmonary hypertension
B. Acute chest syndrome
C. Cardiomyopathy
D. High output heart failure
E. Atrial septal defect

26. A 65-year-old man is in the hospital awaiting liver transplant for liver failure secondary to autoimmune hepatitis. Two days prior, he began to develop a progressive anemia despite absence of obvious blood loss. He has had a deterioration of neurologic function, an increase in ascites, and worsening coagulopathy during the same time period. He is currently Childs Class C. His laboratory studies are as follows:

Hgb	6.7 g/dL
Hct	20%
WBC	11,500 × 10⁹/L
Platelets	27,000 × 10⁹/L
Tbili	15.2 mg/dL
Direct	7.8 mg/dL
Albumin	1.2 g/dL
PT	22 s

What finding would you expect on his peripheral smear?
A. Microcytes
B. Acanthocytes
C. Echinocytes
D. Drepanocytes
E. Dacryocytes

27. A 42-year-old woman with a 20-year history of celiac disease presents with anemia. The patient has been somewhat compliant with a gluten-free diet. She has tried oral iron without a change in her degree of anemia. She reports fatigue and occasional bouts of diarrhea. Her weight is 110 pounds (50 kg); BP is 100/70; pulse is 105. Her exam is otherwise only significant for conjunctival pallor. Her laboratory studies are as follows:

Hgb	7.2 g/dL
Hct	22%
Iron	2 µg/dL
Ferritin	0.2 µg/L

Assuming a target hemoglobin of 12, what is her intravenous iron requirement?
A. 500 mg
B. 600 mg
C. 1100 mg
D. 1500 mg
E. 200 mg

28. A 45-year-old man presents for evaluation of mild pancytopenia. Three years ago, he was successfully treated for aplastic anemia with antithymocyte globulin (ATG) and cyclosporine with normalization of his blood counts, but was subsequently lost to follow-up. For the three days prior to presentation, he complained of significant right upper quadrant pain and was diagnosed with hepatic vein occlusion. Prior personal and family history is negative for any hematologic disorders. His BP is 130/75, pulse 100, and temperature 99°F. He has a diffusely tender abdomen without guarding or rebound. His laboratory studies are as follows:

Hgb	8.7 g/dL
Hct	26%
WBC	1200 × 10⁹/L
Platelets	87,000 × 10⁹/L

Which of the following tests is most likely to lead to the proper diagnosis?
A. FLAER testing
B. Factor V Leiden testing
C. Cytogenetics
D. Protein electrophoresis
E. Antiphospholipid antibody testing

29. A 43-year-old construction worker is referred to you for evaluation of blistering skin lesions over his arms and hands for the past 4 years. The patient wears short-sleeved shirts and spends much of the day working in the sun. His medical history is significant only for previous intravenous drug use when he was in his 20s. He has no family history of liver disease. He takes no medications and consumes two to three beers each day. Physical examination is significant for multiple well-healed skin lesions over his hands and arms. A few fresh blisters are noted on his hands bilaterally. His complete blood count is normal. Iron studies are as follows:

Serum iron	195 µg/dL
Serum TIBC	389 µg/dL
Transferrin saturation	40%
Serum ferritin	632 ng/mL

Which of the following is most appropriate laboratory evaluation for this patient at this time?
A. Urine PBG and ALA
B. Hepatitis serologies
C. HFE testing
D. Liver MRI for iron

30. A 55-year-old man underwent orthotopic liver transplant for end-stage liver disease secondary to chronic hepatitis C 10 days prior. You are asked to see the patient to evaluate hemolytic anemia that began 24 hours after surgery. The patient had an uneventful operative course and received 11 units of red cells in addition to platelets and plasma. He is currently receiving prednisone and tacrolimus. The patient is blood type A positive and received a liver from an O positive donor. The patient left the operating room with a hemoglobin of 11.2 g/dL. One week later, the patient was noted to have a hemoglobin of 5.4 g/dL. The patient is hemodynamically stable, afebrile, and there is no evidence of excessive bleeding. His other laboratory studies are only significant for total and unconjugated bilirubin of 7.5 mg/dL and 6.2 mg/dL, respectively; a platelet count of 10,000 × 10⁹/L; and an LDH of 672 IU/dL.

What is the most likely etiology of this patient's hemolytic anemia?
    A. ABO-mismatched red cells received during surgery
    B. ABO-mismatched plasma received during surgery
    C. Transplanted lymphocytes
    D. Tacrolimus
    E. EBV infection

31. A 20-year-old woman with a history of kidney transplant 5 years previously for renal failure secondary to ureteral reflux presents with erythrocytosis. The patient was diagnosed 2 weeks prior when she underwent routine laboratory testing. She is taking tacrolimus and prednisone. Her renal function was normal. She is asymptomatic. Her BP is 120/80, pulse 88, and temperature 98°F. She has no hepatosplenomegaly. Her laboratory studies are as follows:

Hgb	17.3 g/dL
Hct	52%
Erythropoietin	18.4 mIU/mL (2.6–18.5 mIU/mL)

What treatment would you recommend at this time?
    A. Hydroxyurea
    B. Phlebotomy
    C. Enalapril
    D. Change tacrolimus to cyclosporine

32. A 23-year-old man presents to the emergency department with liver failure and hemolysis. The patient has an unknown past medical history but was brought in by a neighbor who was worried. His BP is 120/70, pulse is 88, and temperature is 98°F. He is markedly jaundiced. He has a dark ring that appears to encircle the iris where the cornea meets the sclera. His liver is enlarged two finger breadths below the costal angle. He has no splenomegaly. His laboratory studies are as follows:

Hgb	8.7 g/dL
Hct	21%
Tbili	8.7 mg/dL
LDH	506 IU/L
ALT	57 IU/L
AST	288 IU/L
Coombs	negative
Smear	Spherocytes, polychromatophils and few nucleated RBCs

How should he be managed?
    A. Glucocorticoids
    B. IVIg
    C. Plasmapheresis
    D. Penicillamine
    E. Rituximab

33. A 62-year-old man presents with worsening anemia of 2 years' duration. The patient is otherwise well. He underwent a bone marrow aspirate and biopsy that showed erythroid dysplasia, 3% bone marrow blasts, and 20% ringed sideroblasts. His exam is unremarkable without hepatosplenomegaly. His laboratory studies are shown:

Hgb	8.7 g/dL
Hct	27%
MCV	107 fL
WBC	5100 × 10⁹/L
Platelets	650,000 × 10⁹/L

His condition is most likely secondary to a mutation in which gene?
    A. BCR/ABL
    B. BCL2
    C. CMYC
    D. SF3B1
    E. MYD88

34. An 86-year-old woman is evaluated for a 6-month history of increasing fatigue and paresthesias of her toes. Her past medical history is significant for type 2 diabetes mellitus and hypertension. Current medications are metformin, lisinopril, and aspirin. On physical examination, her temperature is 36.6°C (98.0°F), blood pressure is 127/74 mm Hg, pulse rate is 97/min, and respiration rate is 12/min. Neurologic examination discloses normal vibratory sense and proprioception in the toes and fingers. Monofilament testing for foot sensation is intact. The remainder of the neurologic and general physical examination is normal. Her laboratory studies are shown:

Hgb	11.8 g/dL
Hct	36%
MCV	106 fL
Serum B12	220 pg/mL
Folate	22 ng/mL

Which of the following is the most appropriate next diagnostic test?
    A. Bone marrow biopsy
    B. Erythrocyte folate measurement
    C. Methylmalonic acid and homocysteine measurement
    D. Parietal cell antibody assay
    E. Intrinsic factor antibody assay

35. A 42-year-old woman who had a kidney transplant 4 years ago for focal segmental glomerulosclerosis presents with anemia. The patient reports 1 month of decreased exercise tolerance. She is compliant with all of her medications that include atenolol, lisinopril, prednisone, cyclosporine, and metformin. Her BP is 120/75, pulse 88, and temperature 99°F. Her laboratory studies are shown:

Hgb	8.7 g/dL
Hct	26%
Platelets	42,000 × 10⁹/L
Smear	Scattered schistocytes with occasional nucleated red cells. Mild thrombocytopenia

Which of the following medications is most likely responsible for her findings?
    A. Atenolol
    B. Lisinopril
    C. Prednisone
    D. Cyclosporine
    E. Metformin

36. A 22-year-old black man is evaluated for worsening of chronic anemia over the past 4 months. His medical history is significant for sickle cell anemia complicated by frequent painful crises, cholecystitis, and one episode of acute chest syndrome that occurred 2 years ago with an accompanying stroke. To prevent stroke recurrence, he initially underwent monthly exchange transfusions, which were subsequently stopped owing to noncompliance. His current medications include hydroxyurea, folate, and oxycodone as needed for pain. The patient admits to difficulty remembering to take his medications, particularly since his stroke. On physical examination, the patient has pale conjunctivae. Temperature is 36.6°C (97.9°F), blood pressure is 116/82 mm Hg, pulse rate is 112/min, and respiration is 18/min. Cardiopulmonary examination discloses tachycardia and an S_4; the lungs are clear. Examination of the abdomen shows a healed cholecystectomy scar. Neurologic examination reveals right-sided weakness with dysarthria. Vibratory sensation and position sense are intact. His laboratory studies are shown:

Hgb	4.1 g/dL
Hct	12%
MCV	99 fL
Reticulocyte	0.2%
Absolute reticulocyte	3400/μL

Which of the following is his most likely diagnosis?
A. Anemia of chronic disease
B. Cobalamin deficiency
C. Folate deficiency
D. Hyperhemolysis
E. Iron deficiency

37. A 20-year-old black woman is evaluated in the hospital after admission 5 days ago with acute left hemispheric stroke. Medical history is significant for sickle cell disease complicated by multiple episodes of acute chest syndrome. Current medications are hydroxyurea and folic acid. On physical examination, her temperature is 37.5°C (99.5°F), blood pressure is 166/92 mm Hg, pulse rate is 112/min and regular, and respiration rate is 18/min. The cardiopulmonary examination is unremarkable. There are no carotid bruits. Right upper and lower extremity weakness and dysarthria are noted on neurologic examination. Laboratory studies indicate a hemoglobin of 10.1 g/dL. An MRI shows an acute infarction in the territory of the right middle cerebral artery.
In addition to aspirin, which of the following is the most appropriate secondary prevention of stroke in this patient?
A. Clopidogrel
B. Dipyridamole
C. Angiotensin-converting enzyme inhibitor
D. Monthly red cell transfusion
E. Atorvastatin

38. A 24-year-old woman in the second trimester of an uncomplicated first pregnancy is evaluated during a routine prenatal visit. The patient has mild anemia but no family history of blood disorders or anemia. Her only medication is a prenatal vitamin containing iron and folate. On physical examination, her blood pressure is 105/65 mm Hg and pulse rate is 72/min. No pallor or petechiae are noted. The patient has a gravid uterus appropriate for gestation. Her complete blood count is normal except for a hemoglobin of 10.5 g/dL. Erythrocyte indices are normal. Serum ferritin concentration is 125 ng/mL.
Which of the following is the most likely cause of this patient's anemia?
A. Increased plasma volume
B. Decreased red cell mass
C. Decreased erythropoietin
D. Increased hepcidin
E. Decreased folate utilization

39. A 24-year-old black woman with sickle cell (SS) anemia is admitted to the hospital with a typical painful crisis involving pain in the back and legs present for the past 24 hours. The patient is 12 weeks pregnant with her first child. Her only medication is folic acid and prenatal vitamins. On physical examination, the patient is in obvious discomfort. Her temperature is 38.7°C (101.8°F), blood pressure is 110/64 mm Hg, pulse rate is 112/min, and respiration rate is 22/min. Arterial oxygen saturation on room air is 95%. The patient has a gravid uterus appropriate for gestation. Her lungs are clear, and there is no costovertebral tenderness. Her laboratory studies are shown:

Hgb	7.2 g/dL
Hct	21%
WBC	13,200/cumm

How should her anemia be managed?
A. Transfuse 1 unit PRBC
B. Transfuse 2 units PRBC
C. Exchange transfuse to Hgb 10 g/dL and less than 30% Hgb S
D. No transfusion needed

40. A 21-year-old Filipino woman is evaluated for severe chronic anemia of lifelong duration. The patient's family history is remarkable for α-thalassemia of unclear type in both parents. She takes no medications. On physical examination, vital signs are normal. There is no scleral icterus. A soft, palpable spleen tip is noted on abdominal examination. The remainder of the examination is normal. Her laboratory studies are shown:

Hgb	8.3 g/dL
Hct	24%
Erythrocyte	$4.6 \times 10^6/\mu L$
Ferritin	457 ng/mL
Smear	Microcytes and prominent target cells

Hgb electrophoresis reveals trace hemoglobin A, trace hemoglobin A2, and a fast moving band.
What is her most likely diagnosis?
A. Alpha thalassemia silent carrier
B. Alpha thalassemia trait
C. Hemoglobin H disease
D. Hydrops fetalis

41. Hepcidin is known to be one of the major regulators of iron absorption.
In which of the following conditions would hepcidin levels be expected to be elevated?
A. Hypoxia
B. Hereditary hemochromatosis (HH)
C. Iron deficiency anemia (IDA)
D. B12 deficiency
E. Chronic infection

42. A 40-year-old otherwise healthy Caucasian man is noted to have an elevated ferritin on routine laboratory screening. Laboratory studies are repeated and confirm ferritin 800 ng/mL (normal 25–400 ng/mL) and iron saturation 80% (normal 20%–55%). Hgb is 15 g/dL (normal 13.5–17.5 g/dL). His father died of nonalcoholic cirrhosis.

What is the most appropriate next step in obtaining a diagnosis?
A. T2* MRI of the liver
B. Liver biopsy
C. HFE mutation testing
D. Hepcidin level
E. Thyroid studies

43. A 19-year-old Caucasian man is referred for management of recently diagnosed severe iron overload. In the last year he has been diagnosed with heart failure, diabetes, and sexual dysfunction. Workup of these conditions eventually led to the diagnosis of iron overload. He has no family history of any of these conditions.

Laboratory studies are as follows:

Serum iron	187 µg/dL
Serum TIBC	210 µg/dL
Transferrin saturation	89%
Serum ferritin	2127 µg/L
AST	58 U/L
ALT	89 U/L

On genetic analysis, which of the following is most likely to be detected?
A. Homozygous C282Y mutation (C282Y/C282Y) in HFE gene
B. Homozygous H63D mutation (H63D/H63D) in HFE gene
C. Mutation in transferrin receptor 2 gene (TFR2)
D. Mutation in hemojuvelin gene (HJV)
E. Mutation in ferroportin gene (SLC401A)

44. A 23-year-old woman with sickle cell anemia (Hb SS) and prior ischemic stroke at age 16 has been maintained on a chronic transfusion program. She has never received treatment for iron overload. She takes folic acid daily and oxycodone as needed. She is planning to go to college and will be staying in a dorm and states she will continue transfusions, but will only accept additional therapies if they are oral and minimally affect her daily routine.

Laboratory studies are as follows:

Hemoglobin	8.3 g/dL
Hematocrit	25%
Platelet count	195,000/µL
Leucocyte count	8890/µL
Ferritin	2545/µg/L
Serum creatinine	0.7 mg/dL
Serum electrolytes	Normal
Liver function tests	Mild elevation of AST and ALT

Which of the following is the most appropriate recommendation for treatment of her iron overload?
A. Deferoxamine
B. Simple phlebotomy
C. Deferasirox
D. No treatment
E. Deferiprone

45. A 43-year-old gardener is referred for evaluation of blistering skin lesions over the palms of his hands. He wears short-sleeved shirts and spends much of the day working in the sun. He takes no medications and consumes two beers each day. He has no other current complaints and denies any history of abdominal pain or psychiatric disorders. Physical examination of the skin is shown in Fig. 34.1.

A complete blood count is normal. Iron studies and hepatitis testing are shown below (reference values in parenthesis):

Serum iron	195 µg/dL (normal, 42–135 µg/dL)
Serum TIBC	369 µg/dL (normal, 225–430 µg/dL)
Transferrin saturation	51% (normal, 20%–50%)
Serum ferritin	420 ng/mL (normal, 30–400 ng/mL)
AST	65 U/L
ALT	83 U/L
Chronic hepatitis testing:	Negative
HIV	Negative

Which of the following diagnostic tests should be ordered next?
A. Urine studies for porphobilinogen (PBG)
B. Urine studies for aminolevulinic acid (ALA)
C. HFE genotyping
D. Red cell enzyme levels of porphobilinogen (PBG) deaminase
E. Stool coproporphyrin

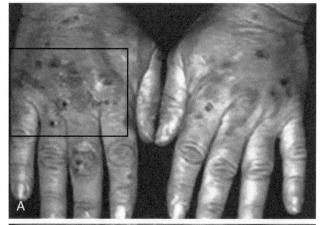
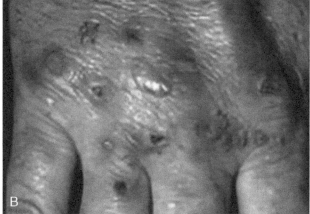

FIG. 34.1

46. A 28-year-old otherwise healthy woman presents to the emergency room with complaints of right arm weakness for 1 week followed by progressive leg weakness. She also describes progressive shortness of breath, as well as abdominal pain and constipation with associated dark urine. She has experienced severe, debilitating abdominal pain in the past without an etiology identified. She reports her symptoms are worse around the time of her menses. On examination she is tachypnic, and weakness is evident in the upper and lower extremities. She is agitated, and her family reports that she has been confused. She experiences a seizure while in the emergency room.
Which of the following laboratory tests should be performed initially to confirm your diagnostic suspicion?
A. Urine porphobilinogen (PBG)
B. Urine coproporphyrin
C. Erythrocyte porphobilinogen deaminase (PBGD)
D. Erythrocyte delta aminolevulinic acid dehydratase (ALAD)
E. Urine uroporphyrins

47. A 34-year-old female in her 26th week of gestation is evaluated for severe anemia. Her pregnancy has been complicated by severe nausea leading to intermittent dehydration. She has also developed gestational diabetes. She complains of dyspnea on exertion, but has no chest pain or shortness of breath. She is able to perform her activities of daily living. She has no other health problems. The fetus is developing normally. Medications include folic acid, multivitamins, and iron sulfate 325 mg once daily, which she takes intermittently when her nausea improves. She is normotensive, and her examination is otherwise unremarkable.
Laboratory data:

Hemoglobin	7.5 g/dL
Hematocrit	23%
MCV	67 fL
Platelet count	465,000 × 10⁹/L
Leukocyte count	7858 × 10⁹/L
Serum creatinine	0.5 mg/dL
Serum electrolytes	Normal
Liver function tests	Normal
Serum iron	15 µg/dL (normal, 42–135 µg/dL)
Serum TIBC	499 µg/dL (normal, 225–430 µg/dL)
Transferrin saturation	3% (normal, 20%–50%)
Serum ferritin	8 ng/mL (normal, 30–400 ng/mL)

Which of the following would you recommend at this time?
A. Erythroid stimulating agent (ESA)
B. Intravenous iron sucrose
C. Oral ferrous sulfate increased to 3 times daily
D. Two units PRBC
E. Oral ferrous gluconate 3 times daily

48. An 82-year-old man with multiple medical problems has severe anemia. His medical history is significant for oxygen dependent COPD, stage IV congestive heart failure with an EF of 20%, a mechanical mitral valve placed 12 years ago, and poorly controlled diabetes mellitus. Up until the last 3 months, he was able to ambulate with a walker and to independently perform his ADLs. Since that time he has mostly been confined to the couch and the bed. His

medications include furosemide, carvedilol, warfarin, and insulin. On examination he appears frail. He is normotensive and has a heart rate of 86 bpm. He has a III/VI systolic ejection murmur over his mitral area. His lung sounds are diminished.
Laboratory data:

Hemoglobin	7.8 g/dL
Hematocrit	25%
MCV	77 fL
Platelet count	465,000 × 10⁹/L
Leukocyte count	4859 × 10⁹/L
Serum creatinine	1.2 mg/dL
AST/ALT	Normal
Serum iron	35 µg/dL (normal, 42–135 µg/dL)
Serum TIBC	469 µg/dL (normal, 225–430 µg/dL)
Transferrin saturation	7% (normal, 20%–50%)
Serum ferritin	23 ng/mL (normal, 30–400 ng/mL)
Haptoglobin	<10 mg/dL
LDH	1234 U/L
Bilirubin	3.8 mg/dL
Bilirubin, direct	0.3 mg/dL

Review of the blood smear reveals 2–3 schistocytes per HPF, hypochromic and microcytic red blood cells.
Echocardiogram: EF 20%, LVH, regurgitant jet around the mitral valve, mitral regurgitation.
Which of the following is the best recommendation for initial treatment?
A. Iron replacement
B. Mitral valve replacement
C. Erythroid stimulating agent (ESA)
D. Therapeutic plasma exchange
E. Eculizumab

49. A 34-year-old man has developed fevers, chills, and sweats over the last month. Despite a good appetite, his weight has decreased 10 pounds. He denies chest pain or shortness of breath and continues to work as an electrician. He has no prior medical history. He admits to a history of frequent intravenous drug use. He is on no medications. Temperature is 38.5°C, blood pressure is 134/65, and heart rate is 95 bpm. Examination is otherwise unremarkable except for needle track marks on his left arm. Blood cultures drawn in the ED are growing methicillin-resistant *Staphylococcus aureus*, and intravenous vancomycin has been started.
Laboratory data are shown below:

Hemoglobin	10.1 g/dL
Hematocrit	30%
MCV	79 fL
Platelet count	235,000 × 10⁹/L
Leucocyte count	8761 × 10⁹/L
Serum creatinine	0.9 mg/dL
AST/ALT	Normal
Serum iron	25 µg/dL (normal, 42–135 µg/dL)
Serum TIBC	169 µg/dL (normal, 225–430 µg/dL)
Transferrin saturation	15% (normal, 20%–50%)
Serum ferritin	439 ng/mL (normal, 30–400 ng/mL)
HIV	Negative
Hepatitis screen	Negative

In addition to continuing antibiotics, which of the following is the best management for his anemia?
A. Erythropoietin stimulating agents (ESA)
B. Two-unit blood transfusion
C. Intravenous iron
D. Repeat CBC in 2–4 weeks
E. Oral iron

50. A 48-year-old man is sent to you for evaluation of anemia. He has been depressed since the unexpected death of his wife 6 months ago. He has been absent from work quite a bit, and his children describe him as being very withdrawn and infrequently leaving the house. He admits to moderate alcohol intake. He has lost 20 pounds over the last 6 months. He appears solemn and disheveled, but physical examination is otherwise unremarkable. The following laboratory data are available:

	Current	6 Months Ago	Reference Values
Hb (males)	10.1 g/dL	14.6 g/dL	12–16 g/dL
Hct (males)	33%	45%	36%–48%
MCV	115 fL	93 fL	80–100 fL
WBC	5.0 K × 10⁹/L	6.8 K × 10⁹/L	4500–10,500 × 10⁹/L
Platelet count	152 K/µL	347 K/µL	150,000–450,000 × 10⁹/L
Reticulocyte count	1.7%	NA	0.5%–1.8%
Methylmalonic acid	Normal	NA	—
Homocysteine	Pending	NA	—

What test should be ordered next in the evaluation of his anemia?
A. B12 level
B. Folate level
C. Bone marrow biopsy
D. Copper level
E. Chromosomal fragility studies

51. A 75-year-old Caucasian man presents for his annual physical examination. He is noted to have pallor of the skin and conjunctiva. Neurologic exam is significant for bilateral distal lower extremity neuropathy with loss of vibration sense and weakness.
Laboratory data is provided below:

White blood cell count	3500 × 10⁹/L
Hemoglobin	9 g/dL
Hematocrit	27%
Platelet	115,000 × 10⁹/L
MCV	116

Which of the following is the most likely diagnosis?
A. Anemia of renal disease
B. Aplastic anemia
C. B12 deficiency
D. Folate deficiency
E. Iron deficiency anemia

52. A 48-year-old man is referred for evaluation of a macrocytic anemia. He has noted a 10-pound weight loss in the last year with periodic fevers and night sweats. He has no prior medical history, takes no medications, and denies ETOH or tobacco use. His physical examination is only significant for mild cyanosis of his fingertips.

Laboratory data:

Hemoglobin	9.8 g/dL
Hematocrit	30%
MCV	151 fL
Platelet count	165,000/µL
Leucocyte count	4761/µL

A blood smear is being prepared for review.
Which of the following tests is most likely to lead to the correct diagnosis?
A. ETOH level
B. Vitamin B12
C. TSH
D. Folate
E. Direct Coombs test

53. A 64-year-old woman has developed fatigue and shortness of breath over the prior 2 months. She was previously well and took no medications.
On physical examination, her temperature is 36.8°C, blood pressure is 134/58, and pulse rate is 112. Pallor is noted. Cardiopulmonary examination is normal. There is no lymphadenopathy. The spleen is palpable 3 cm below the left costal margin. Hepatomegaly is absent. The remainder of the physical examination is normal.
Laboratory data:

Hemoglobin	5.8 g/dL
Hematocrit	17%
MCV	104 fL
Platelet count	210,000 × 10⁹/L
Leukocyte count	5671 × 10⁹/L
Reticulocyte count	0.1%
Absolute reticulocyte count	2000 × 10⁹/L

High power view of the blood smear is shown in Fig. 34.2.
What test would most likely identify the cause for the severe anemia?
A. CT scan of the neck and chest
B. T-cell receptor gene rearrangement
C. PCR for parvovirus DNA
D. Bone marrow cytogenetics
E. HIV testing

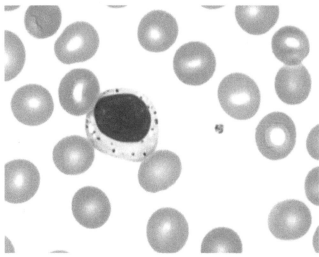

FIG. 34.2 Peripheral smear for patient in question 53.

54. A 48-year-old man with advanced cirrhosis is admitted to the hospital with encephalopathy. His health has been declining over the last 2 years, and he has had several admissions for encephalopathy and ascites. He has been noted to have worsening anemia. Currently he is confused, but afebrile with normal vital signs. He has obvious stigmata of end-stage liver disease. Splenomegaly is noted on examination. There has been no recent alcohol consumption.
Laboratory data:

	Patient Result (Now)	Patient Result (1 Year Ago)	Reference Values
Hbg	7.1 g/dL	11.6 g/dL	12–16 g/dL
Hct	22%	33%	36%–48%
MCV	106 fL	94 fL	80–100 fL
WBC	4000×10^9/L	6100×10^9/L	$4500–10,500 \times 10^9$/L
Platelet count	$92,000 \times 10^9$/L	$176 K \times 10^9$/L	$150,000–450,000 \times 10^9$/L
Reticulocyte count	6.7%	2.8%	0.5%–1.8%

Peripheral blood smear is shown in Fig. 34.3.
Which of the following treatments would be most successful in treatment of his worsening anemia?
A. Rituximab
B. Splenectomy
C. IVIg
D. Prednisone
E. Liver transplantation

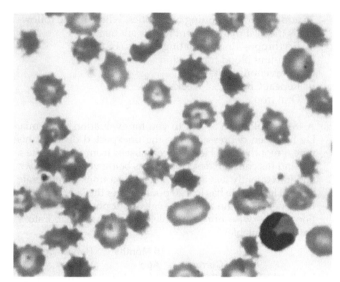

FIG. 34.3 Peripheral smear for patient in question 54.

55. A 16-year-old boy has been referred to hematology for moderate chronic anemia. He was first noted to be anemic at age 9, but had no further evaluation. He has never received a blood transfusion. He is fatigued and has not been able to keep up with his peers in athletic activities, but has been able to attend school and work a part-time job.
Laboratory studies:

Hemoglobin	7.9 g/dL
Hematocrit	24%
MCV	78 fL
Platelet count	175,000/µL
Leucocyte count	5261/µL
Serum creatinine	0.8 mg/dL
AST/ALT	Normal
Transferrin saturation	50% (normal, 20%–50%)
Ferritin	634 ng/mL

Genetic analysis:
No mutations noted in the HFE gene
Mutation noted in the erythroid-specific 5-aminolevulinate synthase (ALAS2) gene
A Prussian blue stain on a bone marrow aspirate specimen is shown in Fig. 34.4.
Which of the following treatments would is most appropriate for initial therapy?
A. Bone marrow transplantation
B. Therapeutic phlebotomy
C. Vitamin B6
D. Zinc
E. Azacytidine

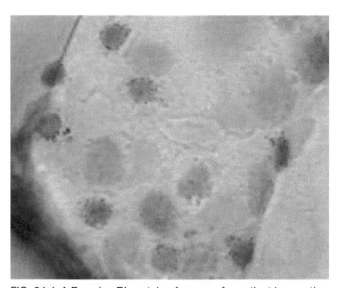

FIG. 34.4 A Prussian Blue stain of marrow for patient in question 55.

is 81/46, and heart rate is 112 bpm. She has poor dentition, thin hair, dry skin, and puffy cheeks. There is no hepatosplenomegaly or lymphadenopathy.
Laboratory studies:

Hemoglobin	8.8 g/dL
Hematocrit	24%
MCV	88 fL
Platelet count	65,000/µL
Leucocyte count	961/µL
ANC	781/µL

Bone marrow biopsy shows the following (Fig. 34.5):
Which of the following is the most appropriate management at this time?
A. PRBC transfusion
B. Platelet transfusion
C. G-CSF
D. Psychiatric referral
E. Bone marrow transplant referral

56. An 18-year-old woman is evaluated for pancytopenia. She appears withdrawn and does not answer many questions. On examination her weight is 42 kg, blood pressure

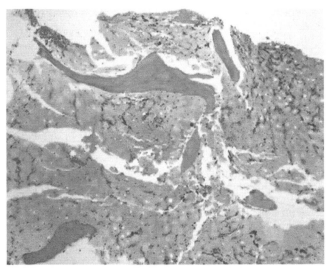

FIG. 34.5 A marrow biopsy for patient in question 56.

57. A 71-year-old woman is evaluated for anemia. In the last 6 months she has noted fatigue, cold intolerance, and increasing constipation. She eats a normal diet consisting of meats, grains, fruits, and vegetables. She takes no medications and denies the use of alcohol. Blood pressure is 164/88, heart rate is 42 bpm, and she is afebrile. On examination she has dry skin. There is no hepatosplenomegaly or lymphadenopathy. A CBC 1 year ago was normal. Review of the peripheral blood smear is unremarkable.
Current laboratory data:

Hemoglobin	10.3 g/dL
Hematocrit	31%
MCV	107 fL
Platelet count	155,000 × 10⁹/L
Leukocyte count	5643 × 10⁹/L
Serum creatinine	0.9 mg/dL
AST/ALT	Normal
Reticulocyte	1.1%
Absolute reticulocyte count	33,000/µL
LDH	194 U/L
Bilirubin	0.8 mg/dL
Vitamin B12	756 pg/mL

What test would most likely identify the cause of the anemia?
A. Thyroid function tests
B. Folate
C. Bone marrow aspirate and biopsy
D. Methylmalonic acid
E. Direct Coombs

58. A patient with advanced human immunodeficiency virus (HIV) infection is referred for evaluation of anemia. She has been compliant with "triple HIV therapy," but her last CD4 count remained low at 39/µL. A high viral load was also detected. She has been complaining of periodic fevers, sweats, and a 20-pound weight loss for the last 3 months. Additional medications include trimethoprim sulfamethoxazole, fluconazole, and pantoprazole, none of which were started within in the last year. On examination, she appears chronically ill and is febrile at 101.5°C. Examination is otherwise unremarkable.
Laboratory evaluation:

Hemoglobin	9.3 g/dL
Hematocrit	28%
MCV	104 fL
Platelet count	151,000 × 10⁹/L

Leucocyte count	4231 × 10⁹/L
Serum creatinine	0.5 mg/dL
AST/ALT	Normal
Reticulocyte	1.7%
Absolute reticulocyte count	45,000 × 10⁹/L
LDH	204 U/L
Bilirubin	0.8 mg/dL
Vitamin B12	756 pg/mL
Folic acid	Normal

Peripheral blood smear shows tear drop cells and nucleated red blood cells. No early myeloid cells are appreciated.
Which of the following is the next best step in the evaluation of this patient?
A. ADAMTS-13
B. Osmotic fragility test
C. Direct Coombs test
D. Bone marrow aspirate and biopsy
E. G-6PD level

59. You are preparing a lecture for your medical school's second year hematology course on human hemoglobin structure and function.
Which of the following would be accurate information to include in your lecture?
A. A shift to the left of the hemoglobin-oxygen dissociation curve reflects decreased oxygen affinity.
B. At birth fetal hemoglobin (Hb F, α2γ2) represents less than 10% of total hemoglobin.
C. Fetal hemoglobin has higher oxygen affinity than does adult hemoglobin.
D. Hb A2 (α2δ2) is elevated in alpha thalassemia.
E. Two copies of the beta globin gene and a single copy of the alpha globin gene exist on their respective chromosomes.

60. A 35-year-old African-American woman is referred for evaluation of refractory iron deficiency anemia. She has been treated with oral iron intermittently for the last 10 years. She denies menorrhagia or melena. Her physical exam is normal.
Laboratory data is provided below:

WBC	5.5 µL (normal 4–10 µL)
Hemoglobin	12 g/dL (normal 13.8–17.2 g/dL)
Hematocrit	36% (normal)
Platelets	Normal
MCV	70 fL (normal 80–96 fL)
RBC	6.2 million (normal 4–5.2 million)
RDW	Normal

Which of the following is the most likely diagnosis?
A. Iron deficiency anemia
B. Alpha-thalassemia carrier (−α/αα)
C. Alpha-thalassemia trait (−α/−α)
D. Beta-thalassemia major (β⁰/β⁰)
E. Anemia of chronic inflammation

61. A 28-year-old Asian woman seeks care for a moderate chronic anemia. She is unaware of her definitive diagnosis and has required three transfusions throughout her life. Her mother, father, and brother have mild anemia. On physical examination mild splenomegaly is noted.
Laboratory studies:

Hemoglobin	7.8 g/dL
Hematocrit	24%
MCV	64 fL
Platelet count	146,000/µL
Leucocyte count	4981/µL
Reticulocyte	4.7%
Absolute reticulocyte count	150,000/µL

Peripheral blood smear shows target cells and microcytic red blood cells with occasional inclusion bodies.

Hemoglobin electrophoresis results: Hb A 75% and 22% of a band to be determined.

What is the most likely diagnosis?

A. B-thalassemia major (Cooley anemia)
B. Alpha-thalassemia minor
C. Hb H disease
D. B-thalassemia minor
E. Hydrops fetalis

62. A 43-year-old Greek woman presents for evaluation of anemia. She had been diagnosed with anemia many years ago and had been placed on oral iron on multiple occasions. She has never required a blood transfusion. She complains of mild fatigue but is otherwise asymptomatic. There is no hepatosplenomegaly.
Laboratory studies:

Hemoglobin	11.3 g/dL
Hematocrit	34%
MCV	71 fL
Platelet count	296,000/μL
Leucocyte count	8231 × 10⁹/L
Reticulocyte	2.9%

Peripheral blood smear shows target cells and microcytic red blood cells.
Hemoglobin electrophoresis reveals:

Hb A	91%
Hb A2	6%
Hb F	3%

What is the most likely diagnosis?

A. Beta-thalassemia major
B. Alpha-thalassemia trait
C. Alpha-thalassemia minor
D. Beta-thalassemia minor
E. Hereditary persistence of fetal hemoglobin

63. A 26-year-old woman with Hb S-beta⁺ thalassemia is currently 13 weeks gestation in her first pregnancy and was admitted to the hospital for a typical painful crisis. Her history is significant for an episode of acute chest syndrome 2 years ago, chronic pain, and hospital admissions for acute painful episodes 1–2 times annually. She has never had a stroke. She has received packed red blood cell transfusion on four occasions. Outpatient medications include folic acid and a prenatal vitamin. She is prescribed oxycodone, which she requires occasionally for more severe pain. On physical examination, temperature is 37.8°C (98.4°F), blood pressure is 113/69 mm Hg, pulse rate is 108/min, and respiratory rate is 12/min. She is sitting up in the bed with her hands over her face and complaining of pain. She has mild scleral icterus.
Laboratory studies:

Hemoglobin	10.1 g/dL
Leukocyte count	5230 × 10⁹/L
Platelet count	349,000 × 10⁹/L
Mean corpuscular volume	76 fL
Total bilirubin	1.9 mg/dL
Direct bilirubin	0.8 mg/dL
Ferritin	668 ng/mL
Type and screen	O+ with no alloantibodies
CXR	No infiltrates
Urinalysis	Negative

Which of the following would you recommend at this time?

A. Hydroxyurea
B. Narcotic analgesia
C. Deferoxamine
D. PRBC
E. Antibiotic

64. A 28-year-old man is noted to be anemic on a pre-employment examination. His prior history is remarkable for multiple episodes of bone pain as a child, which were thought secondary to rapid growth. He does take NSAIDs frequently for joint aches and pains. He was treated for pneumonia at ages 8 and 18. He has no other prior medical history and takes no other medications. He denies alcohol, tobacco, and illicit drug use. His mother is known to have mild microcytic anemia; his father is healthy and has a normal CBC. His brother is known to have sickle cell trait.
The pre-employment CBC is as follows:

WBC	5100 × 10⁹/L
Hb	10.4 g/dL
Hematocrit	31%
Platelet	238,000 × 10⁹/L
MCV	68 fL
Reticulocyte count	3.8%
Absolute reticulocyte count	125,000 × 10⁹/L

Which of the following results on hemoglobin electrophoresis would be most consistent with this patient's clinical and laboratory data (Fig. 34.6)?

	Hb S (%)	Hb F (%)	Hb A2 (%)	Hb A (%)
A.	97	2	1	0
B.	49	3	0	58
C.	87	6	7	0
D.	68	4	5	27
E.	0	3	2	95

65. A 20-year-old woman with Hb SS will be transitioning to an adult hematology practice. Her history includes frequent vasoocclusive pain crisis, iron overload, and avascular necrosis of the left hip. She has received a moderate amount of red blood cell transfusion throughout her life. Medications include MS Contin 30 mg twice daily, oxycodone 5 mg prn, deferasirox 1500 mg daily, and lisinopril 5 mg daily. She is afebrile; her blood pressure is 105/56 and

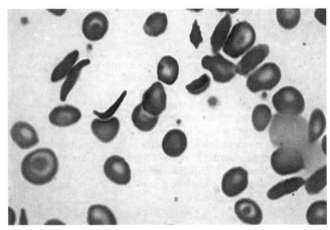

FIG. 34.6 Photo used with permission: Dr. Neil Harris. Department of Pathology, University of Florida.

heart rate 76 bpm. Mild scleral icterus is noted. She states that her pain is reasonably well controlled on her current regimen, but she had seven ED visits and was admitted to the hospital 5 times in the last year.

Laboratory data:

Hemoglobin	7.3 g/dL
Leukocyte count	7453 × 10⁹/L
Platelet count	284,000 × 10⁹/L
Mean corpuscular volume	85 fL
Ferritin	788 ng/mL
Urinalysis	Trace protein
Creatinine	0.8 mg/dL
LFTs	Normal

Your recommendations at this time include:
A. Start monthly partial manual red blood cell exchange
B. Start hydroxyurea
C. Start penicillin prophylaxis
D. Stop Lisinopril
E. Stop MS Contin

66. A 24-year-old male with hemoglobin SS is seen in the emergency room for a sustained painful erection lasting over 6 hours. He reports similar episodes in the past that have been managed successfully at home with warm compress and massage. This is the first time he has had to come to the ED for this complaint. He denies other complications of his sickle cell anemia except for occasional pain crisis typically managed at home with oral NSAIDs and opioid analgesia. He has no history of stroke, acute chest syndrome, or pulmonary hypertension.

Laboratory studies:

Hemoglobin	7.9/dL
Leukocyte count	8953 × 10⁹/L
Platelet count	164,000 × 10⁹/L
Mean corpuscular volume	85 fL
Creatinine	0.6 mg/dL

In addition to fluids, narcotic analgesia, and oxygen, which of the following is the best management?
A. Penile aspiration and irrigation
B. PRBC simple transfusion
C. Penile distal shunt
D. PRBC exchange transfusion
E. Hydroxyurea

67. A 20-year-old woman with hemoglobin SS presents to your clinic after being discharged from the hospital. She was admitted for a vasooclussive pain episode and required IV narcotics for pain management. She has been admitted to the hospital 5 times this year for pain management and was diagnosed with acute chest syndrome during a previous hospital admission. Her outpatient pain management regimen includes both short- and long-acting opioids. She takes folic acid daily and is up-to-date on all of her health maintenance. Which of the following medications should be considered at this time?
A. Aspirin
B. Multivitamin
C. Vitamin D
D. Hydroxyurea
E. Vitamin B12

68. A 21-year-old woman is referred for evaluation for anemia. She reports being easily fatigued for much of her life, but her symptoms have worsened since beginning college. She has never sought medical attention for these complaints. Her only medication is a daily multivitamin. Her family history is significant for a sister who had a

cholecystectomy at age 24 and a mother who has had life-long anemia. On physical examination she has mild scleral icterus and a spleen tip that is palpated 3 cm below the costal margin.

Laboratory data:

Hemoglobin	9.1 g/dL
Leukocyte count	4530/μL
Platelet count	169,000/μL
Mean corpuscular volume	106 fL
Reticulocyte count	5%
Total bilirubin	2.4 mg/dL
Direct bilirubin	0.8 mg/dL
LDH	743 IU/mL

Peripheral blood smear is shown in Fig. 34.7.
Which protein is most likely to be abnormal in this patient?
A. Phosphatidylinositol glycan
B. Ankyrin
C. Rhesus D (Rh D)
D. Pyruvate kinase
E. Glucose-6 phosphate dehydrogenase (G-6PD)

69. A 21-year-old man with a known history of hereditary spherocytosis is seen in the emergency room for a 1-week history of increased lethargy, fatigue, and low-grade fevers. He does not recall any sick contacts, but works full-time in a daycare facility. He has no pets and denies recent travel. He is compliant with folic acid 2.5 mg daily. His baseline hemoglobin is 10–11 g/dL. On examination he is afebrile and has pale sclera. His BP is 105/65 and heart rate is 112 bpm. There is no lymphadenopathy. The spleen tip is palpated two finger breadths below the costal margin.

Laboratory studies:

Hemoglobin	4.2 g/dL
Hematocrit	13%
MCV	95 fL
WBC count	4900 × 10⁹/L
Platelet count	164,000 × 10⁹/L
Reticulocyte count	0.1%

In addition to the consideration of a blood transfusion, which of the following should be recommended?
A. Splenectomy
B. Acyclovir
C. Supportive care
D. IVIg
E. Prednisone

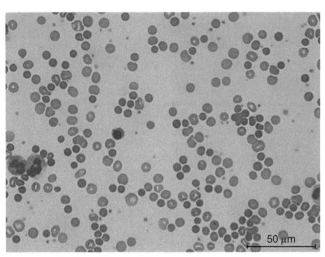

FIG. 34.7 Peripheral smear for patient in question 68.

70. An 18-year-old African-American man was diagnosed with acute lymphocytic leukemia (ALL). Aggressive hydration and rasburicase was started prior to beginning combination chemotherapy. Five days after initiating chemotherapy he developed yellowing of his eyes, and on CBC his anemia had worsened. Further laboratory evaluation revealed a low haptoglobin, an increase in LDH, and an increased indirect bilirubin. A G6PD level sent 72 hours after these events was normal. The patient went on to finish his first induction cycle without incident. A recovery bone marrow biopsy last week showed no residual disease. His PMH is unremarkable except for a similar episode of jaundice at age 14 while taking trimethoprim-sulfamethoxazole for a URI. Family history is unremarkable.

Current laboratory data 3 weeks after induction chemotherapy:

Hemoglobin	12.1 g/dL
Leukocyte count	3930 × 10⁹/L
Platelet count	149,000 × 10⁹/L
Mean corpuscular volume	89 fL
Reticulocyte count	1.8%
Total bilirubin	0.9 mg/dL
Direct bilirubin	0.5 mg/dL
LDH	193 IU/mL

Review of the peripheral blood smear reveals no blasts and normal red blood cell and platelet morphology.

What is the most likely etiology for the episode of acute hemolytic anemia during induction chemotherapy?

A. Autoimmune hemolytic anemia
B. Hereditary spherocytosis
C. Hemolytic uremic syndrome
D. G6PD deficiency
E. Cold agglutinin disease

71. A 21-year-old African-American man is diagnosed with a urinary tract infection, which is treated with trimethoprim-sulfamethaxazole. Approximately 1 week after initiating antibiotics he presents with jaundice, scleral icterus, and anemia. Additional labs are ordered, including haptoglobin (low), LDH (elevated), and indirect bilirubin (increased). Supravital stain on the peripheral blood smear confirms the presence of Heinz bodies.

What is the mode of inheritance of the most likely cause for his clinical and laboratory presentation?

A. X-linked recessive
B. X-linked dominant
C. Autosomal dominant
D. Autosomal recessive
E. Sporadic mutations

72. A 19-year-old woman is referred for further evaluation of anemia. She has been known to be anemic since childhood but has never had a proper evaluation. She reports becoming fatigued with moderate exertion but has been able to participate in athletics and has been successful in school. She is on no medications and denies alcohol or drug use. She has no family history of anemia. Her spleen tip is palpable 2 cm below the costal margin.

Laboratory data:

Hemoglobin	10.1 g/dL
Leukocyte count	5340 × 10⁹/L
Platelet count	189,000 × 10⁹/L
Mean corpuscular volume	103 fL
Reticulocyte count	3.8%

Absolute reticulocyte count	144,000 × 10⁹/L
Total bilirubin	2.1 mg/dL
Direct bilirubin	0.6 mg/dL
LDH	643 IU/mL
Hemoglobin electrophoresis	Normal
Direct Coombs test	Negative

Peripheral blood smear (Fig. 34.8):
What is the most likely diagnosis?
A. G-6PD deficiency
B. Hereditary spherocytosis
C. Autoimmune hemolytic anemia
D. Alpha-thalassemia
E. Pyruvate kinase deficiency

73. A 34-year-old Caucasian woman with rheumatoid arthritis is sent for evaluation of new onset anemia. She recently presented to her primary care physician complaining of fatigue, dark urine, and yellowing of her skin. A CBC 1 year ago was normal. On examination she has scleral icterus, jaundice, and a spleen palpated 2 cm below the costal margin.

Laboratory data:

Hemoglobin	7.9 g/dL
Leukocyte count	7678 × 10⁹/L
Platelet count	204,000 × 10⁹/L
Mean corpuscular volume	106 fL
Reticulocyte count	6.8%
Total bilirubin	2.3 mg/dL
Direct bilirubin	0.5 mg/dL
LDH	876 IU/mL

Peripheral blood smear reveals: spherocytes, macrovalocytes, and normal white blood cell and platelet morphology. A Coombs test is sent.

Which of the following is the most likely result on the Coombs test?

	IgG	Complement
A.	−	−
B.	+++	+
C.	Not interpretable	Not interpretable
D.	−	++

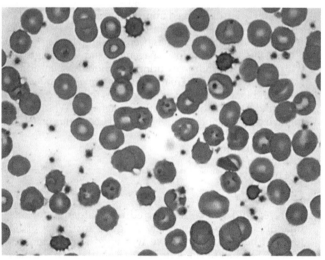

FIG. 34.8 Photo used with permission: Dr. Neil Harris. Dept. of Pathology, University of Florida. Pyruvate kinase deficiency.

74. A 65-year-old woman with CLL presents with worsening fatigue and dyspnea on exertion. She was recently treated with fludarabine, cyclophosphamide, and rituximab (FCR) for disease progression. On physical exam she is pale and has scleral icterus. She is normotensive and has a heart rate of 85 bpm. Her spleen tip is palpable 3 cm below the costal margin. Laboratory data are provided below:

WBC	8500/μL
Hemoglobin	8.5 g/dL
Platelet	175,000/μL
Mean corpuscular volume	104 fL
Reticulocyte count	8.0%
Total bilirubin	4.0 mg/dL
Direct bilirubin	1.0 mg/dL
LDH	750 IU/mL

Review of the peripheral blood smear is significant for spherocytes, occasional reticulocytes, normal white blood cell morphology, and normal platelet morphology.
What is the most appropriate treatment?
A. PRBC transfusion
B. Prednisone
C. IVIg
D. Rituximab
E. Splenectomy

75. A 68-year-old man presents to the emergency department complaining of left-sided chest pain. An EKG reveals ST elevation in the anterior leads, and a cardiac catheterization subsequently reveals triple vessel disease. Emergent coronary artery bypass is recommended within the next 24 hours. The patient reports that he has felt poorly over the last few months with increasing fatigue and dyspnea on exertion. Laboratory studies reveal a macrocytic anemia with hemoglobin of 8.4 g/dL, MCV of 145 fL, and reticulocyte count of 5%. Peripheral blood smear is shown in Fig. 34.9.
A Coombs test is negative for IgG, but positive for C3.
In addition to consideration of blood transfusion, which of the following should be recommended?
A. Prednisone
B. Rituximab
C. Splenectomy
D. Plasmapheresis
E. Eculizumab

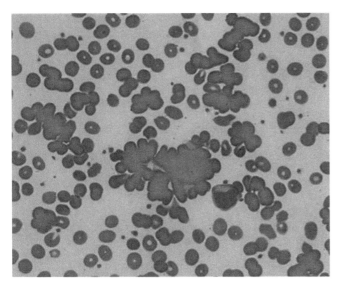

FIG. 34.9 Peripheral smear for patient in question 75.

76. A 75-year-old previously healthy woman complains of worsening fatigue and shortness of breath for the last month. She had previously been healthy and denied any recent illness or new medications. On physical examination she appears pale and is mildly dyspneic. No hepatosplenomegaly is appreciated.
Laboratory data are provided below:

WBC	5000/μL
Hemoglobin	8.0 g/dL
MCV	135 fL
Reticulocyte count	4%
Direct Coombs test	C3 +++, IgG –
SPEP	M spike 0.2 g/dL

What is the next most appropriate step in management?
A. Prednisone
B. Splenectomy
C. Rituximab
D. Erythropoietin
E. Fludarabine

77. A patient who presented with a symptomatic Coombs negative nonspherocytic hemolytic anemia and mild pancytopenia has recently been diagnosed with paroxysmal nocturnal hemoglobinuria (PNH). Eculizumab therapy is considered.
Which of the following is the most likely consequence of treatment with eculizumab in this patient?
A. Normalization of hemoglobin
B. Development of *Neisseria meningitidis*
C. Increase in the percentage of type III (totally deficient of GPI-linked proteins) cells
D. Thrombosis
E. Stabilization of LDH

78. A 25-year-old man presents with jaundice, pallor, and left lower extremity swelling. Ultrasound confirms the presence of a left popliteal DVT. Laboratory studies are consistent with a Coombs negative hemolytic anemia. FLAER testing confirms the diagnosis of paroxysmal nocturnal hemoglobinuria. Given the degree of hemolysis and concomitant thrombotic event, eculizumab therapy is considered.
Which of the following should this patient receive prior to initiating eculizumab?
A. *Neisseria meningitidis* vaccination
B. Haemophilus influenza type B vaccination
C. Hepatitis B series
D. Hepatitis A series
E. Varicella vaccination

79. A 34-year-old previously healthy man is admitted to the hospital with fatigue, abdominal pain, and mild confusion. Based on his laboratory studies (shown below), plasma exchange is initiated. After 5 days he feels a little better and is no longer confused. However, his labs show no significant improvement.

	Current Labs	Admission Labs
Hemoglobin	7.1 g/dL	7.5 g/dL
Leukocyte count	7543 × 10⁹/L	6545 × 10⁹/L
Platelet count	41,000 × 10⁹/L	38,000 × 10⁹/L
Reticulocyte count	3.8%	3.1%
Total bilirubin	4.1 mg/dL	3.6 mg/dL
Direct bilirubin	0.5 mg/dL	0.8 mg/dL

	Current Labs	Admission Labs
LDH	1023 IU/mL	1295 IU/mL
Creatinine	4.8 mg/dL	3.2 mg/dL
ADAMTS-13	NA	44%
Escherichia coli culture and shiga toxin	NA	Not detected
Blood smear	4–5 schistocytes/ per HPF	4–5 schistocytes/ per HPF

At this time, which is the most appropriate action?
A. Addition of rituximab
B. Switch to eculizumab
C. Increase to twice daily plasma exchange
D. Addition of prednisone
E. Continue plasma exchange, but switch to cryopoor plasma as replacement

80. A 45-year-old previously healthy woman presents to the emergency department complaining of fevers, weakness, and bleeding from her gums. Her medical history is significant for a recently resolved viral syndrome. Her family states she has been confused during the last 24 hours. Prior to your arrival she experiences a seizure.
Laboratory data are provided below:

WBC	$5600 \times 10^9/L$
Hemoglobin	5.3 g/dL
Platelet	$21,000 \times 10^9/L$
Creatinine	1.6 mg/dL
LDH	3000 U/L
Total bilirubin	3.2 mg/dL
Direct bilirubin	0.3 mg/dL
Haptoglobin	<10 mg/dL
Reticulocyte count	8%

Review of the peripheral blood smear confirms schistocytes, decreased platelets, and normal WBC morphology.
What is the most effective next step in the management of this patient?
A. Initiate plasmapheresis
B. Administer rituximab
C. Administer eculizumab
D. Transfuse 2 units FFP
E. Administer prednisone

81. A 22-year-old African-American man has Hgb-SS disease, which has been complicated by cholelithiasis requiring cholecystectomy; bilateral avascular necrosis of the femoral heads; two episodes of acute chest; and a stroke at 16 years of age, with minimal right-sided weakness. He was started on simple exchange transfusion, but due to nonadherence to oral iron chelation, the patient developed iron overload, characterized by a ferritin level of 2481 (11 - 209). As a result, he was transitioned to monthly erythrocytapheresis, with goal Hgb-S levels ≤50%. He has now transitioned to the Adult Hematology Clinic, and since he has experienced no recurrent episodes of stroke, he is now inquiring about stopping his monthly sessions of red cell exchange.
Given that he is now an adult, which of the following is the best recommendation?
A. Continue regular red cell exchange
B. Reduce the interval of red cell exchange to obtain a goal Hgb-S of ≤75%
C. Start hydroxyurea and titrate to maximally tolerated dose
D. Stop therapy all together

82. A 57-year-old African-American woman with hypertension, hyperlipidemia, gastroesophageal reflux disease, and hypothyroidism on replacement recently established care with a local primary care physician upon moving to a new area. At her initial visit, routine laboratory testing was performed, which included a CBC, complete metabolic panel, lipids, TSH, and an Hgb-A1c. This was remarkable for the following:

WBC	$5500 \times 10^9/L$
Hemoglobin	12.8 g/dL
Hematocrit	38%
MCV	72 fL
MCH	24.0 pg/cell
MCHC	33.5 g/dL
RDW	20.8 (11.5–14.5)
Platelets	$212,000 \times 10^9/L$
Reticulocyte%	1.53
Absolute reticulocytes	$82,500 \times 10^9/L$

She was referred to gastroenterology, who performed an EGD, colonoscopy, and video capsule endoscopy, all of which failed to show any masses, hemorrhagic sources, or any overt cause for her microcytosis. She is placed on oral iron supplementation, and after 3 months of therapy, her CBC and iron panel shows the following:

WBC	$4400 \times 10^9/L$
Hemoglobin	12.3 g/dL
Hematocrit	37.5%
MCV	73 (80–98) fL
MCH	23.8 pg/cell
MCHC	32.7 g/dL
RDW	21.4
Platelets	$214,000 \times 10^9/L$
Iron	78 µg/dL
TIBC	321 µg/dL
%Saturation	24%
Ferritin	178 ng/mL

The patient is sent to hematology for evaluation of an occult hemorrhagic diathesis. She mentions that her sister and mother were on chronic iron supplementation for iron deficiency anemia, and believes that her family does not absorb iron well. At her initial visit, a hemoglobin electrophoresis is performed and shows the following:

Hgb-A	97.5%
Hgb-A2	2.5%
Hgb-F	<1%

Which of the following laboratory tests will confirm the most likely diagnosis?
A. Bone marrow biopsy to show the presence of ringed sideroblasts
B. Copper level
C. Lead level
D. Sequencing of α-globin genes
E. Zinc level

83. A 65-year-old man presents to his family medicine physician with progressive fatigue, weakness, and dyspnea on exertion. On physical examination, he is noted to be pale, with pale conjunctiva. A CBC is performed and shows:

WBC	$9400 \times 10^9/L$
Hemoglobin	5.2 g/dL
Hematocrit	16.1%
MCV	101 fL
Platelets	$178,000 \times 10^9/L$
Reticulocyte%	6%
Absolute reticulocytes	$310,000 \times 10^9/L$

This is a marked decrease from prior CBC done 8 months previously, which showed a hemoglobin level of 15.4 g/dL. The patient is sent to the emergency room, where a type and screen is sent for transfusion. The blood bank requests additional time in obtaining an appropriate 2 units, as the cross-match is "positive" and a direct antiglobulin test shows 3+ IgG. Since this is going to take longer than expected, the patient is admitted to Medicine for further evaluation and treatment. Additional testing shows the following:

B12	48 pg/mL
Folate	>25.6 ng/mL
Haptoglobin	<10 mg/dL
Iron	62 µg/dL
Lactate dehydrogenase	698 U/L
Transferrin	234 mg/dL

A peripheral blood smear shows microspherocytes and polychromasia:
Which of the following is the most appropriate recommendation at this time?
A. Glucocorticoids
B. Rituximab
C. Transfusion warmed red cells
D. Splenectomy
E. Therapeutic plasma exchange

84. A 78-year-old Caucasian woman with osteoporosis, hypertension, glaucoma, and osteoarthritis is noted to have a progressive, albeit mild, anemia. There are no nutritional deficiencies, and her renal and thyroid functions are noted to be within the normal ranges. She has been sent to a rheumatologist, as she has also noted symptoms consistent with Reynaud phenomenon. Upon further examination, she reveals a slight decrease in her usual level of activity but is otherwise completely able to perform her activities of daily living. At the family's insistence, a consult is placed to hematology, where a hyperbilirubinemia and elevated LDH is noted, prompting a Coombs test. This shows deposition of C3, but not IgG. A cold agglutinin titer returns positive at 1:2560 (<1:20). Cold avoidance is recommended.
In addition, which of the following should be performed next for this patient?
A. Bone marrow biopsy
B. Flow cytometry for CD55/CD59 red cell expression
C. Cryoglobulin titers
D. Donath-Landsteiner antibody testing
E. Serum protein electrophoresis

85. A 67-year-old Caucasian man was admitted with jaundice and acute renal failure 21 months ago. During this admission, he underwent an extensive serologic evaluation, in which elevated serum iron levels were noted. Eventually he underwent genetic testing and was found to be homozygous for the *HFE* C282Y mutation. A liver biopsy showed iron deposition consistent with iron overload, and the patient was started on serial phlebotomy over the course of 5 months, wherein he reportedly reached his goal. His last ferritin was checked 1 month after reaching the goal ferritin level, and he has had no subsequent follow-up since that time. He denies any increase in skin pigmentation, uncontrolled diabetes, or metacarpal osteoarthralgias. There have been no signs consistent with cardiac dysfunction. He denies any chest pain or palpitations. There is no jaundice, ascites, or lower extremity edema.

A hematology consultation is obtained, and at this visit, the following laboratory values show:

WBC	7600 × 10⁹/L
Hemoglobin	15.4 g/dL
Hematocrit	42%
MCV	87 fL
Platelets	144,000 × 10⁹/L
Reticulocytes	1.54%
PT	11.3 sec
aPTT	24.9 sec
D-dimer	0.21
Iron	142 µg/dL
TIBC	285 µg/dL
Transferrin	211 µg/dL
%Saturation	50%
Ferritin	76 ng/mL
Total protein	8.0 mg/dL
Albumin	4.0 mg/dL
Total bilirubin	0.8 mg/dL
Alkaline phosphatase	40 mg/dL
AST	31 U/L
ALT	31 U/L
Alpha-fetoprotein	1.8 ng/mL
HAVAb	Nonreactive
HBsAg	Negative
HbsAb	Nonreactive
HCVAb	Nonreactive

Which of the following is the most appropriate recommendation at this time?
A. No phlebotomy at this time
B. Avoidance of raw seafood
C. Avoidance of iron containing supplements
D. Consuming black tea
E. All of the above

86. A 37-year-old Caucasian woman was noted to have a slight elevation in her transaminases. Further testing included an abdominal ultrasound that showed the presence of cholelithiasis, without evidence of cholecystitis or common bile duct obstruction, and the presence of splenomegaly, ~20 cm. In retrospect, the patient recalled that that she was told she had a "big spleen" many years earlier, which was apparently attributed to an episode of infectious mononucleosis. Given this history and the splenomegaly, she is referred to hematology due to a concern for lymphoma.
The patient denies any fevers, chills, sweats, night sweats, or weight loss. She does admit to increasing symptoms of early satiety and vague feelings of left-sided abdominal pain. She denies any left-shoulder pain. Otherwise, she is without complaints.
As part of her evaluation, a CBC with a differential and peripheral blood smear is ordered (Fig. 34.10) and shows the following:

WBC	8400 × 10⁹/L
Hemoglobin	12.1 g/dL
Hematocrit	34%
MCV	85 fL
MCH	31.7 pg/cell
MCHC	37.3 g/dL
RDW	17.1
Platelets	204,000 × 10⁹/L
Reticulocyte %	9.03
Absolute reticulocyte count	353,100 × 10⁹/L
LDH	191 U/L
DAT	Negative
Haptoglobin	212 mg/dL

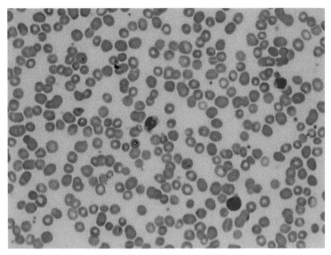

FIG. 34.10 Smear for patient in question 86.

Which of the following is the most appropriate test at this time ?
A. Bone marrow biopsy and flow cytometry
B. Cryoglobulins
C. Acidified serum test
D. Osmotic fragility
E. Serum protein electrophoresis

87. A 47-year-old woman with hypothyroidism on replacement therapy and seasonal allergies has developed progressive fatigue over the course of several months. When she presented to her primary care physician, a standard evaluation was remarkable for the following:

WBC	3400 × 10⁹/L
Hemoglobin	11.2 g/dL
Hematocrit	33.8%
MCV	104 fL
Platelets	151,000 × 10⁹/L
Reticulocyte %	0.8
Reticulocytes	30,000 × 10⁹/L
Iron	61 mcg/L
TIBC	345 mcg/L
%Saturation	26.6%
Ferritin	395 ng/mL
Folate	>25 ng/mL
B12	304 pg/mL
TSH	2.68 U/mL

She is sent to hematology for evaluation of her hypoproliferative anemia and possible bone marrow biopsy. Her referring physician notes that her CBC was normal 2 and 4 years ago during routine annual laboratory testing. However, because of a lapse in insurance, she does not keep her appointments. She is eventually able to keep her clinic visit several months later. At that time, she notes worsening fatigue, dyspnea on exertion, and a painful burning in her feet. Your physical examination is notable for a chronically ill-appearing, pale-appearing woman in mild distress. She had difficulty with walking and getting up on the exam table. You note that there is a loss of vibratory sensation of joint position.
Further laboratory testing shows the following:

WBC	2200 × 10⁹/L
Hemoglobin	8.9 g/dL
Hematocrit	27.1%
MCV	122 fL
Platelets	117,000 × 10⁹/L
Folate	>25 ng/mL

B12	280 pg/mL
TSH	3.57 U/mL
EtOH	Negative
AST	31 U/L
ALT	28 U/L
Total bilirubin	3.4 mg/dL
Total protein	6.9 mg/dL
Albumin	3.8 mg/dL
LDH	4498 U/L

Which of the following is the most appropriate next test to send?
A. Bone marrow biopsy
B. Methylmalonic acid
C. Paraneoplastic antibody panel
D. PET-CT to evaluate for a primary lung cancer
E. Sequencing of *TERT* and *TERC*

88. A 22-year-old African-American graduate student presents to student health for a possible urinary tract infection and is prescribed trimethoprim/sulfamethoxazole, for what is later shown to be pan-sensitive *Escherichia coli*. In addition, it is recommended that he take over-the-counter phenazopyridine. He completes his course of therapy without difficulty and notes symptomatic improvement in his urinary symptoms. However, he soon notes that the red-tinged urine has now become dark-colored, and he is fatigued with marked exercise intolerance. He returns to student health, where the following labs are noted:

WBC	13,100 × 10⁹/L
Hemoglobin	8.1 g/dL
Hematocrit	24.7%
MCV	101 fL
Platelets	239,000 × 10⁹/L
Reticulocyte %	7.8
Reticulocytes	436,000 × 10⁹/L
LDH	2761 U/L
DAT	Negative

He is sent to the emergency room for a blood transfusion, and hematology is consulted. The patient is a fatigued, pale-appearing gentleman who appears his stated age, with scleral icterus and pale conjunctiva. Review of his peripheral smears shows normal appear white cells, without any blasts. The red cells show marked anisopoikilocytosis, characterized by macrocytes that are polychromatic and rare nucleated red cells, along with "bite cells."
Which of the following is the most appropriate next step?
A. Methemoglobin level
B. G6PD level
C. Hexokinase level
D. P50
E. Supportive care

89. A 41-year-old African-American woman with a history of morbid obesity, status post gastric bypass maintained on an iron-containing multivitamin; GERD on PPI therapy; and psoriasis is sent for evaluation of a new onset microcytic anemia. She was referred back to her bariatric surgeon for evaluation for an anastomotic bleed, wherein none was noted on upper endoscopy. Fecal occult blood testing was negative, and she is sent to GI for colonoscopy, where only mild sigmoid diverticulosis is noted. Her iron supplementation is increased to ferrous sulfate 325 mg 3 times daily, but after 3 months of treatment, she

remains with a microcytic anemia. She adamantly denies noncompliance with her iron pills and is sent to hematology for further evaluation and treatment. Which of the following is the most appropriate recommendation at this time?

A. Continued use of ferrous sulfate, 325 mg TID

B. Continued use of ferrous sulfate, 325 mg TID, along with ascorbic acid 500 mg

C. Continued use of ferrous sulfate, 325 mg TID, ascorbic acid 500 mg TID, and stop the PPI

D. Infusion of iron dextran

E. Transfusion of red cells

90. A 24-year-old African-American woman with sickle cell disease is admitted for an acute vasoocclusive crisis. She had been in her usual state of health, when she developed joint pains consistent with her usual pain crises. She stayed home from work, where she is interning to obtain her teaching certificate, and tried her usual regimen of oral narcotics. When her pain threshold became greater than she could tolerate, she presented to the ER and was admitted for hydration and initiation of pain control with patient-controlled analgesia. Her admission labs are remarkable for the following:

WBC	14,200 × 10⁹/L
Hemoglobin	4.1 g/dL
Hematocrit	13.3%
MCV	86 fL
Platelets	589,000 × 10⁹/L
Reticulocyte %	0.5%
Absolute reticulocyte count	3000 × 10⁹/L

She is not transfused acutely. Her chest x-ray shows no infiltrates, and although her temperature is only 37.8°C, blood and urine cultures are drawn, and she is empirically started on ceftriaxone and azithromycin. Twenty-four hours after admission, she is noted to have a progressive increase in her oxygen requirement to the point where she has to be placed on 100% oxygen via a nonrebreather. A rapid-response is called, and she is transferred to the MICU, where hematology is consulted emergently for consideration of red cell exchange.

Which of the following is the most appropriate next step to diagnose the cause of her acute decompensation?

A. Bone marrow biopsy and aspiration

B. CT angiogram of the chest

C. Direct antiglobulin test

D. Donath-Landsteiner antibody

E. Parvovirus antibody titers

91. A 29-year-old African-American man with no significant past medical history, who is to hematology clinic for refractory iron deficiency anemia. He was married 2 years prior and is expecting his first child at the end of the year. He established primary care in order to obtain life and disability insurance, wherein CBC, lipid panel, liver function panel, and electrolytes were checked. This was remarkable for showing the following:

WBC	8500 × 10⁹/L
Hemoglobin	13.0 g/dL
Hematocrit	36%
MCV	61 fL
RDW	39.3
Platelets	425,000 × 10⁹/L

He is started empirically on iron replacement, and when his urease breath test is negative, he is sent to GI. Upper

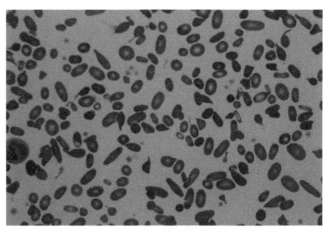

FIG. 34.11 Peripheral smear for patient in question 91.

and lower endoscopies show no abnormalities, and since the patient has noted no GI bleeding or abdominal pain, he does not keep his appointment for video capsule endoscopy. After 6 months of continued thrice-daily oral iron supplementation, there have been no appreciable changes to his CBC. His primary care physician suspects either intolerance or noncompliance with iron supplementation and sends him to clinic for additional treatment options.

On exam, he is a very pleasant man who appears his stated age in no apparent distress. There is no scleral icterus, palpable splenomegaly at least four finger breadths below the costal margin, and he remains guaiac-negative. Laboratory studies reveal the following:

Iron	60 mg/dL
TIBC	276 mg/dL
%Saturation	22%
Ferritin	39.1 ng/mL
Sickle prep	Negative

Hemoglobin electrophoresis migrates as normal Hgb-A and Hgb-A2.

Peripheral smear is as shown in Fig. 34.11.

Given the impending birth of his child, the patient asks for definitive testing to be performed.

Which of the following is the best test to perform in this circumstance?

A. α-Spectrin sequencing

B. β-Globin sequencing

C. Bone marrow biopsy

D. Osmotic fragility

E. Eosin-5-maleimide test

92. A 48-year-old Caucasian man with a history of hypertension, hyperlipidemia, and HIV-infection, with an undetectable viral load and most recent CD4 count of 584 presents for evaluation of macrocytosis. His HIV has been well controlled with zidovudine-lamivudine, without any AIDS-defining illnesses. As part of his New Year's resolution to maintain his health, he has been controlling his dietary intake and exercising regularly, and feels that he is in the best health he had been in a very long time. Therefore he is rather anxious that he has been sent to your clinic for further evaluation. He has been reading on the Internet that HIV infection can be associated with lymphoma and is concerned that is the reason for the referral.

The laboratory studies that prompted this referral are as follows:

WBC	$7600 \times 10^9/L$
Hemoglobin	13.4 g/dL
Hematocrit	40.3%
MCV	112 fL
Platelets	$317,000 \times 10^9/L$
Reticulocyte %	1.86
Reticulocytes	$85,000 \times 10^9/L$
EtOH	<5 mg/dL

Chemistries, liver function, thyroid function, iron, B12, and folate are within reference ranges.

A repeat CBC performed in your office shows near identical results. Review of the peripheral smear normal appearing white cells with neutrophils that were appropriately lobated and granulated. No bilobed or hypersegmented neutrophils were noted. Red cells appeared normal in size, shape, and color, without rouleaux formation, nucleated red cells, or intracellular inclusions. The platelets are normal in size, shape, and color without any clumping evident.

Which of the following is the most appropriate next step in management?

A. Bone marrow biopsy
B. Lead level
C. Methylmalonic acid level
D. Reassurance

93. A 58-year-old African-American man was admitted to the neurology step-down unit for an urgent evaluation of weakness. He presented to his primary care physician for the same symptoms and was sent to the ER for concern for a stroke. A code-stroke was called, where a CT scan and MRI of the brain were negative for an acute process. Rather, he admitted to symptoms of diplopia, dysphagia, nasal-speech, and generalized weakness to the point where he has lost over 30 pounds over the past 6 weeks. Upon admission to the neurology service, single-fiber EMG showed an abnormal jitter, prompting further serologic testing for acetylcholine and muscarinic receptor antibodies. However, it was noted on his admission labs that there is a marked normocytic anemia (see below), which is a marked change from a normal CBC 13 months prior. A consult is placed to hematology to address this. Initial laboratory studies show:

WBC	$12,400 \times 10^9/L$
Hemoglobin	6.1 g/dL
Hematocrit	18.5%
MCV	88
Platelets	$212,000 \times 10^9/L$
Reticulocyte %	0.5%
Absolute reticulocyte count	$4500 \times 10^9/L$

Bone marrow biopsy is performed, showing a hypercellular bone marrow with trilineage hematopoiesis including left-shifted myeloid maturation but significant erythroid hypoplasia and mild megakaryocytic hyperplasia, with no evidence of high-grade dyspoiesis, significant blast populations, metastatic malignancy, or lymphoproliferative disorder. There was abundant stainable iron, with normal cytogenetics and flow cytometry.

Which of the following is the next best test to perform at this time?

A. CT scan of the chest
B. Flow cytometry for CD55/CD59

C. T-cell receptor gene rearrangement
D. Tissue transglutaminase IgA

94. A 53-year-old African-American woman with systemic lupus erythematosus, which was diagnosed during an episode of nephritis, requiring intravenous cyclophosphamide and pulsed methylprednisolone is sent for evaluation of anemia. She now has hypertension, chronic kidney disease (stage III), diabetes mellitus-II (last Hgb-A1c of 12.3), osteoporosis, and hyperlipidemia, which are all being treated with medication. For her SLE, the patient has been treated with azathioprine, mycophenolate, and rituximab, interspersed with pulses of methylprednisolone for flares. She is currently maintained on hydroxychloroquine and prednisone 10 mg/day. A recent CBC and laboratory testing has shown the following:

WBC	$3400 \times 10^9/L$
Hemoglobin	10.2 g/dL
Hematocrit	30.8%
MCV	85 fL
Platelets	$161,000 \times 10^9/L$
Reticulocyte %	1.1
Reticulocytes	$84,000 \times 10^9/L$
Sodium	141 mEq/L
Potassium	4.4 mEq/L
Chloride	109 mEq/L
CO_2	21 mEq/L
BUN	28 mg/dL
Creatinine	2.1 mg/dL
Glucose	181 mg/dL
Erythropoietin	29 U/L
Iron	23 µg/mL
TIBC	202 µg/mL
%Saturation	8%
Ferritin	488 ng/mL

Based upon her history and the available data, what is the most probable explanation for these findings?

A. Alpha-thalassemia
B. Anemia of chronic disease
C. Autoimmune hemolytic anemia
D. Iron deficiency anemia
E. Pure red cell aplasia

95. A 41-year-old African-American man is brought in by EMS to the ER for a syncopal episode at work, where he is involved in the manufacturing of acetaminophen. Upon arrival, he is noted to be tachycardic with a pulse oximetry of 80%. He is placed immediately on 100% FiO_2, followed by an arterial blood gas that shows:

pH	7.41
pCO_2	27
paO_2	197
% O_2 arterial	27.9%

Which of the following is the most appropriate next test to send?

A. Carboxyhemoglobin level
B. Glucose-6 phosphate dehydrogenase level
C. Methemoglobin level
D. Sulfhemoglobin level

96. A 27-year-old African-American woman is referred by her primary care provider for evaluation of anemia. She was treated with oral iron therapy for 1 year without

response. Her family history is notable for anemia in her father. Laboratory values include the following:

Laboratory Test	Patient's Result	Reference Range
Hemoglobin	11.0 g/dL	12–16 g/dL
Hematocrit	32%	35%–48%
MCV	67 fL	80–100 fL
White blood cell count	4.8×10^9/L, with normal differential	4.0–10×10^9/L
Platelet count	198×10^9/L	150–450×10^9/L
Red cell distribution width	11%	11.5%–15.5%
Hemoglobin electrophoresis	—	—
Hemoglobin A	95.5%	96.0%–98.0%
Hemoglobin A2	5.2%	2.3%–3.4%

Peripheral blood smear shows significant microcytosis and increased target cells.
Which of the following is most likely responsible for these findings?
A. Impaired beta-globin chain production
B. Decreased iron utilization secondary to inflammation
C. Decreased dietary iron absorption
D. Sickle cell trait

97. A 22-year-old African-American man undergoes a routine physical examination. Laboratory results reveal:

Laboratory Test	Patient's Result	Reference Range
Hemoglobin	11.0 g/dL	12–16 g/dL
Hematocrit	32%	35%–48%
MCV	67 fL	80–100 fL
Hemoglobin Electrophoresis		
Hemoglobin A	26%	>97.5%
Hemoglobin A2	6.0%	<2.5%
Hemoglobin F	5.0%	0%
Hemoglobin S	63%	0%

A peripheral blood smear reveals hypochromic microcytic red cells. Iron studies are normal.
Which of the following is the most appropriate diagnosis?
A. Sickle cell trait
B. Hemoglobin SS disease
C. Sickle/B+ thalassemia
D. Sickle/B^0 thalassemia
E. Hereditary persistence of fetal hemoglobin

98. A 32-year-old African-American man with sickle cell disease (Hb SS) is admitted for an uncomplicated vasoocclusive pain crisis. He has a history of iron overload from multiple prior transfusions for which he is on nightly deferoxamine, gallstones, s/p cholecystectomy, priapism, and approximately four admissions per year for vasoocclusive pain crises. He has no history of excessive alcohol use, obesity, or illicit drug use. He has not received a recent blood transfusion. Over the course of 4 days he developed worsening abdominal pain, jaundice, and fever. On exam he is hypotensive, tachycardic, jaundiced with scleral icterus, and has severe abdominal pain with hepatomegaly present on palpation. His laboratory results are as follows:

Laboratory Test	Results on Hospital Day 5	Reference Range
Hemoglobin	9.6 g/dL	12–16 g/dL
Hematocrit	28.8%	35%–48%
White blood cell count	13×10^9/L, with normal differential	4–10×10^9/L
Platelet count	159×10^9/L	150–450×10^9/L
Reticulocyte count	16%	0.5%–1.8%
Lactate dehydrogenase	425 U/L	100–240 U/L
Creatinine	2.8 mg/dL	0.7–1.3 mg/dL
Aspartate transaminase (AST)	98 U/L	0–37 U/L
Alanine transaminase (ALT)	150 U/L	0–41 U/L
Total bilirubin	14.5 mg/dL	0.0–1.0 mg/dL
Direct bilirubin	10.5 mg/dL	0.0–0.2 mg/dL
Alkaline phosphatase	250 U/L	35–129 U/L
Prothrombin time (PT)	17.0 s	11–15 s
Activated partial thromboplastin time (aPTT)	37 s	29–36 s
Serum ferritin	1500 ng/mL	25–400 ng/mL

A computed tomography and Doppler ultrasound of the abdomen revealed hepatomegaly with intrahepatic dilatation, normal enhancement of the liver, patent vessels. Viral serologies for hepatitis and HIV were negative. Screening tests for autoimmune hepatitis were negative.
The next best diagnostic or therapeutic step in this patient is:
A. Perform a liver biopsy
B. Perform exchange blood transfusion
C. Initiate hydroxyurea therapy
D. Start ursodeoxycholic acid

99. A 29-year-old Caucasian female is referred to you for worsening anemia. She has a history of chronic anemia since childhood that was intermittently treated with iron supplementation without improvement. She has required packed red blood cell transfusions on two separate occasions in her life. She has a history of gallstones at the age of 25. Her family history is significant for anemia in her mother and a history of gallstones requiring a cholecystectomy in her brother. On physical exam her vital signs are stable, but she has mild splenomegaly, visible pallor, and mild jaundice. Her laboratory results are as follows:

Laboratory Test	Results on Hospital Day 5	Reference Range
Hemoglobin	9.0 g/dL	12–16 g/dL
Hematocrit	27.0%	35%–48%
White blood cell count	8×10^9/L, with normal differential	4–10×10^9/L
Platelet count	202×10^9/L	150–450×10^9/L
Mean corpuscular volume (MCV)	78 μm^3	80–100 μm^3

Laboratory Test	Results on Hospital Day 5	Reference Range
Mean corpuscular hemoglobin concentration (MCHC)	40 pg	26.0–34.0 pg
Reticulocyte count	11%	0.5%–2.5%
Absolute reticulocyte count	380,000/µL	—
Lactate dehydrogenase	300 U/L	100–240 U/L
Haptoglobin	<10 mg/dL	30–200 mg/dL
Aspartate transaminase (AST)	35 U/L	0–37 U/L
Alanine transaminase (ALT)	38 U/L	0–41 U/L
Total bilirubin	3.4 mg/dL	0.0–1.0 mg/dL
Direct bilirubin	0.2 mg/dL	0.0–0.2 mg/dL
Alkaline phosphatase	120 U/L	35–129 U/L

Serum iron studies, vitamin B12, and folate are normal. A direct Coombs test is negative.
Which of the following treatments is most likely to lead to an improvement in symptoms?
A. Splenectomy
B. Prednisone
C. Eculizumab
D. Rituximab

100. A 70-year-old man with a history of osteoarthritis complains of increasing fatigue over the last 6 months. He has required red blood cell transfusions twice over the last 4 months. His last transfusion was 4 weeks ago. He denies any signs of bleeding. His exam is negative for pallor, jaundice, or splenomegaly. Family history is notable for his father who died of colon cancer at the age of 55. His laboratory results are as follows:

Laboratory Test	Patient's Results	Reference Range
Hemoglobin	9.8 g/dL	12–16 g/dL
Hematocrit	24.6%	35%–48%
White blood cell count	6.6 × 10⁹/L, with normal differential	4–10 × 10⁹/L
Platelet count	280 × 10⁹/L	150–450 × 10⁹/L
MCV	119 µm³	80–100 µm³
Reticulocyte count corrected	8%	Varies
Vitamin B12	380 pg/mL	243–894 pg/mL
Folate	9.0 ng/mL	4.4–19.9 ng/mL
Lactate dehydrogenase	425 U/L	100–240 U/L
Haptoglobin	<10 mg/dL	30–200 mg/dL
Total bilirubin	2.3 mg/dL	0.0–1.0 mg/dL
Direct bilirubin	0.3 mg/dL	0.0–0.2 mg/dL
Direct antiglobulin test	C3 positive, IgG negative	Negative
Serum protein electrophoresis/immunofixation	M spike 0.3 g/dL IgM-kappa restricted	No monoclonal Mspike
Flow cytometry	Small clonal population of B cells	Negative

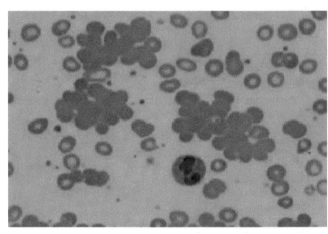

FIG. 34.12

A peripheral blood smear is shown in Fig. 34.12. Which of the following is the best treatment for this patient?
A. Splenectomy
B. Prednisone
C. Plasmapheresis
D. Rituximab

101. A 30-year-old man with sickle cell disease (HbSS) presents to clinic for routine follow-up of sickle cell care. He has a history of priapism 2 years ago that required urological intervention and acute chest syndrome 1 year ago that required red blood cell exchange transfusion. He is admitted approximately once per year in the winter for acute vasoocclusive pain crisis. He does not have a history of stroke, pulmonary hypertension, or iron overload. He is not on hydroxyurea therapy. Today he feels well. His physical exam is notable for some mild scleral icterus, but is otherwise negative. He is scheduled for an elective cholecystectomy in 3 weeks for a history of recurrent cholecystitis. His current laboratory results are as follows:

Laboratory Test	Patient's Results	Reference Range
Hemoglobin	9.1 g/dL	12–16 g/dL
Hematocrit	27.3%	35%–48%
White blood cell count	12 × 10⁹/L, with normal differential	4–10 × 10⁹/L
Platelet count	390 × 10⁹/L	150–450 × 10⁹/L
Reticulocyte count	3%	0.5%–1.8%
Lactate dehydrogenase	425 U/L	100–240 U/L
Creatinine	1.2 mg/dL	0.7–1.3 mg/dL
Aspartate transaminase (AST)	98 U/L	0–37 U/L
Alanine transaminase (ALT)	150 U/L	0–41 U/L
Total bilirubin	1.8 mg/dL	0.0–1.0 mg/dL
Direct bilirubin	0.3 mg/dL	0.0–0.2 mg/dL
Alkaline phosphatase	110 U/L	35–129 U/L

Which of the following is the best recommendation for preoperative management?
A. Red blood cell exchange transfusion
B. Hydroxyurea
C. No preoperative transfusion
D. Venous thromboembolism prophylaxis

102. A 72-year-old previously healthy woman presents to her primary care provider with fatigue, dyspnea on exertion, and intermittent dizziness. She has had worsening lack of energy for 3 months and has noticed her fingertips turn a bluish color in the winter. She denies any fever, chills, night sweats, unintentional weight loss, or lymphadenopathy. Family history is significant for coronary artery disease. A routine CBC drawn 1 year ago was normal. She is taking no medications and does not recall any recent illness. Lab results are as follows:

Laboratory Test	Patient's Results	Reference Range
Hemoglobin	8.6 g/dL	12–16 g/dL
Hematocrit	25.8%	35%–48%
White blood cell count	9×10^9/L, with normal differential	$4–10 \times 10^9$/L
Platelet count	390×10^9/L	$150–450 \times 10^9$/L
MCV	112 μm^3	80–100 μm^3
Reticulocyte count corrected	7%	0.5%–1.8%
Vitamin B12	450 pg/mL	243–894 pg/mL
Folate	6.2 ng/mL	4.4–19.9 ng/mL
Lactate dehydrogenase	375 U/L	100–240 U/L
Haptoglobin	<10 mg/dL	30–200 mg/dL
Creatinine	0.9 mg/dL	0.7–1.3 mg/dL
Aspartate transaminase (AST)	25 U/L	0–37 U/L
Alanine transaminase (ALT)	32 U/L	0–41 U/L
Total bilirubin	1.8 mg/dL	0.0–1.0 mg/dL
Direct bilirubin	0.3 mg/dL	0.0–0.2 mg/dL
Alkaline phosphatase	110 U/L	35–129 U/L
Direct antiglobulin test	C3 positive, IgG negative	Negative

As part of the workup for this disorder the next best diagnostic test is:
A. Serum protein electrophoresis (SPEP)
B. Cryoglobulin testing
C. Osmotic fragility testing
D. Antinuclear antibody testing (ANA)

103. A 24-year-old African-American man with sickle cell anemia (HbSS) was admitted to the hospital for a vasoocclusive pain crisis 2 days ago. He describes this pain crisis as worse than usual. Eight days ago at local hospital where he was admitted for another vasoocclusive pain crisis, he received 2 units of packed red blood cells for a hemoglobin of 7.5 g/dL. His main complaint is back, leg, and abdominal pain that is not being well controlled by intravenous opiates.
Laboratory values are as follows:

Laboratory Test	Patient's Results Today	Patient's Baseline Labs	Reference Range
Hemoglobin	4.8 g/dL	8–9 g/dL	12–16 g/dL
Hematocrit	14.4%	24%–27%	35%–48%
White blood cell count	11×10^9/L, with normal differential	9–12	$4–10 \times 10^9$/L
Platelet count	380×10^9/L	300–400	$150–450 \times 10^9$/L

Laboratory Test	Patient's Results Today	Patient's Baseline Labs	Reference Range
Mean corpuscular volume (MCV)	86 μm^3	85–95	80–100 μm^3
Reticulocyte count corrected	0.2%	3%–6%	0.5%–1.8%
Lactate dehydrogenase	3600 U/L	250–300 U/L	100–240 U/L
Creatinine	1.5 mg/dL	0.9–1.2	0.7–1.3 mg/dL
Aspartate transaminase (AST)	35 U/L	30–40 U/L	0–37 U/L
Alanine transaminase (ALT)	39 U/L	20–40 U/L	0–41 U/L
Total bilirubin	4.8 mg/dL	1.2–2.3 mg/dL	0.0–1.0 mg/dL
Direct bilirubin	0.3 mg/dL	0.1–0.4 mg/dL	0.0–0.2 mg/dL

A hemoglobin electrophoresis revealed the presence of no hemoglobin A.
As part of the workup for this disorder, which of the following is the next best diagnostic test?
A. Chest x-ray
B. Abdominal ultrasound
C. Direct antiglobulin test and type and screen
D. Urine drug toxicology screen

104. A 24-year-old African-American college student presents to the emergency room with fatigue, dyspnea, dark urine, and yellow skin. She has a history of sickle cell trait, polycystic ovary disease, and deep vein thrombosis, which occurred 2 years ago while the patient was on combined oral contraceptives. She is on nitrofurantoin for a recently diagnosed urinary tract infection and progesterone oral contraception. On exam she has scleral icterus, mild jaundice, and no splenomegaly.
Laboratory findings are shown below:

Laboratory Test	Patient's Results Today	Reference Range
Hemoglobin	9.5 g/dL	12–16 g/dL
Hematocrit	29%	35%–48%
White blood cell count	10×10^9/L, with normal differential	$4–10 \times 10^9$/L
Platelet count	320×10^9/L	$150–450 \times 10^9$/L
Mean corpuscular volume (MCV)	104 μm^3	80–100 μm^3
Reticulocyte count corrected	7%	0.5%–1.8%
Lactate dehydrogenase	600 U/L	100–240 U/L
Creatinine	1.0 mg/dL	0.7–1.3 mg/dL
Aspartate transaminase (AST)	35 U/L	0–37 U/L
Alanine transaminase (ALT)	39 U/L	0–41 U/L

Laboratory Test	Patient's Results Today	Reference Range
Total bilirubin	3.8 mg/dL	0.0–1.0 mg/dL
Direct bilirubin	0.3 mg/dL	0.0–0.2 mg/dL
Direct antiglobulin test	Negative	Negative

Which of the following is most likely to be found on the patient's peripheral smear?
A. Bite cells
B. Schistocytes
C. Target cells
D. Spherocytes

105. A 39-year-old man with history of HIV is diagnosed with *Pneumocystis* pneumonia (PCP). He has been noncompliant with his antiretroviral therapy and his CD4 count is <50. He is started on dapsone for treatment of PCP pneumonia. About 10 days later he develops worsening fatigue, dyspnea, dark urine, and yellow skin. Laboratory findings were consistent with a Coombs negative hemolytic anemia.
His peripheral blood smear is shown in Fig. 34.13.
Dapsone is stopped, and he is switched to an alternative therapy for PCP pneumonia. He returns to your clinic 4 weeks later with normalization of his hemoglobin.
The next diagnostic test to order is:
A. Hemoglobin electrophoresis
B. Flow cytometry to detect reduced/absent CD55 and CD59
C. Osmotic fragility testing
D. Fluorescent spot test for NADPH generation

106. A 57-year-old woman reports a 1-year history of gradually worsening fatigue, painful paresthesias of her lower legs and arms, and, more recently, ataxia. Her medical history is significant for hiatal hernia, gastroesophageal reflux disease, and gastric bypass surgery for morbid obesity 10 years ago. She is on a proton pump inhibitor. Physical examination reveals pallor, impaired position and vibration sense, and hyperpigmentation of the skin.
Her laboratory results are as follows:

Laboratory Test	Patient's Results	Reference Range
Hemoglobin	9.8 g/dL	12–16 g/dL
Hematocrit	24.6%	35%–48%
White blood cell count	3.2×10^9/L, with normal differential	$4–10 \times 10^9$/L
Platelet count	140×10^9/L	$150–450 \times 10^9$/L
Mean corpuscular volume (MCV)	105 μm³	80–100 μm³
Lactate dehydrogenase	2600 U/L	100–240 U/L
Haptoglobin	<10 mg/dL	30–200 mg/dL
Direct antiglobulin test	Negative	Negative

Which of the following is the most likely diagnosis?
A. Autoimmune hemolytic anemia
B. Vitamin B12 deficiency
C. Hypothyroidism
D. Monoclonal paraproteinemia

107. A 32-year-old female presents with gradually worsening shortness of breath and fatigue. She has a history of systemic lupus erythematosus (SLE). Her only medication is hydroxychloroquine. On physical exam she is mildly

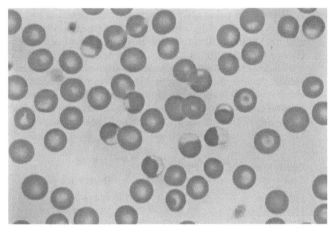

FIG. 34.13

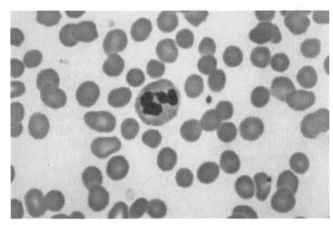

FIG. 34.14

jaundiced and her spleen is palpable. She is hemodynamically stable.
Her laboratory results and peripheral blood smear are shown below:

Laboratory Test	Patient's Results	Reference Range
Hemoglobin	8.0 g/dL	12–16 g/dL
Hematocrit	24.0%	35%–48%
White blood cell count	3.0×10^9/L, with normal differential	$4–10 \times 10^9$/L
Platelet count	162×10^9/L	$150–450 \times 10^9$/L
Mean corpuscular volume (MCV)	105 fL	80–100 fL
Reticulocyte count	7%	0.5%–1.8%
Lactate dehydrogenase	725 U/L	100–240 U/L
Haptoglobin	<10 mg/dL	30–200 mg/dL
Direct antiglobulin test	Positive for IgGco	Negative

Peripheral smear is shown in Fig. 34.14. Which of the following is the best explanation for the patient's positive direct antiglobulin test?
A. Red blood cell (RBC) agglutination due to the presence of autoantibodies bound to the patient's red blood cells
B. RBC agglutination due to the presence of antibodies in the patient's serum that target the donor's red blood cells

C. RBC agglutination due to the presence of alloantibodies bound to the patient's red blood cells

D. RBC agglutination due to the presence of complement fixation on the patient's red blood cells

108. A 32-year-old African-American female with heavy menstrual bleeding is referred for iron deficiency anemia. She describes her menstrual cycles as occurring every 4 weeks but lasting 10 days, requiring changing her pad or tampon ever hour for the first 2 days. Her laboratory results are below. She was given a 6-month trial of oral iron therapy and her ferritin normalized. However, she is still mildly anemic.

Laboratory Test	Patient's Results Before Oral Iron Therapy	Patient's Results After Oral Iron Therapy	Reference Range
Hemoglobin	9.0 g/dL	11 g/dL	12–16 g/dL
Hematocrit	27.0%	33%	35%–48%
White blood cell count	4.5 × 10⁹/L	5.2 × 10⁹/L	4–10 × 10⁹/L
Platelet count	460 × 10⁹/L	310 × 10⁹/L	150–450 × 10⁹/L
Mean corpuscular volume (MCV)	64 fL	70 fL	80–100 fL
Serum ferritin	<5 ng/mL	150 ng/mL	25–400 ng/mL

What is the next best diagnostic test?

A. Hemoglobin electrophoresis to evaluate for sickle cell anemia (HbSS)

B. Hemoglobin electrophoresis to evaluate for sickle cell trait

C. Hemoglobin electrophoresis to evaluate for alpha thalassemia trait

D. DNA analysis to evaluate for alpha thalassemia trait

109. A 20-year-old man presents to hematology clinic to establish care. He reports he has a history of sickle cell disease. Records are obtained from his previous physician, and his hemoglobin electrophoresis was as follows:

	Patient Result	Reference Interval
Hb A	60%	≥95%
Hb S	40%	Absent
Hb A2	<3.5%	≤3.5%
Hb F	0	≤2.1%

Based upon his hemoglobin electrophoresis, what is the most likely diagnosis?

A. Hemoglobin SS

B. Sickle cell trait

C. Hemoglobin SC

D. Sickle beta⁺ thalassemia

E. Hemoglobin SD

110. A 23-year-old man is referred for microcytic anemia, which was noted on routine labs completed by his primary care physician. A CBC is repeated and confirms a normal WBC and platelet count, hemoglobin 10 g/dL (normal 13.8–17.2 g/dL), MCV 66 fL (normal 80–96 fL), and normal RBC count. The peripheral smear reveals target cells and basophilic stippling. A hemoglobin electrophoresis shows the following: Hb A 91.6%, Hb F 0.1%, Hb A₂ 8.3% (nl < 3.5%). Which of the following is the most likely diagnosis?

A. Alpha-thalassemia carrier (α-/αα)

B. Beta-thalassemia minor (β/β⁺ or β/β°)

C. Alpha-thalassemia minor or trait (α–/α–)

D. Beta-thalassemia major (β°/β° Cooley anemia)

E. Hemoglobin H disease (β⁴, –α/––)

111. A 20-year-old Greek woman is referred for evaluation of incidentally discovered microcytic anemia. She has a history of anemia that corrected with vitamin supplementation. CBC shows a normal WBC and differential, normal platelet count, and a hemoglobin of 10.6 mg/dL with MCV 80 and RDW 18. Peripheral blood smear shows normal WBCs and platelets with a dimorphic RBC population. Some of the RBCs appear normal while others are hypochromic microcytes. Siderocytes are present with iron staining. She denies abnormal bleeding. She has no siblings and is unsure of a family history of anemia, but is certain that neither of her parents have required blood transfusions. She feels well and continues to run 1.5 miles 3 times per week. She has no weight loss nor night sweats. She takes only an oral contraceptive; she previously took a vitamin supplement, but discontinued last year when she learned they were not FDA regulated. Physical examination is normal; there is no hepatosplenomegaly and no rash.

Other laboratory studies show:

Ferritin—upper limit of normal
Iron studies—normal

Hemoglobin Electrophoresis:

Hgb A1	97% (95%–98%)
Hgb A2	2% (1.5%–3.5%)
Hgb F	1% (<2%)

No additional Hgbs detected

What is the most likely diagnosis?

A. Beta-thalassemia

B. Alpha-thalassemia intermedia

C. Myelodysplastic syndrome

D. X-linked sideroblastic anemia

112. A 25-year-old with sickle cell anemia is admitted for a sickle pain crisis and is treated with IV narcotic medications. On hospital day 2, the patient develops a fever to 101.4°F and the SpO₂ is 92% on room air. A chest x-ray is performed showing a new RML infiltrate. Blood and sputum cultures are obtained.
WBC 10.4 with slight predominance of neutrophils. Hgb 8.2 g/dL (baseline 8.9 g/dL). Platelets 350,000/μL. The absolute reticulocyte count is 120. The patient has a history of red blood cell alloantibodies.
What is the most likely cause of the patient's fever?

A. Acute chest syndrome

B. Aspiration pneumonitis

C. Sickle pain crisis

D. Pneumococcal pneumonia

113. A 19-year-old man with hemoglobin SC disease presented with left thigh pain consistent with pain crisis. His baseline hemoglobin is 10.9 g/dL and on presentation was 9.1 g/dL. He was afebrile, normotensive, and with sinus tachycardia to 106 bpm. He was administered

IV fluids and IV narcotics with some relief. On hospital day 2, his hemoglobin was found to be 7.2 g/dL and the platelet count fell from 352,000/μL on admission to 72,000/μL. He remains hemodynamically stable and afebrile, but has new left upper quadrant pain. Physical examination reveals clear lung fields; the spleen is palpated four fingerbreadths below the costal margin and is tender to touch. Chest x-ray shows no infiltrate. Peripheral blood smear shows several sickled cells and hemoglobin C crystals. Creatinine is 0.74 mg/dL. AST, ALT, and total bilirubin are within the limits of normal.

What is the most likely cause of the acute drop in hemoglobin and platelet counts?

A. Parvovirus B19 infection
B. IV hydration
C. Hemolysis
D. Acute splenic sequestration
E. Heparin-induced thrombocytopenia

114. A 67-year-old African-American man was admitted for evaluation of left lower quadrant pain, low-grade fevers, and a 20-pound unintentional weight loss of several months' duration. Evaluation revealed an aggressive DLBCL, with significant abdominal adenopathy. He was started on pre-phase chemotherapy with prednisone and cyclophosphamide, and given a rasburicase because of a high risk for tumor lysis syndrome. He was then placed on allopurinol twice daily. On hospital day 4, he noted tea-colored urine. The laboratory testing showed:

On admission:

WBC	11.4 × 10*9/L (4.5–11.0 × 10*9/L)
Hgb	12.6 g/dL (12.0–16.0 g/dL)
Platelets	450,000 × 10^9/L
Creatinine	1.5 mg/dL (baseline 0.8 mg/dL)
Uric acid	12 mg/dL (4–9 mg/dL)
AST	54 (14–38 U/L)
ALT	67 (15–48 U/L)
Alkaline phosphatase	154 U/L (38–126 U/L)
Total bilirubin	1.0 mg/dL (0.0–1.2 mg/dL)
LDH	600 U/L (338–610 U/L)

On day 4:

WBC	11.4 × 10*9/L
Hgb	10.6 g/dL
Platelets	404,000/μL
Creatinine	1.0 mg/dL
Uric acid	6 (4–8)
AST	54
ALT	67
Alkaline phosphatase	154
Total bilirubin	3.5
LDH	1200

Direct antiglobulin testing is negative for IgG or complement.
The peripheral blood smear is shown in Fig. 34.15.
Which of the following is the most likely explanation for the patient's hyperbilirubinemia?

A. Rasburicase
B. Allopurinol
C. Warm autoimmune hemolytic anemia
D. DLBCL liver involvement

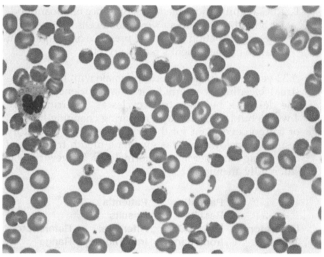
FIG. 34.15 Peripheral smear for patient in question 114.

115. A 45-year-old Greek woman is referred to you for evaluation of microcytic anemia, with hemoglobin 7.4 g/dL (12.0–14.0 g/dL), MCV 70 fL (80–100 fL), and RDW 13% (12.0%–15.0%). She is G2P2 and does not recall prior mention of anemia. Over the last year, she has become increasingly fatigued, with myalgias, intermittent abdominal pain, and diminished libido. She has no ice pica and denies abnormal bleeding; her last menstrual period was at the age of 43. Her fatigue has now started to limit her hobby of making stained glass. She does not consume alcohol. Physical examination is normal and without hepatosplenomegaly.

Additional laboratory studies:

WBC	7.6 × 10*9/L (4.5 – 11 × 10*/L) with a normal differential
Platelet count	238,000/μL (150,000–400,00/μL)
Creatinine	0.85 mg/dL (0.60–1.00 mg/dL)
AST	34 U/L (14–38 U/L)
ALT	54 U/L (15–48 U/L)
Absolute reticulocyte count	90 × 10*9/L (27 – 100 × 10*9/L)
LDH	495 U/L (338–610 U/L)
Total bilirubin	1.0 mg/dL (0.0–1.2 mg/dL)
Ferritin	50 (3–151 ng/mL)

Iron indices within normal limits.
Peripheral blood smear showed microcytic RBCs with basophilic stippling present.
Which of the following is the next best step in evaluating her anemia?

A. Colonoscopy
B. Bone marrow biopsy
C. Hgb electrophoresis
D. Serum lead level

116. A 58-year-old man is evaluated for painful, blistering lesions on the dorsum of his hands bilaterally. He drinks two beers per weekend. There is no family history of blistering skin lesions. Laboratory testing shows:

WBC	7600 × 10^9/L with normal differential
Hgb	14.3 g/dL
Platelets	270,000 × 10^9/L

Creatinine	0.9 mg/dL
AST	90 U/L
ALT	65 U/L
Total bilirubin	1.4 mg/dL
Ferritin	350 ng/mL (40–200 ng/mL)
%Transferrin saturation	50% (20%–45%)

You suspect porphyria cutanea tarda. Which of the following is the next best step in the diagnostic evaluation?
A. Total plasma porphyrins
B. Total erythrocyte porphyrins
C. Sequence UROD gene
D. HFE gene mutation testing

117. A 50-year-old African-American man with Ph+ ALL undergoes busulfan-based conditioning followed by allogeneic stem cell transplantation from an 8/8 matched sibling donor. The posttransplant course has been relatively uneventful, requiring blood and platelet transfusion support but without fevers or signs of infection. He fully engrafted and was discharged to home on day +40. On day +60, he returned for routine visit and was noted to be hypoxic with SpO$_2$ 90% on room air. He feels well and denies lightheadedness, headache, cough, fever, pleuritic chest pain, and dyspnea. Physical examination showed no sign of respiratory distress with clear lung fields and cyanosis of the fingertips and lips. Arterial blood gas showed pH 7.36, paO$_2$ 95 mm Hg, paCO$_2$ 42 mm Hg, HCO$_3$ 24 mEq/L, and methemoglobin of 15%. His medications are acyclovir, dapsone, cyclosporine, amlodipine, and dasatinib. His medical problems include Ph+ ALL in remission after the stem cell transplantation, hypertension, and G6PD deficiency.
Laboratory data:

WBC	7600 × 10^9/L
ALC	1300 × 10^9/L
Hgb	10.7 g/dL
Platelets	210,000 × 10^9/L
Creatinine	0.79 mg/dL
AST	34 U/L
ALT	45 U/L

Which of the following is the next best step in managing this patient's low SpO$_2$?
A. Administration of methylene blue
B. Withhold dapsone
C. Heparin drip
D. Prednisone

118. A 56-year-old man is found to have hereditary hemochromatosis (homozygosity for C282Y) after evaluation for mild fatigue revealed a serum ferritin of 500 μg/L. He smokes cigarettes 1 pack per day, has an occasional glass of wine with dinner, and has no current nor past use of illicit drugs. Testing for HIV, hepatitis B, and hepatitis C are negative. He has no evidence of heart failure, no skin bronzing, and no hypogonadism. Liver function testing is normal. Hemoglobin is 13.4 g/dL. BMI is 23.
Which of the following is the next best step in the management of this patient?
A. Therapeutic phlebotomy
B. Liver biopsy
C. Iron chelation
D. Bone marrow biopsy

119. A 29-year-old man of Italian descent is found to have new onset diabetes and heart failure with EF of 20%. Physical examination reveals skin hyperpigmentation, hepatosplenomegaly, and hypogonadism. Laboratory findings showed AST 63 U/L, AKT 76 U/L, hemoglobin 12.6 g/dL, platelets 100,00/μL, serum iron 41 μM, transferrin saturation 100%, and serum ferritin 1981 μg/L. Liver biopsy was performed which showed severe hepatocellular siderosis and cirrhosis.
A mutation in which of the following genes is most likely to be responsible for the patient's symptoms?
A. HFE1
B. TTR
C. TFR2
D. HJV

120. A 25-year-old law student with paroxysmal nocturnal hemoglobinuria has been managed with eculizumab for 3 years. Prior to beginning eculizumab, he was vaccinated for *Neisseria meningitidis*. Over the last few weeks, several of his classmates have been diagnosed with influenza. He now presents with a headache, fever, and neck stiffness × 1 day. Influenza testing will be delayed due to reagent backorder. In the interim, what is the next best step in the management of this patient?
A. Supportive measures
B. Oseltamivir
C. Lumbar puncture, ceftriaxone, vancomycin
D. Zanamivir

121. A 37-year-old white woman who lives in Minnesota presents in February with 3 days of increasing fatigue, dyspnea, and purplish fingertips when exposed to cold. Three weeks previously, she had onset of fevers, cough, and coryza for "bronchitis" and was prescribed antibiotic treatment, of which she cannot recall the details. Her physical examination is notable for acral cyanosis and mild tachycardia. Laboratory evaluation shows:

WBC	11,400 × 10^9/L
Hgb	8.2 g/dL
MCV	105%
Platelets	210,000 × 10^9/L
Absolute reticulocyte count	120,000 × 10^9/L
LDH	900 U/L
Total bilirubin	4.5 mg/dL
Indirect bilirubin	3.8 mg/dL
AST	34 U/L
ALT	45 U/L
Creatinine	0.89 mg/dL
Haptoglobin	<7 mg/dL

Urinalysis with no hemoglobinuria.
DAT: IgG – no reactivity, complement C3 – positive reactivity
Cold agglutinin titer of 1:1000
Over the next 2 days, the hemoglobin level remains in the 7.5–8.0 g/dL range.
The patient is advised to stay warm.
What additional therapy is recommended?
A. Supportive care
B. Prednisone
C. Rituximab
D. Eculizumab

122. A 19-year-old woman is evaluated for persistent normocytic anemia. She is adopted, and her family history is unknown. She has had episodes of "eye yellowing" following infections since childhood. She has never required

a blood transfusion. She denies menometrorrhagia. On physical examination she is noted to have splenomegaly to 2 cm below the left costal margin; no hepatomegaly. There is faint scleral icterus. Laboratory studies show:

WBC	$7600 \times 10^9/L$
Hgb	10.5 g/dL
MCV	99 fL
RDW	17%
MCHC	38 g/dL
Absolute reticulocyte count	$145 \times 10^*9/L$
Creatinine	0.9 mg/dL
AST	34 U/L
ALT	43 U/L
Total bilirubin	1.5 g/dL
LDH	705 U/L

A peripheral smear shows normal white cell and platelet morphology. Among the red blood cells, a few microspherocytes are seen in addition to polychromasia. Direct antiglobulin testing is negative for both IgG and C3. Which of the following laboratory tests has the highest sensitivity and specificity for the suspected condition?
A. Eosin-5'-maleimide flow cytometry
B. Osmotic fragility
C. Spectrin mutational analysis
D. Serum protein electrophoresis

123. A 35-year-old G4P4 has developed iron deficiency anemia after her most recent pregnancy. She has no chronic medical conditions. She denies menometrorrhagia, hematochezia, or melena. She endorses ice pica. Laboratory studies show:

Hgb	10.8 g/dL
MCV	74 fL
RDW	14.7%
Ferritin	3 ng/mL
Creatinine	0.89 mg/dL

Which of the following patterns of iron regulatory proteins would be expected?
A. Increased hepcidin, increased ferroportin
B. Decreased hepcidin, decreased ferroportin
C. Increased hepcidin, decreased ferroportin
D. Decreased hepcidin, increased ferroportin

124. An 18-year-old African-American woman with known sickle cell trait presents for recommendations regarding beginning a "boot camp" exercise program, as she has heard that such intense exercise regimens can lead to sudden death in persons with sickle cell trait. She has no other medical conditions, is physically fit, and has no family history of sudden death.
Which of the following is the most appropriate recommendation?
A. Avoid intense exercise
B. Hydroxyurea prophylaxis
C. Aspirin prophylaxis
D. Proceed with frequent water and rest breaks

125. A 25-year-old African-American woman is evaluated for microcytic, hypochromic anemia. She denies menometrorrhagia. She denies ice pica. She feels well and denies gastrointestinal pain, melena, and hematochezia. She has one brother with no anemia. Neither her mother nor father is anemic. Laboratory studies reveal:

WBC	$7600 \times 10^9/L$
Hgb	11.6 g/dL
MCV	72 fL
RDW	13.6%
Platelets	$245,000 \times 10^9/L$

Peripheral blood smear shows microcytic and hypochromic red blood cells. Target cells are present.
Ferritin 72 ng/mL (3–151 ng/mL), total iron binding capacity is normal.
Hemoglobin electrophoresis shows a normal pattern.
Which of the following is the next best step in evaluating her microcytic, hypochromic anemia?
A. DNA analysis
B. Serum lead level
C. Kidney function
D. CRP

126. A 40-year-old woman presents with fever, oral ulcers, and a rash over her ears. She has no medical history and takes no prescribed medications. She admits to using illicit substances "occasionally." Physical examination reveals a toxic-appearing woman. Her temperature is 40°C, heart rate is 120 bpm, BP is 100/55, and RR is 20. Her oropharynx reveals deep erythematous aphthous ulcers over gums, cheeks, and tongue. Her ears show a serpiginous, necrotic, vasculitic rash over the pinnae bilaterally. Laboratory studies show an absolute neutrophil count of 0. Hgb is 11.9, and platelets are $455,000 \times 10^9/L$.
Which of the following substances is most likely responsible for the patient's condition?
A. Cocaine adulterated with levamisole
B. Cocaine adulterated with quinine
C. Marijuana contaminated with phencyclidine
D. Oxymorphone extended release (Opana ER)
E. Phencyclidine

127. A 35-year-old woman is seen for evaluation of severe neutropenia of 1 month's duration. She has a history of morbid obesity and underwent bariatric surgery with Roux-en-Y procedure 8 months ago. Her surgery was uncomplicated, and her postoperative course was smooth. She has lost approximately 60 pounds. She has been noticing paresthesias of the hands and feet, as well as some fatigue. She has been iron deficient in the past, but not since she had placement of a levonorgestrel-releasing intrauterine system 3 years ago. Personal and family history are negative for autoimmune disease. Physical examination shows lack of position and vibration sense in the feet. Laboratory data show a hemoglobin of 10.3, MCV of 81, WBC $1300 \times 10^9/L$, and platelet count $198,000 \times 10^9/L$. ANC is $200 \times 10^9/L$; ALC is $1100 \times 10^9/L$. B12 level is >1000 pg/mL.
Which of the following is the most likely diagnosis for the patient's clinical findings?
A. B12 deficiency
B. Chromium deficiency
C. Copper deficiency
D. Selenium deficiency
E. Zinc deficiency

128. A 42-year-old woman with h/o hyperthyroidism presents with 2 days of fever, sore throat, and tender cervical adenopathy. She had been started on methimazole 4 weeks earlier by her endocrinologist. She has no other medical problems and takes only propranolol, oral contraceptives,

and a multivitamin in addition to her methimazole, which she takes 20 mg tid. Family history is negative for blood disorders. Travel history is notable for a trip to Cancun, Mexico, 2 months ago, and she stayed only on resort property. She works as a radiation safety officer for a major university and reported no unusual exposures, and her dosimetry badge has shown radiation exposure within safe limits.

Physical examination reveals a toxic-appearing woman. Her temperature is 39.0°C, BP is 100/64, HR is 110, and RR is 18. Her oropharynx is raw with ulcerated areas over throat and gums. The tonsils are enlarged and inflamed without exudate. Her lungs are clear, and a cardiac exam shows a regular tachycardia with no murmur. Her thyroid is slightly enlarged without bruit, and she has shotty tender cervical adenopathy. There are no supraclavicular or axillary nodes. Her abdomen is benign without organomegaly.

Laboratory studies: WBC: 300×10^9/L, Hg 12 g/dL, Hct 36%, platelets $300,000 \times 10^9$/L, ANC 0.0, ALC 300×10^9/L
Methimazole is stopped, and the patient is treated with antibiotics and G-CSF.

In addition to continuing her propranolol, which of the following is the best option to treat her hyperthyroidism at this point?
A. Methimazole, 5 mg tid
B. Methimazole, 20 mg tid with G-CSF
C. Propylthiouracil, 100 mg tid
D. Propylthiouracil, 100 mg tid with G-CSF
E. Radio-iodine ablation

129. A 60-year-old woman is referred to you for evaluation of leukopenia. She has a history of "arthritis," for which she takes over the counter ibuprofen. Her past medical history is otherwise unremarkable. Physical examination reveals a woman in no acute distress. Her heart rate is 80, BP 120/75, temperature is 36.9°C, and RR 16. She has a normal cardiac and pulmonary exam. There is no adenopathy and no hepatomegaly. The spleen tip is felt three fingerbreadths below the left costal margin. A joint exam shows nodules and ulnar deviation of the fingers bilaterally. CBC shows Hgb 11.4, Hct 32, MCV 85, RDW 12, WBC 3500×10^9/L, and platelets $180,000 \times 10^9$/L. Reticulocyte count is 1%, with an absolute reticulocyte count of $60,000 \times 10^9$/L. ANC 400×10^9/L, ALC 2500×10^9/L, and AMC 200×10^9/L. Flow cytometry of peripheral blood reveals a population of cells that express CD3+CD8+CD57+.

What is the most appropriate treatment for this patient?
A. Alemtuzumab
B. Fludarabine
C. Methotrexate
D. Rituximab
E. Stem cell transplant

130. A 19-year-old female patient with AIDS presents with malaise, fever, loose stool, and unintentional weight loss of 2 months' duration. Physical examination showed erythematous plaques on her face, cervical adenopathy, and splenomegaly to 2 cm below the left costal margin. She had recently been in a homeless shelter in Arizona.

WBC	$1.1 \times 10^*9$/L
Hgb	5.6 g/dL
Platelets	$89,000 \times 10^9$/L

A bone marrow biopsy to evaluate for pancytopenia is shown in Fig. 34.16:

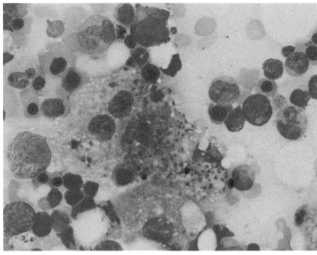

FIG. 34.16 Bone marrow aspiration for patient in question 130.

Which of the following is the most likely diagnosis?
A. Tuberculosis
B. Cryptococcal infection
C. Coccidiomycosis
D. Histoplasmosis

131. A 36-year-old woman presents for evaluation of neutropenia identified by her dentist. She has had "terrible gums" for as long as she can remember, despite good oral hygiene. She has had flares of mouth sores nearly monthly for years. Her mother also has "bad gums." She has never had any serious infections.

WBC	$0.8 \times 10^*9$/L
ANC	$0.3 \times 10^*9$/L
Hgb	14.2 g/dL
Platelets	$346,000 \times 10^9$/L

Monitoring of the CBC over the next month shows a vacillating pattern in the neutrophil count.
Which of the following is the best management?
A. G-CSF given 1–2 days of each cycle
B. G-CSF (in long-acting form) administered weekly
C. Antibiotic prophylaxis
D. Methotrexate

132. A 43-year-old Caucasian woman presents for evaluation of neutropenia found after a recent hospitalization for MRSA cellulitis. At the time of hospitalization, her WBC was $1.8 \times 10^*9$/L, ANC was $0.2 \times 10^*9$/L, Hgb was 13.1 g/dL, and platelets were 410,000/μL. The cellulitis was treated with vancomycin and resolved promptly; vancomycin was discontinued after 1 week. Now, 3 weeks later, she is noted to have persistent neutropenia, ANC $300 \times 10^*9$/L. She has no prior history nor family history of recurrent infections. She has poor general dentition, but has no history of recurrent oral ulcers.

Physical examination shows a somewhat anxious woman with no splenomegaly nor rashes.

Urine toxicology is positive for cocaine. Neutropenia is related to levamisole contamination of the cocaine is suspected.
How long after ceasing levamisole is neutrophil recovery expected?
A. 1–2 days
B. 5–10 days
C. 10–30 days
D. No recovery without intervention

133. A 5-year-old boy from Puerto Rico is evaluated for recurrent epistaxis. An ENT evaluation showed no exposed vessels. On history, his mother also tells you that he has had several skin "boils." He has one brother and one sister, both of whom are healthy. There is no history of bleeding diathesis nor immunodeficiency in his extended family.

Physical examination is notable for partial oculocutaneous albinism and a silvery sheen to his hair. There is no hepatosplenomegaly. There is no lymphadenopathy.

Complete blood count shows normal numbers of leukocytes, erythrocytes, and thrombocytes. PT and aPTT are within the limits of normal.

A peripheral blood smear is shown. Platelet electron microscopy shows absence of dense granules in some platelets (Fig. 34.17).

Which of the following genes is expected to be mutated?
A. LYST
B. HPS1
C. HPS3
D. MYH9

134. A 55-year-old African-American man presents for evaluation of incidentally discovered neutropenia. He has felt well without recurrent infection; no constitutional symptoms are present. His chronic medical conditions include hypertension and hyperlipidemia for which he has taken aspirin, Lisinopril, and atorvastatin for 5 years. He takes no other medications, herbal supplements, nor vitamins. He denies use of illicit drugs and drinks 2–3 beers per weekend. Physical examination shows no lymphadenopathy, splenomegaly, joint deformity, nor synovitis.

WBC	11,000 × 10*9/L
ANC	800 × 10*9/L
ALC	8 × 10*9/L
Hgb	14.5 g/dL
Platelets	249,000 × 10⁹/L
Creatinine	0.89 mg/dL
AST	34 U/L
ALT	43 U/L

Peripheral blood smear shows lymphocytes, which are approximately twice as large as RBC and have abundant cytoplasm-containing azurophilic granules and a round

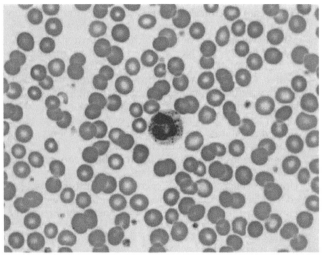

FIG. 34.17 A peripheral blood smear from patient in question 133.

nucleus. Flow cytometry of the peripheral blood demonstrates a population of lymphocytes expressing CD3 CD8, CD16, CD57, alpha/beta T-cell receptor and negative for CD4, CD56, and CD28. T-cell gene rearrangement studies are positive. EBER-ISH is negative. Further studies include negative: ANA, ENA, anticitric citrullinated peptide antibodies, HIV screen, HTLV 1-2 PCR, EBV, and CMV PCR.

Which of the following is the best management of this patient?
A. Observation
B. Low-dose methotrexate
C. Cyclophosphamide
D. G-CSF

135. Which of the following patients would be expected to have the lowest free thrombopoietin levels?
A. A 25-year-old woman with thrombotic thrombocytopenic purpura and a platelet count of 22
B. A 35-year-old man with acute lymphoblastic leukemia and a platelet count of 17
C. A 28-year-old woman with aplastic anemia and a platelet count of 42
D. A 50-year-old man with cirrhosis and portal hypertension from hepatitis C, and a platelet count of 17
E. A 60-year-old man with heparin-associated thrombocytopenia and a platelet count of 35

136. Which of the following represents the correct order of erythroid development?
A. Basophilic erythroblast, polychromatophilic erythroblast, pronormoblast, normoblast, reticulocyte
B. Pronormoblast, normoblast, basophilic erythroblast, polychromatophilic erythroblast, reticulocyte
C. Pronormoblast, basophilic erythroblast, polychromatophilic erythroblast, normoblast, reticulocyte
D. Pronormoblast, polychromatophilic erythroblast, basophilic erythroblast, normoblast, reticulocyte
E. Pronormoblast, normoblast, basophilic erythroblast, polychromatophilic erythroblast, reticulocyte

137. Which of the following is most important for committing primitive multipotent progenitors to the erythroid–megakaryocyte pathway?
A. GATA-1
B. MYH9
C. NF-E2
D. RUNX1
E. TPO

138. A 55-year-old woman presents with severe erosive rheumatoid arthritis. She takes only extra strength aspirin for the pain. Past history is otherwise unremarkable. She neither drinks nor smokes. Physical examination reveals a woman with severely deformed hand and wrist joints that are red and swollen. No organomegaly is present. Stools are guaiac negative. Laboratory evaluation shows Hemoglobin 10.2 g/dL, WBC 14,300 × 10⁹/L, and platelets 685,000 × 10⁹/L. Sedimentation rate is 95.

Which of the following is most responsible for the thrombocytosis?
A. IL-3
B. IL-6
C. IL-11
D. Stem cell factor
E. Thrombopoietin

139. Which of the following represents the correct order of maturation of the myeloid progenitor cells?
    A. Metamyelocyte, myeloblast, promyelocyte, myelocyte, band
    B. Myeloblast, promyelocyte, metamyelocyte, myelocyte, band
    C. Myeloblast, promyelocyte, myelocyte, metamyelocyte, band
    D. Promyelocyte, myelocyte, myeloblast, metamyelocyte, band
    E. Promyelocyte, myeloblast, myelocyte, metamyelocyte, band

140. Which three cytokines are critical for stimulation of bone marrow production of eosinophils?
    A. IL-3, IL-5, and IFN-gamma
    B. IL-3, IL-6, and IFN-gamma
    C. IL-3, IL-5, and GM-CSF
    D. IL-3, IL-6, and GM-CSF
    E. IL-5, IL-6, and GM-CSF

141. A 39-year-old Caucasian woman who is transferred to the MICU for continued care of bleeding. She had been in her usual state of health when, several days prior to her transfer, she developed noted worsening ecchymoses than usual. Thinking this was just clumsiness, she ignored these symptoms until she began to experience symptoms of menorrhagia to the point where she had a syncopal episode. She was found by a neighbor to be incoherent, and EMS were summoned and she was taken to the local ER. There, her CBC was noted to be:

WBC	1.3 (3.2–9.8)
Hgb	4.1 (12.0–15.5)
Hct	13.2 (35–45)
MCV	83
Platelets	23 (150–450)

She is transfused with packed red cells and platelets, with a posttransfusion CBC showing an hemoglobin of **9.6** (12.0–15.5) and platelets of **113** (150–450).
She denies any new medications, including herbs, remedies, or over-the-counter supplements. She denies any environmental or occupational exposures, stating that overall, she had considered herself to be in excellent health, save for an episode of marked transaminitis that was attributed to food poisoning.
Given her history, which of the following is the most appropriate test to perform now?
    A. Bone marrow biopsy
    B. Flow cytometry for CD55/CD59
    C. HIV PCR
    D. T-cell receptor gene rearrangement assay
    E. Viral serologies

142. A 41-year-old Caucasian man, with a history of progressive dyspnea, culminating in end-stage pulmonary disease, who is now oxygen dependent, is referred for evaluation of pancytopenia prior to lung transplantation. His chest imaging is concerning for pulmonary fibrosis, which is confirmed on transbronchial biopsy. On exam, he is a pleasant man wearing oxygen in mild respiratory distress, who appears older than his stated age due to his grey hair, hyperkeratotic palms, and dystrophic nails. His CBC is remarkable for the following:

WBC	6000×10^9/L
Hgb	13.2 g/dL
Hct	39%
MCV	108 fL
Platelets	$126,000 \times 10^9$/L
Reticulocyte%	0.53%
Absolute reticulocytes	$18,200 \times 10^9$/L

Which of the following will be most likely to confirm the diagnosis?
    A. Bone marrow biopsy
    B. Diepoxybutane clastogen analysis of cultured lymphocytes
    C. Sequencing of *MPL*
    D. Sequencing of *SBDS*
    E. Measurement of telomere length

143. A 31-year-old man presents for evaluation of pancytopenia of unknown duration discovered during a pre-employment evaluation. He has no chronic medical conditions and has felt well. He has no history of recurrent infection nor any need for transfusion. He does not drink alcohol and denies illicit drug use. He has not traveled outside of the United States.
Laboratory studies show:

WBC	1300×10^9/L
ANC	600×10^9/L
ALC	500×10^9/L
AMC	100×10^9/L
Hgb	11.1 g/dL
MCV	122 fL
RDW	18.1%
Platelets	$51,000 \times 10^9$/L
AST	27 U/L
ALT	37 U/L
Total bilirubin	0.5 mg/dL

Peripheral blood smear shows macrocytosis, leukopenia and thrombocytopenia with no blasts present.
Physical examination reveals short stature (height 162.5 cm = 5′3″, weight 48 kg = 105 pounds) and a hyperpigmented macule on the abdomen (Fig. 34.18). There is no hepatosplenomegaly. The remainder of the physical examination is normal.
Bone marrow biopsy and aspiration show a hypocellular marrow with mild dyserythropoiesis. Routine cytogenetics reveals a normal male karyotype 46,XY[20].
He has no siblings. His family history is notable for breast cancer in his mother (diagnosed at age 41) and ovarian cancer in his maternal grandmother (at age 43).
Which of the following is the next best step in evaluation?
    A. FANCG gene mutation testing
    B. Chromosomal breakage testing
    C. Telomere size
    D. SBDS mutation testing

144. A 73-year-old woman presents for evaluation of pancytopenia new since her last CBC 5 years previously. She has felt well, without complaint. She is status post gastric bypass 10 years previously. Her medications include aspirin, amlodipine, simvastatin, and fish oil. She uses zinc lozenges to help prevent colds. She receives IV iron replacement approximately once per year. She smokes one pack of cigarettes per day, denies EtOH use, and denies illicit drug use. She is edentulous and wears

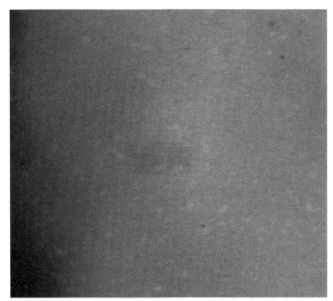

FIG. 34.18

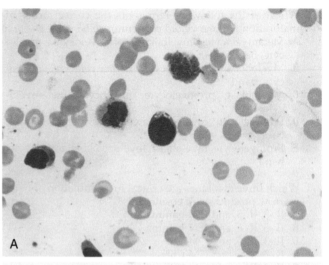

A

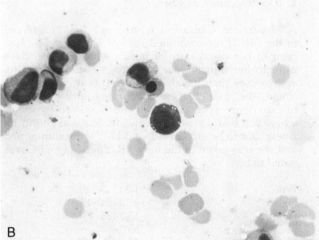

B

FIG. 34.19

dentures. On physical examination, there is no hepatosplenomegaly.

WBC	2.4 × 10*9/L
ANC	1.2 × 10*9/L
Hgb	9.9 mg/dL
MCV	120 fL
Platelets	110,000/μL
LDH	Normal
AST/ALT/creatinine	Normal

Peripheral blood smear shows macrocytosis without other abnormality.

ANA negative. SPEP/IFE with a trace IgG kappa monoclonal band. Serum free light chain testing with normal kappa and lambda levels and ratio.

Bone marrow biopsy revealed a hypocellular marrow with cells shown below. There was no excess in blasts nor plasma cells. Routine cytogenetics showed a normal female karyotype 46,XX[20]. MDS FISH panel is without abnormality (Fig. 34.19A and B).

Which of the following is a likely explanation of her pancytopenia?

A. Oligosecretory multiple myeloma
B. Zinc deficiency
C. Myelodysplastic syndrome
D. Copper deficiency

145. A 62-year-old man is found to have acquired aplastic anemia with bone marrow cellularity of <20% and normal cytogenetic analysis. A small PNH clone is identified. He has a remote history of DVT after immobilization for leg fracture 10 years previously, but no other thromboses. No hemolysis is present.

He is initiated on immunosuppressive therapy.

In light of the coexistent PNH clone, what statement best represents his prognosis?

A. He is likely to develop paroxysmal nocturnal hemoglobinuria.
B. He is likely to have a favorable response to immunosuppressive therapy.
C. He is unlikely to respond to immunosuppressive therapy.
D. He is likely to develop acute leukemia.

146. A 45-year-old is evaluated for chronic pancytopenia first recognized 5 years previously. His medical problems include idiopathic pulmonary fibrosis and hypertension. His only medication is metoprolol. Physical examination is significant only for fine bibasilar crackles. CBC shows WBC 2.4 × 10*9/L, ANC 1.2 × 10*9/L, Hgb 10.6 g/dL, and platelets 99,000/μL. LFTs and creatinine are within the limits of normal.

Bone marrow aspirate and biopsy show a hypocellular marrow without morphologic abnormalities and no increased blasts. Cytogenetics show 46,XY[20] and FISH for MDS probes is normal.

He works as a sports writer and has no international travel. He has no known radiation exposures. He is a current smoker but denies alcohol or illicit drugs.

Viral testing for EBV, CMV, HIV, hepatitis B, and hepatitis C are all negative.

ANA is negative.

Chromosomal breakage analysis with mitomycin C is normal.

He has no known family history of a hematologic malignancy or low blood counts.

Which of the following is the next best diagnostic test?

A. Measurement of leukocyte telomere content
B. DKC gene mutation analysis
C. JAK2 V617F mutation analysis
D. Whole exome sequencing

147. A 25-year-old primigravid woman develops aplastic anemia beginning in the second trimester. She is given supportive care with transfusions as needed. She asks about the usual course of pregnancy-associated aplastic anemia. Which of the following is expected after delivery?
    A. Nearly all women will have a spontaneous recovery.
    B. About half will have a spontaneous recovery.
    C. Almost none will have a spontaneous recovery.
    D. The baby will likely require transfusion support.

148. A 25-year-old woman presents for evaluation of mild pancytopenia. PMHx is significant for multiple dysplastic cervical and vaginal wall lesions. Testing for human papilloma virus (HPV) has been negative. Physical examination reveals a reticulated rash over the patient's neck and whitish striations on her buccal mucosa. She has painted nails. Laboratory studies show an hemoglobin of 7.3 g/dL, MCV 101, WBC 3500 × 10⁹/L, platelets 135,000 × 10⁹/L, ANC 1200 × 10⁹/L, ALC 1900 × 10⁹/L, and AMC 400 × 10⁹/L. Absolute reticulocyte count is 14,000 × 10⁹/L. B12 and folate are within normal limits. A bone marrow biopsy shows a hypoplastic marrow with no evidence of dysplasia and cellularity of 12%.
    Which of the following is the test most likely to yield the correct diagnosis?
    A. Antiintrinsic factor antibodies
    B. CD55/CD59 flow cytometry
    C. Chromosomal breakage testing
    D. Isoamylase
    E. Telomere length

149. A 25-year-old man presents with fever and bleeding from his mouth and nose. He has no PMHx, has never traveled outside the United States, and takes no medications or illicit substances. His family history is unremarkable. He is an only child. He works as a computer engineer and has no history of exposure to ionizing radiation or organic solvents. Physical examination reveals a pale young man in NAD. His heart rate is 100, BP is 120/75, temperature is 38.9°C, and RR is 16. He has a normal cardiac and pulmonary exam, no adenopathy, and no hepatosplenomegaly. He has bleeding gums and oral petechiae. The CBC shows Hgb 6.4, Hct 22, MCV 105, WBC 1.5, and platelets 18. His reticulocyte count is 0.1%, with an absolute reticulocyte count of 6000; ANC is 0.3, ALC is 1.2, and AMC is 0. A bone marrow examination reveals a hypocellular marrow without dysplastic features. Cytogenetics are normal; 2% of peripheral white cells show absence of CD55 and CD59. He is frightened of contracting HIV from a blood transfusion and requests that all transfusions come from his parents, if possible.
    In addition to administration of appropriate antibiotics, what is the most appropriate therapy for this patient?
    A. ATG and cyclosporine
    B. Eculizumab
    C. IVIg and prednisone
    D. Platelet transfusion from his father
    E. Red cell transfusion from his mother

150. A 25-year-old man presents for evaluation of mild pancytopenia. PMHx is significant for episodes of pancreatitis and pancreatic dysfunction. Physical examination shows no somatic abnormalities. Laboratory studies show an hemoglobin of 7.3 g/dL, MCV of 101, WBC 3500 × 10⁹/L, and platelets 135,000 × 10⁹/L. ANC 1200 × 10⁹/L, ALC 1900 × 10⁹/L, and AMC 400 × 10⁹/L. Absolute reticulocyte count is 14,000 × 10⁹/L. B12 and folate are within normal limits. A bone marrow biopsy shows a hypoplastic marrow with no evidence of dysplasia and cellularity of 12%. Isoamylase levels are abnormal.
    Which of the following is the most likely diagnosis
    A. Amegakaryocytic thrombocytopenia
    B. Dyskeratosis congenita
    C. Fanconi anemia
    D. Paroxysmal nocturnal hemoglobinuria
    E. Shwachman-Diamond syndrome

151. A 35-year-old man presents for evaluation of mild pancytopenia. PMHx is significant for episodes of severe abdominal pain diagnosed as esophageal spasm. He has also had complaints of erectile dysfunction. Physical examination shows no somatic abnormalities. Laboratory studies show an hemoglobin of 7.3 g/dL, MCV of 101, WBC 3500 × 10⁹/L, and platelets 135,000 × 10⁹/L. ANC 1200 × 10⁹/L, ALC 1900 × 10⁹/L, and AMC 400 × 10⁹/L. Absolute reticulocyte count is 14,000 × 10⁹/L. B12 and folate are within normal limits. A bone marrow biopsy shows a hypoplastic marrow with no evidence of dysplasia and cellularity of 12%.
    Which of the following is most likely to be abnormal?
    A. CD55/CD59 flow cytometry
    B. Chromosomal breakage testing
    C. Isoamylase
    D. Osmotic fragility
    E. Telomere length

152. A 25-year-old man presents with fever, and bleeding from his mouth and nose. He has no PMHx, has never traveled outside of the United States, and takes no medications or illicit substances. His family history is unremarkable. He is an only child. He works as a computer engineer and has no history of exposure to ionizing radiation or organic solvents. Physical examination reveals a pale young man in NAD. His heart rate is 100, BP is 120/75, temperature is 38.9°C, and RR is 16. He has a normal cardiac and pulmonary exam, and no adenopathy nor hepatosplenomegaly. He has bleeding gums and oral petechiae. The CBC shows an Hgb of 6.4 g/dL, Hct of 22%, MCV of 105, WBC of 1500 × 10⁹/L, and platelets 18,000 × 10⁹/L. Reticulocyte count is 0.1%, with an absolute reticulocyte count of 6000 × 10⁹/L, and ANC is 100 × 10⁹/L, ALC 1200 × 10⁹/L, and AMC 0. Flow cytometry shows IFN-gamma expression on CD8+ T cells. Bone marrow examination reveals a hypocellular marrow without dysplastic features. Cellularity is 5%, and cytogenetics are normal.
    He is treated with ATG and cyclosporine (ATG/CSA).
    Which of the following represents the best predictor of response to this therapy?
    A. ALC < 2000 × 10⁹/L
    B. ANC < 300 × 10⁹/L
    C. Absolute reticulocyte count <25,000 × 10⁹/L
    D. Bone marrow cellularity <5%
    E. IFN gamma on T cells

ANSWERS

1. D

Many patients suspected of having acute porphyria do not have the disease. Such patients frequently have underlying psychiatric disorders. Patients with acute porphyria can experience neuropsychiatric findings during acute attacks. The hallmark laboratory feature of acute porphyria is elevation in the 24-hour urine PBG and ALA. Patients with acute porphyria have elevations in heme metabolites that are several orders of magnitude greater than normal. Trivial elevations in coproporphyrin, as seen in this patient, in the setting of a normal PBG is indicative of secondary coproporphyrinuria, which is not a porphyric state and does not require intervention.

2. E

The constellation of hemoglobin values in the 7–10 g/dL range with normal to low iron, low TIBC, and elevated ferritin is diagnostic of inflammatory anemia. Inflammatory anemia is modulated by the small peptide hepcidin that is increased in the setting of inflammation. Hepcidin causes internalization and proteolysis of ferroportin, the membrane protein in the enterocyte and macrophage that allows for iron release. Patients with inflammatory anemia do not require specific therapy. A ferritin of 565 is incompatible with iron deficiency and supplemental iron should be avoided. Although supplemental erythropoietin may increase the hemoglobin in inflammatory states, it is seldom necessary, especially not in asymptomatic patients.

3. A

The bite of the brown recluse spider (loxoscelism) contains sphingomyelinase D that causes local necrosis at the site of envenomation and hemolytic anemia. Occasionally, the bite is accompanied by DIC. Patients bitten by a brown recluse spider can also have renal injury. There is no antivenom available, and the treatment is supportive. MRSA and lyme do not cause hemolysis. Rhus dermatitis is related to contact with poison ivy, oak, or sumac. Pyoderma gangrenosum can result from a number of underlying disorders but is not associated with hemolysis.

4. C

The peripheral smear is often more sensitive than cardiac ECHO in detecting small paravalvular leaks and valve hemolysis. Similarly, the presence of an audible murmur is not a reproducible finding in small paravalvular abnormalities. The constellation of hemolytic anemia and schistocytes in the setting of an artificial valve should alert the clinician to this possibility. Surgery is the treatment of choice for significant valvular hemolysis. The patient has no signs or symptoms suggesting TTP or DIC. Schistocytes are not present in cold agglutinin disease or warm antibody hemolysis.

5. A

G6PD deficiency is found in Mediterraneans and Africans. About 10% of American Americans have mild G6PD deficiency. G6PD deficiency is X-linked so occurs predominantly in male patients. The patient in question likely developed oxidative hemolysis in response to antibiotic therapy. In African Americans the G6PD variant is unstable, and thus levels fall in older cells but are normal in younger red cells. Measuring G6PD levels in African Americans in the setting of acute hemolysis often produces normal levels as the enzyme-deficient older cells are already destroyed. As such, G6PD levels are best checked after an acute hemolytic episode. PNH is excluded in this patient by the flow cytometry studies. Although bite cells can be seen in G6PD deficiency, this is not a universal finding. Normal Coomb's test excludes other immune causes of hemolysis.

6. B

Serous atrophy of the marrow, also known as gelatinous transformation, occurs in severely malnourished individuals. It has been reported in patients with anorexia, bulimia, HIV, and malignancy-induced cachexia. In the setting of severe malnutrition, the marrow accumulates hyaluronic acid and undergoes fat atrophy and gelatinous transformation. Although the marrow is technically aplastic, the accumulation of hyaluronic acid and the absence of fat exclude aplastic anemia. Similarly, the patient described did not have fibrosis, tumor, or dysplastic features in the marrow.

7. D

The drug metformin can decrease cobalamin levels by almost 20%. This may be due to metformin's effects on Ca^{2+} dependent membrane action where cobalamin/intrinsic factor absorption is Ca^{2+} dependent at the ileal membrane surface. In one study, 7.2% more patients taking metformin had cobalamin deficiency compared with age-matched controls. Metformin-induced cobalamin deficiency can be accompanied by the same neuropsychological findings as other cobalamin deficient states. It can be corrected by supplementing with calcium carbonate 1.2 g daily. The Schilling test is seldom performed as it involves the use of radioactivity and this test, like antibody testing, would not lead to a correct diagnosis.

8. B

The patient described has hereditary spherocytosis, which can be undiagnosed into adulthood. The best test to make the diagnosis is an analysis for E5MI binding that carries a sensitivity of 0.93 and a specificity of 0.98. In contrast, osmotic fragility carries a sensitivity of 0.68 and specificity of 0.53. Analysis of spectrin and protein 4.1 may be useful in the diagnosis of hereditary elliptocytosis or hereditary pyropoikilocytosis. CD55 and CD59 are deficient in patients with PNH.

9. E

Copper is needed to convert ferric iron to ferrous iron. Zinc competes with copper for absorption. As such, copper deficiency and zinc excess can both lead to iron deficiency that is resistant to supplemental iron supplementation. Zinc is a common element in over-the-counter cold medications. The other mentioned supplements are not associated with iron deficiency.

10. B

Hyperparathyroidism can lead to marrow fibrosis and can also lead to decreased erythropoietin synthesis. Additionally, erythroid colonies show suppressed growth in response to the parathyroid hormone, and red cells have shortened survival in the setting of hyperparathyroidism. For all of these reasons, patients who are on dialysis who are not responding to erythropoietin should be checked for elevations in PTH. The treatment for these patients is parathyroidectomy that can restore the hematocrit. Interestingly, calcitriol does not appear to improve erythropoiesis in patients with elevated PTH levels.

11. B

Patients with low oxygen affinity hemoglobin have a physiologic anemia due to increased oxygen delivery by the abnormal hemoglobin. In contrast, patients with a high O_2 affinity hemoglobin present with erythrocytosis. The p50 represents the partial pressure of oxygen at 50% hemoglobin saturation. This normally occurs a 26.6 mm Hg. Patients with low oxygen affinity hemoglobin will have a high p50 due to increased oxygen release by the abnormal hemoglobin. Hemoglobin electrophoresis is abnormal in a very small percentage of such patients who have mutations in the oxygen-binding region of hemoglobin. Pulse oximetry is often not sensitive nor specific in the diagnosis of altered O_2 affinity hemoglobin. Carboxyhemoglobin is useful in the detection of carbon monoxide exposure. E5MI is useful in the diagnosis of spherocytosis.

12. E

Acute megaloblastosis and marrow suppression can occur rapidly after recreational or anesthetic use of nitrous oxide. N_2O oxidizes B12 cobalt from the monovalent to trivalent state rendering methylcobalamin inactive. In this setting, acute neurological effects and delirium can be seen. Treatment is immediate initiation of B12 and folate, which often produce dramatic resolutions of symptoms and improve hematopoiesis within hours.

13. B

The Mentzer index can be useful in differentiating beta thalassemia from iron deficiency. The Mentzer index is the ratio between the MCV (in fL) and the red blood cell count (in 10^{12} cells/L). A value of less than 13 is suggestive of iron deficiency, whereas a value of greater than 13 is more likely iron deficiency. This is the case because in iron deficiency, the erythrocyte count is decreased, whereas in thalassemia, the red cells are small but produced in sufficient or even increased quantity. In hgb SC disease, the erythrocyte count is decreased. Sideroblastic anemia is associated with decreased erythrocytes, as is lead poisoning.

14. E

The patient described has cold agglutinin disease as evidenced by his laboratory studies and peripheral smear, which shows agglutinated red cells in a slide performed at room temperature. Cold agglutinin disease develops when IgM antibodies bind red cells and cause complement mediated hemolysis and destruction in the liver. Cold agglutinin disease is treated by keeping the patient and infusates at body temperature and rituximab administration is considered front-line therapy. Glucocorticoids are typically ineffective, and hemolysis occurs in the liver rendering splenectomy of limited utility. Plasmapheresis and IVIg similarly have not been shown to be particularly effective.

15. D

Ferric, iron sucrose, and ferumoxytol all are generally well tolerated. Ferrous sulfate is frequently not absorbed well in patients with inflammatory bowel disease and typically worsens symptoms, but only rarely causes allergic reactions. Iron dextran may be given as a single dose infusion but has a higher complication rate, especially anaphylaxis.

16. C

The patient described has paroxysmal cold hemoglobinuria, an immune hemolysis that is associated with syphilis and results from complement-mediated hemolysis with antibody to the P-antigen on red cells. The antibody attaches at colder temperatures, but fixes complement in warmer areas of the body. Diagnosis requires analysis for the presence of the Donath Landsteiner antibody. This requires collecting and maintaining a patient blood sample at body temperature. Patient serum is mixed with P antigen positive type O RBC and donor serum. The sample is chilled to 32°F and then warmed. The tube is centrifuged and supernatant assessed for hemolysis. E5MA is used to detect spherocytes in hereditary spherocytosis. PK levels are useful in patients suspect of having PK deficiency. Such patient would present in infancy with Coombs negative hemolysis. ANA and sucrose hemolysis would not be useful.

17. C

The patient described has methemoglobinemia, a condition caused by excessive ferric (Fe^{3+}) rather than ferrous (Fe^{2+}) hemoglobin in the blood. In this case, the use of benzocaine cream lead to the disorder. Ferric hemoglobin has a decreased ability to bind oxygen and leads to decrease release of oxygen by the other three ferrous heme sites on the hemoglobin molecule. Patients with acquired methemoglobinemia respond rapidly to intravenous methylene blue that provides an artificial electron receptor for NADPH methemoglobin reductase. Vitamin C may also be used. The other treatments listed in the question would not provide such an electron receptor and would not reverse methemoglobinemia.

18. C

Hemoglobin E is one of the world's most common hemoglobin mutations. Patients who coinherit Hgb E with beta^0 thalassemia have a variable phenotype ranging from lack of symptoms to transfusion dependence. The patient in question has a moderate anemia. His electrophoretic pattern is classic for Hgb E/beta^0 thalassemia with over 50% Hgb E and the remainder being Hgb F. The etiology of elevated Hgb F in this condition is obscure but may be related to mutations in the gamma promoter region of chromosome 11. The other hemoglobinopathies listed in the question would have very low percentages of Hgb F.

19. B

The patient described most likely has atypical hemolytic uremic syndrome due to a defect complement regulation. Such patients respond to the C5 antibody, eculizumab that is FDA approved for this indication. The patient does not have TTP due to normal ADAMTS13 levels and the absence of and ADAMTS13 inhibitor. As such, treatment for TTP including plasmapheresis, rituximab, and steroids would not be appropriate. Similarly, IVIg, sometimes useful in the treatment of ITP, would not be the appropriate management.

20. B

Patients homozygous for the H63D mutation in the HFE gene seldom have problems with iron overload despite increases in transferrin saturation and mild increases in ferritin. Additionally, premenopausal women have fewer problems with iron overload due to regular iron losses. In contrast, patients who are homozygous for the C282Y HFE mutation or compound heterozygotes for C282Y/H63D are more likely to suffer end-organ complications of iron overload. Phlebotomy is generally reserved for these patients to maintain a ferritin of less than 50 ng/mL.

Liver biopsy and MRI are commonly used methods to detect the amount of iron overload in such patients but would not be appropriate for the patient in question due to her mutational status. Oral iron chelators are indicated for patients with thalassemia or transfusional iron overload as such patients cannot typically tolerate phlebotomy due to baseline anemia.

21. D

The McLeod phenotype is characterized by the absence of the Kell antigen on red cells and is one of the neuroacanthocytosis syndromes. The others include choreaacanthocytosis, Huntington disease-like 2, and pantothenate kinase–associated neurodegeneration. In all of these, patients present as the patient in question with progressive neurologic deterioration. Degeneration of the basal ganglia is a key finding. These are X-linked conditions. The red cell abnormalities are thought to arise from alterations in the red cell membrane due to abnormal phosphorylation of cytoskeletal proteins.

22. D

The patient described has a secondary erythrocytosis based on a "normal" erythropoietin level in the setting of a markedly elevated hemoglobin level. Absence of the JAK2(V617F) mutation makes a myeloproliferative disorder unlikely and in the setting of an erythropoietin level that is not suppressed rules out polycythemia vera. One important secondary cause of erythrocytosis is an underlying neoplasm. Hepatocellular carcinoma and kidney cancer are two such neoplasms that would be revealed on abdominal imaging. Red cell mass would be expected to be increased in any individual with a Hgb of 19.6 and is currently a very difficult to test to obtain. Red cell survival would not be useful, and with a low likelihood of a myeloproliferative disorder a bone marrow biopsy would not be helpful. Flow cytometry would similarly not be useful in this clinical setting.

23. D

The patient described likely has ferroportin disease characterized by a mutation in the ferroportin gene encoded by SLC40A1. Classical ferroportin disease is characterized by elevated ferritin with a normal iron and transferrin saturation. As ferroportin allows efflux of iron from macrophages, enterocytes, and hepatocytes, patients with ferroportin disease have excess iron deposition in these tissues but not in the blood. Hence iron levels and transferrin saturations are normal. In contrast, hemochromatosis due to mutations in HFE or HJV is associated with elevations in ferritin, transferrin saturation, and iron.

24. C

The TMPRSS6 gene encodes the protein matriptase-2 that is able to bind and degrade hemojuvelin that is needed to promote hepcidin production. Hepcidin causes internalization of the membrane protein ferroportin, which allows for iron absorption in the gut and iron release from macrophages. As a result of dysfunctional matriptase-2, patients with mutations in TMPRSS6 have very high hepcidin levels and, as a result, are unable to absorb oral iron. Mutations in TMPRSS6 are responsible for the majority of iron refractory iron deficient anemia. Patients with ferroportin disease of hemojuvelin mutations have hereditary hemochromatosis due to very low hepcidin levels. The porphyric states are not associated with iron deficiency refractory to iron therapy.

25. A

The physical exam described is classic for pulmonary hypertension. A loud P2, right-sided S3 (louder with inspiration) and peripheral edema are all found in patients with elevated pulmonary artery pressures. Patients with sickle cell disease develop pulmonary hypertension at alarming frequency due to both decreased NO levels and decreased arginine, a substrate for NO. The treatment for this disorder is unclear and the prognosis poor. Acute chest syndrome presents as a constellation of fever, chest pain, hypoxia, and pulmonary infiltrate. Cardiomyopathy would most likely present as S3 heard with both inspiration and expiration. ASD is associated with a fixed split S2. High output heart failure may produce a systolic flow murmur but would not produce the cardiac findings in the case.

26. B

The patient described has spur cell hemolytic anemia due to his end-stage liver disease. Chronic liver disease is thought to impair the liver's ability to esterify cholesterol causing free cholesterol to bind to the red cell membrane increasing its surface area and causing bizarre projections. The resulting cells are spur cells or acanthocytes. Microcytes would be expected in iron deficiency or thalassemia, and most patients with liver disease have some degree of macrocytosis. Echinocytes, or burr cells, are found in renal disease. Drepanocytes are sickled cells and dacryocytes are teardrop cells found in myelofibrosis and other marrow abnormalities.

27. C

In evaluating an iron-deficient patient for intravenous replacement, it is important to be able to estimate the iron requirement. To calculate replacement doses of iron, it is important to remember that 1 mL of blood contains about 1 mg of iron. Further, total blood volume is 65 mL/kg and hemoglobin contains about 0.34% iron by weight. Therefore:

Iron deficit (g) = (target Hb-actual Hb[g/dL])/100 × weight (kg) × 65 × 0.0034

Iron deficit (mg) = (target Hb-actual Hb) × weight (kg) × 2.2

Iron deficit (mg) = (target Hb-actual Hb) × weight (pounds)

This represents the amount of iron needed to make up the extra RBC mass. To this amount, storage iron must be added, which is about 600 mg for women and 1000 mg for men. For the above patient, this represents:

(12–7.2) × 110 + 600 = 1128 or about 1100 mg.

If this patient were replaced with oral iron (and if she could absorb oral iron), she would need much more since only about 5%–10% of oral iron is absorbed.

28. A

This patient has a prior history of aplastic anemia and is now found to have pancytopenia and newly diagnosed Budd Chiari syndrome. PNH should be suspected based on its known association with AA and MDS as well as hepatic vein occlusion. Flow cytometry FLAER testing is the most specific and sensitive test to make the diagnosis of PNH. Factor V Leiden would not explain pancytopenia and is only rarely associated with hepatic vein occlusion. Cytogenetics are typically normal in PNH. Protein electrophoresis and APA testing would also not be helpful in this setting.

29. B

This patient presents with blistering skin lesions, a prior history of IV drug use, and current alcohol use. A high suspicion for the diagnosis of porphyria cutanea tarda should be entertained. Many patients with the genetic mutations leading to PCT only become symptomatic when exposed to excessive iron through as can occur with infection with hepatitis C. In fact, patients with hepatitis C have a 66% higher likelihood of developing PCT. This patient should have liver function and hepatitis serologies sent. Patients with AIP do not have skin lesions, and therefore testing for urine AIP and PBG is not necessary. HFE mutations are less likely in the absence of family history and with a transferrin saturation of less than 50%. A liver MRI for iron content would also not be helpful.

30. C

Passenger lymphocytes in transplanted organs can cause hemolysis several days following transplant. This is typically due to antibodies against ABO antigens, but can occur with mismatch of other red blood cell antigens. In the case described, the recipient was type A and received a transplant from a type O donor. The donor lymphocytes expressed anti-A, which reacted against the recipient type A blood cells. Typically, hemolysis due to passenger lymphocytes is short lived and does not require specific treatment. Transfusion should be with type O positive red cells. In contrast, major ABO mismatch causes life-threatening hemolysis and shock. An ABO mismatch causes symptoms immediately during the transfusion. In the case described, the patient remained asymptomatic, which is not indicative of an ABO mismatch. Tacrolimus, and other calcineurin inhibitors, can cause microangiopathic hemolysis. EBV infections can cause cold agglutinin disease or warm antibody mediated hemolysis. In neither of these two cases, would anti-A antibodies be present.

31. C

Patients who have undergone renal transplant can develop a posttransplant erythrocytosis that is responsive to ACE inhibitor or ARB treatment. This typically occurs up to 2 years following transplant and occurs more commonly in patients receiving normal native kidneys, in smokers, in patients with renal artery stenosis, and in patients treated with cyclosporine. This patient does not have a polycythemia vera based on a normal erythropoietin level and would not need hydroxyurea or phlebotomy. Changing to cyclosporine would not correct the problem.

32. D

The patient described has Wilson disease as evidenced by liver disease and the presence of a Keyser-Fleischer ring on exam. This is caused by excessive copper accumulated due to a mutation in ATP7B, which leads to low ceruloplasmin levels and copper accumulation in the brain and liver. Copper also accumulates in the red cell membrane and may damage the cell membrane and inactivate enzymes of the pentose phosphate and glycolytic pathways. Coombs negative hemolytic anemia with spherocytosis can be the presenting feature of Wilson disease. Neurologic disease can also be present. Copper chelation with penicillamine can reverse the hemolytic process. The other treatments mentioned (glucocorticoids, IVIg, plasmapheresis, rituximab) may be effective for some types of immune hemolysis, but would not be useful in a patient with Wilson disease.

33. D

The patient described has refractory anemia with ringed sideroblasts with thrombocytosis. Over 80% of patients with RARS have a mutation in the ribosomal SF3B1 gene that strongly correlates with the presence of ringed sideroblasts in the marrow. The presence of an additional JAK2 mutation produces thrombocytosis in some patients as in the one described. This myelodysplastic disorder has a low likelihood of leukemic progression. BCR/ABL mutations are found in CML, BCL2 mutations in follicular lymphoma, CMYC mutations in Burkitt lymphoma, and MYD88 mutations in Waldenstrom macroglobulinemia.

34. C

Levels of methylmalonic acid and homocysteine become elevated in patients with vitamin B12 deficiency before serum vitamin B12 levels decrease below the normal range (200–800 pg/mL [148–590 pmol/L]). In contrast, only homocysteine is elevated in folate deficiency. Subclinical vitamin B12 deficiency in patients with subtle signs and symptoms of vitamin B12 deficiency, as in this case, can be detected by identification of elevated methylmalonic acid levels. This is particularly true for patients whose vitamin B12 levels are in the "low-normal" range. Additionally, pancytopenia can occur in vitamin B12-deficient patients. Malabsorption, independent of pernicious anemia, is the most likely cause of vitamin B12 deficiency in an older patient. Although bone marrow biopsy can be suggestive of vitamin B12 deficiency, it is not a specific test for confirming this disorder because there are other potential causes of megaloblastic marrow, including myelodysplasia. Erythrocyte folate levels have been touted as a better indication of folate stores than are serum folate levels, but are subject to problems of defining normal values and may not be that helpful clinically. Erythrocyte folate levels can also be depressed in patients with vitamin B12 deficiency. Additionally, folate deficiency would not cause the neurologic symptoms present in this patient. Parietal cell or intrinsic factor antibodies are elevated in patients with pernicious anemia, but may not be elevated in patients whose vitamin B12 deficiency is due to malabsorption.

35. D

The patient described has microangiopathic hemolysis as evidenced by the presence of schistocytes on peripheral smear. This is most likely secondary to cyclosporine, the only drug on her medication list that is associated with microangiopathy. Other drugs commonly associated with this condition include quinine and tacrolimus. Treatment involves stopping the offending drug.

36. C

Patients with hemolytic anemia, such as that in sickle cell disease, have an increased requirement for folate because of excessive cell turnover. This is also true for patients with desquamative skin disorders. In this case, the patient probably has not been taking supplemental folate, perhaps due to an oversight or difficulties with medical adherence in the setting of a previous stroke. The diagnosis can be confirmed with a serum folate measurement. The appropriate treatment for patients with folate deficiency is oral folic acid, 1–5 mg daily, for a duration of 1 to 4 months or until the patient achieves complete hematologic recovery. Following repletion, maintenance therapy with folate should continue indefinitely with 1 mg/day. Folate deficiency does not confer the risk for neurologic sequelae but is associated with anemia characterized by an elevated MCV as is demonstrated in this patient. Importantly, patients taking hydroxyurea may also have an elevated MCV that can confuse the diagnosis.

Hyperhemolysis in sickle cell disease is characterized by an increased reticulocyte count, which is not present in this patient. Anemia of chronic disease is typified by a normal or decreased MCV, not an increased MCV as found in this case. Similarly, patients with iron deficiency have a low MCV. Patients can have coexisting cobalamin deficiency with sickle cell disease, although this is not as likely a diagnosis as folate deficiency since cobalamin deficiency takes years to develop and hemolysis leads to increased folate requirements. Additionally, cobalamin deficiency that causes anemia may also be associated with loss of vibratory sense, which was absent in this patient's neurologic examination findings. However, the anemia of cobalamin deficiency can be reversed with folate therapy, necessitating establishment of a firm diagnosis before folate therapy is begun.

37. D

The pathophysiology of stroke in patients with sickle cell disease is complex, involving adherent erythrocyte membranes, constricted arterioles, nitric oxide depletion, and other factors. Strokes recur in up to 70% of patients with sickle cell disease following an initial stroke, if left untreated. Randomized trials have confirmed the ability of monthly erythrocyte transfusions (hypertransfusions) of 2 units per month to decrease stroke recurrence by 50% in patients with sickle cell disease. In fact, in children at risk for stroke based on abnormal cranial Doppler flow measurements, such hypertransfusion therapy is an effective prophylactic treatment. Furthermore, increased stroke risk returns to baseline in children in whom transfusions are stopped once initiated. Dipyridamole, clopidogrel, statins, and angiotensin-converting enzyme inhibitors have a role in stroke prevention in patients with atherosclerotic disease; however, their role in patients with sickle cell disease remains undefined. Hydroxyurea would be continued, although its role in stroke prevention is unclear.

38. A

Normal pregnancy is associated with mild anemia consisting of hemoglobin concentrations during the first and third trimesters of greater than 11.0 g/dL. Normal hemoglobin concentrations during the second trimester are greater than 10.5 g/dL. Anemia is physiological in pregnancy and related to an expansion of both plasma volume and erythrocyte mass. Because plasma volume expands to a greater extent than erythrocyte mass, the hemoglobin concentration decreases. Expansion of both erythrocyte mass and plasma volume results in effective delivery of oxygen to the developing fetus in a lower-viscosity, high oxygen-carrying-capacity state. Plasma volume expands greatest during the second trimester. Erythropoietin levels reach 150% of prepregnancy levels at delivery. Alterations in hepcidin have not been described in pregnant patients, but as hepcidin decreases iron absorption, elevated hepcidin levels produce iron deficiency over time. The patient described has normal iron levels inconsistent with increased hepcidin levels. The developing fetus needs folate and, as such, folate requirements increase in pregnancy.

39. D

Patients with either sickle painful vasoocclusive crisis or pregnancy do not require routine transfusions unless there are signs and symptoms of lack of oxygen delivery. Sickle cell patients often suffer from iron overload, which is exacerbated by inappropriate transfusion. The patient in question has no indication for blood. She should receive hydration and appropriate analgesia.

40. C

Each copy of chromosome 16 contains two α genes. The normal genotype is (α/α), (α/α). Patients with α-thalassemia can have several genotypes and phenotypes. This patient has a moderate microcytic anemia with an extra band found on hemoglobin electrophoresis. This extra band corresponds to hemoglobin H, which is composed of polymerized β chains, which migrate faster than hemoglobin A on a starch gel. The peripheral blood smear in this case shows target cells and microcytic indices, which are characteristic findings in patients with a three-α-gene defect responsible for hemoglobin H disease. There is a spectrum of disease severity in Hgb H, ranging from moderate anemia to more severe anemia with transfusion dependence, heart failure, and premature mortality. This mutation is more common in Southeast Asians. The history of thalassemia in both parents was responsible for this patient's genotype. Patients with a single-gene abnormality [(−−/α), (α/α)] are silent carriers of α-thalassemia and have normal hematologic indices and hemoglobin electrophoresis results. A two-gene defect in *cis* or *trans* produces α-thalassemia trait, which is characterized by a mild microcytic anemia with a preserved or increased erythrocyte count and normal hemoglobin electrophoresis results. Hydrops fetalis is not compatible with life and results from complete deletion of all alpha genes.

41. E

Hepcidin, a small peptide with antimicrobial properties, has been proven to be the major **negative** regulator of iron absorption. Hepcidin is produced by the liver and inhibits the intestinal absorption, macrophage release, and placental passage of iron. Hepcidin levels typically rise with infection and inflammation (states where the body's response is to conserve iron), and thus levels would be high (although possibly inappropriately) in the anemia of chronic disease (answer E) and fall with hypoxia or iron deficiency anemia (answers A and C). In hereditary hemochromatosis, interactions with the mutated HFE gene, lead to decreased hepcidin levels and therefore chronically increased iron absorption (answer B). B12 deficiency does not affect iron absorption, and thus hepcidin levels should not be significantly altered (answer D).

42. C

HFE hemochromatosis is the most common form of hereditary hemochromatosis. In Caucasians, the most common genotype is homozygous C282Y; however, clinical expression is low, and over 50% of individuals do not develop clinical signs of the disease. HFE mutation testing is thus the most appropriate next step in diagnosis. T2* MRI of the liver and liver biopsy would aid in quantification of iron overload in the liver, but would not be the initial step in the evaluation, and might not be necessary unless ferritin is greater than 1000 ng/mL or liver function tests were abnormal. Laboratory testing for hepcidin levels is not routinely available and although expected to be decreased in HFE hemochromatosis would not be sufficient to make the diagnosis. Thyroid studies also would not aid in making a diagnosis.

43. D

This patient has biochemical and clinical evidence of significant iron overload at a young age. Patients with HFE (type 1) related hemochromatosis rarely present before the fourth decade (answers A and B). Other genetically driven diseases of iron overload are becoming increasingly recognized. Juvenile hemochromatosis (type 2) typically presents at a young age with severe signs of iron overload including heart failure and polyendocrinopathies, while liver dysfunction may be less pronounced. Juvenile hemochromatosis is due to a recessive loss-of-function mutation in the hemojuvelin (HJV) or hepcidin genes (answer D). Type 3 hemochromatosis is typically due to a mutation in the transferrin receptor 2 (TFR2) gene, and its clinical presentation may mimic HFE-related disease, although patients are usually younger and iron overload may be more severe (answer C). Type 4 hemochromatosis is due to mutations in the ferroportin gene. Overall, the clinical manifestations are limited, and in the type 4A variant, transferrin saturation is low (answer E). The type 4B variant presents similar to HFE and type 3 hemochromatosis.

44. C

Transfusional iron overload is a significant problem in SCD patients on chronic transfusion therapy. The aim of iron chelation is to maintain body iron stores below levels that would cause tissue damage. Iron chelation is recommended when serum ferritin is >1000 μg/L, or liver iron content on liver biopsy is >7 mg/g dry weight, or when >120 cc of packed RBC/kg has been transfused. Deferoxamine (answer A) and Deferasirox (answer C) are both reasonable options as an iron chelator. Deferoxamine is given subcutaneously through a pump or intravenously, and adherence to this therapy is typically poor. In this patient who is about to start college and live in a dorm room, an oral iron chelator is a more reasonable first answer and is in accordance with her request. Simple phlebotomy (answer B) would not be an option given her anemia and the fact that she is on a chronic transfusion program. As her AST and ALT are already elevated and ferritin is significantly increased, some form of treatment would be indicated (answer D). Deferiprone, another oral iron chelator, is not yet approved in sickle cell disease but may be another option for oral iron chelation as more data become available (answer E).

45. C

This patient presents for evaluation of blistering skin lesions secondary to PCT. He consumes moderate amounts of alcohol. Both hereditary hemochromatosis and alcohol can increase hepatic iron content, which can precipitate the clinical manifestations of PCT. In fact, many patients with a genetic predisposition to PCT only become symptomatic when exposed to excess iron. Hereditary hemochromatosis has been reported to occur with increased frequency in patients with PCT and should be evaluated in this patient based on his iron studies (answer C). Blistering skin lesions do not occur in acute intermittent porphyria. Neurovisceral findings are typically seen with variegate and coproporphyria. Thus laboratory testing such as urine PBG, ALA, red cell PBG levels, and stool coproporphyrins, all of which are useful in diagnosing and differentiating between the acute porphyrias, is not indicated in this case (answers A, B, D, and E).

46. A

AIP, variegate porphyria, and coprophyria are considered acute neurovisceral porphyrias. Acute intermittent porphyria, the most common form, is caused by a deficiency of the enzyme porphobilinogen deaminase/hydroxymethylbilane synthase needed for heme biosynthesis. Deficiency of the enzyme results in overproduction of aminolevulinic acid and porphobilinogen. Clinical criteria include paroxysmal neurovisceral symptoms, such as abdominal pain, autonomic dysfunction, acute peripheral neuropathy, muscle weakness, hyponatremia, and psychiatric symptoms. Patients may also experience seizures. Rapid screening in the ER includes spot urine for PBG, ALA, and total porphyrins. Urine PBG will be markedly elevated in the acute setting in all the acute porphyrias and would be the initial diagnostic test of answer. Erythrocyte PBG deaminase determination can confirm deficiency of the enzyme, but many asymptomatic carriers exist and evidence of accumulation of porphyrin precursors would be required. Additionally, some patients express the mutated PBG deaminase only in the liver and not in peripheral blood, so testing can be falsely normal. Erythrocyte delta ALAD is decreased in ALA dehydratase porphyria. High levels of urine uroporphyrins are found in PCT. Once the diagnosis of an acute porphyria is made by elevated urine PBG, further studies including coproporphyrins can be evaluated to delineate between the types.

47. B

Anemia during pregnancy remains an important public health problem. Recent clinical trials have shown the safety and efficacy of different formulations of intravenous iron in pregnancy, although iron sucrose appears to be the best studied (answer B). In this patient with severe nausea and dehydration, neither increasing oral ferrous sulfate nor substituting ferrous gluconate are likely to be tolerated (answers C and E). As she does not have any underlying chronic illness and her iron studies are consistent with iron deficiency anemia and not anemia of chronic disease, an erythroid stimulating agent would not be indicated (answer A). In addition, she would have to be iron replete for an ESA to be most effective. She is hemodynamically stable, able to perform most of her ADLs, and the fetus is developing normally, so there is no current indication for PRBC, although she should be followed closely and transfusion could be considered if there were evidence of maternal or fetal compromise (answer D).

48. A

In patients with chronic intravascular hemolysis, iron is lost in the urine and can lead to IDA, which has been shown to worsen the hemolytic process. In this patient with likely heart valve mediated hemolytic anemia and IDA on laboratory evaluation, iron replacement either orally or intravenously would be a first-line treatment option (answer A). Although mitral valve replacement would be a more definitive treatment option in decreasing chronic intravascular hemolysis and iron loss, his overall poor health and significant comorbidities make him a poor surgical candidate (answer B). An ESA is less effective in the setting of iron deficiency, but might be considered as an adjunct therapy after he becomes iron replete (answer C). Therapeutic plasma exchange would be indicated in TTP, which is unlikely given the normal platelet count (answer D). Heart valve mediated hemolysis is much more likely in this patient with a murmur over the mitral area and an echocardiogram revealing regurgitant flow. There is currently no evidence of PNH or HUS; therefore, eculizumab would not be indicated (answer E).

49. D

The anemia of chronic disease/inflammation is a common multifactorial anemia. Typically cytokines and other inflammatory mediators lead to upregulation of hepcidin and subsequently sequestration of iron and suppression of erythropoiesis. The anemia is often normocytic but can be microcytic in up to a third of cases. The iron studies presented in this case are typical with a high or normal ferritin in the setting of a low or low normal total iron binding capacity and a low percent iron saturation. The anemia typically improves with treatment of the underlying disease. Further treatment can be aimed at the anemia if it is severe, symptomatic, or limits activities of daily living (answer D). CBC should be followed to document improvement as the infection is treated and inflammatory cytokines decrease. ESAs, oral iron, or IV iron might all be options if treatment was indicated (answers A, C, and E). Transfusion would also not be indicated with an Hgb of 10.1 g/dL and no cardiopulmonary disease (answer B).

50. B

This patient has an acquired macrocytic anemia in the setting of weight loss and poor oral intake. Folic acid deficiency should be suspected in this clinical scenario (answer B). Folate deficiency is typically due to impaired dietary intake or absorption. Given his depression, reclusive behavior, alcohol consumption, and weight loss, he likely has poor nutrition. In folate deficiency, homocysteine, but not methylmalonic acid is typically elevated. Vitamin B12 deficiency would take longer to develop, given greater body stores, and methylmalonic acid would likely be elevated (answer A). A bone marrow biopsy may be indicated if folate levels are normal and no other etiology identified, but would not be the initial diagnostic answer (answer C). The clinical history and lack of leukopenia make copper deficiency less likely (answer D). Chromosomal fragility studies would be indicated if there was a suspicion of Fanconi anemia, which is unlikely due to lack of supportive clinical history, physical findings, and recent normal CBC (answer E).

51. C

B12 is essential for normal DNA synthesis, and deficiency results in ineffective erythropoiesis with resultant macrocytic anemia and pancytopenia. The neuropathy secondary to B12 deficiency is symmetrical and is associated with posterior column degeneration resulting in loss of vibration and position sense. Both B12 and folate deficiency result in macrocytic anemia and pancytopenia; however, neurologic deficits do not occur in folate deficiency. Anemia of renal disease typically results in a normocytic, normochromic anemia. Aplastic anemia typically causes pancytopenia but would not typically cause neuropathy. Iron deficiency anemia is typically microcytic.

52. E

The patient presented in this vignette had a very high MCV, which is most likely to be a laboratory artifact. In addition, he had recently developed weight loss, fevers, night sweats, and peripheral cyanosis is noted on physical examination. This is highly suggestive of cold agglutinin disease, and the very high MCV is due to agglutination of RBCs as blood cools during testing. Review of the blood smear would show agglutination of RBCs that would likely abate with warming of the sample. A direct Coombs test should be sent and would be expected to be positive for complement and negative for IgG (answer E). The clinical scenario and markedly elevated MCV would be unusual for other causes of macrocytic anemia including chronic ETOH, vitamin B12 deficiency, folate deficiency, or hypothyroidism (answers A–D).

53. B

This patient has a severe acquired hypoproliferative anemia. Pure red cell aplasia (PRCA) is characterized by severe anemia, lack of reticulocytes, and an absence of erythroid precursors in the bone marrow. PRCA may be idiopathic or develop secondary to other diagnoses. The findings on the peripheral blood smear in this case demonstrate lymphocytes with prominent basophilic granules, which is highly suggestive of large granular lymphocytosis (LGL). LGL can be diagnosed by flow cytometry and T-cell receptor gene rearrangement studies (answer B). The great majority of T-cell LGL express CD3, CD8, CD16, CD57, and have a rearrangement of the alpha/beta TCR, but do not usually express CD4 and CD56. Although parvovirus B19 infection, thymoma, and myelodysplasia are potential causes, the peripheral blood smear in this patient reveals a classic-appearing large granular lymphocyte with abundant cytoplasm and azurophilic granules, making these other etiologies less likely (answers A, C, and D). HIV is a known cause of pure red cell aplasia, but large granular lymphocytes would not be expected in the peripheral blood (answer E).

54. E

The patient presented in this vignette has end-stage liver disease and worsening anemia. The peripheral blood smear shows an abundance of spur cells. The presence of spur cell anemia (Zieve syndrome) portends a very poor prognosis. Liver transplantation is the only effective treatment when spur cell anemia is associated with ESLD (answer E). This syndrome may also be seen with acute ETOH and may be reversible with cessation. Answers A–D are all potential treatments for autoimmune hemolytic anemia, but the finding of acanthocytosis makes this diagnosis much less likely.

55. C

The sideroblastic anemias are a heterogeneous group of disorders characterized by anemia (micro/normo/macrocytic) with ring sideroblasts (as shown) on Prussian blue staining, representing iron accumulation in the mitochondria. Both hereditary and acquired forms exist and differentiation is important as treatments differ. The classic X-linked inherited sideroblastic anemia (XLSA) occurs in males and is due to a mutation in the erythroid-specific 5-aminolevulinate synthase (ALAS2) gene. As opposed to the acquired sideroblastic anemias, XSLA is very responsive to oral vitamin B6 (pyridoxine) at doses of 50–100 mg daily (answer C). Bone marrow transplantation or azacytidine may be indicated in the myelodysplastic syndrome variants with ring sideroblasts (answers A and E). Iron unloading would be reasonable, but his symptomatic anemia likely precludes therapeutic phlebotomy (answer B). Zinc excess can lead to copper deficiency, which is a cause of acquired sideroblastic anemia (answer D).

56. D

The patient presented in this vignette had multiple physical findings consistent with the diagnosis of anorexia nervosa including low body weight, poor dentition, dry skin, brittle hair, and puffy cheeks (due to parotid inflammation). Isolated cytopenias as well as pancytopenia have been well described in patients with anorexia nervosa. In advanced stages of anorexia, bone marrow atrophy with a gelatinous appearance on biopsy can be seen. The patient in this vignette should be referred to psychiatry for definitive diagnosis and treatment (answer D). At the current levels of hemoglobin and platelet count, PRBC and platelet transfusion are not indicated (answers A and B). Although the ANC is 781/μL, there is no obvious infection, making G-CSF unwarranted (answer C). Bone marrow transplant referral is not needed at this point as the pancytopenia is less likely to be due to a primary bone marrow disorder and would be expected to improve with improved nutrition (answer E).

57. A

The patient in this vignette has an acquired hypoproliferative macrocytic anemia. Her symptoms of cold intolerance, fatigue, and constipation are classic for hypothyroidism, as is bradycardia and dry skin. Hypothyroidism should be considered in any evaluation of macrocytic anemia, and in this case thyroid function studies will likely be diagnostic (answer A). Folate deficiency is quite uncommon in the western world where foods are fortified with folic acid. In addition, this patient eats a balanced diet and has no other risk factors for folate deficiency (answer B). A primary bone marrow disorder should be in the differential of an unexplained macrocytic anemia, and bone marrow biopsy should be considered if laboratory evaluation is unrevealing. In this case, however, hypothyroidism is much more likely and should be evaluated first (answer C). B12 level is well within the normal range and methylmalonic acid level is unlikely to identify subclinical B12 deficiency (answer D). Coombs test would not likely identify the cause of anemia as the reticulocyte count is low and LDH and bilirubin are normal, making hemolysis much less likely (answer E).

58. D

Anemia is the most common hematologic abnormality in late stage HIV, affecting up to 80% of patients. In many cases, the etiology of the anemia is multifactorial. Malignancy, infection (fungal, viral, mycobacterial), autoimmune hemolytic anemia, and thrombotic microangiopathies should all be considered in the differential diagnosis. The patient in this vignette has advanced HIV with a low CD4 count. She has systemic symptoms of weight loss and fever. Nucleated red blood cells and teardrop-shaped red blood cells are noted on review of the peripheral blood smear. Assessment of the bone marrow looking for fungal infection, mycobacterial infection, or hematologic malignancy is warranted (answer D). There is no evidence of thrombotic thrombocytopenic purpura with a low reticulocyte count, normal platelet count, LDH, and blood smear without schistocytes, and therefore ADAMTS-13 testing is not warranted (answer A). As there is no evidence of hemolysis osmotic fragility, Coombs test and G-6 PD testing would not currently be indicated (answers B, C, and E).

59. C

The structure and function of hemoglobin is essential for human life. Fetal hemoglobin has substantially higher oxygen affinity then does adult hemoglobin, allowing the transport of oxygen across the placenta and to the fetus (answer C). A shift of the hemoglobin-oxygen desaturation curve to the left, as seen with decreased levels of 2.3 BPG leads to increased binding of oxygen (answer A). At birth fetal hemoglobin still represents 60% of total hemoglobin, decreasing to 1% in the adult (answer B). Hb A2 ($\alpha_2\delta_2$) is elevated in beta-thalassemia, not alpha-thalas-

semia (answer D). Two copies of the alpha globin gene and only one copy of the beta globin chain exist on their respective chromosomes (answer E).

60. C

Patients with alpha-thalassemia trait (two alpha gene deletion) exhibit mild microcytic, hypochromic anemia. The hemoglobin electrophoresis is usually normal, and this is often a diagnosis of exclusion. Individuals with one gene deletion usually have a normal hemoglobin and are not microcytic. In iron deficiency anemia the RDW is typically elevated, and the RBC count would be expected to be decreased. Beta-thalassemia major results in more severe anemia and clinical sequelae of ineffective erythropoiesis. The anemia of chronic inflammation is typically normocytic or mildly microcytic and would also be expected to have a decreased RBC count.

61. C

The patient in this vignette has moderate microcytic symptomatic anemia, occasionally requiring transfusion. Both parents have a milder form of anemia. Of the answers listed Hb H disease (α-/--) is the best option (answer C). The clinical manifestations of Hb H disease are more severe than alpha- and beta-thalassemia minor, which usually present with mild asymptomatic microcytic anemia (answers B and D). The clinical course is less severe than in hydrops fetalis, which presents in utero or at birth with severe life-threatening anemia and is usually fatal. In hydrops fetalis, no hemoglobin A, F, or A2 can be made given the lack of production of any alpha chain (answer E). Beta-thalassemia major/Cooley anemia also presents with a more severe course. Typically life-long transfusions are required, growth retardation is noted, and hepatosplenomegaly is appreciated, along with other sequela beginning after around 6 months of life when gamma chain production is significantly decreased (answer A).

62. D

The patient in this vignette has a mild microcytic anemia and target cells on the peripheral blood smear, which could be consistent with either alpha-thalassemia minor or beta-thalassemia minor. Her Mediterranean heritage is classic for beta-thalassemia, and the elevated A2 band ($\alpha_2\delta_2$) is diagnostic (answer D). Beta-thalassemia major (Cooley anemia) is a severe life-threatening transfusion dependent anemia (answer A). Alpha-thalassemia trait does not lead to microcytic red blood cells or anemia (answer B). An elevated A2 band would not be seen in alpha-thalassemia minor (answer C). In hereditary persistence of fetal hemoglobin Hb F would be much higher and Hb A2 would not be elevated (answer E).

63. B

The care of patients with sickle cell disease during pregnancy is complex and should involve a multidisciplinary team consisting of high-risk obstetricians, hematology, and anesthesia. Although most pregnancies result in a live birth, the rates of both maternal and fetal complications are higher as compared with age-matched peers. Narcotic analgesia should be minimized during pregnancy, but is safe to use and should be prescribed during acute painful episodes (answer B). This patient is writhing in pain and will likely require intravenous opioid analgesia. The use of hydroxyurea (answer A) is relatively contraindicated during pregnancy and should not be initiated at this time. Deferoxamine is a Category C drug and should only be used during pregnancy when the benefits outweigh the risks, which it does not in the patient in this vignette who only has a moderate increase in her ferritin (answer C). Prophylactic red blood cell transfusion (answer D) is controversial during pregnancy, but might be considered in Hb SS patients with severe anemia (below 6 g/dL) or with significant morbidities. If there were preconception indications for chronic transfusion, then continuation during pregnancy would be indicated. However in the patient presented in this vignette has Hb S-beta thalassemia, a hemoglobin concentration of 10.1 g/dL and no end organ complications, and thus transfusion is not currently indicated. The routine use of antibiotics without signs of infection is discouraged (answer E).

64. D

The patient in this vignette had mild bone pain throughout life, two episodes of pneumonia, a moderate microcytic anemia, and a blood smear showing target and sickle cells. In addition, one parent has a mild anemia (likely beta$^+$-thalassemia) and another parent had a normal CBC (likely sickle cell trait, given a brother with sickle trait). The course of beta$^+$-thalassemia can be quite variable, and the diagnosis is occasionally delayed into adulthood. The hb electrophoresis in beta$^+$-thalassemia always shows more hb S than A, and the A2 band is typically elevated (answer D). The electrophoretic pattern in answer A is consistent with Hb SS sickle cell anemia. The electrophoresis in answer B is typical of sickle cell trait in which the Hb A is typically higher than Hb S. Sickle cell trait would not be associated with pain crisis, microcytosis, anemia, or the blood smear shown in this vignette. Answer C is consistent with beta^0-thalassemia where no Hb A is produced. The anemia is typically more severe and the clinical course typically worse than presented in this vignette. Answer E represents a normal hemoglobin electrophoresis.

65. B

The time of transition from pediatric to adult care can be very difficult for both the patient and adult provider. This is especially true in complex diseases such as sickle cell anemia. The time of transition is a good time to review current therapies and set up long-term treatment plans. Changing therapy plans that have been in place for long periods of time can be difficult for the patient, but may be necessary. Given her frequent pain crises and hospital admissions, she should be placed on hydroxyurea, based on the results of the randomized MSH trial, which showed a reduction in the median rate of painful vasoocclusive events by almost 50% (2.5 vs. 4.5 crises per year). Hydroxyurea was also associated with a decreased incidence of acute chest syndrome and a reduction in the need for transfusions (answer B). As she does not have a history of stroke, abnormal transcranial Dopplers, or other end-organ complications, chronic transfusion therapy is not indicated (answer A). Penicillin prophylaxis is indicated for children less than 5 years of age, but its role has not been proven in adults (answer C). Lisinopril is indicated given the proteinuria noted on urinalysis (answer D). Although narcotic analgesics should always be used with extreme caution, based on her history of frequent pain crisis and hospital admissions, chronic long acting opioids are currently indicated in this patient (answer E). If hydroxyurea is successful in decreasing the frequency of painful episodes, then weaning off narcotics should be attempted in the future.

66. A

Priapism, defined as a sustained penile erection in the absence of sexual stimulation, should be considered a medical emergency, as impotence and chronic sexual dysfunction can occur if left untreated. Urgent urologic evaluation for aspiration and irrigation of the corpus cavernosum is indicated and is considered the standard of care for priapism lasting more than 4 hours (answer A). Unfortunately, neither simple nor exchange RBC transfusion has proven beneficial, but may be considered in refractory cases (answers B and D). In addition, exchange transfusion in patients with priapism has been associated with headaches, seizures, and other neurologic sequela (ASPEN syndrome), and care should be taken to keep the posttransfusion Hb below 10 g/dL. A distal penile shunt might be necessary in cases refractory to aspiration and irrigation, but should not be initial therapy (answer C). Proximal shunting may be required if distal shunting fails, but is associated with higher rates of impotence. Hydroxyurea would not be beneficial in the acute setting, but could be considered as secondary prophylaxis of stuttering priapism, although randomized data supporting its efficacy is lacking (answer E). Pseudoephedrine, other alpha- and beta-adrenergic agonists, antiandrogens, and phosphodiesterase-inhibitors have also been used for secondary prophylaxis based on limited data.

67. D

Hydroxyurea (HU) is a ribonucleotide reductase inhibitor that increases fetal hemoglobin and hydration of erythrocytes. HU has been shown to decrease painful episodes, hospitalizations, acute chest syndrome, and improve survival in randomized studies of patients with hemoglobin SS and hemoglobin S-beta^0 thalassemia. Thus it is indicated for patients with sickle cell anemia with three or more moderate to severe painful episodes per year, recurrent sickle cell disease associated pain that interferes with daily activity and quality of life, history of recurrent or severe acute chest syndrome, or symptomatic anemia. None of the other answers have shown to reduce mortality or vasoocclusive episodes in individual with sickle cell anemia.

68. B

The patient presented in this vignette has chronic fatigue, jaundice, and splenomegaly. Her labs are consistent with a hemolytic anemia. The peripheral blood smear shows spherocytes, which can be seen in both HS and warm autoimmune hemolytic anemia. The positive family and chronicity of symptoms make HS the much more likely diagnosis. The molecular pathophysiology of HS can be quite diverse with mutations occurring in ankyrin, spectrin, or band 3 (answer B). As in this vignette, the most common form of HS follows a autosomal dominant pattern of inheritance. A PIG A mutation would be seen in PNH, which would typically present with an acquired intravascular hemolysis. In addition, there would not be a positive family history, splenomegaly, or spherocytes on the blood smear (answer A). A mutation in an Rh associated glycoprotein may lead to Rh null disease, which is a cause of hereditary stomatocytosis, which was not seen on the blood smear (answer C). Pyruvate kinase deficiency typically follows an AR mode of inheritance and echinocytes are classically seen on the blood smear (answer D). G-6PD deficiency typically follows an X-linked inheritance, leads to episodic hemolysis, and in the acute phase would present with blister or bite cells on the peripheral smear (answer E).

69. C

The patient presented in this vignette has a known chronic hemolytic anemia. He now presents with acute worsening of his chronic anemia along with symptoms of a recent viral syndrome. He works in a kindergarten and was likely exposed to parvovirus B 19, leading to an aplastic crisis. As the red cell life span in patients with chronic hemolytic anemias is markedly reduced, even brief periods of decreased red cell production can lead to significant anemia. In immunocompetent individuals the infection and suppression of erythropoiesis typically resolves on its own and supportive care is all that is necessary (answer C). Although splenectomy may be very effective in treating symptomatic chronic anemia secondary to hereditary spherocytosis, this patient has a baseline hemoglobin of 10–11 g/dL, and splenectomy would not be indicated, especially at the current time (answer A). There is no effective antiviral agent for parvovirus B 19, and acyclovir or IVIg can be effective at treating chronic parvovirus B 19 infection in immunosuppressed individuals, but is typically not necessary in immunocompetent patients (answer D). Steroids would not be effective in treating aplastic crisis secondary to parvovirus B 19 (answer E).

70. D

The African-American man patient presented in this vignette has an acquired hemolytic anemia after exposure to rasburicase, an oxidant drug known to induce hemolysis in G-6PD deficient individuals. He also describes a similar event after exposure to trimethoprim-sulfamethoxasole. His G-6PD level was normal, but was measured during the acute hemolytic period. In the African American variant of G-6PD deficiency, levels of G6PD are higher in young reticulocytes, and enzyme levels may be normal if measured during an acute hemolytic event. In addition, the lack of bite or blister cells on the blood smear 3 weeks after the hemolytic event is to be expected. These classic blood smear findings are typically seen only during an acute hemolytic episode after which these damaged RBCs are quickly removed from circulation. A G-6PD level sent after recovery from the acute event could confirm the suspected diagnosis (answer D). There is no information provided in the vignette suggesting AIHA, HS, HUS, or CAD as a more likely diagnosis (answers A–C and E).

71. A

G6PD deficiency is inherited in an X-linked recessive pattern. The clinical and laboratory values presented in the stem are classic for the diagnosis, and patients with G6PD develop hemolytic anemia after exposure to oxidant drugs, such as trimethoprim-sulfamethoxazole.

72. E

PK deficiency is the most common enzymopathy of the glycolytic pathway and accounts for greater than 80% of all such defects. The clinical course of PK deficiency is quite heterogeneous, but patients usually have only mild to moderate symptoms secondary to elevated 2,3 DPG levels and a shift of the hemoglobin-oxygen dissociation curve to the left. In pyruvate kinase deficiency, echinocytes (secondary to RBC dehydration as shown in the accompanying blood smear) may be seen on the peripheral blood smear (answer E). A pyruvate kinase level should be ordered to confirm the suspected diagnosis. The patient's blood smear would not be consistent with the other diagnoses listed. In G-6 PD deficiency bite or blister cells would be seen in the acute phase of hemolysis (answer A). In hereditary spherocytosis or autoimmune hemolytic anemia, spherocytes would be seen on the blood smear (answers B and C). In alpha-thalassemia target cells would be expected (answer D).

73. B

The patient presented in this vignette presents with new onset hemolytic anemia. Her history of rheumatoid arthritis, in conjunction with spherocytes on the peripheral blood smear, makes warm autoimmune hemolytic anemia (WAIHA) the most likely diagnosis. In WAIHA anemia the Coombs test is either strongly + for IgG and negative for complement (not listed as a answer) or strongly + for IgG and weakly + for complement as IgG does not fix complement strongly (answer B). Answer A would represent a negative Coombs test. There is no reason to expect the Coombs test should not be interpretable in WAIHA (answer C). The pattern in answer D is one you might expect in cold agglutinin disease as the antibody is an IgM, which fixes complement efficiently.

74. B

In patients with CLL, previous exposure to fludarabine based chemotherapy regimens is associated with an increased risk of developing warm autoimmune hemolytic anemia (WAIHA). Steroids are first-line therapy for WAIHA as they interfere with the ability of macrophages to clear IgG or complement coated erythrocytes and reduce autoantibody production. Although there is emerging data supporting use of rituximab as first-line therapy, published trials thus far have limitations such that rituximab is considered second-line therapy. Splenectomy is also considered second line therapy. IVIg is much less effective in WAIHA as compared with ITP and would not be considered first (or even second) line therapy. PRBC transfusion is given judiciously given the expected hemolysis of transfused blood, as well as difficulty obtaining crossmatch compatible units, and is thus reserved for severe or life threatening anemia. Given her normal vital signs and hemoglobin of 8.5 g/dL, PRBC transfusion would not be indicated.

75. D

The patient presented in this vignette has an acute coronary syndrome, and emergent coronary revascularization is recommended. He is also noted to have anemia with a markedly elevated MCV and RBC agglutination on the peripheral blood smear. The Coombs test is + for C3 only, supporting the diagnosis of cold agglutinin disease. As cardiac bypass is typically performed with cold cardioplegia, plasmapheresis should be performed preoperatively to markedly decrease the causative IgM antibody (answer D). Plasmapheresis is not a definitive treatment in and of itself, but is useful in emergent situations. It efficiently lowers the IgM, which is primarily intravascular, and is thus useful prior to surgical procedures with prolonged cold exposure. Another option for surgery would be to avoid cold cardioplegia if possible, but this was not listed as a answer. Prednisone is not typically affective in cold agglutinin disease as opposed to WAIHA, unless an underlying lymphoproliferative disorder is present (answer A). Rituximab is considered among the first-line treatments in cold agglutinin disease, but would not work quickly enough to be effective prior to bypass surgery scheduled in the next 24 hours (answer B). Splenectomy is typically not effective in cold agglutinin disease, as opposed to WAIHA, and would be contraindicated in the setting of an acute coronary syndrome (answer C). Eculizumab would be indicated as first-line therapy in paroxysmal nocturnal hemoglobinuria or atypical hemolytic uremic syndrome, but is not considered first-line therapy for cold agglutinin disease (answer E).

76. C

Cold agglutinin disease is due to a complement fixing IgM antibody directed towards polysaccharides on the RBC surface. Direct lysis or clearance of C3b coated cells occurs primarily through the Kupffer cells of the liver. Cold agglutinins may be produced in response to infection or in patients with underlying lymphoproliferative disorders. In fact in most patients a small B-cell clone can be identified by flow cytometry or suggested by a small monoclonal band on a serum protein electrophoresis. Treatment should be initiated for symptomatic anemia, transfusion dependence, and/or disabling circulatory symptoms. Rituximab therapy is considered pharmacologic first-line therapy as greater than 50% of patients will respond. Steroids have not been found to be effective in treatment of CAD. Splenectomy is also ineffective given that the liver is the predominant site of sequestration. Erythropoietin could be considered; however, given her degree of anemia and symptoms, she requires more aggressive treatment. Fludarabine and rituximab have been shown to result in response in ~75% of patients; however, fludarabine as a single agent has not been studied.

77. C

Treatment of eculizumab has revolutionized the treatment of PNH. Eculizumab, a humanized monoclonal antibody that acts as an inhibitor of terminal complement, has led to markedly improved quality of life, decreased hemolysis, decreased thrombosis, and potentially increased survival in patients with PNH. Eculizumab binds to the complement component C5 and prevents its cleavage, thus preventing activation of the membrane attack complex. In patients with PNH, the lack of surface GPI anchored proteins on the RBC surface renders the cells more susceptible to complement-mediated lysis. With inhibition of lysis, the percentage of GPI-deficient RBCs actually increases after treatment with eculizumab (answer C). Most PNH patients treated with eculizumab become transfusion independent, because the hemoglobin often fails to normalize as some degree of extravascular hemolysis continues (answer A). Although the incidence of *Neisseria meningitidis* is increased with terminal complement blockade, the incidence still remains quite low (answer B). Vaccination is strongly recommended prior to initiation of eculizumab. The risk of thrombosis has been shown to decrease after use of eculizumab (answer D). LDH markedly decreases and often normalizes after treatment with eculizumab and has been followed as a surrogate marker for hemolysis in patients (answer E).

78. A

Paroxysmal nocturnal hemoglobinuria leads to the absence of two GPI-anchored proteins, CD55 and CD59, which leads to uncontrolled complement activation resulting in hemolytic anemia, thrombosis, and cytopenias. Eculizumab is a monoclonal antibody that inhibits terminal complement by binding to C5. The most serious risk of terminal complement blockade is life-threatening *Neisseria* infections; thus all patients treated with eculizumab should be vaccinated against *Neisseria*. The use of eculizumab has not been associated with HiB, hepatitis A or B, or varicella.

79. B

The differentiation between TTP, atypical HUS (aHUS), and other thrombotic microangiopathies can be difficult. As opposed to other thrombotic microangiopathies, TTP is associated with levels of ADAMTS-13 typically below 5%–10%. Levels that are decreased, but above this range, are nonspecific and can be seen a variety of conditions. In addition, a markedly elevated creatinine is unusual in TTP, while expected in atypical HUS. The degree of thrombocytopenia is often marked in TTP, while more variable and modest in aHUS. The lack of response to plasma exchange is typical in aHUS, while unusual in TTP. Given this patient's laboratory results, which include a moderate decrease in ADAMTS-13, moderate thrombocytopenia, and significant acute renal failure that has worsened with plasma exchange, aHUS is the more likely diagnosis. Eculizumab should be promptly initiated in hopes of preserving renal function (answer B). The additions of rituximab, steroids, or switching to cryopoor plasma are all reasonable answers for refractory TTP (answers A, D, and E). Twice daily plasma exchange is very labor intensive but can be considered in refractory TTP patients with worsening neurologic status or clinical course, although efficacy remains unproven (answer C).

80. A

This patient presents with the classic pentad of TTP: microangiopathic hemolytic anemia, thrombocytopenia, fever, renal failure, and mental status changes. TTP is caused by an inhibitor to ADAMTS-13 leading to accumulation of high-molecular-weight von Willebrand multimers causing small vessel thrombosis and microangiopathic hemolytic anemia. First-line treatment of TTP is plasma exchange utilizing FFP as replacement fluid, thus removing the offending antibody and supplying deficient ADAMTS-13. Rituximab is considered adjunct first- or second-line therapy. Eculizumab could be considered if aHUS was thought to be the diagnosis. In this case, the severe neurologic sequela and only mild renal insufficiency make aHUS less likely. An ADAMTS-13 level can be sent, and if normal this diagnosis can be reconsidered. However, initiation of therapeutic plasma exchange can be life-saving and should not be delayed while awaiting ADAMTS results. FFP could be transfused in a setting in which plasmapheresis is not available, but 2 units would not be considered an effective dose. Prednisone may also be utilized as an adjunct to plasmapheresis, but its efficacy remains uncertain.

81. A

It is recognized that there are risks and costs that are associated with transfusion therapy, be it simple or exchange. This includes iron overload; financial costs; need for intravenous access; risk for alloimmunization; and inconvenience for the patient and/or their family. Nonetheless, transfusion therapy is still considered the treatment of choice for secondary prevention of stroke and is preferred over hydroxyurea therapy. There is no known benefit to allowing the Hgb-S level to rise >50%, and it would not be expected to provide any benefit to the patient.

82. D

Based upon her history physical examination and the available laboratory data, the patient most likely has α-thalassemia trait. The definitive diagnosis would entail analysis of her α-globin genes, either by a multiplex ligation-dependent probe amplification assay or by direct sequencing of the α-globin genes. In this case, α-globin sequencing showed homozygosity for a rightward single α-globin gene deletion (−α3.7/−α3.7). The presence of two α-globin gene deletions is known as "trans alpha-thalassemia" or "alpha-thalassemia-2," which is a chronic and overall clinically silent condition. It is important to recognize this as a cause of chronic and constant microcytosis so that patients and their family members are not misdiagnosed and/or mistreated.

While copper deficiency, usually stemming from zinc toxicity, or lead poisoning can cause a microcytosis, this is coupled with anemia. Similarly, the presence of sideroblasts, either congenital or acquired, is accompanied by anemia, which this patient does not have.

83. A

This patient's presentation and laboratory data are consistent with a warm autoimmune hemolytic anemia (WAIHA). As a result, initial treatment with high-dose steroids is considered to be first-line therapy.

While WAIHA can be treated with rituximab, this is not considered first-line therapy. The absence of complement deposition noted on the DAT does not support a cold autoimmune hemolytic anemia, making the use of warming interventions superfluous. While splenectomy can be used either as first-line therapy for hereditary spherocytosis or as second-line therapy for WAIHA, this is not indicated at this time. Even though there is evidence of hemolysis, the CBC and peripheral smear do not support the presence of a microangiopathy, making plasma exchange an incorrect choice.

84. E

The overwhelming majority of cold agglutinin disease is mediated by an IgM antibody, which is often associated with an underlying condition, which can be discerned in part by the clonality of the IgM autoantibody. Specifically, a monoclonal IgM would result from either MGUS or Waldenström macroglobulinemia. Polyclonal IgM is seen following an infection, typically in children.

A bone marrow biopsy would be indicated if there was concern for lymphoplasmacytic lymphoma, but a SPEP should be considered first. There is no reason to suspect paroxysmal nocturnal hemoglobinuria, making flow cytometry for CD55/CD59 testing an incorrect choice. Cryoglobulins can be associated with anemia and symptoms worsened by exposure to cold temperatures; however, this is not associated with a Coombs(+) hemolytic anemia. The Donath-Landsteiner antibody is present in cases of paroxysmal cold hemoglobinuria, which is not associated with markedly elevated cold agglutinin titers and is typically restricted to an IgG autoantibody.

85. E

A ferritin level of 50–100 μg/L is the goal range to reach with serial phlebotomy and the goal range to maintain total iron body stores.[4] In this case, it is not uncommon to observe that patients may not re-accumulate iron, but periodic assessments of iron status are indicated. As patients with liver disease are susceptible to water-borne illnesses, such as *Vibrio*, raw shellfish should be avoided. Finally, avoiding iron supplementation and preventing iron absorption, as with black tea, are simple maneuvers that are recommended to help avoid iron (re-)accumulation.

86. D

The clinical case and the peripheral smear are consistent with hereditary spherocytosis. Specifically, the el-

evated MCHC, reticulocytosis, and the appearance of spherocytes are supportive of this diagnosis. Although spherocytes can be seen in autoimmune hemolytic anemias, the negative DAT and normal haptoglobin/LDH makes this much less probable. The osmotic fragility test is commonly used to diagnose HS, as the spherocytic, nonbiconcave cells have less surface area:volume and lyse more easily with hypotonic solutions[5], although any condition that weakens the red cell membrane will cause more lysis. This is the initial screen to diagnose HS, which can be followed by more specific tests such as Eosin-5-maleimide binding to Band 3, and ultimately, sequencing the genes for α-spectrin, β-spectrin, ankyrin, and Band 3.

Despite the splenomegaly, there is no reason to suspect either a myelo- or lymphoproliferative disorder, making a bone marrow biopsy and/or SPEP incorrect answers. Cryoglobulinemia would not lead to spherocytes on the peripheral smear, whereas a Ham test has been used for the diagnosis of PNH.

87. B

This patient's presentation is classic for vitamin B12 deficiency, despite the "normal" measured plasma levels of B12. In addition to the marked macrocytic anemia, the neurologic findings are typical for the neuropathy caused by B12 deficiency and are not seen with myelodysplasia or congenital bone marrow failure disorders, such as dyskeratosis congenita. It is well known that "false-positive" levels of B12 occur due to a variety of causes, and plasma levels of B12 do not accurately gauge cellular concentrations of vitamin B12. As a result, testing for methylmalonic acid levels, which are markedly elevated in B12 deficiency, will confirm the diagnosis.

While many lung cancers can lead to neurologic symptoms via a paraneoplastic process, this would not be associated with a pancytopenia with macrocytosis, and evidence of hemolysis.

88. E

The patient is presenting with marked hemolysis from glucose 6-phosphate dehydrogenase deficiency that has been exacerbated by the concomitant use of a sulfa-compound and phenazopyridine. Testing for G6PD activity would provide a falsely normal value and would not be recommended. Standard of care is to remove the offending agent(s) and supportive care. The presence of "bite" or "blister" cells are seen in this setting and would not be noted in methemoglobinemia, unstable hemoglobins, or other enzymatic red cell defects.

89. D

Iron deficiency is a common side effect of gastric bypass, along with other essential elements such as calcium and vitamins B12 and D. While thrice-daily oral iron is associated with side effects that can limit adherence, the patient voiced no issues in regard to this. In her case, despite the 3-month use of oral iron, no benefit has been seen, making the continued use of oral iron unreasonable. In general, transfusion of red cells is unnecessary and will only partially correct the anemia, and even less so correct the iron deficiency.

90. E

Patients with hematologic disorders, such as sickle cell disease or hereditary spherocytosis, are at risk for transient aplastic crisis, as is evident by the marked reticulocytopenia in a patient where a marked reticulocytosis should be present. Viral PCR or culture can be performed, but the presence of IgM antibodies are present in the majority of cases during a transient aplastic crisis.[10] A bone marrow biopsy can be performed that will show the presence of erythroid hypoplasia, but this will not be specific for parvovirus.

Venous thromboembolism is a major cause of morbidity in the sickle cell population, but is not associated with acute anemia and reticulocytopenia. The presence of paroxysmal cold hemoglobinuria should be considered in a patient with hemolytic anemia; however, this is also not associated with reticulocytopenia, and thus checking the Donath-Landsteiner antibody test would not be correct in this case.

91. A

The marked anisocytosis, microcytosis, appearance on the peripheral smear (elliptocytes with marked microcytes) is consistent with hereditary pyropoikilocytosis, which is invariably caused by either homozygous or compound heterozygous mutations in the gene for α-spectrin, *SPTA1*.

Beta-thalassemia in its more severe forms presents with a microcytosis, but not with elliptocytes on the smear and a normal hemoglobin electrophoresis. An osmotic fragility and EMA binding will certainly be abnormal, but this can be seen in hereditary spherocytosis or any other condition that affects red cell membrane integrity, including autoimmune hemolytic anemia(s).

92. D

The most likely cause for the patient's persistent macrocytosis (without anemia) is due to the presence of zidovudine. There are numerous medications, such as hydroxyurea, azathioprine, and methotrexate, that lead to a drug-induced macrocytosis and can be used as a proxy-marker for medication compliance. Given that the other causes of macrocytosis are not supported by the data (cytopenia, ethanol toxicity, B12/folate deficiency, and hypothyroidism), bone marrow biopsy is not indicated. In B12 deficiency, homocysteine levels are also elevated, which makes methylmalonic acid testing an incorrect choice. Lead toxicity is associated with a microcytosis and basophilic stippling of red cells, neither of which are present.

93. A

The findings on the bone marrow biopsy are consistent with pure red cell aplasia, which, when coupled with the symptoms of myasthenia gravis, raises the possibility of a thymoma, wherein CT and/or MRI is recommended as a screen.[13] There is no evidence to support the presence of PNH, which would be diagnosed via flow cytometry for CD55/CD59 expression. The reported normal differential makes a large granular lymphocyte leukemia unlikely, particularly in context with the myasthenia-like symptoms. The history does not support celiac disease, making testing for tTG an incorrect choice.

94. B

The presence of a normocytic anemia, inappropriate reticulocyte count, elevated ferritin with pan-decreased iron panel, in the setting of a patient with multiple medical problems, makes this consistent with the anemia of chronic disease. Certainly thalassemia can lead to a chronic anemia, but a microcytosis would be expected. Patients with lupus are at risk for developing an autoimmune hemolytic anemia, but this is not supported by the history and available laboratory data. The elevated fer-

ritin and low TIBC is inconsistent with iron deficiency. While PRCA remains possible, the mild normocytic anemia in the setting of the numerous medical conditions makes anemia of chronic disease more likely.

95. C

Acetaminophen manufacturing involves agents such as nitrobenzene and aniline, which are known to cause methemoglobinemia (Fig. 34.20). In this case, the patient's methemoglobin level was 70.4% (0.4–1.5), which is considered a medical emergency. Immediate infusion of methylene blue led to a symptomatic improvement, but a paradoxical increase in met-Hgb levels to 81.5% (0.4–1.5), prompting emergent erythrocytapheresis, where his plasma was noted to be markedly discolored (**RED ARROW**) compared with normal plasma (**GREEN ARROW**). This was found to be from continued exposure on his skin, prompting immediate removal and extensive skin scrubbing. After additional doses of methylene blue and the erythrocytapheresis, his met-Hgb level was measured at 17.7 (0.4–1.5). Carboxyhemoglobin levels are measured in individuals suffering carbon monoxide poisoning, which does not lead to this constellation of findings. Patients with G6PD deficiency may have hemolysis following methylene blue administration, but the life-threatening nature of this case mandates methylene blue use, despite potential risk of hemolysis. Sulfhemoglobinemia is a rare condition leading to cyanosis after sulfa exposure. Symptoms include a bluish or greenish discoloration of the blood, skin, and mucous membranes

96. A

The differential for microcytic anemia includes iron deficiency, thalassemia, or anemia of chronic inflammation. A history of anemia unresponsive to iron and a family history of anemia support a diagnosis of thalassemia. Furthermore, the normal red cell distribution width also favors thalassemia over iron deficiency. The patient has no history to suggest anemia of chronic inflammation, which results in disrupted normal iron utilization secondary to an increased level of hepcidin. The mild degree of anemia in this patient favors thalassemia trait rather than a more severe form of thalassemia. When

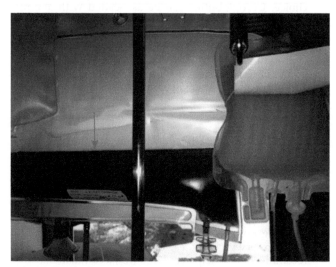

FIG. 34.20 Bradberry SM. Occupational methaemoglobinaemia. Mechanisms of production, features, diagnosis, and management including the use of methylene blue. *Toxicol Rev.* 2003;22(1):13–27.

thalassemia is suspected, a hemoglobin electrophoresis should be obtained. In cases of alpha-thalassemia trait, the hemoglobin electrophoresis results will be normal. However, beta-thalassemia trait can be detected on hemoglobin electrophoresis by the presence of an elevated hemoglobin A2, as is the case here. This abnormal hemoglobin results from the pairing of alpha globin chains with delta globin chains secondary to the reduced production of beta globin chains. In addition, microcytosis is usually out of proportion to the degree of anemia in beta-thalassemia trait. Thalassemia trait does not require treatment. However, patients should receive genetic counseling and should avoid taking iron supplementation unless he/she develops iron deficiency. The absence of hemoglobin S on electrophoresis eliminates sickle cell trait as a possible explanation. In addition, the complete blood count is normal in patients with sickle cell trait.

97. C

Beta-thalassemia can result from more than 150 different mutations of the β-globin gene complex while Hb S production results from a valine substituted for glutamic acid in the β-globin chain. In beta-thalassemia, decreased β-chain synthesis leads to impaired production of the α2β2 tetramer of normal Hb A. In sickle cell anemia (Hb SS) Hb A is not detectable since the normal β-chain is not produced. Also, the Hb F level is often elevated (up to 10%), and Hb S levels are usually greater than 80%. In sickle cell trait, hemoglobin A is found in greater proportion than hemoglobin S, and hemoglobin A2 is not increased. Instead, Hb S and Hb C are usually present in equal proportions on Hgb electrophoresis (45%–50% each) and Hb F is present 7%8%. In HbS/beta⁰ thalassemia, Hb A is again undetectable since there is no production of β-chains. Hb S is approximately 80%, Hb A2 5%–8%, and Hb F 10%–20%. However, this patient has some evidence of Hb A production. With the presence of Hb S and increased Hb A2, this patient has HbS/B⁺ thalassemia.

98. B

Sickle cell hepatopathy describes a variety of pathologies seen in sickle cell disease including gallstone disease, hypoxic liver injury, hepatic sequestration, liver injury due to iron overload, venous outflow obstruction, viral hepatitis (especially in the multitransfused patient), hepatic crises, and sickle cell intrahepatic cholestasis (SCIC). SCIC is an uncommon but severe form of sickle hepatopathy with high mortality rates. The pathophysiology involves sickling in the hepatic sinusoids, which leads to hypoxic injury and swelling of hepatocytes causing a direct back-pressure effect and resultant intracanalicular cholestasis. SCIC presents with acute right upper quadrant abdominal pain, jaundice, severe conjugated hyperbilirubinemia, moderately elevated liver enzymes, acute kidney injury, and occasionally coagulopathy. SCIC can progress rapidly to acute liver failure. In SCIC exchange transfusion is the preferable treatment of choice although this has not been rigorously studied. Maintaining HbS levels of less than 20%–30% is recommended by experts. While other causes of liver disease not specific to sickle cell patient should be excluded, a liver biopsy is a relative contraindication because of risk of bleeding and liver rupture. Hydroxyurea therapy has not been shown to be beneficial for the prevention or treatment of SCIC. In cholestasis, the bile acid ursodeoxycholic acid can improve biliary flow; however, in this patient, exchange transfusion is the more urgent treatment of choice.

99. A

This patient likely has previously undiagnosed hereditary spherocytosis (HS) based on her chronic hyperproliferative anemia, personal and family history of gallstones, and Caucasian race. The pathophysiology of HS is caused by a deficiency or dysfunction of one of the constituents of the red cell cytoskeleton whose role is to maintain the shape, deformability, and elasticity of the red cell. The laboratory features of HS include a normocytic or microcytic anemia, elevated MCHC, signs of hemolysis with increased LDH and decreased haptoglobin, increased spherocytes on peripheral blood smear, and a negative Coombs test, which rules out autoimmune hemolytic anemia. Spherocytes are destroyed solely in the spleen, and therefore splenectomy is very effective in controlling the anemia but does not correct the underlying red blood cell defect. Prednisone would be treatment of choice in warm autoimmune hemolytic anemia. Rituximab can be used in both warm and cold autoimmune hemolytic anemia but has no role in HS. Finally, eculizumab is indicated for paroxysmal nocturnal hemoglobinuria with symptomatic hemolytic anemia.

100. D

This patient has hemolytic anemia as evidenced by an increased LDH, decreased haptoglobin, and indirect bilirubinemia in the setting of anemia. His direct antiglobulin test indicates that he has hemolytic anemia of the cold agglutinin subtype. In primary cold agglutinin disease, the majority of patients are found to have a small monoclonal paraprotein on SPEP/IFE due to a small monoclonal B cell population. The treatment of choice in these patients is rituximab-based therapy. A proportion of patients will respond to single agent rituximab. Splenectomy and prednisone are treatments for warm autoimmune hemolytic anemia. Since hemolysis of C3b-coated red blood cells in cold agglutinin disease occurs outside the spleen, splenectomy is not useful. Prednisone has also not been shown to be effective in cold agglutinin disease. Plasmapheresis can be used in the acute setting of cold agglutinin disease to remove acutely, for example preoperatively, in patients undergoing operations requiring thermal cooling.

101. A

Patients with sickle cell disease who require surgery are at risk for perioperative complications. Preoperative transfusion decreases sickle-cell-related perioperative complications but can be associated with acute transfusion reactions, alloimmunization, and delayed hemolytic transfusion reactions. The Transfusion Alternatives Preoperatively in Sickle Cell Disease (TAPS) Study evaluated a preoperative transfusion strategy versus no preoperative transfusion in HbSS and Hb S-beta⁰ thalassemia patient undergoing low-risk or medium-risk operations. Patients randomized to the transfusion arm received either a conservative transfusion (if baseline hemoglobin was <9 g/dL) to target goal Hb 10 g/dL or red blood cell exchange transfusion (if baseline hemoglobin was >9 g/dL) to target HbS less than 60%. Preoperative transfusion resulted in less preoperative complications, particularly acute chest syndrome. While this patient should be started on hydroxyurea for long-term management of his sickle cell disease given his history of acute chest syndrome, it is not indicated to decrease perioperative complications. Sickle cell disease patients are considered at higher risk for venous thromboembolism than the general population. While aggressive postoperative VTE prophylaxis should be employed, there is no role for preoperative VTE prophylaxis in this setting.

102. A

This patient has laboratory findings consistent with cold agglutinin disease. Her hemolysis testing is positive, her MCV is high, and a direct antiglobulin test detects C3-coated red blood cells. Cold agglutinin disease is a form of autoimmune hemolytic anemia in which the autoantibodies, or cold agglutinins (CA), are defined by the ability to agglutinate RBCs at cold temperatures. The CA are directed against the I or i antigens on red blood cells. Most CA are monoclonal IgM, which can be picked up on routine SPEP testing. The IgM then fixes complement, and these C3b-coated red blood cells are removed from circulation by the liver's reticuloendothelial system. In primary cold agglutinin disease, no underlying systemic disorder explains the autoantibodies. However, the majority of primary cold agglutinin disease is associated with a monoclonal paraprotein (usually IgM) and a monoclonal B-cell clone identified on flow cytometry. Secondary cold agglutinin disease is associated with infections and lymphoproliferative disorders, such as lymphoplasmacytic lymphoma. Cryoglobulin testing is used to diagnose cryoglobulinemia. In cryoglobulinemia, immunoglobulins become insoluble at room reduced temperatures as compared with cold agglutinin disease in which agglutination of red blood cells occur. Osmotic fragility testing is used to diagnose hereditary spherocytosis. ANA testing may be indicated in warm autoimmune hemolytic anemia, as systemic lupus erythematosus is associated with this disorder.

103. C

Alloimmunization to RBC antigens is a major complication of transfusion and the underlying cause of the majority of delayed hemolytic transfusions reactions (DHTR). DHTR presents within 5–10 days following a transfusion of RBC. In patients with sickle cell disease, racial differences between recipient (predominantly African Americans) and donor (predominantly Caucasians) expression of RBC antigens are thought to contribute to the increased risk of alloimmunization. DHTR often presents similarly to a vasoocclusive pain crisis and therefore is often underdiagnosed. In addition to symptoms of a pain crisis, sickle cell patients with DHTR will present with reticulocytopenia and a lower hemoglobin compared with before transfusion. The worsening anemia represents a combination of hemolysis of previously transfused cells (hence the lack of HbA on electrophoresis), "bystander hyperhemolysis" from an immune response causing hemolysis of the recipient's red blood cells, and suppression of erythropoiesis. While a direct antiglobulin test and indirect antiglobulin test (antibody screen) are recommended to evaluate for new alloantibodies or autoantibodies causing a hemolytic reaction, these serologic studies are sometimes equivocal. If DHTR is suspected, treatment consists of minimizing further red blood cell transfusion, high-dose steroids, high doses of erythropoietin stimulating agents, and intravenous immunoglobulin.

104. A

Glucose 6-phosphate dehydrogenase (G6PD) deficiency, an X-linked disorder, is the most common enzymatic disorder of red blood cells. The clinical phenotype of G6PD deficiency varies considerably, with a significant portion of patients being clinically silent. The likelihood of developing hemolysis and the severity of disease are determined by the magnitude of the enzyme deficiency based on the underlying genetic variant (class I–IV) and degree of oxidative challenge. The hallmark of the most common variant is acute hemolytic crisis after exposure to a variety of drugs (e.g., nitrofurantoin) or oxidant stressors. G6PD deficiency should be considered in any patient with non-immune (i.e., Coombs negative) hemolysis. On the acute hemolytic setting, oxidative denaturation of hemoglobin leads to the crosslinking of the denatured globin to the red cell membrane. This results in accumulation of hemoglobin to one side of the cell adjacent to unstained nonhemoglobin-containing portion within the rest of the cell. On a peripheral blood smear, these changes manifest as "bite cells" or "blister cells." Cresyl blue supravital stains of the peripheral blood may also reveal the denatured globin as Heinz bodies during hemolytic episodes.

105. D

The method used to establish the diagnosis of G6PD deficiency is based upon testing the normal function of the enzyme. G6PD catalyzes the initial step in the hexose monophosphate (or pentose phosphate) shunt, which is the only red cell source of reduced NADPH, a cofactor important in glutathione metabolism. Screening tests for G6PD deficiency include the florescent spot test, which is based on the fluorescence of NADPH as the end product. More definitive quantitative assays are available for confirmation. Of note, false-negative results can occur if the most severely deficiency red cells have already been removed from circulation via hemolysis. Therefore diagnostic tests should be postponed until the patient recovers from the acute hemolytic episode. Hemoglobin electrophoresis would be sent if an underlying hemoglobinopathy is suspected as a cause of hemolysis. Paroxysmal nocturnal hemoglobinuria is detected by showing that peripheral blood cells are deficient in glycophosphatidylinositol (GPI)-linked proteins such as CD55 and CD59, by flow cytometry. Osmotic fragility testing is used to diagnose hereditary spherocytosis.

106. B

This patient has classic signs and symptoms of vitamin B12 deficiency. Gastric bypass surgery is a known cause of iron, vitamin B12, and copper deficiency. Absorption of vitamin B12 requires gastric acid for peptic digestion of the food-B12 complexes. Further, absorption of vitamin B12 in the terminal ileum requires the presence of intrinsic factor produced by the parietal cells of the stomach. Vitamin B12 deficiency causing anemia can present several years after bypass surgery since vitamin B12 storage depletion takes many years and high-dose oral vitamin B12 supplementation is very effective for prevention of this micronutrient deficiency. Severe vitamin B12 deficiency can present with pancytopenia, significantly elevated LDH levels, and bone marrow biopsy findings can mimic findings of myelodysplastic syndrome. This patient was not taking oral vitamin B12 supplementation after her surgery. To restore vitamin B12 levels in the acute setting, intramuscular or subcutaneous vitamin B12 should be prescribed for this patient.

107. A

This patient has features of autoimmune hemolytic anemia as evidence by a macrocytic hyperproliferative anemia and positive hemolysis markers. The peripheral smear shows increased spherocytes, which is consistent with warm autoimmune hemolytic anemia (WAIHA). The patient has SLE, a disease that is associated with WAIHA. The diagnostic workup for suspected hemolytic anemia includes a direct antiglobulin test (also known as the direct Coomb test). In a patient with autoimmune hemolytic anemia, the blood sample containing red blood cells with attached human anti-RBC antibodies is washed and then incubated with antihuman antibodies (the Coomb reagent). RBC agglutination occurs because the antihuman antibodies form links between RBCs by binding to the human antibodies on the RBCs. In WAIHA the DAT is typically positive for IgG and negative for C3. In cold agglutinin disease, the DAT is positive for C3 only. Answer B describes an indirect Coombs test.

108. D

Initially, the patient likely had a combination of alpha thalassemia trait and iron deficiency anemia. Her ferritin improved to normal range with oral iron therapy. She still has a mild microcytic anemia. This should prompt investigation for alpha-thalassemia trait (two gene deletions). Alpha-thalassemia trait cannot be identified on hemoglobin electrophoresis, and instead, DNA analysis must be ordered. She likely does not have sickle cell anemia (Hb SS) since these patients are not usually microcytic and baseline hemoglobin is usually lower. She does not have sickle cell trait as these patients have neither anemia nor microcytosis (assuming no other concurrent causes of anemia).

109. B

Sickle cell trait is characterized by Hb A 60% and Hb S 40% on hemoglobin electrophoresis. Patients with hemoglobin SS typically have >90% Hb S, <3.5% Hb A_2, and <10% Hb F on electrophoresis. In Sickle beta$^+$-thalassemia, Hb S is >60%, Hb A is 10%–30%, and A2 is >3.5%. In patients with hemoglobin SC, Hb S is 50% and C and A_2 migrate to the same position on alkaline electrophoresis, so it likely will be reported as A_2 = 50%.

110. B

Patients with beta-thalassemia minor (one normal beta globin allele) are noted to have mild anemia, microcytosis, target cells, and basophilic stippling on the peripheral blood smear. Hemoglobin electrophoresis will confirm an elevated A_2 fraction. The alpha-thalassemia carrier state is clinically silent, and hemoglobin electrophoresis is normal for both the 1 and 2 gene deletions (alpha thalassemia minor). Patients with beta-thalassemia major are typically transfusion dependent and have a higher hemoglobin F fraction on hemoglobin electrophoresis. Hemoglobin H disease is incorrect, as hemoglobin H was not reported on the hemoglobin electrophoresis, and individuals with this condition are often transfusion dependent by the second decade of life.

111. D

X-linked sideroblastic anemia is the most common of the nonsyndromic congenital sideroblastic anemias. Females are affected in approximately 30% of cases. Although the peripheral smear could also be suggestive of severe iron deficiency or thalassemia, the iron studies and hemoglobin electrophoresis do not support either diagnosis in this case. Myelodysplastic syndrome remains on the differential diagnosis; however, her history of "vitamin responsive" anemia and young age make XLSA more likely. The anemia of XLSA is pyridoxine-responsive in the majority of cases.

112. A

The acute chest syndrome (ACS) in a sickle cell patient is characterized by the presence of fever and/or respiratory distress with a new infiltrate on CXR. The etiology of ACS is multifactorial, with pulmonary infection identified in many cases. In adults, the most common bacterial cause identified is *Chlamydophila pneumoniae*. ACS should be recognized and treated promptly.

113. D

Acute splenic sequestration is a serious complication that is generally seen in childhood in patients with sickle cell anemia, but may present in adulthood in patients with "milder" disease forms, such as hemoglobin SC disease. In many cases, LUQ pain and fever are absent, with patients instead complaining of pain elsewhere. The drop in both hemoglobin and platelet count coupled with tender splenomegaly and acute onset argue against bone marrow suppression by parvovirus B19 infection. IV hydration is unlikely the culprit given that his values are dropping well below his known baseline levels along with the tender splenomegaly. There is no evidence of hemolysis by laboratory assessment or peripheral blood smear. Heparin-induced thrombocytopenia is less likely given the drop in both hemoglobin and platelets.

114. A

This man developed progressive anemia and hyperbilirubinemia over the course of 4 days, with concomitant improvement in his serum creatinine and uric acid. He received rasburicase to help prevent tumor lysis syndrome. Blister cells and bite cells are demonstrated on the peripheral blood smear. This finding is characteristic of hemolysis due to G6PD deficiency. Rasburicase is well known to cause both an oxidative hemolytic anemia and methemoglobinemia in patients with underlying G6PD deficiency. The management of oxidative hemolysis secondary to a drug is removal of the offending agent and supportive care, including folic acid and red blood cell transfusion as needed.

115. D

Although basophilic stippling is not pathognomonic for lead poisoning, the constellation of fatigue, myalgias, abdominal pain, and history of lead exposure (stained glass) with basophilic stippling make lead toxicity a primary consideration. That she does not recall previously having anemia makes thalassemia a less likely cause of her microcytic anemia with basophilic stippling. Her serum ferritin does not indicate iron deficiency. The normal platelet and WBC count make the marrow less likely to be revealing.

116. A

First line testing for patients with suspected porphyria cutanea tarda is to evaluate for elevated porphyrin levels. This can be done from the blood or spot urine. Testing erythrocyte porphyrins would be a reasonable first step if erythropoietic protoporphyria or X-linked protoporphyria (nonblistering skin lesions) were suspected, but they are not in this case. While approximately 20% of PCT cases will harbor a UROD gene mutation, the mutation in itself is not diagnostic of PCT; it is just indicative of an underlying susceptibility to develop PCT.

PCT is often associated with mutations in the HFE gene, alcohol use, smoking, and hepatitis C infection. Evaluation for these associated issues is warranted if PCT is identified.

117. B

This patient has dapsone-induced methemoglobinemia as evidenced by the mismatch between the pulse oximetry and arterial blood gas oxygenation coupled with the increased methemoglobin level. Dapsone is a well-recognized cause of methemoglobinemia. This patient presents with asymptomatic methemoglobinemia with a methemoglobin level of 15%. In this scenario, simply withholding further dapsone is reasonable management. Patients with symptoms or methemoglobin levels greater than 20% are primarily considered for acute treatment, generally with methylene blue. However, methylene blue can further exacerbate anemia in patients with underlying G6PD deficiency, and thus in this nonemergent case, simply discontinuing dapsone is the primary consideration.

118. A

Although previously an integral part of the evaluation of hereditary hemochromatosis, liver biopsy for measurement of hepatic iron concentration and morphology was used prior to the availability of genetic testing for HFE gene mutations. Presently, serum ferritin is used as a surrogate for the presence of cirrhosis, noting that patients with a serum ferritin of greater than 1000 µg/L have an increased risk of cirrhosis. Patients with other reasons for underlying liver dysfunction (metabolic syndrome, hepatitis C) also have an increased risk. In general, only those patients at highest risk are recommended to undergo initial liver biopsy to evaluate underlying cirrhosis.

This patient will likely benefit from therapeutic phlebotomy to reduce the serum ferritin, with a goal of less than 50 µg/L. In general, each phlebotomy of 500 mL can lower the serum ferritin by 30 µg/L.

119. D

This patient is suspected to have juvenile hemochromatosis as evidenced by (1) iron overload; (2) early symptom onset; and (3) presentation with cardiomyopathy, diabetes, and hypogonadism rather than liver disease. Mutations within the HJV gene are primarily responsible for this disease and appear to result in decreased levels of hepcidin. HFE1 gene mutations lead to classic hemochromatosis, which can also arise from mutations within TFR2 (transferrin receptor 2). Mutations within TTR (transthyretin) lead to amyloidosis.

120. C

Note that the meningococcal vaccine only covers serovariant B, and meningococcal infection may occur despite vaccination.

121. A

Cold agglutinin disease is characterized by hemolytic anemia, indirect hyperbilirubinemia, reticulocytosis, and direct antiglobulin testing positive for complement (anti-C3) and negative for IgG. The underlying antibody is generally IgM as opposed to paroxysmal cold hemoglobinuria in which an IgG is present. Additionally, the cold agglutinin titer is typically elevated in cold agglutinin disease and only mildly so in PCH. Hemoglobinuria, if present, is typically mild in CAD as opposed to PCH. The most common causes of cold agglutinin disease are infections (such as *Mycoplasma*) and underlying hematologic disorders. In this case, the patient is young and presented with an infection (possibly *Mycoplasma*) approximately 3 weeks before the onset of hemolytic symptoms, classic for infectious-associated CAD. It is expected that full recovery will occur within 4 weeks. If the patient was older, has more serious hemolysis, does not have a preceding infection, or has hemolysis that is not resolving, investigation of underlying disorders in addition to rituximab ± corticosteroids should be considered.

122. A

Although osmotic fragility testing is expected to be positive in cases of hereditary spherocytosis, it lacks specificity, as spherocytes resulting from any cause are expected to have abnormal fragility. The eosin-5'-maleimide binding test is a flow cytometric based assay that evaluates the interaction between the dye eosin-5'-maleimide and the band 3 protein. It has a reported 89%–96% sensitivity and 94%–99% specificity and has largely supplanted osmotic fragility testing. Spectrin mutations will be present in some cases of hereditary spherocytosis; however, mutations in band 3 and ankyrin are also found.

123. D

Hepcidin is a key regulator in iron homeostasis. Hepcidin (a bacteriocidal protein) is expected to be increased in inflammatory states leading to anemia of chronic disease. In iron deficiency resulting from iron losses (in this case, a multiparous woman), hepcidin is expected to be suppressed, thereby allowing increased iron absorption. Ferroportin, the hepcidin receptor, is expected to be normal to increased when hepcidin decreased, as it is not internalized in the absence of hepcidin.

124. D

While persons with the sickle cell trait do not have the overt sickling manifestations and complications as those with sickle cell anemia, they do have an underlying predisposition to venous thromboembolism, chronic kidney disease, and rhabdomyolysis with intensive exercise. The risk of rhabdomyolysis with intensive exercise led the NCAA to institute a policy of screening for sickle trait among its athletes, a policy that was not endorsed by the American Society of Hematology. Strategies to mitigate the development of rhabdomyolysis (such as hydration and rest) among all individuals have been used successfully in intensive training regimens, such as that utilized in the US Army, with success. Thus this patient should be advised of maintaining adequate hydration and taking rest periods to help prevent complications from extreme exercise in the setting of the sickle cell trait, but need not completely avoid such activities.

125. A

This patient has microcytic, hypochromic anemia with a normal RDW, peripheral smear showing target cells and normal iron indices. Further, her hemoglobin electrophoresis pattern is normal. Taken together, a high likelihood of alpha-thalassemia minor exists. A thorough family history is warranted in cases of alpha-thalassemia minor to better assess genetic risks to offspring. In general, alpha-thalassemia minor in patients of African descent is inherited in the *trans* configuration dominates, posing little risk of hydrops fetalis. In non-African patients with alpha-thalassemia minor, *cis* configurations are more common, and there is an increased risk for both hemoglobin H disease and hydrops fetalis.

126. A

Levamisole was formerly paired with 5-fluorouracil as a treatment for colon cancer, but its only legal use now is a deworming agent for livestock. Illicitly, it is used to cut cocaine. Levamisole adds bulk and weight to powdered cocaine and makes the drug appear purer. Additionally, it is felt to possibly potentiate cocaine's stimulant effects. It has a similar appearance to cocaine, and an ability to pass street purity tests. It can lead to agranulocytosis and a necrotizing vasculitis as well as a glomerulonephritis. Quinine has been used to adulterate cocaine, but does not typically lead to agranulocytosis. Phencyclidine has not been associated with hematologic adverse effects, and intravenous abuse of oxymorphone extended release can lead to a thrombotic microangiopathy.

127. C

Copper deficiency can lead to a demyelinating myelopathy resembling that of B12 deficiency. Hematologic complications of copper deficiency include neutropenia and anemia (either microcytic, macrocytic, or normocytic). Bone marrow examination can mimic myelodysplastic syndrome with vacuolated cytoplasm of erythroid precursors as well as ringed sideroblasts. Gastric bypass surgery is a risk factor for the development of copper deficiency. In a case series of 136 patients with gastric bypass surgery, 9.6% had hypocupremia. Two other case series of 64 and 141 bariatric surgery patients reported substantial hypocupremia in 23% at 6 months and 70% at 3 years, respectively, and a progressive reduction in average serum copper concentrations over 5 years. B12 deficiency does not cause neutropenia to this degree, and the measured B12 level does not support a diagnosis of B12 deficiency. While patients after bariatric surgery can develop deficiencies of other trace elements, such as selenium, chromium, and zinc, none of these produce the constellation of neurologic and hematologic findings in this patient.

128. E

Agranulocytosis is the most feared side effect of antithyroid-drug therapy. In the largest series, agranulocytosis occurred in 0.35% receiving methimazole. Development of agranulocytosis may be dose-related and is less common when methimazole is started at 15 mg tid or less. It is important to note that agranulocytosis can develop after a prior uneventful course of drug therapy, a finding that is important since renewed exposure to the drug frequently occurs when patients have a relapse and undergo a second course of antithyroid therapy. The mechanism of agranulocytosis is development of antineutrophil antibodies, and patients may not be rechallenged with the same drug once their counts recover. Moreover, cross-reactivity between propylthiouracil and methimazole for agranulocytosis has been well documented, so the use of the alternative antithyroid drug is contraindicated.

129. C

T-cell large granular lymphocyte leukemia is a rare disorder characterized by expansion of a population of cells expressing the markers CD3, CD8, and CD57. It can be associated with rheumatoid arthritis and splenomegaly, as well as neutropenia. Treatment usually relies on immunosuppression, and methotrexate or cyclosporine are the preferred agents. The use of weekly methotrexate is recommended over cyclosporine as initial treatment for Felty syndrome, which is the triad of splenomegaly, rheumatoid arthritis, and neutropenia. Cyclosporine may also be used, but may also be more toxic. Use of other lymphocytotoxic agents is not recommended as first-line therapy.

130. D

Within a monocyte are numerous intracellular yeast-like organisms 2–4 μm in diameter with eccentric chromatin, surrounded by an artifactual pseudocapsule caused by

cytoplasmic shrinkage. This is characteristic of *Histoplasma capsulatum*. These findings may also be seen on a Wright-Giemsa-stained peripheral blood smear. TB, cryptococcus, and coccidiomycosis may be seen on examination for the bone marrow but typically need special stains to be visualized.

131. A

This patient has cyclic neutropenia, which is likely present since childhood given the history of gingival disease in childhood. G-CSF given just prior to the anticipated lowest days in the neutropenic cycle can limit the number of days of profound neutropenia and improve gingival symptoms. G-CSF does not need to be administered continuously, because, due to the cyclic nature of the condition, she will have normal or near normal neutrophil counts for much of the cycle. Antibiotic prophylaxis could be considered in cases with a history of severe infection; however, it would not be expected to be helpful in the case of gingival disease, and chronic antibiotic therapy is not without its risk. Methotrexate could be considered in the adult form of cyclic neutropenia, which is caused by large granular leukemia, but not in congenital forms, which are caused by genetic mutations.

132. B

Levamisole adulteration of cocaine is prevalent within the United States. Levamisole contamination can lead to agranulocytosis or vasculitis. Typically, the neutrophil count will recover within 5–10 days after cessation of levamisole exposure and G-CSF administration is not necessary.

133. A

Chediak-Higashi syndrome is a rare autosomal recessive disorder that generally presents in childhood with partial oculocutaneous albinism with affected persons have a peculiar silver sheen to their hair. It is characterized by recurrent pyogenic infections, mild mucocutaneous bleeding diathesis, and progressive neurologic deficits. The pathognomonic finding in Chediak-Higashi syndrome is the finding of giant inclusions in polymorphonuclear neutrophils on peripheral blood smear seen using routine staining techniques. In approximately 90% of cases a LYST (lysosomal trafficking) gene mutation is present, and this is presently the only gene known to be associated with the disease.

HPS1 and HPS3 are mutations associated with Hermansky-Pudlak syndrome. While HPS is characterized by oculocutaneous albinism with mucocutaneous bleeding associated with the absence of platelet dense granules, giant neutrophil inclusions are not associated with HPS. Mutations in the HPS3 gene are found in about 25% of affected people from Puerto Rico and in approximately 20% of affected individuals from other areas.

MYH9 gene defects characterize a group of macrothrombocytopenias, which is not present in this case.

134. A

T-cell large granular leukemia is a clonal disorder of large granular lymphocytes, which often results in neutropenia. Some cases may be found on evaluation for recurrent bacterial infections and fever, others incidentally due to evaluation of neutropenia. T-LGL is often associated with an underlying rheumatologic disorder, especially rheumatoid arthritis. The diagnosis is usually made on the morphologic and immunophenotypic findings from peripheral blood, with the presence of clonal LGLs of T-cell lineage.

In general, treatment is recommended for those with ANC 0.5 × 10*9/L, constitutional symptoms, treatment of accompanying rheumatologic disorder, or recurrent infections. Front-line treatment is typically low-dose methotrexate, cyclophosphamide, or cyclosporine.

135. D

Unlike erythropoietin production, which is regulated by increased gene transcription induced by hypoxia, thrombopoietin (TPO) production by the liver is static and not regulated. Platelets and megakaryocytes have high-affinity TPO receptors that bind and internalize TPO. Thus the platelet mass negatively regulates free TPO levels. Additionally, patients with viral hepatitis and cirrhosis have TPO levels that are low. Moreover, patients with thrombocytopenia due to splenic sequestration have a large platelet mass in the spleen, which, unfortunately, are quite capable of binding and internalizing TPO, and thus the lowest TPO levels are found in patients with thrombocytopenia due to hepatitis C cirrhosis and splenomegaly. Patients with ITP also have TPO levels that are lower than expected, but other thrombocytopenic disorders are associated with elevated TPO levels.

136. C

It is important to know the normal stages of erythroid development to properly interpret bone marrow aspirates done for purposes of identifying the cause of an unexplained anemia. The earliest identifiable red cell precursor is the pronormoblast, characterized by a deeply basophilic cytoplasm and a large N:C ratio. The nucleus starts to condense, but the cytoplasm remains basophilic in the basophilic erythroblast, then as the cytoplasm becomes more hemoglobinized, the cell becomes a polychromatophilic erythroblast, then finally a normoblast once the cytoplasm is fully pink/red. Once the cell extrudes it nucleus, it becomes a reticulocyte.

137. A

Multipotent hematopoietic stem cells differentiate into common myeloid progenitor cells, but their commitment to the erythroid-megakaryocyte pathway relies on the action of GATA-1, GATA-2, and FOG-1. GATA-1 then plays a role in later megakaryocyte development as well. *Gata1* knockout mice show erythroid maturation arrest at the proerythroblast stage and severe anemia, as well as megakaryocyte maturation defects with a proliferation of low ploidy cells and the formation of large hypogranulated platelets. Runx1 is a transcription factor whose loss leads to familial thrombocytopenia and a tendency toward the development of myeloid leukemia. It does not appear to be necessary for erythropoiesis. TPO plays a critical role in erythropoiesis and maintenance of the primitive stem cell niche, but it does not act to commit the multipotent stem cell to the erythroid-megakaryocyte pathway. NF-E2 is essential for the final differentiation of megakaryocytes and for platelet formation, and NF-E2 null mice are thrombocytopenic but have abundant immature megakaryocytes. *MYH9* encodes the heavy chain of myosin IIA, which is active in the organization of the demarcation membrane system and in proplatelet formation.

138. C

Rheumatoid arthritis is an inflammatory condition, leading to thrombocytosis in its active state. Interleukin-6 is the major cytokine driving the inflammation in RA, and is a megakaryocytic differentiating factor, leading to platelet production in vivo. This cytokine is associated with reactive thrombocytosis in a number of conditions, and is the major cytokine associated with the thrombocytosis seen in RA. IL-3 leads to proliferation of immature megakaryocytes, not platelets. IL-11 and TPO are required for platelet production, but its role in RA is less well defined. The stem cell factor is needed for the early stages of megakaryocytopoiesis, but does not appear to play a major role in inflammatory conditions.

139. C

The earliest identifiable myeloid cell in the bone marrow is the myeloblast, characterized by a large N:C ratio and open chromatin. The promyelocyte stage is next and shows development of a few dark azurophilic granules in the slightly more abundant cytoplasm. These granules become more abundant, as does the cytoplasm; the nucleus starts to move to one end of the cell, and there is a perinuclear clear area known poetically as the "dawn of neutrophilia," which represents the Golgi apparatus. The metamyelocyte is characterized by a kidney-bean-shaped nucleus that becomes more elongated as it develops into a band form.

140. C

Hematopoietic progenitors differentiate upon exposure to a network of cytokines and chemokines to become committed to the eosinophil/basophil (Eo/B) lineage. Transcription factors, including GATA-1PU.1, and C/EBP members regulate the production of eosinophils in the bone marrow. Cytokines and chemokines are generated under appropriate stimulation from T cells in the bone marrow. The three key cytokines that are critical for stimulation of bone marrow production of eosinophils are IL-3, IL-5, and granulocyte-macrophage colony-stimulating factor (GM-CSF). Though other cytokines such as IL-4, IL-6, IL-11, IL-12, SCF also play a role in eosinophil genesis. IFN-gamma prolongs eosinophil survival but is not necessary for synthesis.

141. A

This patient's presentation is concerning for hepatitis associated aplastic anemia, as based upon the insidious onset of symptoms, reported transaminitis (i.e., hepatitis) and pancytopenia.[14] In these cases, testing for the known hepatitis viruses is often negative. The patient provides no risk factors for HIV exposure, and there is no reason to suspect LGL leukemia. While PNH exists in the setting of aplasia, this is may be more typically accompanied by thrombosis and there are no other findings to support this diagnosis.

142. E

The clinical scenario is compatible with DKC, which is a disease characterized by shortened telomere length, nail dystrophy, pulmonary fibrosis, and laboratory findings of bone marrow failure.[15,16] A bone marrow biopsy typically shows no overt findings, whereas DEB exposure to lymphocytes is used in the diagnosis of Fanconi anemia. Mutations in MPL are the cause for congenital amegakaryocytic thrombocytopenia, which is associated with a markedly decreased platelet count and eventual bone marrow failure, but not the described cutaneous findings or pulmonary fibrosis. Similarly, Shwachman-Diamond syndrome is not associated with pulmonary fibrosis.

143. B

The case is one of Fanconi anemia presenting in adulthood as evidenced by pancytopenia in the absence of leukemia or MDS, short stature, and café au lait spots (pictured). Many genes have been associated with development of Fanconi anemia, not just FANCA. For this reason, chromosomal breakage analysis with mitomycin C or diepoxybutane are the initial diagnostic testing modalities, showing an increased sensitivity to DNA strand breakage in FA patients. Patients with FA are at high risk of developing hematologic malignancy and solid tumors, and exposure to alkylating agents and radiation should be limited.

144. D

Copper deficiency can be confused with myelodysplastic syndrome given the cytopenias and dysplastic features in the bone marrow. In the setting of gastric bypass (in which trace nutrients may not be adequately absorbed) and coupled with the presence of vacuolated erythroids (pictured) in the bone marrow as well as normal cytogenetics, a micronutrient deficiency is suspected. In this case, the copper deficiency may be due to malabsorption with the gastric bypass or zinc toxicity (from zinc lozenges and zinc-containing denture paste). Decreasing zinc intake and supplementing copper should result in improvement in peripheral counts in approximately 6 weeks.

Though there is a monoclonal IgG kappa present by serum immunofixation, there are no other diagnostic criteria for multiple myeloma, and there are no excess plasma cells identified in the bone marrow.

Zinc deficiency would manifest as diarrhea, skin disorders, disturbed olfaction, and predisposition to infection.

145. B

The presence of a small PNH clone in the context of aplastic anemia is associated with a favorable response to immunosuppressive therapy.

146. A

This patient has the combination of a chronic bone marrow failure state plus idiopathic pulmonary fibrosis. The main organs subject to dysfunction in telomeropathies are the bone marrow, lung, and liver. It is important to establish the diagnosis, as the presence of a telomeropathy can affect treatment decisions, as patients are expected to have a heightened sensitivity to high-dose chemotherapy and radiation.

147. B

Aplastic anemia developing during pregnancy has been reported for over a century. The pathogenesis is not well understood at this time. Aplastic anemia during pregnancy can result in significant complications to both the mother and fetus, largely due to maternal anemia and thrombocytopenia. Of the cases reported in the literature, roughly half will have spontaneous recovery after delivery. A handful of subsequent pregnancies have been reported with a return of aplastic anemia. It is advised that a woman with aplastic anemia not become pregnant due to the high likelihood of maternal and fetal complications.

148. E

It is important to understand that a young adult with aplastic anemia could have a congenital bone marrow failure syndrome. This patient has the triad of features characteristic for dyskeratosis congenital (DKC) including (1) a reticulated or mottled skin hyperpigmented rash involving the face, neck, shoulders, and trunk; (2) nail dystrophy involving both hands and feet; and (3) mucosal leukoplakia. Patients with DKC are at increased risk for squamous carcinomas and dysplasia of the mucosal surfaces. Other features may include early greying of the hair, tooth abnormalities, pulmonary fibrosis, and eye abnormalities. It is diagnosed by finding abnormal telomere length. These findings are not characteristic of paroxysmal nocturnal hemoglobinuria, and a CD55/CD59 flow cytometry assay would therefore be unlikely to be diagnostic. Chromosomal breakage in response to either mitomycin C or depoxybutane (DEB) can diagnose Fanconi anemia, which may be characterized by a number of somatic abnormalities including misshapen or missing thumbs, café-au-lait spots, short stature, and developmental delay. Isoamylase is helpful for patients over the age of 3 who may have Shwachman-Diamond syndrome, which this patient is unlikely to have. Lastly, with a normal B12 level, antiintrinsic antibodies would be unlikely to be found.

149. A

This patient has aplastic anemia with a small clone of paroxysmal nocturnal hemoglobinuria cells. These patients have a much better response to immunosuppression, usually with ATG and cyclosporine. Transfusions from family members should be strictly avoided, since they can lead to transfusion-related graft versus host disease. Despite the small PNH clone, there is no role currently for eculizumab, which should be used only for hemolysis. IVIg and prednisone provides insufficient immunosuppression for this patient.

150. E

Of the congenital bone marrow failure syndromes, SDS is the most rare and usually presents with a combination of bone marrow failure and pancreatic abnormalities. DKC classically presents with the triad of (1) a reticulated or mottled skin hyperpigmented rash involving the face, neck, shoulders, and trunk; (2) nail dystrophy involving both hands and feet; and (3) mucosal leukoplakia. Patients with DKC are at increased risk for squamous carcinomas and dysplasia of the mucosal surfaces. Other features may include early greying of the hair, tooth abnormalities, pulmonary fibrosis, and eye abnormalities. It is diagnosed by finding abnormal telomere length. Fanconi anemia may be characterized by a number of somatic abnormalities including misshapen or missing thumbs, café-au-lait spots, short stature, and developmental delay, although some patients may have no somatic mutations. Neither paroxysmal nocturnal hemoglobinuria nor amegakaryocytic thrombocytopenia is associated with pancreatic disease.

151. A

PNH is an acquired clonal disorder of hematopoietic stem cells. In addition to hemolytic anemia, thrombosis, and peripheral blood cytopenias, PNH patients may also have disorders of smooth muscle dystonia, including esophageal spasm and erectile dysfunction, presumably due to nitric oxide scavenging. PNH patients have a hematopoietic clone lacking GPI-linked surface proteins such as CD55 and CD59. Neither of the congenital bone marrow failure syndromes: Fanconi anemia (diagnosed with chromosomal sensitivity to diepoxybutane), Shwachman-Diamond syndrome (which may present with abnormal isoamylase in adults), nor dyskeratosis congenital (diagnosed by abnormally short telomere length) present with smooth muscle dystonia. Hereditary spherocytosis may sometimes present with smooth muscle dystonia, but is not characterized by bone marrow failure.

152. E

Subsets of patients with aplastic anemia may vary in their response to different therapies. A good predictor of response to ATG/CSA is the expression of IFN-gamma on CD8+ T cells. One study showed a response rate of 96 versus 32% in such patients. A higher absolute reticulocyte count (>25,000 × 10⁹/L) is also a good predictor of response to ATG/CSA. A low ANC is a poor prognostic sign in those treated with ATG/CSA, and neither the ALC nor the degree of bone marrow hypocellularity has been correlated with response rates.

REFERENCES

Question 1

1. Anderson KE, Bloomer JR, Bonkovsky HL, et al. Recommendations for the diagnosis and treatment of the acute porphyrias. *Ann Intern Med.* 2005;142:439–450.

Question 2

1. Weiss G. Anemia of chronic disorders: new diagnostic tools and treatment strategies. *Semin Hematol.* 2015;52:313–320.

Question 3

1. Malaque CM, Santoro ME, Cardoso JL, et al. Clinical picture and laboratorial evaluation in human loxoscelism. *Toxicon.* 2011;58:664–671.

Question 4

1. Shapira Y, Vaturi M, Sagie A. Hemolysis associated with prosthetic heart valves: a review. *Cardiol Rev.* 2009;17:121–124.

Question 5

1. Luzzatto L, Seneca E. G6PD deficiency: a classic example of pharmacogenetics with on-going clinical implications. *Br J Haematol.* 2014;164:469–480.

Question 6

1. Mehta K, Gascon P, Robboy S. The gelatinous bone marrow (serous atrophy) in patients with acquired immunodeficiency syndrome. Evidence of excess sulfated glycosaminoglycan. *Arch Pathol Lab Med.* 1992;116:613–619.

Question 7

1. Bauman WA1, Shaw S, Jayatilleke E, Spungen AM, Herbert V. Increased intake of calcium reverses vitamin B12 malabsorption induced by metformin. *Diabetes Care.* 2000;23(9):1227–1231.

Question 8

1. Bianchi P, Fermo E, Vercellati C, et al. Diagnostic power of laboratory tests for hereditary spherocytosis: a comparison study in 150 patients grouped according to molecular and clinical characteristics. *Haematologica.* 2012;97:516–523.

Question 9

1. Imataki O, Ohnishi H, Kitanaka A, Kubota Y, Ishida T, Tanaka T. Pancytopenia complicated with peripheral neuropathy due to copper deficiency: a clinical diagnostic review. *Intern Med.* 2008;47:2063–2065.

Question 10

1. Brancaccio D, Cozzolino M, GAllieni M. Hyperparathyroidism and anemia in uremic subjects: a combined therapeutic approach. *J Am Soc Nephrol.* 2004;15:S21–S24.

Question 11

1. Verhovsek M, Henderson MP, Cox G, Luo HY, Steinberg MH, Chui DH. Unexpectedly low pulse oximetry measurements associated with variant hemoglobins: a systematic review. *Am J Hematol.* 2010;85:882–885.

Question 12

1. Carmel R. How I treat cobalamin (vitamin B12) deficiency. *Blood.* 2008;112:2214–2221.

Question 13

1. Mentzer WC. Differentiation of iron deficiency from thalassemia trait. *Lancet.* 1973;1:882.

Question 14

1. Barcellini W. Immune hemolysis: diagnosis and treatment recommendations. *Semin Hematol.* 2015;52:304–312.

Question 15

1. Abhyankar A, Moss AC. Iron replacement in patients with inflammatory bowel disease: a systematic review and meta-analysis. *Inflamm Bowel Dis.* 2015;21(8):1976–1981.

Question 16

1. Shanbhag S, Spivak J. Paroxysmal cold hemoglobinuria. *Hematol Oncol Clin North Am.* 2015;29:473–478.

Question 17

1. Tush GM, Kuhn RJ. Methemoglobinemia induced by an over-the-counter medication. *Ann Pharmcother.* 1996;30:1251–1254.

Question 18

1. Vichinsky E. Hemoglobin E syndromes. *Hematology Am Soc Hematol Educ Program.* 2007:79–83.

Question 19

1. Mannucci OM, Cugno M. The complex differential diagnosis between thrombotic thrombocytopenic purpura and atypical hemolytic uremic syndrome: laboratory weapons and their impact on treatment and monitoring. *Thromb Res.* 2015;136:851–854.

Question 20

1. Cherfane CE, Hollenbeck RD, Go J, Brown KE. Hereditary hemochromatosis: missed diagnosis or misdiagnosis? *Am J Med.* 2013;126:1010–1015.

Question 21

1. Frey BM, Gassner C, Jung HH. Neurodegeneration in the elderly—when the blood type matters: an overview of the McLeod syndrome with focus on hematological features. *Transfus Apher Sci.* 2015;52:277–284.

Question 22

1. Kremyanskaya M, Mascarenhas J, Hoffman R. Why does my patient have erythrocytosis? *Hematol Oncol Clin North Am.* 2012;26:267–283.

Question 23

1. Mayr R, Jaenecke AR, Schranz M, et al. Ferroportin disease: a systematic meta-analysis of clinical and molecular findings. *J Hepatol.* 2010;53:941–949.

Question 24

1. Poggiali E, Andreozzi F, Nava I. The role of TMPRSS6 polymorphisms in iron deficiency anemia partially responsive to oral iron treatment. *Am J Hematol.* 2015;90:306–309.

Question 25

1. Fonseca G, Souza R. Pulmonary hypertension in sickle cell disease. *Curr Opin Pulm Med.* 2015;21:432–437.

Question 26

1. Marks PW. Hematologic manifestations of liver disease. *Semin Hematol.* 2013;50:216–221.

Question 27

1. Alleyne M, Horne MK, Miller JL. Individualized treatment for iron deficiency anemia in adults. *Am J Med.* 2008;121:943–948.

Question 28

1. Brodsky RA, Mukhina GL, Li S, et al. Improved detection and characterization of paroxysmal nocturnal hemoglobinuria using fluorescent aerolysin. *Am J Clin Path.* 2000;114:459–466.

Question 29

1. Dedania B, Wu GY. Dermatologic extrahepatic manifestations of hepatitis C. *J Clin Transl Hepatol.* 2015;3:127–133.

Question 30

1. Romero S, Solves P, Lancharro A, et al. Passenger lymphocyte syndrome in liver transplant recipients: a description of 12 cases. *Blood Transfus.* 2015;13:423–428.

Question 31

1. Almonte M, Velasquez-Jones L, Valverde S, Carleton B, Medeiros M. Post-renal transplant erythrocytosis: a case report. *Pediatr Transplant.* 2015;19:E7–E10.

Question 32

1. Bose S, Sonny A, Rahman N. A teenager presents with fulminant hepatic failure and acute hemolytic anemia. *Chest.* 2015;147:e100–e104.

Question 33

1. Patnaik MM, Tefferi A. Refractory anemia with ring sideroblasts and RARS with thrombocytosis. *Am J Hematol.* 2015;90:549–559.

Question 34

1. Schwartz J, Morstadt E, Dura A, et al. Biochemical identification of vitamin B12 deficiency in a medical office. *Clin Lab.* 2015;61:687–692.

Question 35

1. Al-Nouri ZL, Reese JA, Terrell DR, Vesely SK, George JN. Drug-induced thrombotic microangiopathy: a systemic review of published reports. *Blood.* 2015;125:616–618.

Question 36

1. Yawn BP, Buchanan GR, Afenyi-Annan AN, et al. Management of sickle cell disease: summary of the 2014 evidence-based report by expert panel members. *JAMA.* 2014;312:1033–1048.

Question 37

1. Yawn BP, Buchanan GR, Afenyi-Annan AN, et al. Management of sickle cell disease: summary of the 2014 evidence-based report by expert panel members. *JAMA.* 2014;312:1033–1048.

Question 38

1. Breymann C. Iron deficiency anemia in pregnancy. *Semin Hematol.* 2015;52:339–347.

Question 39

1. Yawn BP, Buchanan GR, Afenyi-Annan AN, et al. Management of sickle cell disease: summary of the 2014 evidence-based report by expert panel members. *JAMA.* 2014;312:1033–1048.

Question 40

1. Turley E, McFarlane A, Halchuk L, Verhovsek M. Hemoglobin H identification by high-performance liquid chromatography in confirmed hemoglobin H disease. *Int J Lab Hematol.* 2015;37:668–672.

Question 41

1. Nemeth E, Ganz T. Anemia of inflammation. *Hematol Oncol Clin North Am.* 2014;28(4):671–681.
2. Ganz T. Hepcidin and iron regulation, 10 years later. *Blood.* 2011;117(17):4425–4433.

Question 42

1. Pietrangelo A. Iron and the liver. *Liver Int.* 2016;36(suppl 1):116–123.

Question 43

1. Bardou-Jacquet E, Brissot P. Diagnostic evaluation of hereditary hemochromatosis (HFE and non-HFE). *Hematol Oncol Clin North Am.* 2014;28(4):625–635.
2. Bardou-Jacquet E, Ben Ali Z, Beaumont-Epinette MP, Loreal O, Jouanolle AM, Brissot P. Non-HFE hemochromatosis: pathophysiological and diagnostic aspects. *Clin Res Hepatol Gastroenterol.* 2014;38(2):143–154.

Question 44

1. Porter J, Garbowski M. Consequences and management of iron overload in sickle cell disease. *Hematology Am Soc Hematol Educ Program.* 2013;2013:447–456.
2. Brittenham GM. Iron-chelating therapy for transfusional iron overload. *N Engl J Med.* 2011;364:146–156.

Question 45

1. Frank J, Poblete-Gutiérrez P. Porphyria cutanea tarda—when skin meets liver. *Best Pract Res Clin Gastroenterol.* 2010;24(5):735–745.
2. Balwani M, Desnick RJ. The porphyrias: advances in diagnosis and treatment. *Blood.* 2012;120(23):4496–4504.

Question 46

1. Karim Z, Lyoumi S, Nicolas G, Deybach JC, Gouya L, Puy H. Porphyrias: a 2015 update. *Clin Res Hepatol Gastroenterol.* 2015;39(4):412–425.
2. Pischik E, Kauppinen R. An update of clinical management of acute intermittent porphyria. *Appl Clin Genet.* 2015 Sep 1;8:201–214.

Question 47

1. Auerbach M. IV iron in pregnancy: an unmet clinical need. *Am J Hematol.* 2014;89(7):789.
2. Devasenapathy N, Neogi SB, Zodpey S. Is intravenous iron sucrose the treatment of choice for pregnant anemic women? *J Obstet Gynaecol Res.* 2013;39(3):619–626.

Question 48

1. Camaschella C. Iron-deficiency anemia. *N Engl J Med.* 2015;372(19):1832–1843.
2. Shapira Y, Vaturi M, Sagie A. Hemolysis associated with prosthetic heart valves: a review. *Cardiol Rev.* 2009;17(3):121–124.

Question 49

1. Nemeth E, Ganz T. Anemia of inflammation. *Hematol Oncol Clin North Am.* 2014;28(4):671–681.
2. Roy CN. Anemia of inflammation. *Hematology Am Soc Hematol Educ Program.* 2010;2010:276–280.

Question 50

1. Savage DG, Ogundipe A, Allen RH, Stabler SP, Lindenbaum J. Etiology and diagnostic evaluation of macrocytosis. *Am J Med Sci.* 2000;319(6):343–352.
2. Savage DG, Lindenbaum J, Stabler SP, Allen RH. Sensitivity of serum methylmalonic acid and total homocysteine determinations for diagnosing cobalamin and folate deficiencies. *Am J Med.* 1994;96(3):239–246.

Question 51

1. Stabler S. Vitamin B12 deficiency. *N Engl J Med.* 2013;368:149–160.

Question 52

1. Berentsen S, Tjønnfjord GE. Diagnosis and treatment of cold agglutinin mediated autoimmune hemolytic anemia. *Blood Rev.* 2012;26(3):107–115.
2. Bessman JD, Banks D. Spurious macrocytosis, a common clue to erythrocyte cold agglutinins. *Am J Clin Pathol.* 1980;74(6):797–800.

Question 53

1. Steinway SN, LeBlanc F, Loughran Jr TP. The pathogenesis and treatment of large granular lymphocyte leukemia. *Blood Rev.* 2014;28(3):87–94.
2. Sawada K, Hirokawa M, Fujishima N. Diagnosis and management of acquired pure red cell aplasia. *Hematol Oncol Clin North Am.* 2009;23(2):249–259.
3. Figure 34.2: This image was originally published in ASH Image Bank. Joseph Jurcic. Large Granular Lymphocyte Leukemia - 2. 11/15/2004; image number-00017942 © the American Society of Hematology. www.ashimagebank.org.

Question 54

1. Alexopoulou A, Vasilieva L, Kanellopoulou T, Pouriki S, Soultati A, Dourakis SP. Presence of spur cells as a highly predictive factor of mortality in patients with cirrhosis. *J Gastroenterol Hepatol.* 2014;29(4):830–834.
2. Vassiliadis T, Mpoumponaris A, Vakalopoulou S, et al. Spur cells and spur cell anemia in hospitalized patients with advanced liver disease: incidence and correlation with disease severity and survival. *Hepatol Res.* 2010;40(2):161–170.
3. Figure 34.3: This image was originally published in ASH Image Bank. John Lazarchick. Spur cell anemia 1. 06/21/2004; image number-00002636 © the American Society of Hematology. http://www.ashimagebank.org.

Question 55

1. Fleming MD. Congenital sideroblastic anemias: iron and heme lost in mitochondrial translation. *Hematology Am Soc Hematol Educ Program.* 2011;2011:525–531.
2. Camaschella C. Recent advances in the understanding of inherited sideroblastic anaemia. *Br J Haematol.* 2008;143(1):27–38.
3. Figure 34.4: This image was originally published in ASH Image Bank. John Lazarchick Ringed sideroblasts. 11/01/2008; image number-00003735 © the American Society of Hematology. www.ashimagebank.org.

Question 56

1. Sabel AL, Gaudiani JL, Statland B, Mehler PS. Hematological abnormalities in severe anorexia nervosa. *Ann Hematol.* 2013;92(5):605–613.
2. Hütter G, Ganepola S, Hofmann WK. The hematology of anorexia nervosa. *Int J Eat Disord.* 2009;42(4):293–300.
3. Figure 34.5: This image was originally published in ASH Image Bank. John Lazarchick; Marvaretta Stevenson. Anorexia Nervosa - Arrow Morphology. 01/18/2004; image number-00002345 © the American Society of Hematology. www.ashimagebank.org.

Question 57

1. Kaferle J, Strzoda CE. Evaluation of macrocytosis. *Am Fam Physician.* 2009;79(3):203–208.

Question 58

1. Redig AJ, Berliner N. Pathogenesis and clinical implications of HIV-related anemia in 2013. *Hematology Am Soc Hematol Educ Program.* 2013;2013:377–381.
2. Belperio PS, Rhew DC. Prevalence and outcomes of anemia in individuals with human immunodeficiency virus: a systematic review of the literature. *Am J Med.* 2004;116(suppl 7A):27S–43S.

Question 59

1. Perutz MF. Molecular anatomy, physiology, and pathology of hemoglobin. In: Stamatoyannopoulos G, Nienhuis AW, Leder PW, Majerus PW, eds. *The Molecular Basis of Blood Disorders.* Philadelphia: WB Saunders; 1987:127.

Question 60

1. Muncie Jr HL, Campbell J. Alpha and beta thalassemia. *Am Fam Physician.* 2009;80(4):339–344.

Question 61

1. Fucharoen S, Viprakasit V. Hb H disease: clinical course and disease modifiers. *Hematology Am Soc Hematol Educ Program.* 2009:26–34.
2. Muncie Jr HL, Campbell J. Alpha and beta thalassemia. *Am Fam Physician.* 2009;80(4):339–344.

Question 62

1. Martin A, Thompson AA. *Thalassemias. Pediatr Clin North Am.* 2013;60(6):1383–1391.
2. Muncie Jr HL, Campbell J. Alpha and beta thalassemia. *Am Fam Physician.* 2009;80(4):339–344.

Question 63

1. Parrish MR, Morrison JC. Sickle cell crisis and pregnancy. *Semin Perinatol.* 2013;37(4):274–279.
2. Naik RP, Lanzkron S. Baby on board: what you need to know about pregnancy in the hemoglobinopathies. *Hematology Am Soc Hematol Educ Program.* 2012;2012:208–214.

Question 64

1. Yawn BP, Buchanan GR, Afenyi-Annan AN, et al. Management of sickle cell disease: summary of the 2014 evidence-based report by expert panel members. *JAMA.* 2014;312(10):1033–1048.

Question 65

1. Wong TE, Brandow AM, Lim W, Lottenberg R. Update on the use of hydroxyurea therapy in sickle cell disease. *Blood.* 2014;124(26):3850–3857.
2. Yawn BP, Buchanan GR, Afenyi-Annan AN, et al. Management of sickle cell disease: summary of the 2014 evidence-based report by expert panel members. *JAMA.* 2014;312(10):1033–1048.
3. Charache S, Terrin ML, Moore RD, et al. Investigators of the Multicenter Study of Hydroxyurea in Sickle Cell Anemia. Effect of hydroxyurea on the frequency of painful crises in sickle cell anemia. *N Engl J Med.* 1995;332(20):1317–1322.

Question 66

1. Anele UA, Le BV, Resar LM, Burnett AL. How I treat priapism. *Blood.* 2015;125(23):3551–3558.
2. Yawn BP, Buchanan GR, Afenyi-Annan AN, et al. Management of sickle cell disease: summary of the 2014 evidence-based report by expert panel members. *JAMA.* 2014;312(10):1033–1048.
3. Olujohungbe A, Burnett AL. How I manage priapism due to sickle cell disease. *Br J Haematol.* 2013;160(6):754–765.

Question 67

1. Charache S, Terrin ML, Moore RD, et al. Effect of Hydroxyurea on the frequency of painful crises in sickle cell anemia. *N Eng J Med.* 1995;332:1317–1322.
2. Ferster A, Vermylen C, Cornu G, et al. Hydroxyurea for treatment of severe sickle cell anemia: a pediatric clinical trial. *Blood.* 1996;88(6):1960–1964.
3. Yawn BP, Buchanan GR, Afenyi-Annan AN, et al. Management of sickle cell disease: summary of the 2014 evidence-based report by expert panel members. *JAMA.* 2014;312(10):1033–1048.

Question 68

1. Da Costa L, Galimand J, Fenneteau O, Mohandas N. Hereditary spherocytosis, elliptocytosis, and other red cell membrane disorders. *Blood Rev.* 2013;27(4):167–178.
2. Barcellini W, Bianchi P, Fermo E, et al. Hereditary red cell membrane defects: diagnostic and clinical aspects. *Blood Transfus.* 2011;9(3):274–277.
3. Figure 34.7: This image was originally published in ASH Image Bank. Michael Low and Gareth Gregory. Passenger lymphocyte syndrome after lung transplant 11/15/2012; image number-00014843. © the American Society of Hematology.

Question 69

1. Kobayashi Y, Hatta Y, Ishiwatari Y, Kanno H, Takei M. Human parvovirus B19-induced aplastic crisis in an adult patient with hereditary spherocytosis: a case report and review of the literature. *BMC Res Notes.* 2014;7:137.
2. Saarinen UM, Chorba TL, Tattersall P, et al. Human parvovirus B19-induced epidemic acute red cell aplasia in patients with hereditary hemolytic anemia. *Blood.* 1986;67(5):1411–1417.

Question 70

1. Luzzatto L, Seneca E. G6PD deficiency: a classic example of pharmacogenetics with on-going clinical implications. *Br J Haematol.* 2014;164(4):469–480.
2. Cheah CY, Lew TE, Seymour JF, Burbury K. Rasburicase causing severe oxidative hemolysis and methemoglobinemia in a patient with previously unrecognized glucose-6-phosphate dehydrogenase deficiency. *Acta Haematol.* 2013;130(4):254–259.
3. Beutler E. Glucose-6-phosphate dehydrogenase deficiency: a historical perspective. *Blood.* 2008;111(1):16–24.

Question 71

1. Verma IC, Puri RD. Global burden of genetic disease and the role of genetic screening. *Semin Fetal Neonatal Med.* 2015;20(5):354–363.
2. Luzzatto L, Seneca E. G6PD deficiency: a classic example of pharmacogenetics with on-going clinical implications. *Br J Haematol.* 2014;164(4):469–480.

Question 72

1. Grace RF, Zanella A, Neufeld EJ, et al. Erythrocyte pyruvate kinase deficiency: 2015 status report. *Am J Hematol.* 2015;90(9):825–830.
2. Zanella A, Fermo E, Bianchi P, Valentini G. Red cell pyruvate kinase deficiency: molecular and clinical aspects. *Br J Haematol.* 2005;130(1):11–25.

Question 73

1. Naik R. Warm autoimmune hemolytic anemia. *Hematol Oncol Clin North Am.* 2015;29(3):445–453.
2. Zantek ND, Koepsell SA, Tharp Jr DR, Cohn CS. The direct antiglobulin test: a critical step in the evaluation of hemolysis. *Am J Hematol.* 2012;87(7):707–709.

Question 74

1. Dierickx D, Kentos A, Delannoy A. The role of rituximab in adults with warm antibody autoimmune hemolytic anemia. *Blood.* 2015;125(21):3223–3229.
2. Salama A. Treatment options for primary autoimmune hemolytic anemia: a short comprehensive review. *Transfus Med Hemother.* 2015;42(5):294–301.

Question 75

1. Berentsen S, Randen U, Tjønnfjord GE. Cold agglutinin-mediated autoimmune hemolytic anemia. *Hematol Oncol Clin North Am.* 2015;29(3):455–471.
2. Swiecicki PL, Hegerova LT, Gertz MA. Cold agglutinin disease. *Blood.* 2013;122(7):1114–1121.
3. Barbara DW, Mauermann WJ, Neal JR, Abel MD, Schaff HV, Winters JL. Cold agglutinins in patients undergoing cardiac surgery requiring cardiopulmonary bypass. *J Thorac Cardiovasc Surg.* 2013;146(3):668–680.
4. Figure 34.9: This image was originally published in ASH Image Bank. John Lazarchick. Cold agglutinin disease - 2 03/01/2010 ; image number-00001053. © the American Society of Hematology. www.ashimagebank.org.

Question 76

1. Liu C, Grossman BJ. Red blood cell transfusion for hematologic disorders. *Hematology Am Soc Hematol Educ Program.* 2015;2015(1):454–461.
2. Berentsen S, Tjonnfjord G. Diagnosis and treatment of cold agglutinin mediated autoimmune hemolytic anemia. *Blood Rev.* 2012;26(3):107–115.

Question 77

1. DeZern AE, Brodsky RA. Paroxysmal nocturnal hemoglobinuria: a complement-mediated hemolytic anemia. *Hematol Oncol Clin North Am.* 2015;29(3):479–494.
2. Brodsky RA. Paroxysmal nocturnal hemoglobinuria. *Blood.* 2014;124(18):2804–2811.
3. McKeage K. Eculizumab: a review of its use in paroxysmal nocturnal haemoglobinuria. *Drugs.* 2011;71(17):2327–2345.

Question 78

1. Brodsky RA. Paroxysmal nocturnal hemoglobinuria. *Blood.* 2014;124(18):2804–2811.

Question 79

1. Legendre CM, Licht C, Loirat C. Eculizumab in atypical hemolytic-uremic syndrome. *N Engl J Med.* 2013;369(14):1379–1380.
2. Wada H, Matsumoto T, Yamashita Y. Natural history of thrombotic thrombocytopenic purpura and hemolytic uremic syndrome. *Semin Thromb Hemost.* 2014;40(8):866–873.
3. Coppo P, Schwarzinger M, Buffet M. Predictive features of severe acquired ADAMTS13 deficiency in idiopathic thrombotic microangiopathies: the French TMA reference center experience. *PLoS One.* 2010;5(4):e10208.

Question 80

1. George J, Nester C. Syndromes of thrombotic microangiopathy. *N Engl J Med.* 2014;371:654–666.
2. Tersteeg C, Verhenne S, Roose E. ADAMTS13 and anti-ADAMTS13 autoantibodies in thrombotic thrombocytopenic purpua-current perspectives and new treatment strategies. *Expert Rev Hematol.* 2015;8:1–13.

Question 81

1. Ware RE, Helms RW, Investigators SW. Stroke with transfusions changing to hydroxyurea (SWiTCH). *Blood.* 2012;119:3925–3932.

Question 82

1. Muncie Jr HL, Campbell J. Alpha and beta thalassemia. *Am Fam Physician.* 2009;80(4):339–344.

Question 83

1. Salama A. Treatment options for primary autoimmune hemolytic anemia: a short comprehensive review. *Transfus Med Hemother.* 2015;42(5):294–301.
2. Lechner K, Jager U. How I treat autoimmune hemolytic anemias in adults. *Blood.* 2010;116:1831–1838.

Question 84

1. Barcellini W. Immune hemolysis: diagnosis and treatment recommendations. *Semin Hematol.* 2015;52(4):304–312.
2. Swiecicki PL, Hegerova LT, Gertz MA. Cold agglutinin disease. *Blood.* 2013;122:1114–1121.

Question 85

1. Bacon BR, Adams PC, Kowdley KV, Powell LW, Tavill AS. American Association for the Study of Liver D. Diagnosis and management of hemochromatosis: 2011 practice guideline by the American Association for the Study of Liver Diseases. *Hepatology.* 2011;54:328–343.

Question 86

1. Da Costa L, Galimand J, Fenneteau O, Mohandas N. Hereditary spherocytosis, elliptocytosis, and other red cell membrane disorders. *Blood Rev.* 2013;27(4):167–178.

Question 87

1. Schwartz J, Morstadt E, Dura A, et al. Biochemical identification of vitamin B12 deficiency in a medical office. *Clin Lab.* 2015;61:687–692.
2. Solomon LR. Cobalamin-responsive disorders in the ambulatory care setting: unreliability of cobalamin, methylmalonic acid, and homocysteine testing. *Blood.* 2005;105:978–985.
3. Stabler SP. Clinical practice. Vitamin B12 deficiency. *N Engl J Med.* 2013;368:149–160.

Question 88

1. Luzzatto L, Seneca E. G6PD deficiency: a classic example of pharmacogenetics with on-going clinical implications. *Br J Haematol.* 2014;164:469–480.

Question 89

1. Malinowski SS. Nutritional and metabolic complications of bariatric surgery. *Am J Med Sci.* 2006;331:219–225.

Question 90

1. Young NS, Brown KE. Parvovirus B19. *N Engl J Med.* 2004;350:586–597.

Question 91

1. Gallagher PG, Tse WT, Marchesi SL, Zarkowsky HS, Forget BG. A defect in alpha-spectrin mRNA accumulation in hereditary pyropoikilocytosis. *Trans Assoc Am Physicians.* 1991;104:32–39.

Question 92

1. Aslinia F, Mazza JJ, Yale SH. Megaloblastic anemia and other causes of macrocytosis. *Clin Med Res.* 2006;4:236–241.

Question 93

1. Sawada K, Fujishima N, Hirokawa M. Acquired pure red cell aplasia: updated review of treatment. *Br J Haematol.* 2008;142:505–514.

Question 94

1. Cullis JO. Diagnosis and management of anaemia of chronic disease: current status. *Br J Haematol.* 2011;154:289.

Question 95

1. Bradberry SM. Occupational methaemoglobinaemia. Mechanisms of production, features, diagnosis and management including the use of methylene blue. *Toxicol Rev.* 2003;22(1):13–27.

Question 96

1. Muncie Jr HL, Campbell J. Alpha and beta thalassemia. *Am Fam Physician.* 2009;80(4):339–344.

Question 97

1. Yawn BP, Buchanan GR, Afenyi-Annan AN, et al. Management of sickle cell disease: summary of the 2014 evidence-based report by expert panel members. *JAMA.* 2014;312(10):1033–1048.

Question 98

1. Gardner K, Suddle A, Kane P, et al. How we treat sickle cell hepatopathy and liver transplantation in adults. *Blood.* 2014;123:2302–2307.

Question 99

1. Bolton-Maggs PHB, Stevens RF, Dodd NJ, et al. Guidelines for the diagnosis and management of hereditary spherocytosis. *Br J Haematol.* 2004;126:455–474.

Question 100

1. Swiecicki PL, Hegerova LT, Gertz MA. Cold agglutinin disease. *Blood.* 2013;122:1114–1121.
2. Berentsen S, Tjonnfjord GE. Diagnosis and treatment of cold agglutinin mediated autoimmune hemolytic anemia. *Blood Rev.* 2012;26:107–115.

Question 101

1. Howard J, Malfroy M, Llewelyn C, et al. The transfusion alternatives preopeartively in sickle cell disease (TAPS) study: a randomized, controlled multicentre clinical trial. *Lancet.* 2013;381:930–938.
2. National Heart, Lung, and Blood Institute (NHLBI). Evidence-Based Management of Sickle Cell Disease: Expert Panel Report, 2014. Available at http://www.nhlbi.nih.gov/guidelines

Question 102

1. Swiecicki PL, Hegerova LT, Gertz MA. Cold agglutinin disease. *Blood.* 2013;122:1114–1121.
2. Berentsen S, Tjonnfjord GE. Diagnosis and treatment of cold agglutinin mediated autoimmune hemolytic anemia. *Blood Rev.* 2012;26:107–115.

Question 103

1. Scheuneman LP, Ataga KI. Delayed hemolytic transfusion reaction in sickle cell disease. *Am J Med Sci.* 2010;339:266–269.
2. Gardner K, Hoppe C, Mijovic A, Thein SL. How we treat delayed hemolytic transfusion reactions in patients with sickle cell disease. *Br J Haematol.* 2015;170:745–756.

Question 104

1. Bain BJ. Diagnosis from the Blood Smear. *N Engl J Med.* 2005;353:498–507.
2. Mason PJ, Bautista JM, Gilsanz F. G6PD deficiency: the genotype-phenotype association. *Blood Rev.* 2007;21:267–283.

Question 105

1. Mason PJ, Bautista JM, Gilsanz F. G6PD deficiency: the genotype-phenotype association. *Blood Rev.* 2007;21:267–283.

Question 106

1. Stabler SP. Vitamin B12 deficiency. *N Engl J Med.* 2013;368:149–160.
2. Chen M, Krishnamurthy A, Mohamed AR, Green R. Hematologic disorders following gastric bypass surgery: emerging concepts of the interplay between nutritional deficiency and inflammation. *Biomed Res Int.* 2013;2013:205467.

Question 107

1. Lechner K, Jager U. How I treat autoimmune hemolytic anemia in adults. *Blood.* 2010;116:1831–1838.

Question 108

1. Harteveld CL, Higgs DR. α-thalassaemia. *Orphanet J Rare Dis.* 2010;5:13.
2. Muncie HL, Campbell JS. Alpha and beta thalassemia. *Am Fam Physician.* 2009;15:339–344.

Question 109

1. Clarke G, Higgins T. Laboratory investigation of hemoglobinopathies and thalassemias: review and update. *Clin Chem.* 2000;46(8 pt 2):1284–1290.

Question 110

1. Clarke G, Higgins T. Laboratory investigation of hemoglobinopathies and thalassemias: review and update. *Clin Chem.* 2000;46(8 pt 2):1284–1290.

Question 111

1. Fleming MD. Congenital sideroblastic anemias: iron and heme lost in mitochondrial translation. *Hematology Am Soc Hematol Educ Program.* 2011;2011:525–531.

Question 112

1. Howard J, Hart N, Roberts-Harewood M, Cummins M, Awogbade M, Davis B. Guideline on the management of acute chest syndrome in sickle cell disease. *Br J Haematol.* 2015;169(4):492–505.

Question 113

1. Koduri PR, Nathan S. Acute splenic sequestration crisis in adults with hemoglobin S-C disease: a report of nine cases. *Ann Hematol.* 2006;85(4):239–243.
2. Naymagon L, Pendurti G, Billett HH. Acute splenic sequestration crisis in adult sickle cell disease: a report of 16 cases. *Hemoglobin.* 2015;39(6):375–379.

Question 114

1. Cheah CY, Lew TE, Seymour JF, Burbury K. Rasburicase causing severe oxidative hemolysis and methemoglobinemia in a patient with previously unrecognized glucose-6-phosphate dehydrogenase deficiency. *Acta haematologica.* 2013;130(4):254–259.

Question 115

1. Cheson BD, Rom WN, Webber RC. Basophilic stippling of red blood cells: a nonspecific finding of multiple etiology. *Am J Ind Med.* 1984;5(4):327–334.
2. Munoz J, Guo Y. Basophilic stippling: a lead to the diagnosis. *Blood.* 2011;118(20):5370.

Question 116

1. Bonkovsky HL, Poh-Fitzpatrick M, Pimstone N, et al. Porphyria cutanea tarda, hepatitis C, and HFE gene mutations in North America. *Hepatology.* 1998;27(6):1661–1669.
2. Liu LU, Phillips J, Bonkovsky H. Porphyria cutanea tarda, type II. In: Pagon RA, Adam MP, Ardinger HH, Wallace SE, Amemiya A, Bean LJH, et al., eds. *GeneReviews(R).* Seattle: University of Washington; 1993. Seattle University of Washington, Seattle. All rights reserved.

Question 117

1. Dunford LM, Roy DM, Hahn TE, et al. Dapsone-induced methemoglobinemia after hematopoietic stem cell transplantation. *Biol Blood Marrow Transplant.* 2006;12(2):241–242.
2. Prchal JT. Clinical features, diagnosis, and treatment of methemoglobinemia UpToDate: UpToDate. *Waltham.* 2016.

Question 118

1. Kanwar P, Kowdley KV. Diagnosis and treatment of hereditary hemochromatosis: an update. *Expert Rev Gastroenterol Hepatol.* 2013;7(6):517–530.

Question 119

1. Camaschella C, Fargion S, Sampietro M, et al. Inherited HFE-unrelated hemochromatosis in Italian families. *Hepatology.* 1999;29(5):1563–1564.
2. Camaschella C, Roetto A, Cicilano M, et al. Juvenile and adult hemochromatosis are distinct genetic disorders. *Eur J Hum Genet.* 1997;5(6):371–375.

Question 120

1. http://soliris.net/resources/pdf/soliris_pi.pdf>; 2016 Accessed 29.01.16.
2. Bouts A, Monnens L, Davin JC, Struijk G, Spanjaard L. Insufficient protection by Neisseria meningitidis vaccination alone during eculizumab therapy. *Pediatric Nephrol.* 2011;26(10):1919–1920.

Question 121

1. Swiecicki PL, Hegerova LT, Gertz MA. Cold agglutinin disease. *Blood.* 2013;122(7):1114–1121.
2. Turtzo DF, Ghatak PK. Acute hemolytic anemia with Mycoplasma pneumoniae pneumonia. *JAMA.* 1976;236(10):1140–1141.

Question 122

1. Bolton-Maggs PH, Stevens RF, Dodd NJ, Lamont G, Tittensor P, King MJ. Guidelines for the diagnosis and management of hereditary spherocytosis. *Br J Haematol.* 2004;126(4):455–474.
2. Girodon F, Garcon L, Bergoin E, et al. Usefulness of the eosin-5'-maleimide cytometric method as a first-line screening test for the diagnosis of hereditary spherocytosis: comparison with ektacytometry and protein electrophoresis. *Br J Haematol.* 2008;140(4):468–470.

Question 123

1. Ganz T. Hepcidin and iron regulation, 10 years later. *Blood.* 2011;117(17):4425–4433.

Question 124

1. Thompson AA. Sickle cell trait testing and athletic participation: a solution in search of a problem? *Hematology Am Soc Hematol Educ Program.* 2013;2013(1):632–637.

Question 125

1. Piel FB, Weatherall DJ. The alpha-thalassemias. *N Engl J Med.* 2014;371(20):1908–1916.

Question 126

1. Lee KC, Ladizinski B, Federman DG. Complications associated with use of levamisole-contaminated cocaine: an emerging public health challenge. *Mayo Clin Proc.* 2012;87:581–586.

Question 127

1. Chhetri SK, Mills RJ, Shaunak S, Emsley HC. Copper deficiency. *BMJ.* 2014;348. g3691.

Question 128

1. Cooper DS. Antithyroid drugs. *N Engl J Med.* 2005;352:905–917.

Question 129

1. Dearden C. Large granular lymphocytic leukaemia pathogenesis and management. *Br J Haematol.* 2011;152(3):273–283.

Question 130

1. Edelman M, Mckitrick J. Histoplasma capsulatum in a peripheral-blood smear. *N Engl J Med.* 2000;342(1):28.
2. Park H, Shafer D. Disseminated histoplasmosis in peripheral blood smear. *Blood.* 2014;123(10):1445.

Question 131

1. Hammond WPt, Price TH, Souza LM, Dale DC. Treatment of cyclic neutropenia with granulocyte colony-stimulating factor. *N Engl J Med.* 1989;320(20):1306–1311.

Question 132

1. Buchanan JA, Lavonas EJ. Agranulocytosis and other consequences due to use of illicit cocaine contaminated with levamisole. *Curr Opin Hematol.* 2012;19(1):27–31.

Question 133

1. Antunes H, Pereira A, Cunha I. Chediak-Higashi syndrome: pathognomonic feature. *Lancet.* 2013;382(9903):1514.
2. Introne WJ, Westbroek W, Golas GA, Adams D. Chediak-Higashi syndrome. In: Pagon RA, Adam MP, Ardinger HH, et al., eds. *GeneReviews(R).* Seattle (WA): University of Washington; 1993. Seattle University of Washington, Seattle. All rights reserved.
3. Teixeira C, Barbot J, Freitas MI. From blood film to the diagnosis of rare hereditary disorders. *Br J Haematol.* 2015;168(3):315.

Question 134

1. Network NCC. *T-cell large granular lymphocytic leukemia;* January 02, 2016. Available from www.nccn.org/professionals/physician_gls/pdf/nhl.pdf.

Question 135

1. Hitchcock IS, Kaushansky K. Thrombopoietin from beginning to end. *Br J Haematol.* 2014;165(2):259–268.
2. Giannini EG, Peck-Radosavljevic M. Platelet dysfunction: status of thrombopoietin in thrombocytopenia associated with chronic liver failure. *Semin Thromb Hemost.* 2015;41(5):455–461.

Question 136

1. Prchal JT, Thiagarajan P. Erythropoiesis. In: Kaushansky K, Lichtman MA, Prchal JT, et al., eds. *Williams Hematology.* 9th ed. New York: McGraw-Hill; 2015. http://accessmedicine.mhmedical.com/content.aspx?bookid=1581&Sectionid=94303394.

Question 137

1. Geddis AE. Megakaryocytes. In: Greer JP, Arber DA, Glader B, et al., eds. *Wintrobe's Clinical Hematology.* 13th ed. Lippincott Williams & Wilkins; 2014.

Question 138

1. Ertenli I1, Kiraz S, Oztürk MA, Haznedaroğlu Ic, Celik I, Calgüneri M. Pathologic thrombopoiesis of rheumatoid arthritis. *Rheumatol Int*. 2003;23(2):49–60.

Question 139

1. Smith C. Production, distribution, and fate of neutrophils. In: Kaushansky K, Lichtman MA, Prchal JT, et al., eds. *Williams Hematology*. 9th ed. New York: McGraw-Hill; 2015. http://accessmedicine.mhmedical.com.libproxy.lib.unc.edu/content.aspx?bookid=1581&Sectionid=101238652.

Question 140

1. Lacy P, Adamko DJ, Moqbel R. The human eosinophil. In: Greer JP, Arber DA, Glader B, et al., eds. *Wintrobe's Clinical Hematology*. 13th ed. Lippincott Williams & Wilkins; 2014.

Question 141

1. Brown KE, Tisdale J, Barrett AJ, Dunbar CE, Young NS. Hepatitis-associated aplastic anemia. *N Engl J Med*. 1997;336:1059–1064.

Question 142

1. Fernandez Garcia MS, Teruya-Feldstein J. The diagnosis and treatment of dyskeratosis congenita: a review. *J Blood Med*. 2014;5: 157–167.
2. Armanios M, Blackburn EH. The telomere syndromes. *Nat Rev Genet*. 2012;13:693–704.

Question 143

1. Soulier J. Fanconi anemia. *Hematology Am Soc Hematol Educ Program*. 2011;2011:492–497.

Question 144

1. Gregg XT, Reddy V, Prchal JT. Copper deficiency masquerading as myelodysplastic syndrome. *Blood*. 2002;100(4):1493–1495.
2. Nations SP, Boyer PJ, Love LA, et al. Denture cream: an unusual source of excess zinc, leading to hypocupremia and neurologic disease. *Neurology*. 2008;71(9):639–643.
3. Prasad AS, Brewer GJ, Schoomaker EB, Rabbani P. Hypocupremia induced by zinc therapy in adults. *JAMA*. 1978;240(20):2166–2168.

Question 145

1. Kulagin A, Lisukov I, Ivanova M, et al. Prognostic value of paroxysmal nocturnal haemoglobinuria clone presence in aplastic anaemia patients treated with combined immunosuppression: results of two-centre prospective study. *Br J Haematol*. 2014;164(4): 546–554.

2. Zhao X, Zhang L, Jing L, et al. The role of paroxysmal nocturnal hemoglobinuria clones in response to immunosuppressive therapy of patients with severe aplastic anemia. *Ann Hematol*. 2015;94(7):1105–1110.
3. Pu JJ, Mukhina G, Wang H, Savage WJ, Brodsky RA. Natural history of paroxysmal nocturnal hemoglobinuria clones in patients presenting as aplastic anemia. *Eur J Haematol*. 2011;87(1):37–45.

Question 146

1. Townsley DM, Dumitriu B, Young NS. Bone marrow failure and the telomeropathies. *Blood*. 2014;124(18):2775–2783.

Question 147

1. Choudhry VP, Gupta S, Gupta M, Kashyap R, Saxena R. Pregnancy associated aplastic anemia—a series of 10 cases with review of literature. *Hematology*. 2002;7(4):233–238.

Question 148

1. Chirnomas SD, Kupfer GM. The inherited bone marrow failure syndromes. *Pediatr Clin North Am*. 2013;60:1291.

Question 149

1. Guinan EC. Diagnosis and management of aplastic anemia. *Hematology Am Soc Hematol Educ Program*. 2011;2011:76–81.

Question 150

1. Chung NG, Kim M. Current insights into inherited bone marrow failure syndromes. *Korean J Pediatr*. 2014;57(8):337–344.

Question 151

1. Brodsky RA. Paroxysmal nocturnal hemoglobinuria. *Blood*. 2014; 124:2804–2811.

Question 152

1. Sloand E, Kim S, Maciejewski JP, Tisdale J, Follmann D, Young NS. Intracellular interferon-gamma in circulating and marrow T cells detected by flow cytometry and the response to immunosuppressive therapy in patients with aplastic anemia. *Blood*. 2002;100:1185.

Transfusion Medicine

Marc J. Khan, Marc Zumberg, Ara Metjian, Anita Rajasekhar, Brandi Reeves, and Molly Weidner Mandernach

QUESTIONS

1. A 65-year-old man with a 7-year history of coronary artery disease with two stents and a 15-year history of CLL presents with severe dyspnea on exertion, substernal chest pain, and fatigue for the past 48 hours. The patient's CLL has required therapy 1 year prior with fludarabine, cyclophosphamide, and rituximab. On exam his BP is 85/60, pulse 120, RR 18, and temp 99°F. He has pale mucous membranes and icteric sclera. His EKG shows flipped T-waves in the anterior leads. His laboratory studies are shown:

Hgb	5.6 g/dL
Hct	17%
WBC	42,000 × 10⁹/L (15% polys, 80% lymphs, 5% monos)
Platelets	89,000 × 10⁹/L
Retic	375,000 × 10⁹/L
Tbili	11.5 mg/dL
LDH	562 IU/L

After 1 hour, the blood bank is unable to find a compatible crossmatch red cell unit.
How should he be managed?
   A. Methylprednisolone
   B. Rituximab
   C. Apheresis
   D. Continue to search for compatible unit
   E. Transfuse ABO-compatible, crossmatch-incompatible red cells

2. A 28-year-old man with homozygous sickle cell disease (SS) presents preoperatively for cholecystectomy. He is currently asymptomatic. The patient's disease has been complicated by acute chest syndrome on two occasions and frequent vasoocclusive crisis. He is taking folate and hydroxyurea. His current laboratory studies are as follows:

Hgb	5.6 g/dL
Hct	17%
Baseline Hgb	5.0–6.0 g/dL
Reticulocyte	59,000 × 10⁹/L

How should his anemia be managed preoperatively?
   A. No transfusion
   B. Simple transfusion to Hgb 10 g/dL
   C. Simple transfusion to Hgb 12 g/dL
   D. Exchange transfusion to 10 g/dL with less than 30% Hgb S
   E. Exchange transfusion to 12 g/dL with less than 30% Hgb S

3. In which of the following clinical scenarios would transfusion of fresh frozen plasma be indicated as first-line therapy?
   A. A 45-year-old woman with severe factor XI deficiency and prior bleeding who requires urgent bowel resection
   B. A 45-year-old man with advanced liver disease and INR of 1.8 requiring a PICC line
   C. A 24-year-old man with severe hemophilia B with an intracranial hemorrhage
   D. A 64-year-old woman with an EF of 5%–10% who is on warfarin with an INR of 3.6 and suffers an intracranial hemorrhage
   E. A 16-year-old woman with severe factor XIII deficiency in need of a cholecystectomy

4. A patient with an unknown bleeding disorder presents to a rural emergency room. Blood products are available, but no specific factor concentrates or specialized hemostatic agents are on formulary, except for DDAVP and tranexamic acid.
   Before transfer to a tertiary referral center, in which clinical scenario is transfusion of cryoprecipitate best indicated?
   A. A man with severe hemophilia B and a large thigh hematoma after trauma
   B. A woman with severe factor XI deficiency and a retroperitoneal bleed after an MVA
   C. A man with hemophilia A who is able to self-infuse factor VIII and has a hemarthrosis
   D. A woman with mild type I von Willebrand disease and a nosebleed
   E. A woman with factor XIII deficiency in need of an emergent appendectomy

5. A 24-year-old African American man with Hgb-S/β⁰-thalassemia is brought in via EMS to the ER for acute right-sided hemiparesis and aphasia. While CT scan shows no acute intracranial pathology, MRI shows infarctions in the left middle cerebral artery territory, with magnetic resonance angiography of the cranial and neck vessels significant for moyamoya in the right posterior circulation. He is admitted to the neuro-ICU for monitoring and permissive hypertension.
   Which of the following is the best recommendation at this time?
   A. Aspirin, 81 mg daily
   B. Dual antiplatelet therapy with aspirin, 81 mg/day, and clopidogrel 75 mg daily
   C. Erythrocytapheresis to goal Hgb-S of less than 30%
   D. Supportive care
   E. Transfusion of 2 units of phenotypically matched packed red cells

TABLE 35.1 Laboratory Results for Patient in Question 6

Laboratory Test	Patient's Result	Reference Range
Hemoglobin	8.0 g/dL	12–16 g/dL
Hematocrit	24%	35%–48%
White blood cell count	11.2×10^9/L	4–10×10^9/L
Platelet count	420×10^9/L	150–450×10^9/L
Mean corpuscular volume (MCV)	91 fL	80–100 fL
Reticulocyte count	1.5%	0.5%–1.8%
Estimated glomerular filtration rate (eGFR)	60 mL/min	> 60 mL/min
Ferritin	550 ng/mL	18–320 ng/mL
Iron	20 µg/dL	33–150 µg/dL
Total iron-binding capacity	180 µg/dL	220–440 µg/dL
% iron saturation	30%	11%–50%

6. A 56-year-old man is admitted to the medical intensive care unit (ICU) for pneumonia and sepsis. He is being treated with intravenous antibiotics. His hemoglobin has gradually trended downward during the hospitalization from 12.5 g/dL on admission to 8.0 g/dL today (reference range, 12–16 g/dL). He is intubated and sedated. He is no longer on vasopressors. The ICU team plans to extubate the patient today. There are no signs of blood loss. He is euvolemic. Laboratory results are in Table 35.1.
   Which of the following is the most appropriate recommendation?
   A. Transfuse 2 units of red blood cells
   B. Proceed with extubation as planned
   C. Give an erythrocyte-stimulating agent and intravenous iron
   D. Begin oral therapeutic iron

7. A 60-year-old man with coronary artery disease and a normal creatinine is admitted to the hospital for treatment of pneumonia. He receives appropriate antibiotics and supportive therapy. His hemoglobin is 10 g/dL on admission and decreases to 9 g/dL during the course of his hospitalization. There is no evidence of bleeding. He is now asymptomatic, and his cough has improved significantly. His blood pressure, pulse, and oxygen saturation are within normal limits.
   Which of the following is the most appropriate next step in management of his anemia?
   A. Administer erythropoietin
   B. Transfuse 1 unit of packed red blood cells
   C. Transfuse 2 units of packed red blood cells
   D. Administer IV iron
   E. No therapy indicated

8. A 65-year-old G2P2 with IgA lambda multiple myeloma being treated with daratumumab complains of increasing palpitations and dyspnea on exertion. This is her third cycle of daratumumab, and she achieved a complete response after cycle 2. Her hemoglobin is trending downward, presently 7.1 g/dL from 8.5 g/dL 2 weeks prior. The WBC and

platelet count are normal. LDH is normal, and liver tests including bilirubin are normal. Serum protein electrophoresis with immunofixation shows a faint IgG kappa monoclonal spike, too low to quantify.
   The patient has never before received a blood transfusion. You are notified by the blood bank that your patient's RBCs are pan-reactive on routine compatibility testing.
   What is the best explanation for this patient's RBC incompatibility?
   A. Multiple myeloma
   B. Pregnancy history
   C. Autoimmune hemolytic anemia
   D. Daratumumab

9. A 25-year-old with sickle cell disease is planned for an elective laparoscopic cholecystectomy. Her hemoglobin is measured to be 7.8 g/dL, and it is recommended that she have red blood cell transfusion. She has no history of red blood cell antibodies. You are notified by the blood bank that there are currently no units of C, E, and Kell negative blood.
   Which of the following is the most appropriate recommendation at this time?
   A. Proceed with surgery; administer available units.
   B. Delay surgery; wait for C, E, Kell negative blood.
   C. Proceed with surgery; do not administer blood.
   D. Proceed with surgery; perform a simple exchange transfusion.

10. A 38-year-old woman presents 7 days following knee replacement surgery with bruising and gum bleeding. The patient has a 25-year history of rheumatoid arthritis. She has been healthy, and aside from the recent knee surgery, she has had three cesarean sections that were not complicated. Her recent surgery required 2 units of transfused blood in the OR and was otherwise uncomplicated. She was discharged on day 3. On exam, she has multiple ecchymosis on her trunk and extremities, bleeding gums, and petechiae on her lower extremities. Her laboratory studies are as follows:

Hgb	10.7 g/dL
Hct	32%
Platelets	4000×10^9/L
Blood type	O+

    What is the best way to manage her condition?
    A. Transfusion of random donor platelets
    B. Methylprednisolone
    C. Intravenous immunoglobulin
    D. Rituximab
    E. Splenectomy

11. A 58-year-old man with a 7-year history of CLL that has not required treatment presents with bleeding gums, epistaxis, hematochezia, and a platelet count of 6000×10^9/L. The patient reports that he has had an allergic reaction to a blood transfusion 5 years prior given during a bout of diverticulosis. The transfusion reaction prompted admission to the ICU due to low blood pressure and difficulty breathing. On exam, the patient has bleeding gums and blood in his nares. He is passing bloody stools. His laboratory studies are shown:

Hgb	11.2 g/dL
Hct	33%
WBC	$19,400 \times 10^9$/L (15% polys, 80% lymphs, 5% monos)
Platelet	6000×10^9/L

What is the best way to manage her condition?
A. Transfusion of pooled random donor platelets
B. Transfusion of single donor platelets
C. Transfusion of irradiated platelets
D. Transfusion of washed platelets
E. Transfusion of platelets from an IgA deficient patient

12. A 38-year-old woman is receiving induction therapy with cytarabine and idarubicin for acute myelogenous leukemia. Her family members very much want to donate blood for direct donation to support her during her leukemia therapy. How should such blood products be prepared prior to transfusion?
A. Leukocyte reduction
B. Irradiation
C. Washing
D. Full serologic crossmatch

13. A 32-year-old woman with SC disease is admitted to the hospital with a vasoocclusive crisis characterized by pain in her back and extremities. She has a history of frequent painful crisis. On initial exam, her temperature is 99°F, BP is 120/70, and pulse is 100. Her O₂ sat is 98% on room air. She is transfused 2 units of PRBC for worsening anemia. Towards the end of her second unit, she reports shortness of breath. On follow-up exam she has an increase in her jugular venous distention, diffuse crackles in both lungs, and an S3 is heard on cardiac exam. A chest x-ray reveals diffuse bilateral fluffy infiltrates.
What is the most likely diagnosis?
A. Transfusion associated circulatory overload
B. Transfusion related acute lung injury
C. Bacterial sepsis
D. Pulmonary embolism
E. Acute chest syndrome

14. A 43-year-old multiparous woman with severe factor XI deficiency and prior postoperative bleeding is brought to the emergency department immediately after she was an unrestrained passenger in a major automobile accident. She has suffered a broken hip and will need nonemergent surgery. The use of packed red blood cells is anticipated, and FFP will be needed secondary to her to her coagulation defect.
Her husband tells the emergency department physician that during a packed red cell transfusion 4 years ago, she developed an anaphylactic reaction and required epinephrine and oral intubation as part of the resuscitation process.
Which of the following products should you recommend at the time of surgery to minimize the risk of anaphylaxis?
A. Irradiated red blood cells
B. Leukoreduced red blood cells
C. Fresh frozen plasma from an IgA deficient donor
D. HLA-matched red blood cells
E. Washed fresh frozen plasma

15. A 53-year-old woman without prior medical history develops shortness of breath, chills, and fever during transfusion of a unit of packed red blood cells for symptomatic postoperative anemia.
On physical examination, temperature is 38.2°C (102.0°F), blood pressure is 136/66 mm Hg, pulse rate is 117, and respiration rate is 23 breaths/min. Oxygen saturation is 86% with the patient breathing oxygen, 2 L/min by nasal cannula. There is no jugular venous distention or peripheral edema. Cardiopulmonary examination discloses tachycardia with a regular rhythm and no S₃ or murmur.

Laboratory studies indicate a hemoglobin level of 7.7 g/dL, a leukocyte count of 7600 × 10⁹/L, and a platelet count of 235,000 × 10⁹/L. A preoperative and postoperative type and screen indicate A-positive blood type with a negative antibody screen. Diffuse bilateral infiltrates are seen on chest radiograph. An electrocardiogram shows sinus tachycardia but no ST changes.
Which of the following is the most likely mechanism leading to this transfusion reaction?
A. ABO incompatibility
B. Development of a new alloantibody
C. T lymphocyte attack against the recipient red blood cells
D. Antileukocyte antibodies
E. Fluid overload

16. A 34-year-old woman with sickle cell anemia (Hb SS) is evaluated for increasing bone pain, dyspnea, and fatigue; which has worsened over the last 2 days. She had been hospitalized 7 days prior for an elective cholecystectomy and received 2 units of preoperative AB-negative and C antigen–negative; leukodepleted erythrocytes, in accordance with her preoperative type and screen; and known anti-C alloantibody.
The operation was uneventful, and she was discharged to home 24 hours later. Current medications include only hydroxyurea and folic acid.
On physical examination, the patient is in obvious pain. Temperature is 37.4°C (99.4°F), blood pressure is 151/88 mm Hg, pulse rate is 111, and respiratory rate is 14 breaths/minute. The patient has jaundice. The cardiopulmonary and neurologic examinations are normal (Table 35.2).
Which of the following laboratory tests/findings would lead to the most likely diagnosis?
A. Type and screen
B. HLA typing
C. IgA level
D. Presence of antineutrophil antibodies
E. Presence of CMV

17. A 35-year-old woman pregnant with her fourth child presents to the emergency department with dyspnea and orthostasis. Hemoglobin is 6 g/dL, MCV 78 fL, and white blood cell count and platelet count are normal. Based upon her symptoms, it is elected to transfuse 2 units of PRBC. Two years ago she received a PRBC transfusion for treatment of severe anemia secondary to menorrhagia and experienced a febrile nonhemolytic transfusion reaction.
Which of the following RBC products should be ordered for this patient?
A. Leukoreduced
B. Irradiated

TABLE 35.2 Laboratory Results for Patientin Question 16

Laboratory Studies	Current Value	Values at Recent Hospital Discharge 7 Days Ago
Hemoglobin	6.9 g/dL	8.9 g/dL
Leukocyte count	11,000/µL	7860/µL
Platelet count	345,000/µL	207,000/µL (207 × 10⁹/L)
Total bilirubin	4.8 mg/dL	1.6 mg/dL
Direct bilirubin	0.6 mg/dL	0.7

C. Washed

D. CMV-negative

E. Phenotypically matched

18. A 27-year-old African American woman with sickle cell disease, which has been characterized by infrequent crises, presents to the ER. She is on hydroxyurea and folate, with as needed oral morphine. Recently, she had developed a pain crisis following an upper respiratory tract infection that was unrelieved by her oral analgesia. She presented to her local ER, where she was noted to be anemic at her baseline hemoglobin of 8.5, treated with 2 units of packed red cells, intravenous fluids, antiemetics, and a PCA for 5 hours. This was effective in providing symptomatic relief, and she was discharged home.

She returns 2 days later with even more severe pain and new onset dyspnea. A repeat CBC and additional labs are sent and show:

WBC	$16,800 \times 10^9$/L (3.2–9.8)
Hemoglobin	3.1 g/dL (12.0–15.5)
Hematocrit	8.9% (35–45)
MCV	91 fL
Platelets	$435,000 \times 10^9$/L
Reticulocyte%	8.5% (0.7–2.0)
Absolute reticulocyte count	$395,000 \times 10^9$/L
Total bilirubin	7.8 (0.5–1.4)
LDH	1737 (100–200)

Upon examination, you find a 27-year-old African American woman in pain that is being somewhat relieved by the use of hydromorphone boluses. She is markedly icteric, with pale conjunctiva. However, she denies chest pain or dyspnea.

Which of the following is the most appropriate next step in management?

A. Continued use of folate

B. Enoxaparin

C. Intravenous immunoglobulins

D. Repeat type and screen and direct Coombs

E. All of the above

19. A 34-year-old Hispanic woman has been admitted for gallstone pancreatitis. Her history is remarkable for moderate obesity, diet-controlled diabetes, and an episode of postpartum bleeding following the delivery of her second child 2 years ago, necessitating transfusion of 2 units of blood. During this admission, she is kept NPO and is treated with adequate analgesia and antiemetics, with daily improvement in her pain and clinical status. Her pancreatic and liver enzymes normalize, but due to issues with childcare, she requests to undergo her cholecystectomy during this admission.

The consulting surgeon agrees, but the operation cannot be performed until Tuesday, due to scheduling issues in the OR, and she has to stay over the weekend. During this time, she is transfused with 2 units packed red cells prior.

The patient does well over the next days and is looking forward to having her surgery. On the day of her surgery, early AM labs show a drop in her hemoglobin of at least 2 units, with an increase in her total bilirubin to 4.1 (0.5–1.4).

Which of the following is the most appropriate next step?

A. Check thin and thick blood smears

B. Clear her for surgery

C. Draw blood cultures, ×2

D. Recheck a type and screen

E. Transfuse another 2 units of blood

20. An 84-year-old man with refractory anemia with excess blasts-2 (RAEB-2) is not considered to be a candidate for high-intensity chemotherapy. Following one cycle of a hypomethylating agent, he has declined any additional therapy with chemotherapy, deciding upon supportive care alone. During the course of his treatment, he has been treated with recombinant erythropoietin, although this has become less effective. As a result, he has received 2 units of packed red cells every month week for the 14 months in order to ameliorate his symptoms of dyspnea and fatigue.

Which of the following is the most appropriate next step in management?

A. Darbepoetin

B. Deferasirox

C. Eltrombopag

D. Romiplostim

21. A 43-year-old man with a mechanical mitral valve, who is maintained on warfarin, and without any other comorbidity, is brought into the ER for an open femur fracture. His INR is measured at 2.8, and due to the emergent nature of his case, he is given 4 units of fresh frozen plasma along with 10 mg IV of vitamin K. Following the completion of his second unit and during infusion of the third unit, he develops the sudden onset of dyspnea and is noted to be markedly hypoxic, despite the use of supplemental oxygen. No evidence for volume overload or chest wall petechiae is noted on physical examination, whereas a STAT chest x-ray shows bilateral infiltrates.

Which of the following is the most appropriate next step in management?

A. CT angiogram of the chest

B. Intravenous immunoglobulin

C. rFVIIa

D. Stopping the red cell infusion

E. Ventilation/perfusion scan of the chest

22. A 58-year-old African American woman, who is G5P3 (G2 and G4 complicated by early second trimester losses), has been admitted to the Gyn-Onc service for an exploratory laparotomy, after an endometrial biopsy showed the presence of adenocarcinoma. She undergoes a hysterectomy, bilateral salpingo-oophorectomy, and pelvic lymphadenectomy, which fortunately shows no evidence of metastatic disease. She receives 2 units of packed red cells intraoperatively and is sent to the step-down floor without incident. The following day, she is started on enoxaparin for thromboprophylaxis, an oral proton pump inhibitor, her home medications, and begins to ambulate with physical therapy. Her postoperative course is complicated by an ileus, which delays the removal of her nasogastric tube, but she is otherwise recovering well. On postoperative day #6, coffee-ground material is noted in the suction canister, and the nurse reports increased ecchymoses with venipuncture. A repeat CBC is drawn and shows the following:

WBC	9.9 (3.2–9.8)
Hemoglobin	11.2 (12.0–15.5)
Hematocrit	33.9 (35–45)
MCV	87
Platelets	3 (150–450)

Review of the peripheral smear shows no schistocytes or platelet clumping.

Which of the following should be performed to correctly diagnose her thrombocytopenia?

A. Antibodies to HPA-1a

B. Heparin/PF4 ELISA

C. Pantoprazole-dependent platelet antibodies
D. PCR for CMV
E. Serotonin release assay

23. A 38-year-old woman with SLE, has been admitted for a relapse of her TTP. She developed fatigue and petechiae, at which point she returned to the ER for a CBC, as this was similar to her prior episodes. This showed a platelet count of 14 (150–450), LDH 896 (100–200), and presence of schistocytes on her peripheral blood smear. The patient is admitted, started on prednisone, and undergoes placement of a right internal jugular hemodialysis catheter for the initiation of daily therapeutic plasma exchange (TPE). She is maintained on this regimen, when during the third session of TPE, she notes persistent perioral "tingling," along with numbness in her fingertips. Repeat labs show the following:

WBC	18.3 (3.2–9.8)
Hemoglobin	9.3 (12.0–15.5)
Hematocrit	28.1 (35–45)
MCV	91
Platelets	31 (150–450)
ANC	13.3 (2.0–8.6)

Which of the following is the most appropriate next step in management?
A. Increase TPE to twice daily
B. Calcium gluconate
C. MRI of the brain to evaluate for a stroke
D. Rituximab

24. A 63-year-old woman with MDS developed worsening cytopenias with increasing blast count. She has no siblings that could serve as a matched related donor. While awaiting the search results for an unrelated donor, the patient has become transfusion-dependent.
    However, her red cell transfusions have become complicated by repeated episodes of fevers and chills. Multiple times her transfusions have been stopped, and a workup by the blood bank has shown no hemolysis, infections, or mismatch as the cause for her symptoms. Invariably, her symptoms resolve in less than an hour after stopping the transfusion.
    Which of the following may help prevent her from experiencing this reaction again?
    A. Pretreatment with dexamethasone
    B. Pretreatment with diphenhydramine
    C. Use of irradiated red cells
    D. Use of leukoreduced packed red cells

25. A 47-year-old man with diffuse large B-cell lymphoma was initially treated with R-CHOP and, following his first relapse, was able to achieve a remission with R-ICE. He then underwent a matched related donor bone marrow transplant, which was initially complicated by delayed engraftment and mucositis, followed by GVHD. He has been treated with methylprednisolone and tacrolimus to control his GVHD, with mycophenolate added later in the course of his treatment. On day 47 following his transplant, he is able to be discharged home, with plans for frequent monitoring visits.
    The patient slowly improves and has persistent skin and gut GVHD, with flares noted when his steroids are tapered. During one of his clinically stable periods, he and his wife are able to take a long overdue vacation. While they are away, he has a lower GI bleed and presents to the local ER. He is noted to be anemic, transfused 4 units of packed red cells, and instructed to return home and

follow-up with his oncologist. He is seen about a week later, and although there are no more episodes of hematochezia, the patient thinks that he has a viral infection. He is noted to be febrile with an erythematous rash that is distinctly different from his skin GVHD. Laboratory testing shows the following:

WBC	1.5 (3.2–9.8)
Hemoglobin	8.7 (13.7–17.3)
Hematocrit	26.8 (39–49)
MCV	101 (80–98)
Platelets	37 (150–450)
Total bilirubin	1.6 (0.4–1.5)
AST	145 (15–41)
ALT	226 (17–63)
Alkaline phosphatase	85

Skin biopsy shows satellite dyskeratosis.
Which of the following is the most likely diagnosis?
A. Acute GVHD
B. CMV reactivation
C. Photosensitivity reaction due to tacrolimus
D. Transfusion-associated GVHD

26. A 43-year-old man with asthma, recurrent sinus infections, and eczema has been brought in by EMS following a fall off a ladder while hanging Christmas lights. An ultrasound examination of his abdomen shows a large fluid collection in the abdominal musculature, consistent with a hematoma. He is noted to have bled at least 4 units and is given 2 units of packed red cells. Within minutes of receiving the blood, the patient becomes hypotensive, tachycardic, tachypneic, with stridor and wheezing noted. The transfusion is stopped, sent to the blood bank, and he is treated emergently with epinephrine, followed by high-dose steroids, antihistamines, and H2-receptor blockade.
    Which of the following is the most appropriate next step?
    A. Direct Coombs
    B. IgA level
    C. Repeat type and screen
    D. Transfusion of matched red cells

27. A 39-year-old patient with ulcerative colitis has been admitted for an acute flare and symptomatic anemia. She is treated with high-dose methylprednisolone, intravenous fluids, and is transfused 2 units of packed red cells. Five minutes into the transfusion, she summons the nurse for rapidly progressive left arm pain and chills. Aside from an increased temperature, her vital signs remain relatively stable.
    Which of the following is the most likely diagnosis?
    A. Acute hemolytic transfusion reaction (AHTR)
    B. Anaphylaxis
    C. Bacterial contamination
    D. Febrile nonhemolytic transfusion reaction
    E. Transfusion-associated lung injury

28. A 28-year-old man with sickle cell disease, complicated by avascular necrosis, pigment cholelithiasis, and recurrent pain crises is routinely treated locally with opioid analgesics, intravenous fluids, antiemetics, and 1–2 units of packed red cells. The patient is now being transferred to another institution because of an inability to provide cross-matched red cells.
    Upon arrival to the ER, the patient is noted to be an adult African American man in moderate distress. He is icteric and splinting his left shoulder, but otherwise there are no other pertinent exam findings. Among the usual labs that

are drawn in the ER, a T&S is performed and shows the following:

ABO and Rh	B POS
Direct Coombs	Negative
Allo (serum) antibody specificity	Anti-C, -Jsa, -Lea, -V, and HTLA
Percentage of units compatible	Less than 1%

What is the most likely diagnosis?
A. Acquired B antigen
B. Alloimmunization
C. Autoimmunization
D. McLeod phenotype

29. A 77-year-old woman with MDS has been maintained on a chronic transfusion program, as she has not responded to growth factor therapy or hypomethylation therapy. While her symptoms are mitigated with routine red cell transfusions, she has noted an increase in bruising, prompting platelet transfusion. Due to the progressive and refractory nature of her disease, she is referred to palliative care for additional options. Despite the platelet transfusions, the patient notes persistent spontaneous bruising. Laboratory testing shows the following:

Pretransfusion

WBC	2400 × 10⁹/L (3.2–9.8)
Hemoglobin	8.9 g/dL (12.0–15.5)
Hematocrit	27.1% (35–45)
MCV	104/L (80–98)
Platelets	17,000 × 10⁹/L (150–450)

Posttransfusion

WBC	2300 × 10⁹/L (3.2–9.8)
Hemoglobin	8.9 g/dL (12.0–15.5)
Hematocrit	26.9% (35–45)
MCV	104/L (80–98)
Platelets	18,000 × 10⁹/L (150–450)

Which of the following is the next best step in management?
A. Direct Coombs test
B. HLA-antibodies measurement
C. Platelet antibodies assay
D. HPA-matched platelet transfusion

30. A 57-year-old man was in his usual state of health when he was hospitalized for the treatment of diverticular bleed while vacationing in Martha's Vineyard. He was treated with ceftriaxone and metronidazole and given 2 units of packed red cells. After a 2-day admission, he was sent home on oral antibiotics. He returned home and had follow-up with his primary care physician, but noted no significant improvement with his fevers or malaise. A CBC was performed and showed the following (Fig. 35.1):

WBC	14.7 (3.2–9.8)
Hemoglobin	7.3 (13.7–17.3)
Hematocrit	22.4 (39–49)
MCV	83
Platelets	124 (150–450)

Which of the following is the most appropriate next step in management?
A. Hepatitis A IgM
B. Macroscopic agglutination with acute and convalescent sera
C. PCR of Babesia 18S rRNA
D. Thin/thick smears

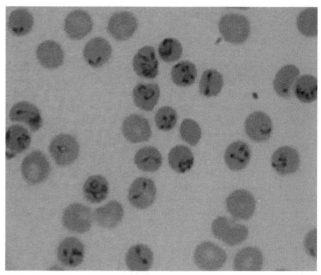

FIG. 35.1 CA peripheral smear.

31. A 57-year-old man with hypertension, diabetes mellitus, chronic kidney disease (stage III), ischemic cardiomyopathy with an ejection fraction of 15%, and atrial fibrillation is maintained on therapeutic anticoagulation with rivaroxaban. He has required increasing diuretic use to control his peripheral edema, resulting in periodic episodes of worsening renal function. He develops symptoms of profound light-headedness and dizziness and is brought to the ER, where he is noted to have a 4-unit drop in his hemoglobin compared with a CBC performed 4 weeks prior. While in the trauma bay, he is noted to have a large melenic bowel movement. A massive transfusion protocol is initiated, which includes an equal amount of fresh frozen plasma to counteract the effects of anticoagulation. He is resuscitated and transferred to the MICU, where he is later noted to suddenly be hypoxic, tachypneic, dyspneic, and orthopneic. The patient is emergently intubated, and the portable chest x-ray to evaluate the position of his endotracheal tube shows diffuse opacities consistent with marked pulmonary edema.
Which of the following is the most likely diagnosis?
A. Air embolism
B. Anaphylaxis
C. Diffuse alveolar hemorrhage
D. Transfusion associated circulatory overload
E. Transfusion-related acute lung injury

32. In the case of question 31, while the patient above is undergoing attempts at correcting his respiratory compromise, an EKG is performed to evaluate for myocardial injury. This is significant for showing the presence of peaked T-waves and shortened QT interval. Which of the following is the cause of his EKG changes?
A. Hyperkalemia
B. Hypocalcemia
C. Hypomagnesemia
D. Iron overload

33. A 37-year-old woman with no significant past medical history was recently diagnosed with acute myelogenous leukemia. She was admitted, underwent placement of a dual-lumen right internal jugular catheter, and started induction chemotherapy with a standard course of 7+3

(cytarabine 200 mg/m^2/day ×7; daunorubicin 60 mg/m^2 ×3). Her D#14 bone marrow shows a markedly aplastic marrow, with an estimated less than 5% blasts. She receives supportive care and is generally doing as well as can be expected, when on day 17 she develops progressive dyspnea with right-sided pleuritic chest pain. A CT-angiogram of the chest shows right middle and upper lobar pulmonary artery filling defects, with a peripheral opacity concerning for infarction. Bilateral upper extremity ultrasounds show thrombosis in the right internal jugular, subclavian, and axillary veins. Due to her discomfort and magnitude of her thromboembolism, she is started on a low-dose unfractionated heparin drip, with twice-daily platelet transfusions. The patient continues with her anticoagulation and platelet transfusions, when on day 23 she is noted to have a change in mental status and a temperature of 38.5°C following her qAM platelet transfusion. She is "pan-cultured," started on cefepime, when her blood cultures show the presence of coagulase negative staphylococcus.

Which of the following is the most likely diagnosis?
A. Bacterial contamination of platelet transfusion
B. Internal jugular vein thrombophlebitis
C. Line infection
D. Transfusion reaction

34. A 48-year-old man has been diagnosed with fistulizing Crohn disease, which is now controlled with a maintenance regimen of infliximab, allowing him to resume his work as the regional sales manager for his corporation. During a business trip to Florida, he had another flare of his inflammatory bowel disease and was hospitalized, where he received 2 units of packed red cells, intravenous methylprednisolone, and antibiotics. He improved and was discharged home a week later.

He returned home, when about 2 weeks later he developed progressive chest pain, dyspnea, and orthopnea. EMS is summoned, and he is brought to the ER, where an EKG shows diffuse ST-segment elevation with depression of the PR interval. Despite serial cardiac enzymes being negative, he is taken to the cardiac catheterization lab, where no flow-limiting coronary disease is noted. A ventriculogram shows a left-ventricle ejection fraction of 25%. A bedside echocardiogram confirms this finding and shows a pericardial effusion.

What is the most likely cause for his presentation?
A. Acute Chagas disease
B. Aortic dissection
C. Postmyocardial infarction injury syndrome
D. Systemic lupus erythematosus

35. A 37-year-old African-American man has Hgb-SC disease and has remained in relatively good health, with a limited number of painful crises. He is admitted with cholelithiasis, and plans are made to proceed with a cholecystectomy. He is noted to have a hemoglobin level of 11.7 (12.0–15.5), which is less than his baseline of hemoglobin of 12.3. The night prior to surgery, he is kept NPO and given a 2-unit red cell transfusion. That morning, he complains of a headache and appears lethargic. A repeat CBC shows no hemolysis; rather, an appropriate rise in the hemoglobin to 14.1 g/dL. A STAT head CT shows no bleed and a MRI reveals no infarction.

Which of the following is the most likely diagnosis?
A. Cerebral vascular accident
B. Diphenhydramine toxicity
C. Hyperviscosity
D. Paradoxical embolism

36. A 38-year-old man has a past medical history of sickle cell disease, complicated by recurrent episodes of acute chest and priapism, along with hypertension and diabetes, which is controlled with the use of enalapril, along with diet and exercise. He has been admitted for chest pain that has worsened despite the use of his narcotics at home. On presentation to the ER, he is noted to be tachypneic, tachycardic, and hypoxic on room air. A chest x-ray is remarkable for new bilateral lower lobe opacities. He is pan-cultured in the ER; started on vancomycin, piperacillin/tazobactam, and ciprofloxacin; and admitted to the Medicine service. It is felt that he is having a recurrent episode of acute chest, and he is prepared for an emergent red cell exchange, using phenotypically matched red cells via the blood bank's sickle cell protocol. A VasCath is placed in the right femoral vein under ultrasound guidance, and when the appropriate amount of blood has been obtained and released by the blood bank, erythrocytapheresis commences.

After the third unit of blood has completed, Mr. Williams is noted to be flushed, stridorous, and hypotensive, wherein he also notes abdominal cramping with an immediate need to have a bowel movement. The procedure is immediately halted, with a resolution of his symptoms within 2 hours. Laboratory testing shows no hemolysis or renal impairment.

Which of the following is the most likely cause for his event:
A. ACE-I associated reaction
B. Anaphylaxis
C. Transfusion mismatch
D. Transfusion reaction

ANSWERS

1. E
Patients with autoimmune hemolytic anemia, as in this scenario, who have life-threatening anemia need to be transfused with the least incompatible blood. When time is of the essence, treating the underlying hemolysis with steroids, apheresis, or rituximab without giving red cells can lead to patient death. Communication between the blood bank and clinician is important, and although the autoantibody will shorten the survival of transfused red cells, this will produce at most a delayed transfusion reaction that is not life-threatening. The bedside team needs to remain vigilant for acute intravascular hemolysis during transfusion.

2. B
Patients with SS disease who require surgery and general anesthesia should be transfused to an Hgb of 10 g/dL preoperatively to avoid pulmonary complications. An older study comparing simple with exchange transfusion found no difference between the two groups, with much less expense and effort in the simple transfusion group. Patients with SS disease are at risk for complications of hyperviscosity when there is greater than 10 g/dL.

3. A

Fresh frozen plasma (FFP) is one of the most overutilized blood products with few proven indications. In the United States, as opposed to Europe, a factor XI concentrate is not available, and FFP would be the product of choice when indicated, as in this patient with prior bleeding history (answer A), in need of urgent surgery. FFP would not be indicated in a nonbleeding patient with advanced liver disease undergoing a minor procedure, especially with an INR only mildly elevated at 1.8 (answer B). In a patient with hemophilia B, factor IX concentrates would be the treatment of choice for a life-threatening bleed (answer C). The volume of FFP to reverse a markedly elevated INR in a patient with severe CHF would likely be prohibitive and one of the prothrombin complex concentrates, such as KCentra, would be a better choice (answer D). In a patient with factor XIII deficiency, a factor XIII concentrate, or if not available, cryoprecipitate, would be a more appropriate choice than FFP, given its higher concentration of factor XIII (answer E).

4. E

Cryoprecipitate was originally developed for use in hemophilia A. As cryoprecipitate is a pooled plasma product without viral inactivation and is associated with adverse events, its use has been replaced in many diseases with more specific factor concentrates. Today cryoprecipitate is most commonly used to replenish fibrinogen in cases of acquired coagulopathy. However, if specific products are not available, it should be remembered that cryoprecipitate also contains factor XIII, factor VIII, vWF, and fibronectin in addition to fibrinogen. Thus cryoprecipitate should be transfused in a factor XIII deficient patient who is bleeding or in need of urgent surgical intervention if factor XIII concentrates are not available (answer E). As there is no significant amount of factor IX or factor XI in cryoprecipitate, it should not be used to treat hemophilia B or factor XI deficiency (answer A). In the patient who can self-infuse factor VIII, he should use his home product to treat his hemarthrosis (answer C). In mild type I vWD, DDAVP should raise vWF and factor VIII three- to fivefold and would be the preferred agent of first choice (answer D).

5. C

In emergency situations in sickle cell disease, such as acute stroke, it is imperative to rapidly lower the Hgb-S concentration, as with an exchange transfusion. A simple transfusion would be indicated only if erythrocytapheresis is not immediately available.

The use of antiplatelet therapy, single or dual, should not be used in this case. Not only is there the risk of hemorrhagic conversion with the current stroke, the presence of moyamoya is another risk factor for intracranial hemorrhage.

6. B

This patient has anemia of inflammation related to his underlying pneumonia and sepsis. He does not have iron deficiency or anemia associated with kidney dysfunction and therefore does not need iron replacement or an erythrocyte-stimulating agent. A multicenter, randomized controlled trial in euvolemic ICU patients with a hemoglobin level of less than 9 g/dL evaluated a restrictive transfusion strategy (transfusion for a hemoglobin of <7 g/dL) versus a liberal transfusion strategy (transfusion for a hemoglobin level of <10 g/dL). No difference in 30-day overall survival was found between the two groups. In addition to lack of benefit, a liberal transfusion strategy is costly and can lead to increased transfusion-related adverse events.

7. E

No transfusion is indicated. The American Association of Blood Banks (AABB) suggests adhering to a restrictive transfusion strategy (7–8 g/dL) in hospitalized, stable patients (Grade: strong recommendation; high-quality evidence). Randomized studies have suggested that critically ill patients who are not actively bleeding and without cardiac compromise do equally well with a hemoglobin transfusion threshold of 7 g/dL, as with 10 g/dL. The AABB also suggests adhering to a restrictive strategy in hospitalized patients with preexisting cardiovascular disease and recommends considering transfusion for patients with symptoms or a hemoglobin level of 8 g/dL or less (Grade: weak recommendation; moderate-quality evidence). We are not given iron studies to determine the appropriateness of IV iron therapy, and he does not have suggestion of renal insufficiency resulting in decreased erythropoietin; thus administration of IV iron or erythropoietin is not indicated.

8. D

Daratumumab, a monoclonal anti-CD38 used to treat multiple myeloma, can bind to CD38 present on RBCs and interfere with in vitro compatibility assays. The blood bank should be alerted when patients are beginning daratumumab for consideration of RBC phenotyping in anticipation of this problem. Other studies, including washing off the daratumumab with DTT or using cord blood, can be used for compatibility testing, although this may be cumbersome for evaluation.

Pregnancy should not cause a pan-reactive antibody. Her multiple myeloma appears to remain in a complete response; the faint IgG kappa monoclonal spike is likely daratumumab, which is an IgG kappa monoclonal antibody (as her myeloma was IgA lambda). The LDH is normal, suggesting there is not a component of autoimmune hemolytic anemia.

9. B

This patient is undergoing a moderate risk procedure in cholecystectomy with a hemoglobin at baseline of 7.8 g/dL. A recent prospective randomized trial evaluating simple transfusion to a hemoglobin of 10 g/dL versus no transfusion was stopped early due to excess adverse events in the nontransfusion arm. Patients with sickle cell disease are at risk of developing alloantibodies and should be given C, E, and Kell negative blood at a minimum. In this patient who is having elective surgery, the surgery should be postponed until the appropriate blood products are available to mitigate the risk of alloimmunization.

10. C

Posttransfusion purpura occurs 5–15 days after transfusion in patients previously sensitized to platelet antigens. PTP occurs most commonly in multigravida women who have been sensitized to fetal platelet antigens. Most commonly, women who are negative for HPA-1a who develop antibodies to this antigen during childbirth can experience the immune destruction of native platelets when transfused blood products from HPA-1a positive donors. The pathophysiology surrounding destruction of the patient's HPA-1a negative platelets is not well understood. If platelet transfusion is indicated, the patient's platelets should be phenotyped, and if HPA-1a negative, only HPA-1a-negative platelets should be used. Otherwise, IVIg and plasmapheresis have shown some efficacy in increasing platelet counts. Transfusion of random donor platelets is contraindicated, as most donors are HPA-1a positive. Methylprednisolone, rituximab, and splenectomy are treatments for ITP, which this patient does not have.

11. E

Patients who are IgA deficient who have received a prior transfusion can become sensitized to IgA and have an anaphylactic response to transfusion of blood products from a donor who is not IgA deficient. The patient in question requires platelets due to severe thrombocytopenia and active bleeding. Although red cells can be washed to remove IgA, platelet washing is difficult and often results in activation and aggregation of the platelet product. Obtaining platelets from an IgA deficient donor is the preferred method of transfusion in patients deficient in IgA.

12. B

Transfusion-associated graft versus host disease (tGVHD) can occur in patients undergoing treatment for hematologic malignancy or in patients who are severely immunosuppressed. tGVHD occurs when donor lymphocytes engraft and a host response leads to severe pancytopenia and mortality approaching 100%. Gamma-irradiation of all blood products protects against tGVHD, whereas leukocyte reduction, washing, or full serologic crossmatch do not. The risk for tGVHD is higher in patients who receive blood from a donor who shares an HLA haplotype, as is seen in family member donation.

13. A

Dyspnea and signs of circulatory overload including increased JVD, lung crackles, and extra heart sound and edema following a blood transfusion represents transfusion associated circulatory overload that should be managed with urgent diuresis. TRALI has a similar presentation but is excluded in the setting of volume overload. Sepsis would present later following a transfusion, and pulmonary embolism would not likely be bilateral and would not present with left heart failure. Acute chest syndrome is a constellation of symptoms and would present more gradually than circulatory overload.

14. C

IgA deficiency is relatively common, affecting approximately in 1 in 500 persons. Up to 40% of these individuals develop anti-IgA antibodies. When such patients are exposed to IgA during a blood transfusion, they are at risk of anaphylaxis due to a reaction between recipient antibodies and donor IgA in the transfused donor blood product. The risk of anaphylaxis is highest with fresh frozen plasma, but it may also occur with transfusion of cellular products, as variable amounts of plasma are found in these products. Washing of red blood cells to remove plasma products can greatly reduce this risk, but it was not listed as a choice. As FFP is not a cellular product, washing is not a viable option (answer E). Plasma can be obtained, however, from an IgA deficient donor to minimize the risk of anaphylaxis (answer C).

Irradiation of donor red cells (answer A) is indicated in severely immunocompromised recipients to decrease the risk of transfusion-associated graft versus host disease. Leukoreduction (answer B) is standard practice at many blood centers and decreases the incidence of transfusion-associated febrile nonhemolytic transfusion reactions and cytomegalovirus (CMV) transmission, but it would not prevent anaphylaxis or allergic-type transfusion reactions. HLA-matched red blood cells (answer D) are not usually required and would not decrease the risk of an anaphylactic reaction. HLA matching of platelets is useful in a subset of patients with immune-mediated platelet transfusion refractoriness.

15. D

The most likely diagnosis in this case is TRALI, the leading cause of transfusion-related mortality in the United States. The patient in this vignette developed fever, dyspnea, diffuse pulmonary infiltrates, and hypoxia during a red blood cell transfusion. This presentation is very consistent with TRALI, a reaction secondary to antileukocyte antibodies in donor plasma directed against recipient leukocytes, which subsequently sequester in the lungs, typically during or within 6 hours of a transfusion (answer D). TRALI can occur with any blood product, even erythrocytes and platelets, which often contain small amounts of plasma. Treatment of TRALI is primarily supportive, and most patients fully recover within days or a week. Deferral of multiparous females from donation of plasma has decreased the incidence of TRALI.

TRALI can be difficult to distinguish from transfusion-associated circulatory overload (TACO). However, this patient, because she had received only a single unit of packed erythrocytes, had no underlying cardiac disease, and had no jugular venous distention, S_3 or peripheral edema was unlikely to develop fluid overload (answer E).

An AHTR is most commonly caused by a human error leading to ABO incompatibility. Very early in the transfusion, an affected patient develops hypotension and often disseminated intravascular coagulation, but this patient is normotensive and presented primarily with hypoxia after the transfusion was complete making an AHTR unlikely (answer A). The development of a new alloantibody may lead to a DHTR several days after the transfusion, leading to worsening anemia, but would not be compatible with the case presented (answer B). In addition, the repeat type and screen did not reveal a new alloantibody. T-lymphocyte attacks against an immunocompromised recipient can lead to transfusion-associated graft versus host disease and presents with fatal pancytopenia and often skin, liver, and GI abnormalities (answer C).

16. A

The presence of a new alloantibody on a repeat type and screen would best explain this patient's current clinical presentation (answer A). She has sickle cell anemia and has received a blood transfusion in the past week. Her worsening anemia and severe pain crisis occurring 5–10 days after receiving a transfusion is classic for a DHTR in a patient with sickle cell anemia. Her clinical course, including jaundice, an elevated indirect bilirubin level, and a hemoglobin level lower than her post transfusion value, combined with a type and screen demonstrating the presence of a new alloantibody, would be diagnostic of a DHTR. In addition, this patient has a known alloantibody against the C antigen and is at greater risk for further alloantibody formation and subsequent DHTR. Transfusion of phenotypically matched red blood cells is indicated for all future transfusions.

HLA alloimmunization can cause platelet refractoriness, but this patient did not receive platelets. In addition, HLA alloimmunization would not explain her current symptoms or worsening anemia (answer B). Anaphylaxis during blood transfusion can occur in a minority of patients with a severe IgA deficiency who develop antibodies, but this patient's symptoms are not consistent with anaphylaxis (answer C). Donor antibodies targeting recipient neutrophils are known to cause TRALI, which may lead to noncardiogenic pulmonary edema. Patients may also develop fever and hypotension, none of which were present in this patient (answer D). Transmission of CMV would be quite unlikely as the patient received leukocyte-depleted red blood cells (answer E).

17. A

Multiparous women and multiply transfused patients develop leukoreactive antibodies that result in nonhemolytic febrile reactions. Thus leukoreduced blood products are given to reduce HLA alloimmunization, reduce the risk of CMV transmission, and reduce the incidence of febrile, nonhemolytic transfusion reactions. Washed blood products are indicated in patients with recurrent, severe allergic transfusion reactions, IgA deficient patients with IgA antibodies, and in those patients with ABO-incompatible bone marrow transplant. Irradiated products are given to prevent transfusion-associated graft versus host disease. CMV-negative and phenotypically matched RBCs would not prevent a febrile nonhemolytic transfusion reaction.

18. E

This case a represents what has been described as "hyperhemolysis" in a patient with sickle cell anemia, wherein the transfused red cells are rapidly hemolyzed, in addition to the patient's own red cells, leading to critically low hemoglobin. Continuing folate is always indicated in patients with hemolysis. While the exact mechanisms still remain unknown, the use of IVIg is commonly employed, along with corticosteroid use. Although patients with hyperhemolysis may not have developed a new allo- or autoantibody to red cells, this has been noted and is prudent prior to any additional blood product exposure. As she is a hospitalized patient, with hemolysis, and receiving IVIg, it is reasonable to ensure thromboprophylaxis.

19. D

The patient's history and laboratory findings are consistent with a delayed hemolytic transfusion reaction several days after transfusion. This is characterized by an anamnestic response to a minor blood group antigen from a prior transfusion or pregnancy. A repeat type and screen and/or a direct Coombs will now show the presence of the alloantibody. Thin and thick smears are useful for the presence of malaria, which is not consistent with this case. Similarly, there is no reason to suspect bacterial infection as the cause for her hemolysis. Given the hemolysis, it would not be prudent to either proceed with surgery or transfuse further red cells.

20. B

As the patient has received more than 25 units of packed red cells, there is a near certainty of iron overload, which is an expected complication of repeated blood transfusions. It is recommended that patients with MDS who have received more than 20 units of packed red cells be considered for chelation therapy. Use of another erythropoiesis agent is not expected to be beneficial, and the use of thrombopoietin reception agonists is not approved for use in MDS.

21. D

The rapid onset of symptoms, hypoxia, and infiltrates following the receipt of plasma is consistent with TRALI. Therefore, the infusion must be stopped and the blood bank alerted immediately. Aggressive supportive care is indicated, including intubation and mechanical ventilation, if required. There is no role for the use of IVIg in the treatment of TRALI.

While there is the chance for a pulmonary embolism, either from a thrombus or from bone marrow infarction, this is not supported by the physical examination. There is no approved indication for the use of rFVIIa in the reversal of warfarin, particularly if four-factor prothrombin complex concentrates are available.

22. A

The sudden drop in the platelet count several days after transfusion in a multiparous patient that is associated with bleeding symptoms is consistent with posttransfusion purpura. This is associated with the development of an alloantibody to one of the human platelet antigens (HPA), most oftentimes HPA-1A, although numerous other types (-2A, -2B, -3A, 3B, etc.) have also been described. Treatment consists of intravenous immunoglobulin.

Although the patient is on enoxaparin, which can be associated with HIT, the marked thrombocytopenia and hemorrhagic manifestations are inconsistent with this diagnosis, raising the chance that checking a heparin/PF4 ELISA and/or SRA might lead to an incorrect diagnosis. Neither CMV viremia nor drug-induced thrombocytopenia is consistent with the case. Proton pump inhibitors are unlikely to cause this presentation.

23. B

Units of red cells and plasma are stored in a citrate-containing solution, which chelates calcium, preventing coagulation. With large enough volumes of either blood products, the plasma level of calcium falls, leading to symptomatic hypocalcemia. This is a common side effect of apheresis involving red cells or plasma, and is readily treated with calcium supplementation.

Although the platelet count has not returned to normal (i.e., >150), it is still early in the disease course and has increased. Increasing the intensity of therapy or immune suppression at this time is not indicated. While patients with TTP are susceptible to CNS damage from their microangiopathy, her symptoms are consistent with hypocalcemia and does not warrant imaging.

24. D

This case represents episodes of febrile nonhemolytic reactions, which may be reduced or prevented by the use of leukoreduced blood, although good data are lacking to support this practice. Since there is not an allergic reaction or hemolytic, there is no role for the use of steroids or antihistamines. As the patient is not immunosuppressed, there is no need for irradiated red cells.

25. D

The constellation of fevers, diffuse erythematous rash, pancytopenia, and transaminitis are suggestive of this process, particularly as the patient was not noted to have received irradiated red cells with his transfusion. The skin biopsy finding of dyskeratosis and satellitosis is diagnostic. Tacrolimus is not known to cause photosensitivity reactions, with GVHD not being associated with pancytopenia. CMV reactivation would not be expected to cause a diffuse erythematous rash.

26. B

The history of recurrent infections, asthma, and atopy is consistent with a patient who may have IgA deficiency. While not occurring in the majority of patients with IgA deficiency, anaphylaxis to blood products can occur. As this case does not represent a DHTR, a DAT and T&S will not be useful. The symptoms are not consistent with a transfusion of mismatched red cells.

27. A

The development of sudden arm pain, fevers, with or without flank pain is consistent with an AHTR, when the wrong blood is transfused to the wrong patient. Treatment includes the immediate cessation of the transfusion, sending all blood and components to the blood bank, hydration, and supportive care. The absence of respiratory findings or hypotension/tachycardia makes this inconsistent with anaphylaxis. Bacterial contamination would be expected to produce vital sign changes. The absence of respiratory symptoms makes TRALI unlikely.

28. B

Unfortunately, this case represents a marked alloimmunization of a multiply transfused patient. In patients with sickle cell disease, great care must be taken to ensure that there is matching to minor antigens, above the usual process for otherwise unaffected individuals, as severe alloimmunization is associated with decreased rates of survival. Acquired B-antigen occurs when a patient with type A blood is modified by infection or malignancy, resulting in the appearance of a B-blood type. There is no reason to suspect this. Similarly, the negative direct Coombs and presence of an Rh-antigen makes autoimmunity and the McLeod phenotype, respectively, incorrect.

29. B

In a multiply transfused patient, the presence of HLA-antibodies can lead to platelet refractoriness, which could have been avoided with the use of leukodepleted products. There is no evidence of hemolysis, which would make checking a DAT pointless. While patients may have platelet antibodies, there is no reason to suspect PTP or transfuse HPA-matched platelets.

30. C

His case is consistent with transfusion-associated babesiosis, which is becoming a growing issue in endemic areas. His visit to a classically endemic area of babesiosis and findings on the peripheral smear are typical for his presentation. There is no liver involvement or travel to areas endemic for malaria, making hepatitis or malaria unreasonable. Macroscopic agglutination with acute and convalescent sera is for the diagnosis of leptospirosis, which is not consistent with this case.

31. D

The patient's decompensation is consistent with TACO, given the findings of his sudden respiratory decompensation, findings on chest x-ray, and symptoms of heart failure. There is no mention of central venous catheterization to account for an air embolism. Likewise, the history is not consistent with anaphylaxis, and no mention is made of either blood in the endotracheal tube or an alveolar pattern on chest x-ray. Finally, TRALI is typically associated with fevers and absence of heart failure symptoms.

32. A

This patient is a prime example of who is most likely to sustain this complication of transfusion. The receipt of multiple blood products, the volume of said transfusions, and the impaired renal function are all risk factors for transfusion-associated hyperkalemia. Hypocalcemia, either from the effects of citrate or from severe hypomagnesemia, would lead to a prolonged QT-interval. There is no reason to suspect iron overload after this event.

33. A

Bacterial infection of platelet transfusions is the most common infectious complication of blood product transfusion. Internal jugular vein thrombophlebitis, while classically associated with *Fusarium* infections, would not be expected following the initiation of anticoagulation. Given the temporal relation with the platelet transfusion, a catheter-associated infection is less likely. Her symptoms, including the culture results, are not consistent with a transfusion reaction.

34. A

Chagas disease can be spread via blood transfusion, with donors in Florida having the highest seroprevalence rate. In immunocompromised patients, the acute phase of infections with *T. cruzi* can present with heart failure-type symptoms and a myopericarditis. Aortic dissection would have been detected during his catheterization, and there was no myocardial infarction for Dressler syndrome. While SLE can manifest with a serositis, there are no other reasons to suspect this.

35. C

Patients with sickling disorders may be at risk for hyperviscosity with their hemoglobin levels are elevated, particularly if transfused to greater than 12 g/dL. The lethargy, malaise, and headache are caused by the effects of transfusion, and in a case such as this, phlebotomy is required.

Given the negative findings on his neurologic imaging, there is no support for the diagnoses of either a stroke, generally or from a paradoxical embolism. Diphenhydramine toxicity would present with anticholinergic symptoms and would not be expected from the usual premedication dosing.

36. A

The presence of an ACE-inhibitor during therapeutic apheresis can cause a number of reactions, as noted in the case. This is due to the increased amount of bradykinin that is generated by the passage of the patient's blood over the negatively charged surface of the apheresis circuit, which cannot be effectively degraded due to the inhibition of ACE.

While anaphylaxis shares similar symptoms, these symptoms are more consistent with that from the ACE inhibition. The absence of groin pain and/or hemolysis rules out a mismatch, and a simple transfusion reaction is associated with mild fevers.

REFERENCES

Question 30

1. Figure 35.1 from Lobo CA, Cursino-Santos JR, Alhassan A Rodrigues M. Babesia: an emerging infectious threat in transfusion medicine. *PLoS Pathog.* 2013;9(7):e1003387. http://dx.doi.org/10.1371/journal.ppat.1003387.

CHAPTER

36

Pain Control and End of Life

Jason Meadows

QUESTIONS

1. A 57-year-old woman with known metastatic breast cancer involving multiple thoracic vertebrae presents to the emergency department complaining of severe back pain. Her pain has increased over the last 3–4 days and is no longer responsive to oral acetaminophen. The pain is currently 9/10, does not radiate, and is worse with movement. She denies weakness or loss of sensation in her trunk, perineum, or lower extremities. She further denies urinary or fecal incontinence.

   On physical exam, she has full strength and a normal sensory exam in all extremities. Serum electrolytes and creatinine are normal. Spinal magnetic resonance imaging (MRI) reveals progression of T4–6 vertebral metastases without evidence of epidural extension.

   You order morphine 2 mg IV and decide to reassess her in 15 minutes at which time she continues to report severe pain with no significant improvement. What is the next most appropriate step in her management?
   A. Administer morphine 2 mg IV
   B. Administer morphine 4 mg IV
   C. Continue to monitor
   D. Administer hydromorphone 0.8 mg IV
   E. Start a patient-controlled analgesia (PCA) pump

2. A 62-year-old woman with breast cancer and known liver metastases presents to the emergency department complaining of severe abdominal pain. Her pain has increased over the last 3–4 days and is no longer responsive to oral acetaminophen. The pain is currently 9/10, does not radiate, and is worse with movement and deep breathing. She denies fever, chills, nausea, vomiting, or changes in bowel habits.

   On physical exam, she her abdomen is severely tender to palpation in the right upper quadrant. Serum electrolytes and lipase are within normal limits. AST and ALT are 86 and 77 U/L, respectively. Creatinine is 2.4 mg/dL, which is her baseline. Abdominal CT shows a dominant 4.5 cm liver mass, which is enlarged compared with a previous CT.

   You see that she was given morphine 5 mg IV in the ER, and she reports that relieved her pain completely for a few hours. You are concerned about continuing to give morphine given her renal function. Which is the most appropriate next order?
   A. Hydromorphone 1.5 mg IV
   B. Fentanyl 50 µg IV
   C. Fentanyl 100 µg IV
   D. Fentanyl 250 µg IV
   E. Fentanyl patch 100 µg/h TD

3. A 59-year-old male with non-small cell lung cancer (NSCLC) who recently completed chemotherapy with cisplatin and etoposide presents to your clinic for follow-up. He reports generally tolerating chemotherapy well with only moderate nausea that he controlled with antiemetics. Since completing chemotherapy, he has noticed burning pain in his feet that has made it difficult to get to sleep at night.

   He denies any similar pain in his hands and denies weakness, any other paresthesias, urinary or bowel incontinence, or back pain.

   His vital signs are within normal limits as are cardiac and respiratory exams. Feet and toes are normal in appearance, but exam is significant for decreased sensation bilaterally. All electrolytes are normal.

   Which is the next best step in management?
   A. Reassurance
   B. Initiate oxycodone 5 mg every 4 hours as needed
   C. Initiate duloxetine 60 mg orally once daily
   D. Initiate gabapentin 300 mg once daily with instructions for dose escalation at home
   E. Refer to pain specialist to initiate transcutaneous electrical nerve stimulation (TENS)

4. A 32-year-old female with diffuse large B-cell lymphoma receiving R-CHOP chemotherapy presents to your clinic with a complaint of pain most pronounced in her low back, both hips, and thighs. Labs 2 days ago were significant for severe neutropenia, and she received pegfilgrastim at that time.

   She denies tingling, numbness, or weakness in the lower extremities and has not lost bowel or bladder control.

Lower extremity strength, sensation, and reflexes are within normal limits.

What is the next best step in management?

A. Add loratadine
B. Add naproxen
C. Add oxycodone
D. Add lidocaine patch
E. Obtain MRI spine

5. A 36-year-old woman with BRCA1+ metastatic breast cancer presents to your clinic for a second opinion after receiving treatment at another institution. She complains of left rib pain from known metastases that was previously controlled with oxycodone 5–10 mg po q4h prn, but the patient says she now needs to take this around the clock.

She reports no relevant past medical history other than ADD, which is well controlled with methylphenidate. Family history is significant for ovarian cancer in her mother and maternal grandmother. On detailed questioning, she reports that her father used cocaine and was sexually abusive to her when she was young. She denies personal alcohol or illicit drug use, but she smokes one pack of cigarettes daily.

Physical exam reveals no abnormal findings.

After discussing your recommendations for her breast cancer treatment, she asks if you can assume prescription of her oxycodone. Which of the above characteristics does NOT increase her risk of aberrant behaviors on opioid medications?

A. Ongoing tobacco abuse
B. History of preadolescent sexual abuse
C. Father's cocaine abuse
D. History of ADD
E. Patient's age

6. Your colleague referred a 68-year-old woman with known ER+/PR+ breast cancer with known metastases to lumbosacral vertebrae from clinic to the ER for a complaint of severe back pain. Her pain has increased over the last 3–4 days and is no longer responsive to her home pain regimen. At home she takes MS contin 15 mg q8h and immediate-release morphine 15 mg q4h prn, which she has taken 3 times in the last 24 hours. The pain is currently 9/10, does not radiate, and is worse with movement. She denies weakness or loss of sensation in lower extremities. She further denies urinary or fecal incontinence.

On physical exam, she has full strength and a normal sensory exam in all extremities. Serum electrolytes and creatinine are normal. Spinal MRI reveals progression of L4, L5, and S1 vertebral metastases with no evidence of pathological fracture or cord compression.

You order morphine 6 mg IV and decide to reassess her in 15 minutes at which time she continues to report severe pain with no significant improvement. What is the next most appropriate step in her management?

A. Administer morphine 6 mg IV
B. Administer morphine 12 mg IV
C. Continue to monitor for 15–30 more minutes
D. Consult the palliative medicine service
E. Consult neurosurgery for surgical decompression

7. A 77-year-old man with hypertension, insulin-dependent diabetes (with longstanding diabetic neuropathy and nephropathy), and colon cancer metastatic to lung and liver presents to your clinic for follow-up. His abdominal pain due to liver metastases and his opioid-induced constipation are well controlled. On detailed questioning, he does admit to "seeing birds flying in the room sometimes" and says that a few times his wife has stopped him while he was carrying on conversations with people who were not really there. He has no personal or family history of dementia, stroke, or brain metastases.

He currently takes long- and short-acting insulin, amlodipine 10 mg daily, morphine ER 100 mg q12h and morphine IR 15 mg q4h as needed, senna 2 tabs nightly, and a multivitamin.

On exam, you note 28/30 on mini-mental status exam (losing points for short-term recall) and normal neurological exam. Labs are notable for creatinine 2.4 mg/dL which has worsened from 2.1 mg/dL measured 3 months ago. Electrolytes are normal.

What is the next best step in management?

A. Stop amlodipine
B. Obtain psychiatry consultation
C. Stop morphine ER and start fentanyl 100 μg/h patch
D. Stop morphine ER and start fentanyl 50 μg/h patch
E. Increase morphine ER dose by 25%–50%.

8. A 59-year-old male with NSCLC who recently completed chemotherapy with cisplatin and etoposide presents to your clinic for follow-up. He reports generally tolerating chemotherapy well with only moderate nausea that he controlled with antiemetics. Since completing chemotherapy, he has noticed moderate to severe burning pain in his hands and feet that has made it difficult to work, run errands, and get to sleep at night. He takes gabapentin 300 mg qhs, which he says has not helped.

He denies any similar pain in his hands and denies weakness, any other paresthesias, urinary or bowel incontinence, or back pain.

His vital signs are within normal limits as are cardiac and respiratory exams. His hands and feet are normal in appearance, but exam is significant for decreased sensation bilaterally. All electrolytes are normal.

Which is the next best step in management?

A. Increase gabapentin to 300 mg BID
B. Stop gabapentin and initiate pregabalin therapy
C. Continue gabapentin and initiate lidocaine 5% patch
D. Refer to pain specialist to initiate TENS
E. Continue gabapentin and initiate oxycodone therapy

9. A 32-year-old female with diffuse large B-cell lymphoma receiving R-CHOP chemotherapy calls your clinic with a complaint of ongoing pain in her low back, both hips, and thighs. Labs 3 days ago were significant for severe neutropenia, and she received pegfilgrastim at that time. She was seen yesterday and started on naproxen for pain, which has provided only partial relief.

She denies tingling, numbness, or weakness in the lower extremities and has not lost bowel or bladder control.

Lower extremity strength, sensation, and reflexes are within normal limits.

What is the next best step in management?

A. Add loratadine
B. Stop naproxen and start ibuprofen
C. Stop naproxen and start acetaminophen
D. Add lidocaine patch
E. Obtain MRI spine

10. A 79-year-old man with a history of insulin-dependent diabetes, chronic obstructive pulmonary disease (COPD), and prostate cancer with lumbosacral metastases is admitted to the inpatient oncology service after presenting with back pain and urinary retention. A urinary catheter was

placed, and he was started on a fentanyl PCA for pain. MRI revealed progression of lumbosacral vertebral metastases without evidence of cord compression.

On the morning of hospital day 3, he reports excellent pain control; but later that day, his nurse notes that he is somnolent and more confused. Prior to this he denied any pain or nausea to his nurse and reported a normal bowel movement in the morning.

Vital signs significant for T 37.9 C, HR 104, RR 24, BP 126/80. His exam shows persistent left basilar crackles that appear to be chronic and some mild hypogastric tenderness. Creatinine this morning was 2.6 mg/dL, which was unchanged from the previous day but worse than his baseline of 1.8 mg/dL.

Which of the following should NOT be included in your initial management?

A. Check fingerstick glucose, serum chemistry, and complete blood count
B. Obtain blood and urine cultures after changing his urinary catheter
C. Stop the fentanyl PCA and administer naloxone 0.4 mg
D. Obtain a chest x-ray
E. Obtain an EKG

11. A 57-year-old woman with known metastatic breast cancer involving multiple thoracic vertebrae presents to the emergency department complaining of severe back pain. Her pain has increased over the last 3–4 days and is no longer responsive to oral acetaminophen. The pain is currently 9/10, does not radiate, and is worse with movement. She denies weakness or loss of sensation in her trunk, perineum, or lower extremities. She further denies urinary or fecal incontinence. Other than her cancer, she has no significant medical history.

On physical exam, she has full strength and a normal sensory exam in all extremities. Serum electrolytes and creatinine are normal. Spinal MRI reveals progression of T4–6 vertebral metastases without pathological fracture or epidural extension of her disease.

You order morphine 2 mg IV and decide to reassess her in 15 minutes at which time she continues to report severe pain with no significant improvement. You order morphine 4 mg IV and 30 minutes later give an additional 6 mg. She reports that her pain is still "moderate" but reports no other symptoms. What is the next most appropriate step in her management?

A. Consult the palliative medicine service
B. Discontinue morphine and initiate hydromorphone therapy
C. Repeat morphine 6 mg IV now
D. Initiate extended release morphine
E. Initiate methadone therapy

12. A 77-year-old man with hypertension, insulin-dependent diabetes (with longstanding diabetic neuropathy and nephropathy), and colon cancer metastatic to lung and liver was admitted to hospital directly from your clinic several days ago. Due to concerns about his evolving diabetic nephropathy, he was rotated off of his home morphine regimen to a fentanyl PCA and is currently on a basal rate of 100 μg/h with demand doses of 50 μg and a 10-minute lockout.

He reports excellent pain controlled with no adverse effects from his current PCA. What is the next best step in management?

A. Transition off the basal rate of his PCA to a fentanyl 50 μg/h patch
B. Transition off the basal rate of his PCA to a fentanyl 100 μg/h patch

C. Transition off the basal rate of his PCA to a fentanyl 150 μg/h patch
D. Transition off the basal rate of his PCA and start morphine ER 100 mg q8h
E. Obtain palliative medicine consultation

13. A 52-year-old male with AML who completed an allogeneic stem cell transplant from a matched, unrelated donor 2 months ago. His hospitalization course was complicated by herpes zoster along the T4 dermatome on the left. Although his rash completely resolved, he continues to describe 5/10 burning pain at that site, which has improved from 9/10 prior to starting gabapentin, which is now at 1200 mg q8h.

He expresses a desire for improved pain control but says "I'm already taking too many pills."

What is the next best step in management?

A. Increase gabapentin to 1500 mg q8h
B. Add lidocaine 5% patch
C. Add oxycodone 5 mg q4h as needed
D. Start diphenhydramine
E. Obtain MRI spine

14. A 32-year-old female with diffuse large B-cell lymphoma receiving R-CHOP chemotherapy calls your clinic with a complaint of ongoing pain in her low back, both hips, and thighs. Labs 3 days ago were significant for severe neutropenia, and she received pegfilgrastim at that time. She was seen yesterday and started on naproxen for pain that has provided only partial relief.

She denies tingling, numbness, or weakness in the lower extremities and has not lost bowel or bladder control.

Lower extremity strength, sensation, and reflexes are within normal limits.

What is the next best step in management?

A. Stop naproxen and start ibuprofen
B. Stop naproxen and start acetaminophen
C. Add lidocaine patch
D. Add oxycodone
E. Obtain MRI spine

15. A 79-year-old man with a history of insulin-dependent diabetes, COPD, and prostate cancer with lumbosacral metastases is admitted to the inpatient oncology service after presenting with back pain and urinary retention. A urinary catheter was placed, and he was started on a morphine PCA for pain. MRI revealed progression of lumbosacral vertebral metastases without evidence of cord compression.

On the morning of hospital day 2, he reports excellent pain control; but later that day, his nurse notes that he is somnolent and more confused. Prior to this, he denied any pain or nausea to his nurse and reported a normal bowel movement in the morning.

Vital signs significant for T 37.0 C, HR 82, RR 8, BP 126/80, SaO2 93%. On exam, his pupils are miotic, breath sounds are clear, and abdomen is soft but with decreased bowel sounds. Creatinine this morning was 2.6 mg/dL, which was unchanged from the previous day but worse than his baseline of 1.8 mg/dL.

What is the next most appropriate step in management?

A. Obtain arterial blood gas
B. Discontinue morphine PCA and transfer the patient to ICU for close monitoring
C. Administer naloxone 0.4 mg IV
D. Administer naloxone 0.08 mg IV
E. Initiate sepsis workup

16. An 82-year-old former attorney with metastatic pancreatic adenocarcinoma who presents to your clinic accompanied by his wife for follow-up. He recently had progression of disease after completing FOLFIRINOX, and he reports worsening fatigue and malaise over the last week. His wife reports that he spends most of his day in bed, eats very little, and needs assistance to get to the bathroom 10 feet away.

    You discuss a plan to forgo further chemotherapy based on his poor performance status and introduce a plan to increase his medical support at home by introducing hospice care.

    Which of the follow is true about hospice enrollment?
    A. Patients are allowed to receive hospice care for 6 months.
    B. A DNR code status is required to enroll in hospice.
    C. A patient can typically expect 24-hour access to the hospice agency by phone.
    D. Patients enrolled in hospice may not present to the ER.
    E. Hospice care does not allow patients to live at home.

17. A 76-year-old woman with metastatic breast cancer you have followed for several years in your clinic. She was discharged 3 weeks ago after a week in hospital for pneumonia. At that time, she was very deconditioned but insisted on going home with physical therapy services. She has excellent family support at home. She has rarely gotten out of bed since discharge and has continued to lose weight. Her son and daughter report distress over her inability to finish even one can of her nutrition supplement shakes in the course of a day. She is now being readmitted to the hospital for extreme fatigue and acutely altered mentation.

    Your inpatient team schedules a meeting with the patient's children. The patient cannot participate in the meeting due to altered mentation.

    You feel that due to her very poor performance status and acute medical condition that further cancer therapy would pose more risk than potential benefit, and you think additional medical support from a hospice service at home would help preserve the patient's wish to avoid hospitalization.

    In presenting this news to her children, which of the following techniques would not be appropriate to include in your family meeting?
    A. Asking the family's perspective on their mother's current condition and plan of care
    B. Using empathic responses to address emotions
    C. Requiring that the patient is present in the room to preserve autonomy
    D. Explaining misunderstandings or misconceptions the family may have
    E. Summarize the conclusions of the meeting at the end

18. A 77-year-old female patient of yours with severe COPD and widely metastatic NSCLC presented to hospital 4 days ago with dyspnea and fevers and was found to have pneumonia and significant progression of disease in her lungs with slight bilateral pleural effusions.

    Despite appropriate antibiotic, steroid, and inhaler management, she continues to require high-flow nasal cannula at 40 L/min and chest x-ray has slightly worsened. She previously stated that she would never want mechanical ventilation, and this was appropriately documented. She has no pain.

    The patient becomes increasingly confused and starts moaning but maintains a normal respiratory rate with unchanged O2 saturation. pCO2 is 90 mm Hg increased from 75 mm Hg yesterday. The family is worried she is in pain.

What is the most appropriate action?
A. Start a fentanyl transdermal pain
B. Administer morphine 5 mg IV now
C. Meet with family to discuss her decline and initiate delirium treatment
D. Call ICU and initiate plans for intubation
E. Discontinue her home SSRI

19. An 82-year-old former attorney with metastatic pancreatic adenocarcinoma who presents to your clinic accompanied by his wife for follow-up. He recently had progression of disease after completing FOLFIRINOX, and he reports worsening fatigue and malaise over the last week. His wife reports that he spends most of his day in bed, eats very little, and needs assistance to get to the bathroom 10 feet away.

    You discuss a plan to forgo further chemotherapy based on his poor performance status and introduce a plan to increase his medical support at home by introducing hospice care.

    Which of the following services would likely require an additional out-of-pocket expense beyond what is covered by the Medicare Hospice Benefit?
    A. 24-hour emergency phone contact with hospice service
    B. Continuous care at home for short-term need
    C. Social work counseling at home
    D. Hospital bed, bedside commode, and other medical equipment
    E. Around-the-clock home nursing or nurse's aide services

20. A 76-year-old woman with metastatic breast cancer you have followed for several years in your clinic. She was discharged 3 weeks ago after a week in hospital for pneumonia. At that time, she was very deconditioned but insisted on going home with physical therapy services. She has excellent family support at home. She has rarely gotten out of bed since discharge and has continued to lose weight. Her son and daughter report distress over her inability to finish even one can of her nutrition supplement shakes in the course of a day. She is now being readmitted to the hospital for extreme fatigue and acutely altered mentation.

    Your inpatient team schedules a meeting with the patient's children. The patient cannot participate in the meeting due to altered mentation.

    You explain that you feel that due to her very poor performance status and acute medical condition that further cancer therapy would pose more risk than potential benefit. You share your concern about further decline in her condition and recommend placing a do no resuscitate (DNR) order to allow natural death if this happens, reassuring them that you plan to continue all other current medical therapies. You introduce the idea of home hospice as a possibility if she stabilizes sufficiently for discharge. Her children state that their mother would "want everything done."
    What is the most appropriate next step?
    A. Acknowledge their wish and document FULL CODE status in your note
    B. Tell them that CPR would be inappropriate in this case and obtain an ethics consultation
    C. Ask the children to explain further what they mean by "everything"
    D. Request that the nurse place an NG tube and start artificial feeding since the patient has not been eating enough
    E. Suggest that you meet with the family again in a few days

21. A 77-year-old female patient of yours with severe COPD and widely metastatic NSCLC presented to hospital 4 days ago with dyspnea and fevers and was found to have pneumonia and significant progression of disease in her lungs with slight bilateral pleural effusions.

Despite optimal medical management, she continues to require high-flow nasal cannula. She expressed a desire to allow natural death, and a DNR order was placed accordingly.

As she continues to decline, the family notes her breathing starts to look like she is "gasping" with long pauses in between and asks if she is "suffocating." She otherwise appears comfortable. RR is 16, O2 sat 91%.

What is the next appropriate action?
A. Explain that this is a normal part of the dying process
B. Increase her high-flow nasal cannula to maximal support
C. Start a morphine continuous infusion
D. Call ICU and initiate plans for intubation
E. Administer nebulized albuterol treatment

22. An 82-year-old former attorney with metastatic pancreatic adenocarcinoma who presents to your clinic accompanied by his wife for follow-up. He recently had progression of disease after completing FOLFIRINOX, and he reports worsening fatigue and malaise over the last week. His wife reports that he spends most of his day in bed, eats very little, and needs assistance to get to the bathroom 10 feet away.

You discuss a plan to forgo further chemotherapy based on his poor performance status and introduce a plan to increase his medical support at home by introducing hospice care. He reports that he wants to spend as much time as possible with his family and avoid "going through any more tests."

Which of the following is important in your discussion?
A. Avoid making a recommendation so as not to bias the patient's decision
B. Say, "There's nothing more we can do"
C. Discuss hospice only with the family out of earshot from the patient
D. Emphasize that hospice care would align with his goal to remain at home and avoid hospitalization
E. Tell the patient that he cannot come to your clinic because chemo is no longer an option

23. A 76-year-old woman with metastatic breast cancer you have followed for several years in your clinic. She was discharged 3 weeks ago after a week in hospital for

pneumonia. At that time, she was very deconditioned but insisted on going home with physical therapy services. She has excellent family support at home. She has rarely gotten out of bed since discharge and has continued to lose weight. Her son and daughter report distress over her inability to finish even one can of her nutrition supplement shakes in the course of a day. She is now being readmitted to the hospital for extreme fatigue and acutely altered mentation.

You are worried about her decline and think she has a poor prognosis measured in weeks to months.

As part of your discussion with her and her children, you want to address code status and recommend a DNR order be placed.

Which of the following should be part of the discussion?
A. Describe CPR in mechanistic terms (e.g., "push on your chest")
B. Ask if she would want her doctors to "do everything"
C. Clarify that code status will not affect any other medical care she receives
D. Use terms like "Pass away" to make the topic of death easier to discuss
E. Ask separately about her preferences for intubation, defibrillation, and CPR.

24. A 65-year-old Chinese-American man with widely metastatic colon adenocarcinoma was admitted to hospital 3 days ago for profound weakness, fatigue, and anorexia. He was discharged 2 weeks ago after a 1-week admission for pneumonia. At that time, the patient decided to enroll in home hospice care. Since then, his daughter reports that it was "getting too hard to watch him starving," adding that he "just won't eat." The patient confirms his lack of desire to eat and fatigue and says he feels frustrated that his daughter pushes him to eat more. He otherwise endorses a good mood.

On exam, you note a severely cachectic man with dry, pale skin who appears lethargic.

What is the next best step in management?
A. Initiate plans for percutaneous endogastric feeding tube placement
B. Initiate parenteral feeding
C. Explain that this is a normal process in advanced cancer and encourage oral feeding of foods he likes
D. Ask the patient about suicidal ideation
E. Increase the rate of IV fluids

ANSWERS

1. B

This patient is suffering from somatic pain related to vertebral metastases. According to NCCN Adult Cancer Pain Guidelines, if severe pain is unchanged 15 minutes after the initial intravenous bolus of morphine or other opioid, escalation by 50%–100% is appropriate. Answers A and C would not achieve adequate analgesia. A rotation to another opioid (D) is unnecessary unless the patient has intolerable adverse effects from morphine. Rapid titration of opioid is acceptable at this time without initiating a PCA (E).

2. B

This patient is in pain crisis due to progression of her liver metastases. Since this patient will likely require rapid

escalation of opioid, the safest management would be to avoid morphine, which relies heavily on renal clearance of active metabolites. Since morphine 5 mg IV was effective, an equianalgesic dose of another opioid would be appropriate. Hydromorphone 0.75 mg and fentanyl 50 µg (answer B) are equianalgesic in this case.

3. C

This patient is suffering from chemotherapy-induced peripheral neuropathy (CIPN) after treatment with cisplatin. The American Society of Clinical Oncology gives a moderate recommendation to initiate duloxetine therapy in this setting. Despite inconclusive evidence, trials of gabapentin, pregabalin, or tricyclic antidepressants are also considered reasonable (answer D). A TENS unit can be an effective nonpharmacological treatment for CIPN, but it is not first-line treatment.

4. B

Nonsteroidal antiinflammatory drugs (NSAIDs) and acetaminophen are considered first-line therapy for treating bone pain associated with colony-stimulating factors such as pegfilgrastim. Antihistamines and opioids (A and C) are part of second-line treatment. A lidocaine patch would not provide benefit for this pain (D). MRI spine is unlikely to provide further information about the pain and is not indicated, as no worrisome neurological signs or symptoms are present (E).

5. A

This patient has a high risk for aberrant behaviors on opioids. This scale includes age 16–45 (answer E) and personal or family history of alcohol, illicit drug (C), or prescription drug abuse. Of note, tobacco abuse is not a risk factor on this scale. Several psychiatric diagnoses including ADD do increase risk of opioid misuse (D). In women, preadolescent sexual abuse also increases this risk and should be part of your routine assessment when prescribing opioids. Patients at higher risk for opioid misuse may require pain specialist referral.

6. B

This patient is suffering from somatic pain related to vertebral metastases. In this opioid-tolerant patient, your initial inpatient opioid dosing should be 10%–20% of the patient's total opioid use in the preceding 24 hours. Her total morphine usage, 90 mg orally, is equivalent to 30 mg IV morphine. Therefore, 6 mg IV is an appropriate initial dose. According to NCCN Adult Cancer Pain Guidelines, if severe pain is unchanged 15 minutes after the initial intravenous bolus of morphine or other opioid, escalation by 50%–100% is appropriate. Answers A and C would not achieve adequate analgesia. While palliative medicine consultation is often helpful (D), a guideline-based increase in opioids is appropriate in this case. The patient has no symptoms suspicious for spinal cord compression, and there is no indication for urgent neurosurgical intervention (E).

7. D

The patient has RUQ abdominal pain that is well controlled. He appears to be suffering visual hallucinations due to morphine in the setting of worsening diabetic nephropathy. It is safest to avoid morphine in this patient, as it relies heavily on renal clearance. It is unlikely that he has developed a primary psychiatric illness (answer B). His current total daily morphine ER is 200 mg, which is equivalent to about 1666 µg of fentanyl per day (69 µg of fentanyl per hour). A dose reduction of 25%–50% to account for incomplete cross-tolerance of opioids is appropriate. As such, a fentanyl 50 µg/h patch would be safe and effective in this patient.

8. A

This patient is suffering from CIPN after treatment with cisplatin. He is receiving gabapentin therapy at low doses, and this should be escalated by 50%–100% every 3 days until pain is adequately controlled. Maximum dosing in a patient with normal renal function is 1200 mg q8h. In this setting, increasing his gabapentin would be more appropriate than adding (answers C and E) another therapy or switching to an alternate agent (B).

9. A

While NSAIDs and acetaminophen are first-line therapy for bone pain secondary to colony-stimulating factors such as pegfilgrastim, there is no evidence for superiority of any of single agent over another (answers B and C). However, there is evidence of benefit for antihistamines. MRI would not be indicated with signs or symptoms of neurological dysfunction. Topical lidocaine will not help treat this pain.

10. C

There are a variety of reasons for the change in this patient's condition including hypoglycemia (answer A), infection (B and D), cardiac ischemia (E), and other causes. If his condition were the result of opioid intoxication, you would expect to see respiratory depression rather than tachypnea. Furthermore, the initial starting dose of naloxone should be 0.04–0.08 mg. Giving an entire 0.4 mg vial would likely cause acute pain crisis and symptoms of withdrawal.

11. A

This patient is suffering from somatic pain related to vertebral metastases. According to NCCN Adult Cancer Pain Guidelines, after 2–3 cycles of rapid titration of opioid, a consultation to palliative care or other pain specialist is appropriate. Since she got inadequate pain relief from morphine 6 mg, further dose escalation is appropriate (C). Since she did not experience any intolerable adverse effects after receiving morphine rotation to another opioid, (B) is not appropriate or necessary. Extended release formulations such as extended-release morphine and methadone are usually initiated after at least 24 hours of treatment with intermittent dosing of short-acting opioid (D and E). Furthermore, due to the unique pharmacological profile of methadone, it should only be initiated by experienced prescribers.

12. B

The conversion of IV to transdermal fentanyl in this patient is 1:1. No dose increase or reduction is necessary if he is reporting good pain control without adverse effects. It is safest to avoid morphine (answer D) in this patient, as morphine relies heavily on renal clearance. Palliative medicine consultation (E) is not necessary in this case, as the patient's pain is controlled with his current PCA.

13. B

Gabapentin, already at maximum dose, (answer A) has shown some benefit in this patient's pain, but he is requesting additional pain relief without additional pill burden (C). Lidocaine patch has been shown to provide relief for postherpetic neuralgia compared with placebo. There is no role for diphenhydramine or additional imaging for postherpetic neuralgia (D and E).

14. D

While NSAIDs and acetaminophen are first-line therapy for bone pain secondary to colony-stimulating factors such as pegfilgrastim, there is no evidence for superiority of any single agent over another (answers A and B). However, there is evidence of benefit for opioids. MRI would not be indicated with signs or symptoms of neurological dysfunction. Topical lidocaine will not help treat this pain.

15. D

This patient has severe respiratory depression in the setting of rapid titration of morphine and acute renal insufficiency. Morphine is glucuronidated in the liver to active metabolites that are renally cleared, and using an agent such as fentanyl that does not dependent on renal function would have been safer in this situation. Transfer to ICU (answer B) may be required but is not the next step as this patient needs urgent opioid reversal. Administering naloxone 0.08 mg is the most appropriate initial dose. Naloxone 0.4 mg (answer C) would only be given in the case of cardiopulmonary arrest. Outside of this setting, high-dose naloxone would likely precipitate acute pain and possibly acute opioid withdrawal in an opioid-tolerant patient. Other workup including ABG and blood cultures (A and E) would be lower priority because of the likelihood of opioid intoxication.

16. C

Medicare guidelines for hospice eligibility require a physician's certification of a "life expectancy of 6 months or less if the terminal illness runs its normal course." This determination can be made based on decline in clinical status (e.g., significant weight loss, intractable symptoms, and decline in performance status) or poor baseline function combined with disease-specific criteria (e.g., metastatic cancer, end-stage liver disease). This patient's poor performance status and metastatic pancreatic cancer are sufficient for hospice enrollment. Hospice care is often performed at home (answer E). In addition to some in-home support, 24-hour phone support is common. Patients can continue to be enrolled in hospice indefinitely as long as they continue to meet criteria for hospice (A); and a DNR code status is not legally required (B), although some institutions may require it. While hospice can help patients avoid unwanted hospital admission, they are allowed to terminate hospice enrollment to present to an acute hospital if they wish.

17. C

Discussing serious news about a very sick patient can be challenging, and it is important to have a routine for these discussions. One commonly-used mnemonic is SPIKES: **S**etting, **P**atient/Family **P**erception, **I**nvitation, **G**iving **K**nowledge, **E**mpathy, **S**ummarize. Conducting meetings in a private, comfortable setting with proper introduction of meeting participants and acknowledgment of potential interruptions (e.g., pagers) is very important but sometimes overlooked when discussing serious news. In cases such as this where the patient's mental status prevents her participation in the meeting, it may be easiest and best to conduct the meeting in a separate conference room or other quiet space.

18. C

This likely represents terminal delirium, a natural part of the dying process. Since she has no history of pain, it is unlikely that this is the reason for her current presentation. Also, although opioids are appropriate to control dyspnea at end of life, this patient's respiratory rate and O_2 saturation are normal (answers A and B). Her wishes to avoid intubation should be honored (D). Although it is important to reevaluate and limit nonessential medications at end of life, stopping certain home medications can also lead to withdrawal and increase risk of delirium (E).

19. E

In most cases, hospice services represent an increase in a patient's current level of medical support at home including 24-hour phone access and some in-person access to an interdisciplinary hospice team including physicians, nurses, nurse's aides, social workers, chaplains, and other providers. Some clinicians who are less familiar with hospice may unintentionally convey that hospice will provide continuous nursing care, leading to patient mistrust and frustration when this expectation is not met. Around-the-clock nursing care, if available, will often come at an additional cost to the patient.

20. C

This is a common scenario, and it is inappropriate to assume that you know what "everything" means or that it means the same thing for all patients. While "everything medically possible" is one interpretation (answers A and D), there are often other worries or emotions underlying these statements that must be investigated. Patients may fear abandonment by their doctor, worry about leaving family behind, fear that symptoms will worsen, or have a variety of other concerns.

21. A

This patient is demonstrating a Cheyne-Stokes breathing pattern characteristic of end-of-life. With a normal RR and O2 saturation, there is no reason to increase her O2 support, start morphine, or give albuterol (answers B, C, and E). Her documented wishes to avoid intubation should be honored.

22. D

Conversations about hospice can be challenging. It is important avoid euphemism, "nothing we can do" is unclear, and statements that suggest abandonment (answers B and E). At the same time, if the patient wishes to be involved in his healthcare decision-making, it is important to involve him in the conversation (C). It is appropriate and does not compromise patient autonomy for the physician to make a recommendation based on his/her best medical judgment (A).

23. C

It is important that patients and their families understand that they will continue to receive excellent medical care regardless of code status, as patients often worry about being abandoned by their physicians. Using euphemisms such as "do everything" or "pass away" (answers B and D) can lead to misunderstanding and prevent informed decision-making. Initially, giving small amounts of information may be easier for the patient to absorb, and it is not necessary to describe mechanistic details of resuscitation. Similarly, presenting code status as a menu incorrectly characterizes them as separate interventions and adds an inappropriate level of detail.

24. C

Anorexia is a common symptom in advanced cancer. While there is a role for medications to stimulate appetite in patients who wish to try them, there is no evidence that alternate modes of feeding with improve survival or quality of life (answers A and B). Depression screening is appropriate in the right clinical situation, but normalizing the symptom of anorexia in cancer is the most likely to help the patient and daughter in this case. Increasing the rate of IV fluids will not affect appetite (E).

REFERENCES

Question 1

1. NCCN Adult Cancer Pain Guidelines.

Question 2

1. NCCN Adult Cancer Pain Guidelines.

Question 3

1. NCCN Adult Cancer Pain Guidelines.
2. Hershman DL, Lacchetti C, Dworkin RH, et al. Prevention and management of chemotherapy-induced peripheral neuropathy in survivors of adult cancers: American Society of Clinical Oncology clinical practice guideline. *J Clin Oncol.* 2014;32(18):1941–1967.

3. Smith EM, Pang H, Cirrincione C, et al. Effect of duloxetine on pain, function, and quality of life among patients with chemotherapy-induced painful peripheral neuropathy: a randomized clinical trial. *JAMA*. 2013;309(13):1359–1367.

Question 4

1. Lambertini M, Del Mastro L, Bellodi A, Pronzato P. The five "Ws" for bone pain due to the administration of granulocyte-colony stimulating factors (G-CSFs). *Crit Rev Oncol Hematol*. 2014;89(1):112–128.

Question 5

1. Webster LR, Webster RM. Predicting aberrant behaviors in opioid-treated patients: preliminary validation of the opioid risk tool. *Pain Med*. 2005;6(6):432–442.
2. NCCN Adult Cancer Pain Guidelines.

Question 6

1. NCCN Adult Cancer Pain Guidelines.

Question 7

1. NCCN Adult Cancer Pain Guidelines.

Question 8

1. NCCN Adult Cancer Pain Guidelines.

Question 9

1. Lambertini M, Del Mastro L, Bellodi A, Pronzato P. The five "Ws" for bone pain due to the administration of granulocyte-colony stimulating factors (G-CSFs). *Crit Rev Oncol Hematol*. 2014;89(1):112–128.

Question 11

1. NCCN Adult Cancer Pain Guidelines.

Question 12

1. NCCN Adult Cancer Pain Guidelines.

Question 13

1. Wolff RF, Bala MM, Westwood M, Kessels AG, Kleijnen J. 5% lidocaine-medicated plaster vs other relevant interventions and placebo for post-herpetic neuralgia (PHN): a systematic review. *Acta Neurol Scand*. 2011;123(5):295–309.
2. NCCN Adult Cancer Pain Guidelines.
3. <http://www.mypcnow.org/#!core-curriculum/vdw7n>.

Question 14

1. Lambertini M, Del Mastro L, Bellodi A, Pronzato P. The five "Ws" for bone pain due to the administration of granulocyte-colony stimulating factors (G-CSFs). *Crit Rev Oncol Hematol*. 2014;89(1):112–128.

Question 15

1. NCCN Adult Cancer Pain Guidelines.
2. Hoffman JR, Schriger DL, Luo JS. The empiric use of naloxone in patients with altered mental status: a reappraisal. *Ann Emerg Med*. 1991;20(3):246–252.

Question 16

1. <http://www.mypcnow.org/#!core-curriculum/vdw7n>.
2. <https://www.cms.gov/medicare-coverage-database/details/lcd-details.aspx?LCDId=33393&ContrId=272&ver=2&ContrVer=1&CntrctrSelected=272*1&Cntrctr=272&name=National+Government+Services%2c+Inc.+(06004%2c+HHH+MAC)&DocType=All&s=56&bc=AggAAAIAAAAAAA%3d%3d&#0>.

Question 17

1. Baile WF, Buckman R, Lenzi R, Glober G, Beale EA, Kudelka AP. SPIKES—a six-step protocol for delivering bad news: application to the patient with cancer. *Oncologist*. 2000;5(4):302–311.

Question 18

1. Ferris FD, von Gunten CF, Emanuel LL. Competency in end-of-life care: last hours of life. *J Palliat Med*. 2003;6(4):605–613.

Question 19

More information on hospice eligibility can be found at the CMS website.
1. <http://www.mypcnow.org/#!core-curriculum/vdw7n>.

Question 20

1. Quill TE, Arnold R, Back AL. Discussing treatment preferences with patients who want "everything." *Ann Intern Med*. 2009;151(5):345–349.

Question 21

1. Ferris FD, von Gunten CF, Emanuel LL. Competency in end-of-life care: last hours of life. *J Palliat Med*. 2003;6(4):605–613.

Question 22

More information on hospice eligibility can be found at the CMS website.
1. <http://www.mypcnow.org/#!core-curriculum/vdw7n>.

Question 23

1. <http://www.mypcnow.org/#!core-curriculum/vdw7n>.

Question 24

1. Ferris FD, von Gunten CF, Emanuel LL. Competency in end-of-life care: last hours of life. *J Palliat Med*. 2003;6(4):605–613.

Survivorship and Treatment-Related Issues

Erin Roesch and Benjamin A. Weinberg

QUESTIONS

1. A 53-year-old woman with history of classical Hodgkin lymphoma was treated in 1980 with mantle radiation and 6 cycles of doxorubicin, bleomycin, vinblastine, and dacarbazine. Her disease is in remission. She has never smoked. Which of the following is true regarding her risk of the development of second solid cancers?
   - **A.** Her overall risk of second solid cancers is the same as patients treated between 1990 and 2000.
   - **B.** She is more likely to develop lung cancer than any other solid malignancy.
   - **C.** After 40 years post-treatment, her risk of developing a solid cancer is equivalent to that of the general population.
   - **D.** Her risk of second solid cancers would be higher if she had received supradiaphragmatic field radiotherapy excluding the axilla rather than mantle-field radiotherapy.
   - **E.** She is not at an increased risk of developing gastrointestinal malignancies compared with the general population.

2. An 83-year-old man who recently completed 6 cycles of adjuvant FOLFOX chemotherapy for colorectal cancer presents to clinic with his daughter who is concerned about his declining cognitive function. She states that he is more forgetful than usual, not remembering appointments, and misplacing items throughout his house. Which of the following is NOT recommended as a strategy for management of cancer-associated cognitive dysfunction?
   - **A.** Assessment of sleep disturbance
   - **B.** Maintain regular physical activity
   - **C.** Stress reduction using meditation
   - **D.** Avoidance of multitasking
   - **E.** Use of organizational strategies such as memory aids and notes

   Manifestations of Advanced Cancer and Its Treatment—paraneoplastic syndromes, renal, infections, fatigue, psychiatry, GI, neurology, endocrinology, musculoskeletal, skin, hematological

3. A 67-year-old man with a history of stage IV lung adenocarcinoma, epidermal growth factor receptors, ALK, and ROS wild-type, 50 pack-year smoking history, returns to clinic with 3 weeks of progressive, worsening pain in his bilateral ankles and knees. A positron emission tomography (PET) scan shows new diffuse uptake in the long bones. The patient's physical exam is unremarkable except for his hands as pictured above. Which of the following does the patient have (Fig. 37.1)?

   - **A.** Dermatomyositis
   - **B.** Trousseau syndrome
   - **C.** Hypertrophic osteoarthropathy
   - **D.** Chronic hypoxia due to COPD
   - **E.** Lambert-Eaton syndrome

4. A 55-year-old woman with pancreatic adenocarcinoma status post a pancreaticoduodenectomy with R0 resection returns for follow-up on month 6 of adjuvant gemcitabine chemotherapy. She has developed weakness, fatigue, abdominal pain, and a purpuric skin rash over the last 2 weeks. Laboratory values are as follows:

   WBC 8000/μL
   Hemoglobin 6.8 g/dL
   Hematocrit 24%
   Platelets 38,000/μL
   INR 1.1 s
   Prothrombin time 13.5 s
   Activated thromboplastin time 38 s
   LDH 852 units/L
   Haptoglobin <8 mg/dL
   Creatinine 3.4 mg/dL (baseline 1.2)

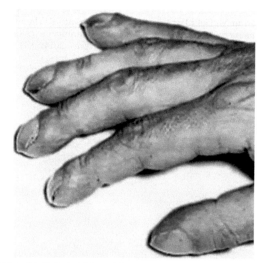

FIG. 37.1 Digital clubbing. (Courtesy R.A. DeRemee, MD, Mayo Clinic, Rochester, Minn.) (Reproduced with permission from: Midthun DE, Jett JR. Clinical presentation of lung cancer. In: Pass HI, et al. [eds.] *Lung Cancer: Principles and Practice.* Philadelphia: Lippincott-Raven; 1996:426. Copyright © Elsevier Science, Inc.)

Which of the following is the most accurate diagnosis?
A. Thrombotic microangiopathy
B. Henoch-Schönlein purpura
C. Progression of pancreatic adenocarcinoma
D. Cryoglobulinemia
E. Acquired factor VIII inhibitor

5. A 62-year-old woman with resected stage I transverse colon adenocarcinoma returns for follow-up 4 years after resection. Her colonoscopy 1 year after resection was normal. If her colonoscopy now is normal, when should she receive her next surveillance colonoscopy?
A. 1 year
B. 2 years
C. 3 years
D. 5 years
E. 10 years

6. Which of the following chemotherapy drugs is deemed to be low risk for the impairment of spermatogenesis?
A. Cyclophosphamide
B. Cisplatin
C. Melphalan
D. Bleomycin
E. Doxorubicin

Manifestations of Advanced Cancer and Its Treatment—paraneoplastic syndromes, renal, infections, fatigue, psychiatry, GI, neurology, endocrinology, musculoskeletal, skin, hematological

7. A 67-year-old woman with stage IV non-small cell lung cancer who began erlotinib 150 mg daily 1 week ago returns with a facial rash. She reports 2 days of a red, pruritic rash across her nose and bilateral cheeks. Physical exam reveals a diffuse, erythematous, papulopustular eruption with crusting without sparing of the nasolabial folds. What is the next best step in management?
A. Hold erlotinib until rash resolves
B. Continue erlotinib and initiate prednisone 40 mg by mouth daily until rash resolves
C. Decrease erlotinib to 100 mg daily and increase back to 150 mg daily once rash resolves
D. Continue erlotinib and initiate minocycline 100 mg by mouth daily, loratadine 10 mg by mouth daily, and topical metronidazole 1% gel daily until the rash resolves
E. Hold erlotinib and initiate isotretinoin 20 mg by mouth daily until rash resolves

8. A 59-year-old man with glioblastoma multiforme returns for follow-up on week 6 of adjuvant temozolomide with concurrent intensity-modulated radiation therapy following an R0 resection. He continues to take dexamethasone 4 mg daily for cerebral edema. For the last 3 days, he reports worsening fatigue, fever, and nonproductive cough. He also has progressively worse shortness of breath, now dyspneic with any ambulation and unable to speak complete sentences without pausing to take a breath. He is sent to the emergency department where his oxygen saturation is 89% on room air, and a chest x-ray reveals diffuse ground-glass opacities and perihilar interstitial and alveolar infiltrates. In addition to supplemental oxygen, what is the next best step in treatment?
A. Initiate piperacillin/tazobactam and vancomycin intravenously
B. Initiate methylprednisolone intravenously
C. Initiate azithromycin and ceftriaxone intravenously
D. Initiate trimethoprim/sulfamethoxazole intravenously
E. Initiate liposomal amphotericin B intravenously

9. A 73-year-old woman with limited stage non-small cell lung cancer returns to your clinic, having just completed 4 cycles of cisplatin and etoposide chemotherapy with concurrent radiation. Baseline MRI brain prior to treatment revealed no brain metastases. She has an excellent performance status (ECOG 0) and normal cognitive function. Which of the following is true regarding the use of prophylactic cranial irradiation (PCI)?
A. She is likely to develop neurocognitive side effects within 12 months after PCI.
B. Adverse effects from PCI occur at the same rates regardless of baseline neurocognitive functioning.
C. Patients treated with 36 Gy have similar rates of neurotoxicity and mortality as patients treated with 25 Gy.
D. PCI is not indicated in extensive stage small cell lung cancer.
E. PCI can be used even if the patient did not have a response to initial chemoradiation.

10. A 60-year-old woman returns for follow-up after completing adjuvant doxorubicin/cyclophosphamide followed by paclitaxel and radiation therapy for a stage III breast cancer. The patient asks what is the chance of a developing a nonbreast cancer due to her prior cancer treatment. She has no family history and no other personal history of malignancy. Which of the following is true?
A. She is not at any increased risk of development of a nonbreast malignancy.
B. Of all nonbreast malignancies, she is at the highest risk of developing acute myeloid leukemia within the next 15 years.
C. Of all nonbreast malignancies, she is at the highest risk of developing a gastrointestinal cancer within the next 15 years.
D. Of all nonbreast malignancies, she is at the highest risk of developing a lung cancer within the next 15 years.
E. Her risk of developing a nonbreast malignancy approaches that of the age-matched general population after 5 years.

11. A 67-year-old woman who received neoadjuvant doxorubicin, cyclophosphamide, and paclitaxel prior to mastectomy presents for follow-up 1 year after completing doxorubicin. She received a total doxorubicin dose of 300 mg/m^2 and has underlying hypertension, type 2 diabetes mellitus, and hyperlipidemia. She has never smoked. She denies difficulty breathing on exertion, at rest, or while laying flat, but she does note lower extremity swelling. Which one of the following is the most appropriate test to perform at this time?
A. Resting electrocardiogram
B. Exercise treadmill stress test
C. Coronary angiography
D. Echocardiogram or multigated acquisition (MUGA) scan
E. Serum B-type natriuretic peptide (BNP)

12. A 45-year-old female is s/p lumpectomy for a hormone receptor-negative, node-negative, invasive ductal carcinoma of the left breast. She elects to pursue adjuvant chemotherapy, and goes on to complete 4 cycles of dose dense Adriamycin/Cyclophosphamide followed by 4 cycles of Paclitaxel administered every 2 weeks. Three years later, she presents with fatigue and anemia and is diagnosed with myelodysplastic syndrome. Which of the following cytogenetic abnormalities is she most likely to harbor?
A. t(11q23)
B. del(7q)

C. t(15;17)
D. inv(16)
E. t(9;22)

13. A 69-year-old male diagnosed with a stage IIIb colon adenocarcinoma underwent surgery and adjuvant chemotherapy with FOLFOX, followed by active surveillance for five years and remains without evidence of disease recurrence. He presents for follow-up and enquires about lung cancer screening with low-dose CT, as he is a former smoker. Which of the following is true regarding eligibility for screening based on the National Lung Screening Trial?
A. Remote history of lung cancer
B. Age of 55-74
C. 20-pack-year smoking history
D. Former smoker, quit within the past 20 years
E. Reported symptom of hemoptysis

14. A 44-year-old female was diagnosed one year ago with a 1.5 cm right-sided invasive ductal carcinoma, hormone receptor-positive, HER2-negative, node-negative with a recurrence score of 24, s/p lumpectomy and sentinel lymph node biopsy. She completed adjuvant chemotherapy and radiation, and is currently receiving endocrine therapy with tamoxifen. Her family history includes the patient's mother diagnosed with breast cancer at the age of 48. In addition to clinic visits with history and physical exam, which item should be included in the follow-up plan for this patient?
A. Breast MRI
B. Monitoring of tumor markers (CA 15-3, CA 27.29)
C. PET/CT
D. Annual screening for endometrial cancer with transvaginal ultrasound
E. Consideration for referral for genetic counseling

15. A 56-year-old postmenopausal female was diagnosed with endometrial cancer and underwent hysterectomy and radiation therapy. She tolerated treatment well overall, and presents for a regularly scheduled follow-up visit. She endorses dyspareunia for the past several weeks, as well as decreased libido and feels as though these symptoms are affecting her quality of life and relationship with her husband. Which of the following is true?
A. Psychological factors have minimal effect on sexual functioning.
B. Providers are more likely, compared to the patient, to initiate a discussion regarding sexuality-related concerns.
C. A provider's experience and/or comfort level may be a barrier to initiating a sexuality-related discussion.
D. A high-risk treatment for decreased sexual function is radiation.
E. Testosterone replacement will help her libido.

16. A 26-year-old female was diagnosed with Hodgkin lymphoma and received two cycles of ABVD (doxorubicin, bleomycin, vinblastine, and dacarbazine) and chest radiotherapy. In addition to history and physical and routine lab studies, which of the following is included in follow-up for this patient?
A. Thyroid function tests
B. Breast MRI
C. Routine bone marrow biopsies
D. Surveillance PET imaging
E. Cardiac MRI

17. A 46-year-old female diagnosed with unfavorable-risk acute myeloid leukemia (AML) achieves a complete remission with induction chemotherapy and then proceeds to a matched sibling allogeneic transplantation. Which of the following is the leading cause of excess deaths in patients who had survived for at least five years after transplant?
A. Infection
B. Pulmonary embolism
C. Recurrent disease or second malignancies
D. Chronic graft-versus-host disease
E. Cardiovascular events

18. A 75-year-old man with metastatic melanoma *BRAF* V600E wild-type returns for follow-up. He started ipilimumab 8 weeks ago and is now having five loose bowel movements a day. Stool studies reveal an absence of fecal leukocytes, negative stool culture, and negative *Clostridium difficile* titer. He is started on prednisone 60 mg by mouth daily, and after no improvement in his diarrhea after 2 days, he is admitted to the hospital and started on methylprednisolone 120 mg intravenously daily. Computed tomography (CT) scan of the abdomen and pelvis with contrast demonstrates pancolitis, and flexible sigmoidoscopy with biopsy supports the diagnosis of immune-related colitis. After 3 days, he now has seven loose bowel movements a day. What is the next best step in management?
A. Loperamide 2 mg by mouth every 3 hours as needed
B. Infliximab 300 mg intravenously and continuation of methylprednisolone
C. Ciprofloxacin 500 mg intravenously twice daily and metronidazole 500 mg intravenously three times daily for 14 days and continuation of methylprednisolone
D. Budesonide 9 mg by mouth every morning for 8 weeks
E. Increase methylprednisolone to 120 mg intravenously twice daily

19. A 53-year-old man returns for follow-up prior to cycle 10 of mFOLFOX6 plus bevacizumab for first-line treatment of metastatic colon adenocarcinoma to the liver. His dose of oxaliplatin was reduced to 75% since cycle 8 due to peripheral neuropathy. He states that for the past 3 weeks, he has noticed worsening numbness in the fingers of both hands and can no longer button his shirt unassisted. What is the next best step in management?
A. Initiate vitamin E 400 international units PO daily
B. Initiate duloxetine 60 mg PO daily
C. Initiate glutathione 500 mg PO twice daily
D. Initiate nimodipine 10 mg PO daily
E. Discontinue oxaliplatin

20. A 78-year-old woman with locally advanced, unresectable pancreatic adenocarcinoma (T4N0M0) and an ECOG performance status of 2 is admitted to the hospital with abdominal pain uncontrolled by oral medications and a fentanyl transdermal patch (300 µg/h). A computed tomography (CT) scan of the abdomen and pelvis without contrast shows a slight interval enlargement a pancreatic head mass but no other significant changes. She is started on a dilaudid patient controlled analgesia (PCA) pump with control of her abdominal pain. What is the next best step in controlling the patient's pain?
A. Refer for celiac plexus blockade
B. Refer to general surgery for a palliative pancreaticoduodenectomy
C. Increase fentanyl transdermal patch to 600 µg/h
D. Initiate FOLFIRINOX chemotherapy
E. Refer for hospice consultation

21. A 68-year-old woman with diabetes mellitus type II and metastatic colorectal cancer to the liver on first-line FOL-FOX plus bevacizumab presents to the emergency room with crushing left-sided chest pressure radiating down her left arm. She has received 3 cycles of chemotherapy, most recently 8 days ago. Her initial serum troponin is elevated to 2.3, and electrocardiogram reveals ST elevation of 2 mm in leads I, V2–V4, and ST depressions in leads II, III, and aVF. The diagnosis of acute anterior ST-elevation myocardial infarction is made. Which of the following agents is likely most responsible for causing the patient's myocardial infarction?
    A. 5-Fluorouracil
    B. Leucovorin
    C. Oxaliplatin
    D. Bevacizumab
    E. None of the above

22. A 53-year-old man is admitted to the hospital for his first cycle of doxorubicin, ifosfamide, and mesna for advanced soft tissue sarcoma. On the second day of treatment, he becomes more confused and is disoriented to location and time. Laboratory studies are as follows:

    WBC 5.5×10^9/L
    Hemoglobin 14.2 g/dL
    Hematocrit 42.9%
    Platelets 205×10^9/L
    Sodium 136 mEq/L
    Potassium 3.9 mEq/L
    Chloride 105 mEq/L
    CO_2 24 mEq/L
    BUN 47 mg/dL
    Creatinine 1.6 mg/dL (baseline 1.0)
    Glucose 93 mg/dL
    Calcium 9.5 mg/dL
    Magnesium 2.0 mEq/L
    Phosphorus 3.2 mg/dL
    Total protein 7.2 g/dL
    Albumin 2.9 g/dL
    Total bilirubin 1.0 mg/dL
    AST 32 IU/L
    ALT 28 IU/L
    Alkaline phosphatase 108 IU/L
    Urinalysis: normal

    Which of the following explains his current symptoms?
    A. Acute renal failure
    B. Ifosfamide encephalopathy
    C. Hemorrhagic cystitis
    D. Doxorubicin encephalopathy
    E. Mesna overdose

23. An 89-year-old man with squamous cell carcinoma of the head and neck is about to begin palliative chemotherapy with weekly cetuximab. Which of the following must be monitored closely during his treatment?
    A. Hemoglobin
    B. Sodium
    C. Absolute neutrophil count
    D. Magnesium
    E. Bilirubin

24. A 60-year-old female with metastatic breast cancer and leptomeningeal disease presents to clinic for planned administration of intrathecal chemotherapy. The indications and risks of a lumbar puncture are explained to the patient and consent is obtained. The patient is placed in a sitting

position, prepped and draped in a sterile fashion. Where is the appropriate location to insert the spinal needle?
    A. T12 and L1 interspace
    B. L1 and L2 interspace
    C. L2 and L3 interspace
    D. L3 and L4 interspace
    E. L5 and S1 interspace

25. A 45-year-old male with a recent diagnosis of HIV-associated DLBCL is being admitted for his first cycle of dose-adjusted R-EPOCH (rituximab, etoposide, prednisone, vincristine, cyclophosphamide, doxorubicin) as well as intrathecal (IT) prophylaxis with methotrexate. He tolerates chemotherapy well, although after lumbar puncture and administration of IT chemotherapy he develops a persistent headache. Brain imaging is performed to rule out an intracranial complication related to the procedure, and he is ultimately diagnosed with a post-LP headache. Which of the following factors has been shown to contribute to the development of headache after lumbar puncture?
    A. Volume of CSF removed
    B. Duration of bed rest after procedure
    C. Replacement of stylet before withdrawing the needle
    D. Positioning of patient
    E. CSF opening pressure

26. A 62-year-old male presents to the emergency room with progressive fatigue and epistaxis. Labs reveal a WBC count of 30,000/μL with 25% blasts, platelet count of 20,000 μL and hemoglobin of 8 g/dl. The diagnosis of acute leukemia is suspected and a bone marrow biopsy is planned. Which of the following regarding this procedure is true?
    A. This patient's thrombocytopenia is a contraindication to biopsy
    B. The anterior iliac crest is the preferred biopsy site
    C. The same skin incision should not be used for aspirate and biopsy
    D. The most common complication is infection
    E. The presence of bony spicules in the aspirate confirms the presence of bone marrow

27. A 63-year-old man with peritoneal carcinomatosis from metastatic pancreatic cancer is admitted to the hospital with abdominal pain due to ascites. An ultrasound-guided therapeutic paracentesis is performed with aspiration of 2 liters of ascitic fluid. One hour after the procedure, the patient becomes tachycardic to 120 beats per minute and hypotensive (blood pressure 83/52). In addition to fluid resuscitation, which of the following is the next best step in management?
    A. Stat abdominal series including an upright abdominal x-ray
    B. Infusion of normal saline into the peritoneal cavity
    C. Stat electrocardiogram
    D. Stat computed tomography study to evaluate for a pulmonary embolism
    E. Send the ascitic fluid for gram stain and culture

28. A 77-year-old woman with metastatic breast cancer with leptomeningeal involvement presents to clinic for scheduled intrathecal injection of liposomal cytarabine via an Ommaya reservoir. Which of the following is **NOT** part of the procedure to administer the chemotherapy?
    A. Clean the skin with a chlorhexidine-based solution and allow it to dry prior to accessing the reservoir.
    B. Use a 19-20 gauge hypodermic needle to access the reservoir and administer the chemotherapy.
    C. Flush the chemotherapy with an equivalent volume of preservative-free normal saline.

D. If CSF is removed during the procedure, the patient should lie flat 30-60 minutes afterwards to prevent a headache.

E. A dressing is applied to where the needle was removed.

29. A 73-year-old man presents to clinic for a scheduled bone marrow biopsy and aspiration to investigate pancytopenia. Which of the following is true about the procedure?

A. The procedure should be delayed if the platelet count is less than 20,000 / μL.

B. If a biopsy is unable to be obtained at the posterior iliac crest, the sternum is an alternative biopsy site.

C. The periosteum should be anesthetized with a 1-2% lidocaine solution in a dime-sized area, as the aspiration and biopsy should be obtained from slightly different sites.

D. Skin breakdown or infection over the biopsy site is not a contraindication to using that site.

E. Sutures should be applied to improve hemostasis after the biopsy needle is withdrawn.

ANSWERS

1. A

The rate of second solid cancers from Hodgkin lymphoma has not changed over time, based on a Dutch study of 3905 patients comparing the population periods 1965–1976, 1977–1988, and 1989–2000. Exposures to both chemotherapy and radiotherapy increased the risk of developing secondary cancers. The most common secondary cancers were breast cancer (20.4%), lung cancer (20.2%), gastrointestinal cancer (19.7%), non-Hodgkin lymphoma (13.1%), and leukemia (5.0%). The most common second cancer for women in this cohort was breast cancer, not lung cancer. Even 40 years after treatment, survivors remain at increased risk of development second solid cancers compared with the general population. Mantle-field radiation carries an increased risk compared with supradiaphragmatic radiation sparing the axilla due to the larger radiation field. Survivors of Hodgkin lymphoma are at an increased risk of developing gastrointestinal malignancies due to exposure to chemotherapy and radiation.

2. D

It is actually recommended that patients try to multitask when their attention and concentration are at the highest to improve cognitive function, based on the 2015 NCCN Guidelines. Other strategies include use of memory aids, relaxation, stress management, minimizing sleep disturbances, physical activity, and limiting alcohol use.

3. C

The patient has hypertrophic osteoarthropathy (HOA, also known as hypertrophic pulmonary osteoarthropathy [HPO]), a paraneoplastic syndrome that affects less than 1% of patients with lung cancer. It is more commonly seen in men with advanced disease, adenocarcinoma histology, and an extensive smoking history. Fig. 37.1A and B depicts nailbed hypertrophy ("clubbing") that can cause a distal enlargement in the fingers of patients with lung cancer. The clinical manifestations of HOA include clubbed fingers, periostitis of the lung bones, and arthritis. Plain films of the bones demonstrate periosteal thickening and new bone formation. Symptoms from HOA can resolve after a lung cancer is resected, but it is usually treated symptomatically with nonsteroidal antiinflammatory agents and bisphosphonates. Dermatomyositis is also a paraneoplastic syndrome that can be associated with lung cancer, but its classic clinical manifestations include muscle weakness and characteristic skin findings such as heliotrope eruptions, Gottron papules, and the shawl sign. Trousseau syndrome is a recurrent phlebitis that is associated with malignancy, most commonly associated with pancreatic adenocarcinoma. The patient may have hypoxia due to lung disease, but this would not directly account for the patient's arthropathy. Lambert-Eaton syndrome is a paraneoplastic myasthenic syndrome due to antibodies directed against the presynaptic voltage-gated calcium channel that prevent the release of acetylcholine.

4. A

The patient has drug-induced thrombotic microangiopathy (TMA) from exposure to gemcitabine. TMA is manifested by a microangiopathic hemolytic anemia with anemia, thrombocytopenia, acute kidney injury, elevated LDH, and depressed haptoglobin, and it is associated with medications including gemcitabine. Henoch-Schonlein purpura (HSP) is a vasculitis more commonly seen in children and is associated with palpable purpura in the absence of thrombocytopenia, arthritis, abdominal pain, and renal dysfunction. Progression of the patient's malignancy would not account for the constellation of laboratory abnormalities. Cryoglobulinemia is an inflammatory syndrome involving small-to-medium vessel vasculitis, commonly seen with hepatitis C viral infection, and would also not cause the microangiopathic process seen in this patient. An acquired factor VIII inhibitor is associated with bleeding and an isolated prolonged activated thromboplastin time.

5. D

If the patient has normal 1- and 4-year postresection colonoscopies, her next surveillance colonoscopy is due in 5 years (9 years postresection); 1–3 years would be too soon, and 10 years (the normal colonoscopy surveillance interval in the general population) is too long for this cancer survivor.

6. D

While bleomycin has a low risk of causing impaired spermatogenesis, cyclophosphamide and melphalan are high risk, and cisplatin and doxorubicin are medium risk. If men are postpubertal prior to starting chemotherapy, sperm banking with cryopreservation should be offered as cytotoxic treatments can cause temporary and sometimes permanent sterility.

7. D

The patient has a grade 2 erlotinib-induced skin rash as manifested by a macular or papular eruption with erythema and pruritus covering less than 50% of the patient's body surface area. Erlotinib inhibits epidermal growth factor receptors (EGFRs) in the skin, causing an inflammatory response. The patient requires an oral tetracycline and topical antibiotic with minocycline and metronidazole respectively. The addition of an oral antihistamine helps control inflammation and is indicated for any erlotinib-induced rash. No dose reduction or treatment interruption is necessary for a grade 2 rash unless it fails to improve with treatment or is causing distressing symptoms affecting the patient's quality of life. In such a case, treatment may be interrupted for 3–5 days and restarted at 150 mg; if it recurs within 15 days, then the dose should be reduced to 100 mg daily. For grade 3 rashes, treatment should be interrupted until the rash improves to at least grade 2, and erlotinib should then be restarted at 100 mg daily. Oral corticosteroids and isotretinoin are not indicated for the treatment of erlotinib-induced rashes.

8. D

The patient has *Pneumocystis jirovecii* pneumonia (PJP) and requires prompt administration of intravenous trimethoprim/sulfamethoxazole. He is at high risk for developing PJP given lymphopenia due to temozolomide, radiation, and chronic corticosteroids. In fact, all patients undergoing adjuvant concurrent chemoradiation with temozolomide should be on prophylactic antibiotics against PJP. Intravenous piperacillin/tazobactam and vancomycin would be effective against hospital-acquired pneumonia including *Pseudomonas aeruginosa* and methicillin-resistant *Staphylococcus aureus* (MRSA) but would not cover PJP. Methylprednisolone may be indicated in patients with PJP who are hypoxic or have an arterial blood gas with a partial pressure of oxygen 70 mm Hg or less or an alveolar-arterial gradient equal to 35 mm Hg or greater; however, corticosteroids alone would not be effective treatment in this patient. Azithromycin and ceftriaxone would be effective treatment against community-acquired pneumonia including *Streptococcus pneumonia* and *Haemophilus influenzae* but also would not cover PJP. Intravenous amphotericin B would be appropriate treatment for a disseminated fungal infection such as histoplasmosis, but the patient's clinical scenario is most consistent with PJP.

9. A

The patient is likely to develop neurocognitive deficits from prophylactic cranial irradiation (PCI), especially due to her age. In the RTOG 0212 trial, 83% of patients above age 60 and 56% of patients under age 60 developed chronic neurotoxicity within 12 months after PCI. PCI is contraindicated in patients with baseline cognitive dysfunction or poor-performance status. Patients treated with 36 Gy have higher rates of mortality and neurotoxicity than those treated with 25 Gy. Patients with extensive stage disease may still be considered for PCI if they have a good response to chemoradiation, whereas patients with stable or progressive disease on chemoradiation are not candidates for PCI.

10. C

The 15-year cumulative incidence of developing a gastrointestinal malignancy in breast cancer patients is 2.48, versus only 0.87 for development of a lung cancer and 0.16 for acute myeloid leukemia, based on a Dutch study of 58,068 patients. Standardized incidence ratios were also elevated for cancers of the uterus, ovary, kidney, and bladder, and for soft tissue sarcomas, melanoma, and non-Hodgkin lymphoma. Patients 60 years or older had a higher association of developing a nonbreast cancer than patients aged 50–59. Breast cancer survivors continue to have a higher rate of nonbreast cancers compared with the age-matched population for at least 15 years after treatment.

11. D

Per the 2015 NCCN survivorship guidelines, the patient should have an echocardiogram or MUGA scan to evaluate left ventricular function given her prior exposure to an anthracycline. In addition, she has other cardiovascular risk factors (hypertension, diabetes, and hyperlipidemia), and her peripheral edema may be related to heart failure.

An electrocardiogram is unlikely to reveal underlying ischemia or arrhythmias, but it may be a useful study if the echocardiogram is unrevealing. Similarly, tests to evaluate myocardial ischemia (stress tests or coronary angiography) should not be performed prior to an echocardiogram. Serum B-type natriuretic peptide (BNP) may be elevated in heart failure but would not reveal the patient's left ventricular function.

12. A

The development of secondary malignancies, including leukemia, has been reported after treatment with chemotherapy. This potential risk is equally as important to discuss with patients as are the more acute, noticeable toxicities such as nausea, vomiting and fatigue. Acute myelogenous leukemia is the most common type of therapy-related leukemia, however acute lymphocytic leukemia, chronic myelogenous leukemia and myelodysplastic syndrome have also been observed. Regarding MDS, the therapy-related subtype accounts for approximately 15% of cases, has the highest rate of progression to acute leukemia, and is difficult to effectively treat. Both DNA topoisomerase-II inhibitors and alkylating agents have been implicated as causative factors in the development of secondary hematologic malignancies. Treatment-related MDS or leukemia following exposure to alkylating therapies including cyclophosphamide, ifosfamide, cisplatin, chlorambucil, melphalan, and procarbazine, generally has a latency period of 4-7 years and is associated with deletions in chromosomes 5 and/or 7. Leukemia development following treatment with topoisomerase-II inhibitors including etoposide and doxorubicin is characterized by a shorter latency period (1-3 years) and translocations usually involving 11q23. Both t(15;17) and inv(16) are favorable risk cytogenetics in AML while t(9;22) is poor risk.

13. B

The National Lung Screening Trial (NLST) was performed to determine whether mortality related to lung cancer could be reduced with low-dose CT screening in high-risk individuals. Over 53,000 participants were randomly assigned to have three annual screenings with either low-dose CT or chest radiography. Eligibility criteria included age 55-74 years, at least 30 pack-year smoking history, and if a former smoker, had quit within the previous 15 years. Exclusion criteria included a previous diagnosis of lung cancer, a chest CT obtained within 18 months before enrollment and symptoms of hemoptysis or unexplained weight loss (>15 lbs) in the preceding year. This trial demonstrated the effectiveness of low-dose CT screening in a high-risk population of patients, with a relative reduction in the rate of death from lung cancer of 20% with this modality. The number needed to screen with low-dose CT to prevent one lung-cancer related death was 320.

14. E

Plans for surveillance and survivorship issues are an important aspect of the care of breast cancer patients. The primary aim of surveillance after adjuvant therapy is to detect any new malignancy at an early, curable stage. The American Society of Clinical Oncology (ASCO) published an evidence-based clinical practice guideline in 1997 on the follow-up and management of breast cancer patients after completion of primary, curative treatment. These guidelines are updated by an expert panel on a periodic basis, which were published in 2013. Regular history and physical examinations should be performed every 3-6 months for the first 3 years, every 6-12 months for years 4 and 5, and annually after this time. In the setting of breast-conserving surgery, mammography should occur 6 months after radiation therapy is completed (which is often about 1 year following diagnosis). Mammogram should then be performed annually, unless otherwise indicated. Breast MRI is not recommended for routine breast cancer surveillance. Of note, in asymptomatic patients without specific findings on physical exam, the use of routine complete blood counts, chemistry panels, tumor markers (CEA, CA 15-3, CA 27.29) and imaging is not recommended. This patient should be considered for referral for genetic counseling based on her own and her mother's diagnosis of breast cancer before the age of 50. Additional criteria to recommend referral include Ashkenazi Jewish heritage, history of ovarian cancer at any age in the patient or any first- or second-degree relative, two or more first- or second-degree relatives diagnosed with breast cancer at any age, patient or relative with diagnosis of bilateral breast cancer, and male relative with history of breast cancer. Regular gynecologic follow-up is recommended for all women. Tamoxifen is associated with an increased risk of endometrial cancer, and patients should be educated to report any vaginal bleeding to their provider. However, screening with transvaginal or pelvic ultrasound is not indicated.

15. C

A diagnosis of cancer and its treatment may have significant impact on an individual's sexual activity, in the form of decreased libido, pain with intercourse, difficulty reaching orgasm, and vaginal dryness. Fatigue, pain, and restriction of movement, fluctuations in weight, scars and radiation treatment may all affect a patient's appearance and the way they perceive themselves. Psychological distress can impact desire to have sex and satisfaction. Certain cancers may have a direct effect on sexual functioning, such as cancers of the genitalia and their relationship to nerve and blood supply to the area. In regards to decreasing sexual function, chemotherapy and radical pelvic surgery appear to be the highest risk treatments. Health care providers are more likely to wait for the patient to ask questions related to sexual issues, and potential barriers to initiating discussion include the following: lack of experience and/or comfort with discussing this issue, and limited proven therapies available for cancer patients who have sexuality-related concerns. Although transdermal testosterone has shown effectiveness in increasing libido in women without cancer, the results of the randomized, double-blind, placebo-controlled trial of transdermal testosterone in women with cancer were negative. A possible explanation for the negative trial in cancer patients is that these women were postmenopausal and did not receive estrogen replacement.

16. B

Hodgkin lymphoma survivors are at risk of developing therapy-related complications that may surface several years after primary treatment. These include second malignancies (hematologic and solid tumor), cardiac, pulmonary and thyroid disease. History and physical exam should be performed every 3-6 months for 1-2 years, then every 6-12 months until year 3, then annually. Labs including CBC, chemistry profile, and ESR (if elevated at the time of diagnosis) should be followed as clinically indicated. Additionally, evaluation of thyroid function (TSH) should occur at one, two and at least five years if radiation to the neck is performed. CT scans should be done to confirm remission status; however, surveillance scans are not indicated unless dictated by clinical symptoms. It is recommended to consider annual breast MRI in addition to mammogram for women who received radiation to the chest between ages 10-35 years. Screening with combined MRI and mammogram among 96 pediatric Hodgkin lymphoma patients who had received chest radiotherapy demonstrated sensitivity and specificity of 100% and 88.6%, respectively. Hodgkin survivors are also at risk for long-term cardiovascular complications related to chemotherapy and/or radiation. Patients should be assessed for any cardiovascular-related symptoms, and well-established risk factors such as smoking, hyperlipidemia, hypertension and diabetes should be addressed and minimized. Furthermore, NCCN recommends considering stress test/echocardiogram at 10 year intervals after completion of treatment and consideration of carotid ultrasound if neck irradiation was administered.

17. C

Mortality rates among patients who have had a hematopoietic cell transplant remain higher than those for the general population for at least 30 years post-transplant, with an estimated 30% lower life expectancy in these individuals. The leading causes of excess deaths in 5-year survivors (in rank order) were recurrent disease, second malignancies, infection, chronic graft-versus-host disease, respiratory diseases, and cardiovascular diseases. Studies have shown that the risk of recurrent malignancy decreases with time after transplantation, and the risk of development of second malignancies increases with time after transplantation. Pond et al showed that recurrent and secondary malignancies were responsible for similar proportions of deaths among survivors beyond six years. Therefore, in the setting of further time from transplantation and increasing age of the patient, secondary malignancies may overcome recurrent disease as the major cause of excess deaths.

18. B

The patient has refractory ipilimumab-related colitis, as confirmed by sigmoidoscopy. He requires emergent treatment with infliximab as his colitis has not improved after 72 hours on intravenous corticosteroids. A high index of suspicion and prompt management of immune-related colitis are necessary as delayed or inadequate treatment can result in death. Loperamide is used for the management of grade 1 diarrhea (an increase in two bowel movements over baseline in 24 hours) but has no role in steroid-refractory colitis. Ciprofloxacin and metronidazole would be appropriate in an infectious colitis, but this has been excluded by stool studies. Budesonide was studied as diarrheal prophylaxis in 115 patients receiving ipilimumab in a phase II study, and there was not a significant difference in the rate of grade 2 or higher diarrhea in the budesonide group (32.7%) compared with the placebo group (35.0%). Increasing methylprednisolone to 120 mg twice daily is unlikely to improve the patient's colitis.

19. E

The patient has platinum-induced neurotoxicity from oxaliplatin. The appropriate clinical decision is to discontinue oxaliplatin given grade 3 motor neuropathy. The other options are all thought to play a role in combating platinum-induced neuropathy, but none have been proven to prevent neurotoxicity or slow the progression of neurotoxicity while continuing platinum-based chemotherapy.

20. A

The patient has abdominal pain due to unresectable pancreatic cancer that is refractory to oral and transdermal opioids. She requires evaluation for a celiac plexus block that has been shown to reduce abdominal pain in this patient population. In a metaanalysis of five randomized controlled trials, patients who received a celiac plexus block were more likely to have decreased pain and decreased opioid requirements compared with patients who received sham procedures and/or the standard of care. A Whipple procedure (pancreaticoduodenectomy) is not indicated as the patient does not have resectable disease; thus, surgery would cause more discomfort without improving survival. The patient is already on a high dose of transdermal fentanyl, so further escalation of opioids is unlikely to achieve better pain control on its own. While chemotherapy may benefit the patient in terms of pain control and survival, FOLFIRINOX would be preferred for borderline resectable disease in patients with an ECOG performance status of 0–1 and not preferred in a patient with unresectable disease and an ECOG performance status of two or more. In addition, chemotherapy should be deferred until the patient's pain can be more effectively managed. Hospice may be appropriate but would not improve the patient's pain control at this point in time.

21. D

The patient has an acute myocardial infarction related to exposure to bevacizumab. Bevacizumab increases the risks of impaired wound healing, hypertension, proteinuria, venous and arterial thrombosis, hemorrhage, gastrointestinal perforation, and congestive heart failure. Her age (above 65) and history of diabetes places her at increased risk of myocardial infarction related to bevacizumab. 5-Fluorouracil also carries an increased risk of myocardial infarction, but it is more often associated with coronary vasospasm during infusion and is less likely to cause a myocardial infarction this far out after an infusion. Oxaliplatin is associated with QT prolongation and ventricular arrhythmias but not myocardial infarction. Leucovorin is not associated with an increased risk of myocardial infarction.

22. B

The patient has ifosfamide encephalopathy, likely secondary to the accumulation of chloroacetaldehyde (a breakdown product of ifosfamide). He is at increased risk for this condition given his hypoalbuminemia and renal dysfunction. While methylene blue can be given to reverse this condition, it typically resolves spontaneously after holding ifosfamide. While his BUN is elevated due to acute renal failure, it is not sufficiently elevated to cause uremic encephalopathy. Hemorrhagic cystitis is another potential side effect of ifosfamide, but the patient's urinalysis is normal and this would not account for his encephalopathy. Doxorubicin and mesna are not associated with encephalopathy.

23. D

Cetuximab is associated with hypomagnesemia and should be monitored (along with calcium and potassium) while patients are receiving cetuximab. Electrolyte levels should be monitored regularly until at least 8 weeks after treatment, and early replacement to keep magnesium levels above 2.0 mEq/L is appropriate. Cetuximab is not associated with anemia, hyper- or hypo-natremia, neutropenia, or hyperbilirubinemia.

24. D

The proper positioning of a patient, site identification, sterile preparation and analgesia are important for the success of a lumbar puncture and to minimize complications. Acceptable positions include lateral recumbent and sitting positions. The patient should be instructed to arch their back "like a cat" to widen the gap between the spinous processes. In terms of landmarks, the individual performing the procedure should imagine a line between the superior aspects of the iliac crests that intersects the midline at the L4 spinous process. The spinal needle should be inserted in the L3 and L4 or L4 and L5 interspace, because these points are below where the spinal cord ends (between L1 and L2).[1]

25. C

Headache after lumbar puncture is a relatively common occurrence (32%), and may be associated with morbidity and rare but serious complications such as seizures and subdural hematomas if left untreated. Various factors have been shown to contribute to the development of post-LP headache, and knowledge of these factors can potentially lead to a reduction in this procedural complication. A lower chance of a post-LP headache occurring can be achieved with smaller needle size, insertion of needle with bevel parallel to dural fibers (as opposed to perpendicular), fewer lumbar puncture attempts, and replacement of the stylet before withdrawing the needle. In a study of 600 patients the incidence of headache was 5% when the stylet was reinserted compared with 16% when the stylet was not replaced.[2] It is hypothesized that if the needle is withdrawn without the stylet in place, a strand of arachnoid may enter the needle and potentially be brought back through the dural defect and create a path for prolonged CSF leakage. The incidence of headache after lumbar puncture has not been shown to depend on volume of CSF removed, CSF opening pressure, duration of bed rest after the procedure, or positioning of patient (upright versus sitting position).[3]

26. E

Bone marrow aspiration and biopsy is performed in the evaluation of hematologic conditions, cancers, metastatic disease, storage disorders and some chronic systemic diseases. The procedure has no absolute contraindications, although relative contraindications include bleeding disorder and active infection at the biopsy site. Thrombocytopenia and other coagulopathies are not absolute contraindications, although the administration of platelets can be considered if platelet count is less than 20,000/μL. The posterior iliac crest is the most common proposed site, however, alternatives that have historically been used include the anterior iliac crest, manubrium of the sternum, tibia (in infants), and vertebral body (rare cases). Upon collecting the aspirate, one can examine for spicules by examining the flow of blood in the syringe or spreading a drop of blood on a slide and allowing it to spread. Bony spicules will appear as small irregularities in the blood sample and confirm the presence of bone marrow. The aspirate and core biopsy may be performed through the same skin incision, however, the needle should be re-directed at a different angle into the bone itself. When performing the core biopsy, after puncturing the periosteum, the needle should be advanced to a depth of approximately 2cm, as this is an adequate length of an adult specimen. Complications are rare, but have been reported, with the most common being hemorrhage. Risk factors for hemorrhage include thrombocytopenia, use of anticoagulants and underlying myeloproliferative disorder.[4]

27. A

The patient likely has a gastrointestinal perforation from the therapeutic paracentesis. The main risks of the procedure include bleeding, pain, ascitic fluid leakage, infection, and gastrointestinal perforation. The patient is hemodynamically unstable and requires immediate fluid resuscitation. To confirm a diagnosis of gastrointestinal perforation, an abdominal series should be ordered to document free intraperitoneal air under the diaphragm or over the liver or spleen while positioned in the right or left lateral decubitus respectively. Fluid resuscitation within the peritoneal cavity would not be of benefit as the patient is intravascularly depleted. Studies to evaluate for myocardial ischemia or pulmonary emboli would lead to delays in diagnosis and treatment. The microbiology of the ascitic fluid may be useful for guiding future antimicrobial therapy but would not be helpful in the acute setting.

28. B

A butterfly needle (23 or 25 gauge) should be used to access an Ommaya reservoir, not a larger needle, in order to prevent CSF leakage. Sterile procedures should be used including a chlorhexidine-based cleaning solution. Chemotherapy should be flushed with normal saline. The patient should lay flat if CSF was removed to prevent a headache. The Ommaya reservoir site only needs a simple dressing after the needle is withdrawn.

29. C

The patient's periosteum requires sufficient anesthesia given its sensitivity to needle puncture, and a large enough area should be prepared as the aspiration and biopsy should be performed at slightly different locations in order to yield high quality specimens. Thrombocytopenia is not a contraindication to the procedure and platelet transfusions are not necessary. The sternum is an appropriate site for bone marrow aspiration if the iliac crest is not suitable, but the sternum is not an appropriate site for a biopsy due to the risk of complications including hemorrhage, cardiac tamponade, and pneumothorax. Biopsy sites should not include skin breakdown or infection due to the increased risk of infection and impaired wound healing from using those sites. Simple manual pressure and a dressing are all that is required after a bone marrow aspiration and biopsy, thus suturing of the puncture site is unnecessary.

REFERENCES

Question 1

1. Schaapveld M, Aleman BM, van Eggermond AM, et al. Second cancer risk up to 40 years after treatment for Hodgkin's lymphoma. *New Engl J Med.* 2015;373(26):2499–2511.

Question 2

1. *National Comprehensive Cancer Network.* Survivorship, version 2. 2015. <http://www.nccn.org/professionals/physician_gls/pdf/survivorship.pdf>. Accessed 06.02.16.

Question 3

1. Ito T, Goto K, Yoh K, et al. Hypertrophic pulmonary osteoarthropathy as a paraneoplastic manifestation of lung cancer. *J Thorac Oncol.* 2010;5(7):976–980.

Question 4

1. Blake-Haskins JA, Lechleider RJ, Kreitman RJ. Thrombotic microangiopathy with targeted cancer agents. *Clin Cancer Res.* 2011;17(18):5858–5866.

Question 5

1. Rex DK, Kahi CJ, Levin B, et al. Guidelines for colonoscopy surveillance after cancer resection: a consensus update by the American Cancer Society and the US Multi-Society Task Force on Colorectal Cancer. *Gastroenterology.* 2006;130:1865–1871.

Question 6

1. Wallace WH, Anderson RA, Irvine DS. Fertility preservation for young patients with cancer: who is at risk and what can be offered? *Lancet Oncol.* 2005;6:209–218.

Question 7

1. Tsimboukis S, Merikas I, Karapanagiotou EM, Saif MW, Syrigos KN. Erlotinib-induced skin rash in patients with non-small-cell lung cancer: pathogenesis, clinical significance, and management. *Clin Lung Cancer.* 2009;10(2):106–111.

Question 8

1. De Vos FY, Gijtenbeek JM, Bleeker-Rovers CP, van Herpen CM. Pneumocystis jirovecii pneumonia prophylaxis during temozolomide treatment for high-grade gliomas. *Crit Rev Oncol Hematol.* 2013;85(3):373–382.

Question 9

1. Wolfson AH, Bae K, Komaki R, et al. Primary analysis of a phase II randomized trial Radiation Therapy Oncology Group (RTOG) 0212: impact of different total doses and schedules of prophylactic cranial irradiation on chronic neurotoxicity and quality of life for patients with limited-disease small-cell lung cancer. *Int J Radiat Oncol Biol Phys.* 2011;81:77–84.
2. Le Péchoux C, Dunant A, Senan S, et al. Standard-dose versus higher-dose prophylactic cranial irradiation (PCI) in patients with limited-stage small-cell lung cancer in complete remission after chemotherapy and thoracic radiotherapy (PCI 99-01, EORTC 22003-08004, RTOG 0212, and IFCT 99-01): a randomised clinical trial. *Lancet Oncol.* 2009;10:467–474.

Question 10

1. Schaapveld M, Visser O, Louwman MJ, et al. Risk of new primary nonbreast cancers after breast cancer treatment: a Dutch population-based study. *J Clin Oncol.* 2008;26(8):1239–1246.

Question 11

1. *National Comprehensive Cancer Network.* Survivorship, version 2. 2015. <http://www.nccn.org/professionals/physician_gls/pdf/survivorship.pdf>. Accessed 06.02.16.

Question 12

1. Rheingold S, Neugut A, Meadows A. Therapy-Related Secondary Cancers. In: Kufe D, Pollock R, Weichselbaum R, Bast R, eds. *Holland-Frei Cancer Medicine.* 6th ed.; 2003.

Question 13

1. The National Lung Screening Trial Research Team, Aberle D, Adams A, Berg C, WC B, Clapp J. Reduced lung-cancer mortality with low-dose computed tomographic screening. *N Engl J Med.* 2011;365(5):395–409.

Question 14

1. Khatcheressian JL, Hurley P, Bantug E, et al. Breast cancer follow-up and management after primary treatment: American society of clinical oncology clinical practice guideline update. *J Clin Oncol.* 2012;31(7):961–965.
2. Tamoxifen and uterine cancer. Committee Opinion No. 601. American College of Obstetricians and Gynecologists. *Obstet Gynecol.* 2014;123(6):1394–1397.

Question 15

1. Katz A. The sounds of silence: sexuality information for cancer patients. *J Clin Oncol.* 2005;23(1):238–241.

2. Barton DL, Wender DB, Sloan JA, et al. Randomized controlled trial to evaluate transdermal testosterone in female cancer survivors with decreased libido; North Central Cancer Treatment Group Protocol N02C3. *J Natl Cancer Inst.* 2007;99(9):672–679.

Question 16

1. Eichenauer DA, Engert A, Andre M, et al. Hodgkin's lymphoma: ESMO clinical practice guidelines for diagnosis, treatment and follow-up. *Ann Oncol.* 2014;25:iii70–iii75.
2. Tieu MT, Cigsar C, Ahmed S, et al. Breast cancer detection among young survivors of pediatric Hodgkin lymphoma with screening magnetic resonance imaging. *Cancer.* 2014;120(16):2507–2513.
3. National Comprehensive Cancer Network. Hodgkin Lymphoma (Version 2.2016). https://www.nccn.org/professionals/physician _gls/pdf/hodgkins.pdf. Accessed June 13, 2016.

Question 17

1. Martin PJ, Counts GW, Appelbaum FR, et al. Life expectancy in patients surviving more than 5 years after hematopoietic cell transplantation. *J Clin Oncol.* 2010;28(6):1011–1016.
2. Rizzo JD, Curtis RE, Sobocinski KA, et al. Solid cancers after allogeneic hematopoietic cell transplantation. *Blood.* 2009;113(5):1175–1183.

Question 18

1. Weber JS, Kähler KC, Hauschild A. Management of immune-related adverse events and kinetics of response with ipilimumab. *J Clin Oncol.* 2012;30(21):2691–2697.
2. Weber J, Thompson JA, Hamid O, et al. A randomized, double-blind, placebo-controlled, phase II study comparing the tolerability and efficacy of ipilimumab administered with or without prophylactic budesonide in patients with unresectable stage III or IV melanoma. *Clin Cancer Res.* 2009;15:5591–5598.

Question 19

1. Avan A, Postma TJ, Ceresa C, et al. Platinum-induced neurotoxicity and preventive strategies: past, present, and future. *Oncologist.* 2015;20(4):411–432.

Question 20

1. Yan BM, Myers RP. Neurolytic celiac plexus block for pain control in unresectable pancreatic cancer. *Am J Gastroenterol.* 2007;102(2):430–438.

Question 22

1. Nicolao P, Giometto B. Neurological toxicity of ifosfamide. *Oncology.* 2003;65(suppl 2):11–16.

Question 24

1. Ellenby MS, Tegtmeyer K, Lai S, Braner D. Lumbar puncture. *N Engl J Med.* 2006;355(13):e12.

Question 25

1. Strupp M, Brandt T, Muller A. Incidence of post-lumbar puncture syndrome reduced by reinserting the stylet: a randomized prospective study of 600 patients. *J Neurol.* 1998;245(9):589–592.
2. Ahmed SV, Jayawarna C, Jude E. Post lumbar puncture headache: diagnosis and management. *Postgrad Med J.* 2006;82(973):713–716.

Question 26

1. Malempati S, Joshi S, Lai S, Braner D, Tegtmeyer K. Bone marrow aspiration and biopsy. *N Engl J Med.* 2009;361. e28.